Mineral Waters and
Pure Mountain Air

Contributions to Southern Appalachian Studies

1. *Memoirs of Grassy Creek: Growing Up in the Mountains on the Virginia–North Carolina Line.* Zetta Barker Hamby. 1998

2. *The Pond Mountain Chronicle: Self-Portrait of a Southern Appalachian Community.* Edited by Leland R. Cooper and Mary Lee Cooper. 1998

3. *Traditional Musicians of the Central Blue Ridge: Old Time, Early Country, Folk and Bluegrass Label Recording Artists, with Discographies.* Marty McGee. 2000

4. *W.R. Trivett, Appalachian Pictureman: Photographs of a Bygone Time.* Ralph E. Lentz II. 2001

5. *The People of the New River: Oral Histories from the Ashe, Alleghany and Watauga Counties of North Carolina.* Edited by Leland R. Cooper and Mary Lee Cooper. 2001

6. *John Fox, Jr., Appalachian Author.* Bill York. 2003

7. *The Thistle and the Brier: Historical Links and Cultural Parallels Between Scotland and Appalachia.* Richard Blaustein. 2003

8. *Tales from Sacred Wind: Coming of Age in Appalachia. The Cratis Williams Chronicles.* Cratis D. Williams. Edited by David Cratis Williams and Patricia D. Beaver. 2003

9. *Willard Gayheart, Appalachian Artist.* Willard Gayheart and Donia S. Eley. 2003

10. *The Forest City Lynching of 1900: Populism, Racism, and White Supremacy in Rutherford County, North Carolina.* J. Timothy Cole. 2003

11. *The Brevard Rosenwald School: Black Education and Community Building in a Southern Appalachian Town, 1920–1966.* Betty J. Reed. 2004

12. *The Bristol Sessions: Writings About the Big Bang of Country Music.* Edited by Charles K. Wolfe and Ted Olson. 2005

13. *Community and Change in the North Carolina Mountains: Oral Histories and Profiles of People from Western Watauga County.* Compiled by Nannie Greene and Catherine Stokes Sheppard. 2006

14. *Ashe County: A History; A New Edition.* Arthur Lloyd Fletcher. 2009 [2006]

15. *The New River Controversy; A New Edition.* Thomas J. Schoenbaum. Epilogue by R. Seth Woodard. 2007

16. *The Blue Ridge Parkway by Foot: A Park Ranger's Memoir.* Tim Pegram. 2007

17. *James Still: Critical Essays on the Dean of Appalachian Literature.* Edited by Ted Olson and Kathy H. Olson. 2008

18. *Owsley County, Kentucky, and the Perpetuation of Poverty.* John R. Burch, Jr. 2008

19. *Asheville: A History.* Nan K. Chase. 2007

20. *Southern Appalachian Poetry: An Anthology of Works by 37 Poets.* Edited by Marita Garin. 2008

21. *Ball, Bat and Bitumen: A History of Coalfield Baseball in the Appalachian South.* L.M. Sutter. 2009

22. *The Frontier Nursing Service: America's First Rural Nurse-Midwife Service and School.* Marie Bartlett. 2009

23. *James Still in Interviews, Oral Histories and Memoirs.* Edited by Ted Olson. 2009

24. *The Millstone Quarries of Powell County, Kentucky.* Charles D. Hockensmith. 2009

25. *The Bibliography of Appalachia: More Than 4,700 Books, Articles, Monographs and Dissertations, Topically Arranged and Indexed.* Compiled by John R. Burch, Jr. 2009

26. *Appalachian Children's Literature: An Annotated Bibliography.* Compiled by Roberta Teague Herrin and Sheila Quinn Oliver. 2010

27. *Southern Appalachian Storytellers: Interviews with Sixteen Keepers of the Oral Tradition.* Edited by Saundra Gerrell Kelley. 2010

28. *Southern West Virginia and the Struggle for Modernity.* Christopher Dorsey. 2011

29. *George Scarbrough, Appalachian Poet: A Biographical and Literary Study with Unpublished Writings.* Randy Mackin. 2011

30. *The Water-Powered Mills of Floyd County, Virginia: Illustrated Histories, 1770–2010.* Franklin F. Webb and Ricky L. Cox. 2012

31. *School Segregation in Western North Carolina: A History, 1860s–1970s.* Betty Jamerson Reed. 2011

32. *The Ravenscroft School in Asheville: A History of the Institution and Its People and Buildings.* Dale Wayne Slusser. 2014

33. *The Ore Knob Mine Murders: The Crimes, the Investigation and the Trials.* Rose M. Haynes. 2013

34. *New Art of Willard Gayheart.* Willard Gayheart and Donia S. Eley. 2014

35. *Public Health in Appalachia: Essays from the Clinic and the Field.* Edited by Wendy Welch. 2014

36. *The Rhetoric of Appalachian Identity.* Todd Snyder. 2014

37. *African American and Cherokee Nurses in Appalachia: A History, 1900–1965.* Phoebe Ann Pollitt. 2016

38. *A Hospital for Ashe County: Four Generations of Appalachian Community Health Care.* Janet C. Pittard. 2016

39. *Dwight Diller: West Virginia Mountain Musician.* Lewis M. Stern. 2016

40. *The Brown Mountain Lights: History, Science and Human Nature Explain an Appalachian Mystery.* Wade Edward Speer. 2017

41. *Richard L. Davis and the Color Line in Ohio Coal: A Hocking Valley Mine Labor Organizer, 1862–1900.* Frans H. Doppen. 2016

42. *The Silent Appalachian: Wordless Mountaineers in Fiction, Film and Television.* Vicki Sigmon Collins. 2017

43. *The Trees of Ashe County, North Carolina.* Doug Munroe. 2017

44. *Melungeon Portraits: Exploring Kinship and Identity.* Tamara L. Stachowicz. 2018

45. *Always Been a Rambler: G.B. Grayson and Henry Whitter, Country Music Pioneers of Southern Appalachia.* Josh Beckworth. 2018

46. *Tommy Thompson: New-Timey String Band Musician.* Lewis M. Stern. 2019

47. *Appalachian Fiddler Albert Hash: The Last Leaf on the Tree.* Malcolm L. Smith with Edwin Lacy. 2020

48. *Junaluska: Oral Histories of a Black Appalachian Community.* Edited by Susan E. Keefe with the Junaluska Heritage Association. 2020

49. *Boone Before Boone: The Archaeological Record of Northwestern North Carolina Through 1769.* Tom Whyte. 2020

50. *From the Front Lines of the Appalachian Addiction Crisis: Healthcare Providers Discuss Opioids, Meth and Recovery.* Edited by Wendy Welch. 2020

51. *Writers by the River: Reflections on 40+ Years of the Highland Summer Conference.* Edited by Donia S. Eley and Grace Toney Edwards. 2021

52. *Wayne Howard: Old Time Music, the Hammons Family and Mountain Lore.* Lewis M. Stern. 2021

53. *Lost Cove, North Carolina: Portrait of a Vanished Appalachian Community, 1864–1957.* Christy A. Smith. 2022

54. *LeConte Lodge: A Centennial History of a Smoky Mountain Landmark.* Tom Layton and Mike Hembree. 2024

55. *D.D. Dougherty, Lillie Dougherty and the Early Years of Appalachian State.* Doris Perry Stam. 2024

56. *Southern Mountain Music: The Collected Writings of Wayne Erbsen.* Wayne Erbsen. 2025

57. *Appalachian Nursing: A History, 1890–1960.* Sharon Loury. 2025

58. *Mineral Waters and Pure Mountain Air: Lesser-Known Health Resorts of Southern Appalachia, 1800–1940.* Mary F. Fanslow. 2025

Mineral Waters and Pure Mountain Air

Lesser-Known Health Resorts of Southern Appalachia, 1800–1940

MARY F. FANSLOW

CONTRIBUTIONS TO
SOUTHERN APPALACHIAN STUDIES, 58

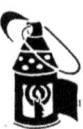

McFarland & Company, Inc., Publishers
Jefferson, North Carolina

This book has undergone peer review.

ISBN (print) 978-1-4766-9728-4
ISBN (ebook) 978-1-4766-5757-8

LIBRARY OF CONGRESS CATALOGING DATA ARE AVAILABLE

© 2026 Mary F. Fanslow. All rights reserved

*No part of this book may be reproduced or transmitted in any form
or by any means, electronic or mechanical, including photocopying
or recording, or by any information storage and retrieval system,
without permission in writing from the publisher.*

Front cover images: top of Roan Mountain, on the dividing line between North Carolina and Tennessee, 1905; "Holston Springs, Scott County, Virginia," Charles Rufus Boyd, *Resources of South-West Virginia: Showing the Mineral Deposits of Iron, Coal, Zinc, Copper and Lead*, 3rd edition (New York: John Wiley & Sons, 1881), 208 (Library of Congress; image courtesy of the Archives of Appalachia, East Tennessee State University); *background* the top of Roan Mountain © Serge Skiba/Shutterstock.

Printed in the United States of America

*McFarland & Company, Inc., Publishers
Box 611, Jefferson, North Carolina 28640
www.mcfarlandpub.com*

To the memory of my father, Bob Fanslow,
high school and university history teacher, and
to my mother, Linda Fanslow, teacher and librarian,
for her encouragement

*"A good teacher affects eternity; he can never tell
where his influence stops."*—Henry Adams

Acknowledgments

The research and writing for this book took seven years, much of it during the pandemic when travel was limited and many institutions closed. I owe thanks to the libraries and archives that provided virtual support. In particular, I would like to thank Daniel Ferkin of the Holston Conference Archives at Tennessee Wesleyan University for church records; Arabeth Balasko of the Greenbrier Historical Society in Lewisburg, West Virginia, for exploring my query on free Black labor at White Sulphur Springs; Stevvi Cook of the Grainger County, Tennessee, Archives for information on Tate Spring; and Lorna Loring of the Stewart Bell, Jr., Archives in Winchester, Virginia, for answering my queries on northern Virginia spas. I enjoyed our phone and email exchanges very much.

Closer to home, I owe thanks to many. The Exchange Place Association's Heather Gilbreath and the late Billie Moore provided me with invaluable insights. The late Lucy Gump introduced me to Austin Springs, driving me to its location and sharing her research and interviews. Ned Irwin, Washington County, Tennessee, archivist, critiqued my initial draft on Austin Springs. Jane Caldwell of Emory & Henry University's Kelly Library spent an afternoon with me to show me useful material at her library and followed up with helpful information. Kenny Stallard oriented me to the Scott County, Virginia, Historical Society's print and online materials. Wayne Steinmetz, retired Pomona College chemistry professor, tutored me in geology and read my initial drafts. The Kingsport, Tennessee, Public Library's Karen Cassell and Genevieve Lively filled more than eighty interlibrary loan requests and queries. East Tennessee State University faculty members Tom Lee and Marie Tedesco lifted my spirits when I despaired of completing this manuscript. Marie, a fellow runner, guided me to background resources and different pathways of thought to enable me to finish this marathon.

Table of Contents

Acknowledgments ... ix

General Introduction ... 1

Alabama ... 7
- Introduction ... 7
- Blount Springs ... 11
- DeKalb County: Mentone, Alabama White Sulphur Springs ... 15
- Monte Sano ... 19
- Talladega County: Chandler Springs, Talladega Springs, and Shocco Springs ... 24
- The Three Resorts: Postbellum Discussion and Aftermath ... 28
- Valhermoso Springs ... 29

Georgia ... 33
- Introduction ... 33
- Catoosa Springs ... 37
- Gainesville: Gower's Spring, New Holland Springs, Oconee White Sulphur Springs ... 43
- Porter's Springs ... 53
- Rowland Springs ... 59

Kentucky ... 66
- Introduction ... 66
- Lewis County: Esculapia and Glen Springs ... 69
- Estill Springs ... 73
- Pulaski County: Rockcastle Springs and Sublimity Springs ... 78

North Carolina	84
Introduction	84
Ashe County: Healing Springs and Shatley Springs	88
Burke County: Piedmont Springs, Glen Alpine Springs, and Connelly Springs	93
Haywood County: Haywood White Sulphur Springs and Eagles Nest	106
South Carolina	117
Introduction	117
Chick Springs	125
Glenn Springs	133
Tennessee	142
Introduction	142
Austin's Springs	146
Cloudland Hotel	153
Montvale Springs	162
Rhea Springs	167
Tate Spring	172
Unaka Springs	178
Virginia	184
Introduction	184
Holston Springs	190
Montgomery County: Yellow Sulphur Springs, Alleghany Springs, Montgomery White Sulphur Springs	196
Shannondale, Jordan White Sulphur Springs, Rock Enon	210
Chapter Notes	219
Bibliography	275
Index	295

General Introduction

Mineral Waters and Pure Mountain Air reflects my interest in the socioeconomic history of Southern Appalachian mountain resorts and health spas, dating from my 2004 master's thesis disputing the image of Appalachian isolation through the lens of five East Tennessee health resorts.[1] I expand upon my thesis by continuing an exploration of the illusion of geographic and socioeconomic isolation through a historical survey of selected Southern Appalachian resorts in eight states. For this exploration, I considered several aspects: the geographic boundaries of Southern Appalachia, my interpretation of a health resort, accessible and impactful information sources to illuminate facets of my topic, and the concept of isolation.

Geographic definitions of Appalachia and its subset of Southern Appalachia abound. Following the lead of many scholars of Southern Appalachia, I used John C. Campbell's definition for the Southern Highlands, his preferred term for Southern Appalachia, or the Mountain South. In his posthumously published 1921 work, *The Southern Highlander and His Homeland*, Campbell includes more than 200 counties in Alabama, Georgia, South Carolina, Tennessee, North Carolina, Kentucky, Virginia, West Virginia, and Maryland, outlining an area extending from northeastern Alabama along the Appalachian Valley and Ridge physiographic province to the Mason-Dixon line. Except for the Mason-Dixon political boundary, Campbell relied on topography—mountains, valleys, and plateaus—for his definition. Campbell's framework therefore fits well with my exploration of resorts as opposed to any reliance on, for example, Appalachian Regional Commission (ARC) maps, which are based on federal political consideration of county economic status.[2]

The selection of lesser-known resorts that I ultimately researched hinged upon two major factors: my access to sufficient information (several unchosen resorts unfortunately appear in only a few newspaper ads) and the resort location within the wide range of topographies on Campbell's map. As I began my project, I penciled in resort sites on topo maps to study their placement within Campbell's region. I wondered if these lesser-known resorts scattered throughout deep river gorges, high plateaus, remote hills, and steep mountain slopes were geographically isolated by their lands' physical features, the terrain limiting linkages to the outside regions.

By limiting my survey to health resorts, whether mineral spring spas or high altitude retreats promising hay fever and other catarrh relief, I eliminated places such as Georgia's Tallulah Falls Gorge that functioned mainly as sight-seeing destinations.[3] For each state, I chose health resorts (for example, Kentucky's Rockcastle

Springs) largely neglected by previous scholars and excluded health resorts (for example, Virginia's White Sulphur Springs and North Carolina's Warm Springs) that scholars have extensively researched. I included West Virginia in my chapter on Virginia because one of the resorts I selected originated before West Virginia became a state in 1861. I excluded the four Southern Appalachian Maryland counties because little accessible information was available on the one resort found within them, Cumberland County's Flintstone Springs.[4]

I researched the selected health resorts largely from newspapers, published diaries and journals, books mainly from the nineteenth century, railroad guides, and, to a lesser extent, easily accessible archival and library holdings of unpublished documents. Newspapers and railroad guides deserve a particular call-out. Newspapers provided interesting commentary on how newspaper editors wished the resorts to be perceived. Resort owners or managers stopped by editorial offices to drum up business; editors might obligingly publish a brief account of that visit in the next issue. Resorts hosted state newspaper associations, whose attendees described the visited resorts' ambiances in their respective papers, providing free publicity as a result. Railroad guides contained resort descriptions and illustrations to bolster passenger travel and provided maps of the rail line network largely in the East. By reading connection timetables and studying guide rail maps published over several years, I gained insight into the growing accessibility of rail service, one factor of many that demonstrates the linkage of these selected resorts to other regions.

If increased post–Civil War rail service to smaller health resorts demonstrates the selected resorts' connectivity to visitors from outside the region, perhaps the concept of Southern Appalachian isolation should have been weakened by now. Yet the perception of isolation persists in recent scholarship and reports. Steven Stoll, for example, in *Ramp Hollow: The Ordeal of Appalachia* (2017), cites a 2007 ARC report that describes the Appalachian mountains "as nearly impenetrable barriers to socioeconomic interaction, commerce, and prosperity.... Appalachia is a place apart, a place where people have long suffered the chronic economic consequences of physical isolation."[5] Alana M. Anton in her 2023 dissertation writes that both "media and scholarship often hide Appalachians' lived cultural experience behind either a culture in decay or a romanticized area with little government oversight and people who care little about the outside world."[6]

In part, the origin of Appalachian isolation evolved after the Civil War from the works of Mary Noailles Murfree; John Fox, Jr.; and other local color writers.[7] Mountaineers in local color romances, for example, inhabited primitive log cabins with their lissome, unsophisticated daughters interacting with "outside" progressive, worldly, educated men. Many readers of popular literature embraced these imaginative writings; indeed, George Vincent acknowledged Murfree and Fox in his 1898 "Retarded Frontier" article for educating an American public ignorant of the "fact" that mountaineers "[live] in practical isolation until this very day."[8] Allen Batteau contends that Murfree and Fox engaged in a "true act of creativity" to shape an insular image of mountainous Appalachia through embellishing and rearranging facts to fit a formulaic framework to sell their writings.[9]

After 1890, works centered on Southern Appalachia shifted from local color writings to explorations of a "problem to be solved" by educators, sociologists, and Christian charity organizations.[10] The year after Vincent's article appeared, William G. Frost, president of eastern Kentucky's Berea College and a leader in the mountain missionary "do good" movement, enhanced the myth of regional isolated backwardness by his description of the local residents as a "simple people" in a "Rip Van Winkle sleep" whom he hoped could be enlightened through education without rendering them "sophisticated."[11] According to Batteau, Frost, more than any other individual, was responsible for inventing the region as a social entity by his resplendent ordination of the area as one of "God's grand divisions.... Appalachian America."[12] As Amanda Fickey and Michael Samers point out, the concept of "a region apart" became further entrenched sixty-five years later through the *President's Appalachian Regional Commission Report of 1964*, which described the region as geographically and topologically isolated.[13]

Stoll dismisses the idea of isolation in his critique that Appalachia has long resided within the capitalist world, from early white hunters to the ARC, acknowledging the groundwork laid by sociologist Wilma A. Dunaway.[14] Dunaway, an advocate of American economist and sociologist Immanuel Wallerstein's world systems approach, deconstructs the myth of an isolated Southern Appalachia in *The First American Frontier* (1996) by demonstrating that Southern Appalachia has always been part of a global capitalism system beginning with its deerskin trade in the 1700s with European urban centers.[15] Through her analysis of large data sets constructed from antebellum records, she shows that the region's production and provision of extractive, agrarian, and other goods and services resulted in inter-regional market trade by the early 1800s. By 1830, she calculates that the most lucrative commercial ventures lay in the region's mineral spas.[16] According to Dunaway, an amount equivalent to 25 percent for every dollar invested in industry in Southern Appalachia was spent at these mountain spas by guests traveling largely from elsewhere.[17]

The most unanticipated linkage or connection disputing the concept of isolation appears in the lesser-known, smaller health resorts' emulation of the well-known, large resorts. I had thought before beginning my research that resorts off the "beaten" path and less popular than, say, Virginia's White Sulphur Springs—considered to be the *crème de la crème* in antebellum society—attracted a limited local clientele and offered a few spartan recreational activities less sophisticated than the ones publicized by the more prestigious resorts. The resorts I researched, however, generally provided similar health offerings: regimens for imbibing the waters or, for several mountainous retreats, respite from pollen and refuge from epidemics. Activities typically included croquet and ten pins, promenades along verandahs with prominently advertised walking lengths, and good "country" food. Genial proprietors ensured hospitable settings for socialization among political and military leaders and other elites and hosted events such as dances or chaperoned outings for the unattached. Fire-eating southern politicians, propagandists for southern independence, discussed states' rights at South Carolina's upstate watering holes as well as at the Virginia springs.[18] Guests cheered for competing knights at chivalrous tournaments not only at White Sulphur but also at northern Virginia's Shannondale Springs, South Carolina health resorts, and Catoosa Springs in Georgia. Southern

Appalachia, as demonstrated through these lesser-known health resorts, interacted with the "outside" world via this service economy. If I were to redact resort names and locations, many readers might not be able to distinguish, for example, South Carolina's Chick Springs or Kentucky's Estill Springs from the Virginia springs resorts, which attracted national figures and Deep South elites.

The long distances traveled to and from smaller resorts also supports Southern Appalachia's connectivity to other regions in the nation. These health resorts, as well as the major Virginia springs resorts, attracted patrons who might travel many miles: the sickly who sought cures and the elites who wished to recreate and engage in social activities. Holston Springs, seventy miles from Cumberland Gap in extreme Southwest Virginia, advertised as early as 1810 in a Lowcountry (South Carolina) newspaper to planters more than 350 miles away. Lowcountry and Delta planters traveled by steamer to the small resort of Rhea Springs via the Tennessee River and to eastern Kentucky resorts via the Ohio River just as they went by boat to Guyandotte, Virginia, to then continue by stage to White Sulphur Springs. Some visitors to the health resorts journeyed there along drover roads used to drive livestock and fowl to markets, which, as Sam Bowers Hilliard shows, provided another link to trade centers outside the region.[19] As David Hsiung demonstrates in *Two Worlds in the Tennessee Mountains*, an exploration of that region's antebellum development, a framework of connectedness can unify the seemingly disparate concepts of community and isolation.[20] In other words, a resort hidden on the banks of a river gorge may be physically isolated but connected to the larger world by its visitors and by its service economy. The service economy might include, for example, the resort's suppliers of foodstuffs, linens, and furniture and its use of musicians and professional hotelmen, often with experience elsewhere in the South, who attracted patrons who knew them from previous hostelries.

During the antebellum period, the slave economy also connected the Mountain South to external southern and mid–Atlantic markets, which, in turn, connected the region to the Caribbean and most of Latin America. "Black birders," who kidnapped Blacks for sale into slavery, and slave traders from within and outside the region organized coffle marches to southern markets.[21] In 1836, for example, an Abingdon, Virginia, firm purchased about 100 enslaved persons in Southwest Virginia and East Tennessee and then drove them to Mississippi markets via Kingsport, Tennessee, about seven miles south of Holston Springs, and Grainger County's Bean Station, a frequent coffle stopping point near the mineral waters of Tate Spring.[22] Two of the largest slaveowners in Southern Appalachia, John Sharpe Rowland of Georgia's Rowland Springs and James Robert Love of North Carolina's Haywood White Sulphur Springs, used enslaved labor at their health resorts. Other hotel proprietors hired enslaved persons or used their own enslaved laborers for such work as tending fields for crops to supply hotel food, cleaning hotels, providing entertainment, and guiding visitors on outdoor excursions.

Enslaved workers traveled from Deep South plantations or farms to Mountain South health resorts both within the well-known Virginia springs circuit and outside the circuit to less exclusive mineral spas such as Kentucky's Sublimity Springs in the wilderness of the Rockcastle River. Primarily, they accompanied their owners to tend to their comfort. Secondarily, some slaveholders sent their ailing enslaved persons to health resorts for treatment to ensure the well-being of their labor "commodity," not necessarily as acts of compassion. The small Virginia spring resorts at Rockbridge and Bath Alum treated at least eight enslaved laborers with pulmonary and rheumatic issues.[23] Likewise, the Tennessee springs at Rhea and Montvale received enslaved patients.[24]

During the Civil War, most Southern Appalachian health resorts I researched closed, received refugees from cities potentially affected by military skirmishes, served as hospitals, or acted as military headquarters. Proprietors such as Montvale Springs' Confederate sympathizer Sterling Lanier fled south to Alabama while Unionist slaveholder Clisbe (Clisby) Austin fled north to upper East Tennessee from his Tunnel Hill, Georgia, hotel, eventually establishing the health resort of Austin Springs near Johnson City.[25] The movement of troops and war refugees across Southern Appalachia again dispels the notion of an impenetrable mountainous fortress.

Southern newspapers demonstrate a linkage from Southern Appalachia to other regions by urging "low country people" to spend their funds at Mountain South health resorts rather "than to run off to the North" just as the pro-southern *De Bow's Review* urged its readership to do the same on behalf of emerging Gulf Coast resorts.[26] Readers asked by the southern press to "cease patronizing our enemies" might instead visit Catoosa Springs, South Carolina's, Chick Springs, and the Gainesville, Georgia, springs, all of which billed themselves at various times as the "Saratoga of the South."[27] After the Civil War, southern newspapers again beseeched their readership to "stay at home" (a popular phrase) to financially support regional businesses, including lesser-known Southern Appalachian health resorts such as Georgia's Rowland, Catoosa, and Cohutta springs.[28]

Several postbellum events also speak to the connectivity of the Southern Appalachian resorts to other parts of the South. Some mineral spring resorts continued to engage in Deep South culture: Virginia's New River Valley health resorts received former Confederate generals Jubal Early and P.G.T. Beauregard as they reminisced about the "Lost Cause," a quasi-religious movement from 1865 to about 1920 seeking to preserve the white identity of the defeated South, "the memory of a dead political nation."[29] Some freed persons employed at a few of the covered health resorts, perhaps knowledgeable of work stoppages outside the region, asserted an independence: Black waiters, for example, struck for better wages in late summer 1898 at both North Carolina's Haywood White Sulphur Springs and at Kentucky's Glen Springs in apparently uncoordinated strikes.[30] Great epidemics such as the 1873 New Orleans cholera outbreak, the 1878 and 1879 Memphis yellow fevers, and the 1888 "Yellow Jax" Jacksonville fever brought trainloads of frightened Delta and Lowcountry refugees to many Southern Appalachian health resorts, particularly those in upper East Tennessee and western North Carolina. Some health resort operators shipped their resort's mineral spring waters outside the region to druggists for resale or to individual consumers, comparing the water, for instance, to that of Saratoga's. These events hint at broader themes emanating from resort activities and culture that merit further research and analysis for a future volume beyond the scope of this book.

Perplexing to me was the relative isolation of some resorts where guests commented on the locals as if they were foreign: how did this fit into a framework of connectivity? To resolve the quandary, I turned to Hsiung. He uses the vivid imagery of "main stream" and "rivulet" respectively to demonstrate that upper East Tennessee's ridge and valley physiographic province's western Holston and Watauga river valley residents were able to plant a variety of crops, develop communities, and engage frequently with trade markets compared to inhabitants struggling to farm on the steep Unaka ridges to the east.[31] The more mountainous resorts such as northwestern Georgia's Porter Springs, upper East Tennessee's Cloudland Hotel, and Sublimity Springs exemplify the "rivulet" concept; travelers commented on nearby mountaineers' poverty and ignorance, the latter generally the result of inaccessible schools. North Carolina residents referred to the northwest corner of their state, home to Shatley Springs and Healing Springs, as the "Lost Province" because of its lack of convenient transportation to the rest of the state.[32]

Most of the health resorts covered in this work no longer exist because improved roads took potential visitors elsewhere; owners failed to invest in infrastructure maintenance; and/or buyers of resorts repurposed hotels for schools or for other uses. A few health resorts, notably Shatley Springs, still shelter potable mineral spring waters. Some bygone resorts, such as the Cloudland Hotel, as well as North Carolina's Piedmont Springs, Sublimity Springs, and Rockcastle Springs, have crumbled and now lie within U.S. national forests. Their grounds and those of other health resorts subsumed into the wilderness are still serving purposes of health. The Japanese concept of *shinrin-yoku* or "forest bathing," for example, has become popular in recent years to relieve stress via meditative walks in the woods. During the Covid-19 pandemic, people sought refuge from a poorly understood contagion, not unlike nineteenth-century persons escaping a cholera epidemic, along the uncrowded, healthy ambiance of Southern Appalachian trails. The goal of restorative health continues in the ambiance of the former Southern Appalachian mineral spring resorts and retreats.

Alabama

Introduction

When one imagines Alabama, a kaleidoscope of images may appear. On the one hand, popular cultural icons such as the eponymous southern rock band and the Crimson Tide come to mind. On the other hand, disturbing images of violent twentieth-century Civil Rights struggles may emerge, including a defiant Governor George Wallace in 1963 calling for segregation forever and police brutality in 1965 against marchers from Selma to Montgomery.

Southern Appalachian Alabama was not immune from the racial violence of the central and more southern areas of the state. Although one postbellum traveler described it as "grand mountains … rapids and noisy waterfalls; vast stretches of forests," the pastoral scenery ironically served as the setting for Jackson County's 1931 "Scottsboro Boys" trial, which wrongly convicted nine young Black males of raping two white women, and the 1963 Ku Klux Klan bombing of a Birmingham church that killed four young Black girls.[1] The construct of an isolated mountainous region apart from societal trends elsewhere does not hold true for northern Alabama.

Alabama's Southern Appalachian region largely falls into the Highland Rim on its northwestern and north central border with Tennessee; the Cumberland Plateau on its northeastern border with Tennessee and Georgia; the Valley and Ridge, above the Piedmont, running northeasterly; and the Piedmont, southeast of the Valley and Ridge and bordering Georgia. The Highland Rim contains the Southern Appalachian counties of Morgan and Madison. The Cumberland Plateau falls completely in Campbell's definition of Southern Appalachia; its counties include Jackson, DeKalb, Marshall, Blount, Cullman, Winston, and Walker and contain the Lookout, Sand, and Blount mountain ridges. Within the Valley and Ridge are the Southern Appalachian counties of Shelby, St. Clair, Etowah, Calhoun, Cherokee, Jefferson, and Talladega, home to Shades Mountain and Blackjack Ridge. Lastly, the Piedmont Upland, including the Ashland Plateau to the east of the Talladega Mountains, contains the Southern Appalachian counties of Clay, Cleburne, and Coosa.[2] If one drives from Rockford in Coosa County westward to Interstate 65 North and then follows it through Birmingham to the Tennessee border, one gains a general sense of Campbell's boundary of Southern Appalachian Alabama. Driving from Birmingham eastward to Chattanooga along Interstate 59 North gives a motorist a view of the

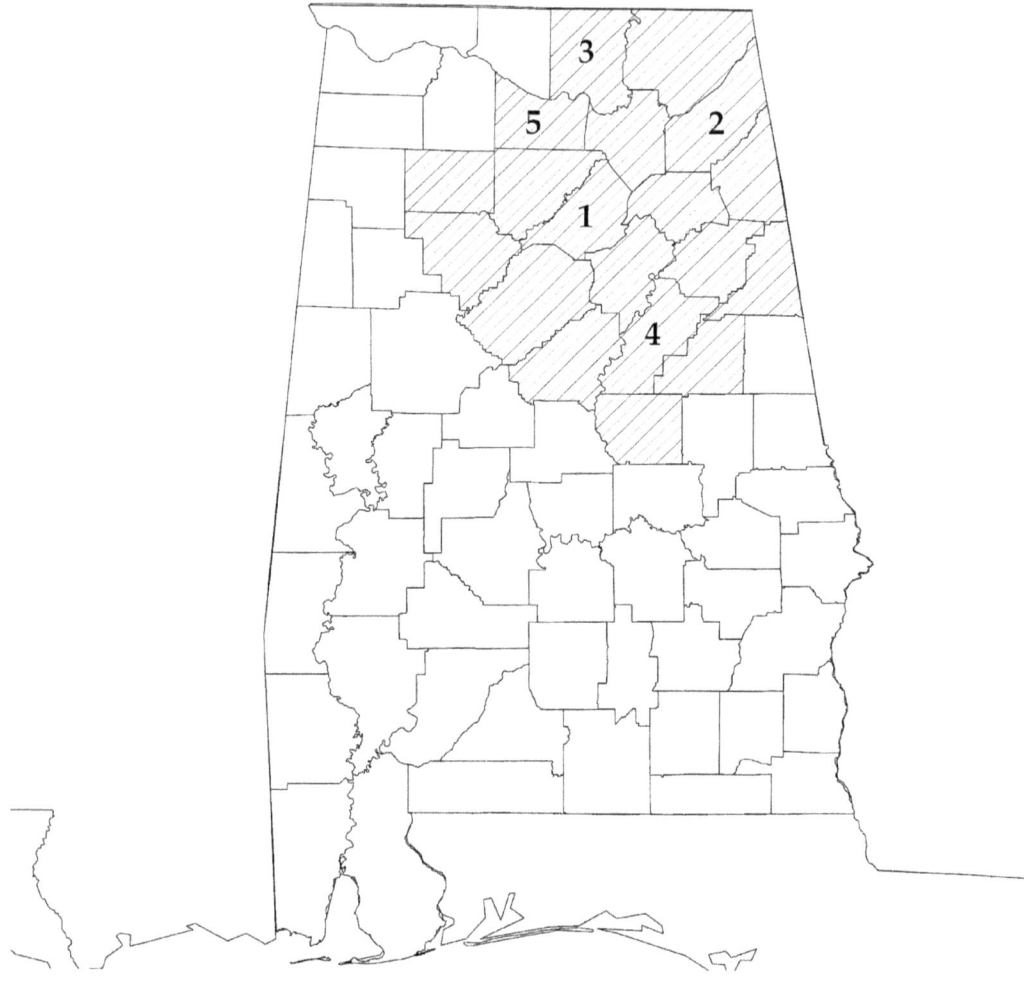

Alabama counties with featured health resorts: (1) Blount County—Blount Springs; (2) DeKalb County—Mentone and Alabama White Sulphur Springs; (3) Madison County—Monte Sano; (4) Talladega County—Chandler Springs, Talladega Springs, and Shocco Springs; (5) Morgan County—Valhermoso Springs (Sources: Esri, NOAA, USGS. Cartographer: Sayona Turner, East Tennessee State University).

mountains of northeast Alabama. Following State Highway 9 from Ashland in Clay County eastward to Heflin in Cleburne County orients a driver to the Piedmont.

Minerals and coal permeate throughout these physiographical provinces. Limestone varies from the dark gray Coosa limestone in Jones Valley to the light gray Chickamauga limestone on the south end of Blount Mountain. Shales, sandstone, and the harder (less erodible) limestone tend to constitute the steep escarpments of the valleys and ridges, including sandstone veined with iron ore found on Blount County's aptly named Red Mountain. In the nineteenth century, industrialists mined northern Alabama's iron ores and thick bituminous coal seams.[3] Less common but highly valued were ores such as gold, silver, and copper. The enterprising minister and academic Benjamin Franklin Riley boasted that his so-called

Mineral Belt, covering much of Southern Appalachian Alabama, contained "almost all the chief minerals known to art, and in many instances in fabulous abundance."[4]

Because limestone crevices allow for the seepage of water containing dissolved minerals, the plentiful mineral springs that dot Southern Appalachian Alabama gave rise to over twenty-five health resorts, some analyzed by state scientists. In 1850, the first state geologist, Michael Tuomey, described the geology of Blount Springs, St. Clair Springs, and Shelby Springs. Blount and St. Clair waters, he observed, flowed out of Silurian rocks in "precisely" the same geological position as the Virginia springs, a prestigious accolade for the former. He classified one of Shelby's springs as calciferous due to its seepage through limestone (calcium carbonate) and another spring as both sulphurous and chalybeate (iron) because of its issue through black shale.[5] By the early 1900s, qualitative and quantitative chemical analysis had advanced to the point that the then state geologist, Eugene A. Smith, could record the mineral content of Chandler Springs and its neighbor two miles away, Chambers' Springs, both on the Talladega Mountains' Hillabee schist, to parts per million.[6]

State residents did not limit their search for good health to such Appalachian Alabama health resorts as described by the state geologists; some Alabama elite traveled extensively. U.S. Senator C.C. (Clement Claiborne) Clay, Jr., who suffered from severe chronic asthma, and his wife owned a cottage at Monte Sano but contemplated a visit to western North Carolina to ease his breathing; friends instead recommended Arkansas or Texas. The Clays also traveled to Minnesota for its air quality; journeyed to a water-cure institute in Brattleboro, Vermont, for hydropathic treatment; sought asthmatic relief in Florida; and sojourned at Virginia's Sweet Springs where Clay appreciatively recorded that he had gained seventeen pounds.[7] Colonel George Strother Gaines of Mobile, federal factor (trade agent) to Native Americans in the region, was ordered by his physician in the summer of 1843 "to the mountains of Virginia for the benefit of the air and mineral waters."[8] A Talladega businessman, despite his proximity to several high elevation local resorts, died suddenly of "hemorrhage from the lungs" the day before he had planned to leave for a two-month stay in Warm Springs (current Hot Springs), North Carolina, for treatment of his consumption (tuberculosis).[9]

Alabama physicians apparently did not routinely endorse the resorts in their state, nor did the resorts regularly engage their services as was common at the Virginia springs. Although some Alabama resorts employed resident doctors (a few were even founded by physicians), newspaper advertisements rarely publicized the concept of a resident physician. Alabama doctors themselves, however, did make the round of resorts, both in and out of Southern Appalachian Alabama. Josiah Nott, cofounder of both the Mobile Medical Society and the Medical Association in the State of Alabama (and infamous racist justifying slavery on "scientific" studies), enjoyed visits to several state resorts, especially Mobile Bay's Point Clear's Battle House. Nott also traveled several times to South Carolina's Upstate resorts. He particularly favored, however, the Virginia springs where he sought relief from rheumatism.[10] Huntsville physician John Y. Bassett, another advocate of white supremacy, sojourned in Florida's genial winter weather for a pulmonary condition yet also rhapsodized that Madison County, home of Monte Sano, supplied "all that is essential to health, comfort, and long life."[11]

Moreover, nineteenth-century Alabama physicians rarely discussed the attributes of mineral waters or the salubrious effects of the mountains at their annual medical meetings, published as the *Transactions of the Medical Association of the State of Alabama*. In the one nineteenth-century *Transactions* paper devoted to mineral water attributes, the author focused parochially on the merits of his Livingston community artesian well in Sumter County on the Mississippi border. For several desperate itinerant patients, the Livingston well water allegedly provided near miraculous cures contrasted to the Virginia springs, Florida, or to northeast Alabama's Hanna Springs ("little to no benefit" for one man who subsequently gained a pound daily from drinking the Livingston water).[12]

Many of the state medical meetings centered on the poorly understood seasonal fevers and epidemics that pervaded cities with an "atmosphere of doom [that] settled upon every heart" and caused streets to become deserted.[13] Bassett, for instance, noted that Madison County from 1830 on experienced epidemics of "bilious intermitting and remitting fevers in the summer and fall" and "typhoid cases of the same, together with inflammation of the thoracic viscera in the winter and spring."[14] "Black jaundice," "cachemia hæmorrhagica," and "yellow disease" were grim synonyms discussed at the 1869 medical meeting for an illness characterized by vomiting of "dark grumous bile," "bronze yellow" skin, an impacted gall bladder, and kidney hemorrhage.[15] Other papers and follow-up discussions at the 1869 session parsed in excruciating detail the perceived differences among "Bloody Chills," "typhomalarial fever," "Typhoid Pneumonia," and "Up-Country Yellow-Fever," all in vain efforts to formulate appropriate treatments.[16]

Attendees across the decades advocated a wide spectrum of treatments for fevers: Thomsonian baths; arsenious acid; ipecac and calomel (a mercury compound); spirits of nitrous ether to clear malarial congestion of the gall-bladder; and sulphites dissolved in orange-peel syrup.[17] One prescient presenter in 1869 exasperatedly ticked off the assorted dubious remedies of the era and then lectured his colleagues from an early evidence-based medicine approach, *"Cure, by the administration of proper doses of quinine, your intermittent fevers, and you ... stop forever, this horrible disease* [italics original]."[18]

An 1869 paper noted with alarm that northern mountainous Alabama, considered exempt from autumnal fevers, had recently seen diseases of malarial origin. For this peculiar situation, the paper's authors blamed the marsh miasma on the Civil War: "During and since the war ... many thousand acres [are] grown up in weeds ... expos[ed] to the action of heat and moisture.... [T]he effluvia from which may have largely contributed to produce so great an increase in the amount of sickness in this section."[19]

After the end of the Civil War, perhaps in part due to the observed rise in seasonal fevers, Southern Appalachian Alabama resorts, which had largely closed during the conflict, reopened. Shelby Springs, for example, had hosted a "very gay and fashionable crowd" during the war, including many displaced New Orleans Creole families, until "much [to the guests'] consternation and disappointment," the

Confederates in 1863 commandeered the resort as a hospital operated by the Catholic order Sisters of Mercy, who served as nurses. After the war, Shelby Springs entertained in 1867 the likes of Lydia Johnston, wife of former Confederate General Joseph E. Johnston.[20] Returning veterans such as Confederate John Washington Inzer, prisoner of war at Johnson's Island in Lake Erie, sought to recover from his "rather poor state of health" at St. Clair County's Cook's Springs.[21] Governor Robert M. Patton, desperate to revive the shattered state economy, exhorted his fellow residents in a letter published in many state newspapers to spend their money at home. The governor called out Blount Springs ("salubrious atmosphere equal[s] the famous Saratoga"), Shelby Springs ("cure of numerous chronic disease"), and Talladega Springs and Chandler Springs ("equal [to] any of the celebrated Virginia Springs").[22]

Postwar railroad construction, while enabling locals to travel elsewhere, also reciprocally encouraged potential northern investors to take note of the southern landscape. A *New York World* correspondent lauded the "valuable mineral waters ... which can be profitably bottled and sent off to market.... Blount Springs [and] Talladega Springs ... are unsurpassed."[23]

The resorts described in this chapter represent antebellum and postbellum watering holes found in various Southern Appalachian Alabama geographies. Mentone, Valhermoso Springs, Alabama White Sulphur Springs, and Monte Sano lie in the northeast corner of the state that skirts both the Highland Rim and the Cumberland Plateau. Blount Springs represents the central Cumberland Plateau section. The Talladega County mineral spring resorts of Chandler, Talladega, and Shocco (Chocco) serve as examples for the southeastern Valley and Ridge section. Blount Springs and Valhermoso Springs catered to guests as early as the 1820s; northerners built Mentone and the Alabama White Sulphur after the Civil War. All hosted in the nineteenth century largely an in-state clientele and to a lesser extent Gulf Coast elite.

Blount Springs

Two hundred years ago, the Alabama territorial legislature carved Blount County out of the territory's north central "rugged and mountainous [terrain] with beautiful valleys."[24] The mountains, according to early surveyor and geologist George Powell, "are all nearly of the same height, being from four to five hundred feet high.... [T]he tops of these long mountains covered densely with tall timber are cooler than the lower portions of the county ... for in hot weather, a person on reaching near their tops is sure to find himself in a cool delightful breeze."[25]

Through one of the mountain gaps lies Sequatchie (Sequatchee) Valley, wedged between the Cumberland Plateau and the Sand Mountain ridge. In this valley flow the mineral waters of Blount Springs. Powell lauded the waters' attributes in 1855:

> The "Blount Springs," are in themselves, one of the greatest natural advantages of our county. At these Springs, within an area of a few rods, are found the White, Red and Sweet-Sulphur, and Freestone water, and at a short distance, the Limestone and Chalybeate.... [T]hey promise at some day, to command great patronage, and to afford of themselves, a market to an incalculable amount of Blount productions.[26]

Huntsville trader and merchant Luther Morgan discovered the springs in the late 1810s; sometime after 1818, he bought the tract around the springs and began to improve the property.[27] By 1826, notable Alabama elites such as plantation owner and politician Clement Comer (C.C.) Clay, Sr., and his family were visiting the "large *Boarding House* [italics original] with more than 30 comfortable cabins," which publicized as early as 1822 in a Huntsville newspaper its liquor and game for "Gentlemen fond of sport."[28] In 1828, John H. Harris and James Perrine purchased the springs property at auction after the Morgan family defaulted on loans.[29] Within seven years, Blount Springs gained prominence as a stagecoach stop along a major route from Huntsville to Tuscaloosa.[30]

In the decades preceding the Civil War, Blount Springs' reputation grew. Travel handbooks such as *Appletons'* noted the springs' popularity ("much resorted to"); other guides praised the "fashionable watering place" with its "several varieties of sulphur fountains, within thirty feet" for the convenience of guests.[31] Shrewd publicists advertised the springs as "Alabama's Fountain of Youth" and boasted that the waters "have been pronounced by competent judges, equal to any in the country."[32]

One flowery notice, published in at least four Alabama and Mississippi newspapers, exalted Blount Springs' waters and its "pure air and delightful climate" for "the afflicted and invalid, the fashionable and the opulent, and the wearied seeker of toil of business."[33] The ad emphasized the resort's "sources of amusement," including its provision of a "Band of Music" (printed in large boldface) to perform at saloon and lawn parties at "hours agreeable to the guests."[34] Even in the resort's early period, management recognized that it could bolster profits by providing social activities (assisted by the "choicest Wines, Liquors, Cordials, Cigars") in addition to catering to sickly guests seeking a cure.[35]

Guests at Blount Springs in the antebellum period, as elsewhere, were those who could afford time away from their livelihoods and therefore typically hailed from the upper crust of society. Deep South plantation owners constituted a large segment of visitors. For example, one aristocratic southern Alabamian in 1844 wrote to his Rhode Island tailor from the resort requesting fifty-three pea jackets for his "servants" (enslaved persons) and twenty for those of his sister-in-law.[36] Sarah Haynsworth Gayle, first wife of future Alabama governor John Gayle, recorded in her journal that regional elites had journeyed 120 miles to Blount Springs. Gayle herself suffered poor health and thought a "trip to the Blount Springs might renew my life" but with her several children thought such a trek was "out of the question" (she instead consumed large amounts of opium, which impaired both her mental and physical health).[37] Other wealthy planters in south Alabama built cottages around the springs to spend the "heated term" with their families.[38]

In the late 1850s, Matthew Duffee, a Louisiana plantation owner and former Mobile hotelier, moved to Blount Springs where he operated the eponymous "Duffee House." Sources vary on whether Duffee bought the hotel from another party or built the structure.[39] Two notable events occurred at the resort during Duffee's ownership during the Civil War. John Bell, 1860 Constitutional Union party presidential candidate turned secessionist, stayed there in 1862, having left his home in Nashville to avoid advancing Union troops and to raise funds in Alabama for the Confederate military.⁴⁰ Bell refused a Federal passport arranged by his wife to return home, choosing to remain at Blount Springs to "patriotically [await] a safe conduct under Confederate auspices."⁴¹ Duffee's daughter, writer and Blount Springs postmistress Mary Gordon Duffee, in 1864 intercepted $100,000 in Confederate bills in the mail intended for the military and spent it in a "Robin Hood" fashion on provisions for the destitute families of Confederate soldiers; Jefferson Davis himself ordered her release without trial. She returned to Blount Springs where one journalist referred to her as a "harmless 'crank,'" who "has never been known to speak well of any one [sic], but when she takes a pen in her hand to write she becomes a changed being."⁴²

After the war, the resort rebounded. Colonel J.F.B. Jackson of Chattanooga bought Blount Springs and several thousand acres in its vicinity and erected in 1878 a new hotel, the New Jackson House, near the depot of the South & North Alabama Railroad, now finished between Birmingham to the south and to the vicinity of Decatur to the north.⁴³ The three-story framed hotel, with wrap-around verandahs on the first two floors, accommodated 500 guests although over 600 visitors at one period in the late 1870s overflowed its grounds.⁴⁴

The resort regained its reputation as a favorite of the regional wealthy white families: The grand ball to celebrate the New Jackson House opening attracted guests from Nashville, Mobile, Montgomery, and Birmingham.⁴⁵ Blount Springs also became a staple for the "best white Creoles" of New Orleans; for example, state legislator Theophile T. Allain, son of a Creole Louisiana planter and an enslaved female, and one of the wealthiest in the Louisiana "colored aristocracy," often vacationed at Blount Springs with his family.⁴⁶

An archaeologist traveling through northern Alabama in 1883 aired a different view of the Jackson House. In April, he tersely wrote that it was a "miserable $2 a day hotel by the R.R. with a saloon. Blount Springs a quiet mountain resort for chronic complaints." Upon his return through the area a few weeks, he evidently found no other lodging as his diatribe continued: "Hotel Jackson here claims to be first class but it is very poor, bad fare poorly cooked & served, waiters indifferent…. Dirt meets the eye inside & out—About the springs it is filthy—A good place for fast people."⁴⁷

The archaeologist's views evidently were in the minority because the emerging national railway system brought in guests from outside the southern region, fulfilling Powell's prediction that "Rail-Roads [will make] our mountains accessible to the seekers of health."⁴⁸ The Fort Wayne, Muncie & Cincinnati Railroad extolled its "Excursion South" rates for parties of ten or more to visit Kentucky's Mammoth Cave, Crab Orchard Springs, and Rockcastle Springs followed by a final stop at Blount Springs.⁴⁹ The Mobile and Ohio Railroad advertised summer tourist tickets to Blount Springs and other regional resorts, reassuring potentially anxious travelers that "[t]hese are all well known resorts, and have been patronized liberally for a number of years by the best people in the Southern States."⁵⁰

Perhaps travelers needed reassurance for their visits to Blount. State troops saved a Black male from a lynch mob that accused him of murdering a judge near Blount Springs.⁵¹ Three men indicted in Huntsville for dealing in counterfeit money recruited "hit men" to deal with the government witnesses. At least four witnesses were poisoned, stabbed, or killed in some other fashion. One of the witnesses was assassinated at Blount Springs.[52] Equally scandalous was the murder of the drunk resident Blount Springs physician by a local farmer who shot the good doctor after the inebriated physician reached into his pocket during their dispute over a medical expense.[53]

Alabamians perceived Blount Springs as a haven from epidemics that swept through the South. In addition to its claim that it was malaria-free, Blount Springs received panicked guests fleeing from cholera and yellow fever. During the 1873 cholera epidemic, however, Birmingham residents both fled to and from Blount Springs. A party of 200 lost seven members to cholera en route to the resort; once the public was advised that the victims had contracted cholera before the resort visit, other Birmingham residents sought refuge at the springs.[54] A case of "cramp cholera" at Blount Springs the same summer caused "men, women, and children [to rush] from their rooms [to take] the midnight train for a place of safety."[55] Partly as a result of the 1873 epidemic, physician Herndon B. Robinson established a hospital near Blount Springs to promote the therapeutic use of the sulphur springs. By the mid-1890s, he had converted the ten-room hospital into a guesthouse where he received several Alabama politicians.[56] In November 1897, a yellow fever epidemic drove all but one of the state supreme court justices to Blount Springs; they returned to Montgomery via a fumigated railcar.[57]

Blount Springs prospered at the turn of the century but then faltered by the Great Depression. In 1903, owners Mack and J.W. Sloss, brothers in the Birmingham steel business, sold the property to Birmingham Mayor Walter Melville "Mel" Drennen, who unsuccessfully gambled that the steel industry would expand into Blount County, bringing more business to the resort.[58] In 1915, fire destroyed most of the resort complex, including the old Blount Springs hotel, the nearby Mountain Hotel, and several private cottages.[59] Some business continued at Blount Springs until Drennen's death in 1926, including sales of bottled water in 1916 and visitors to William Rice's sixteen-room hotel on the main road, built in 1923.[60] William Edward Fitch in his encyclopedic *Mineral Waters of the United States and American Spas* noted that the hotel in the mid-1920s offered only "fair accommodations and bathing facilities" as contrasted to his "excellent" rating accorded to southern Alabama's more opulent Bladon Springs. Fitch complimented the water: The springs "have received the approval and endorsement of the medical profession for more than three-quarters of a century [and] have been used with success in disorders of the digestive apparatus ... [and] certain phases of rheumatism and rheumatic arthritis."[61]

The Blount Springs property today has been subdivided for various uses. In 1989, part of the Blount Springs tract re-emerged as a private gated community near U.S. Highway 31, spearheaded by a Drennen nephew, who bought the property, largely untouched since Drennen's death. A family committed to historic preservation owns land that includes the site of Rice's hotel.[62] And, through the crumbling remnants of the once grand Blount Springs resort, the sulphur water still passes.

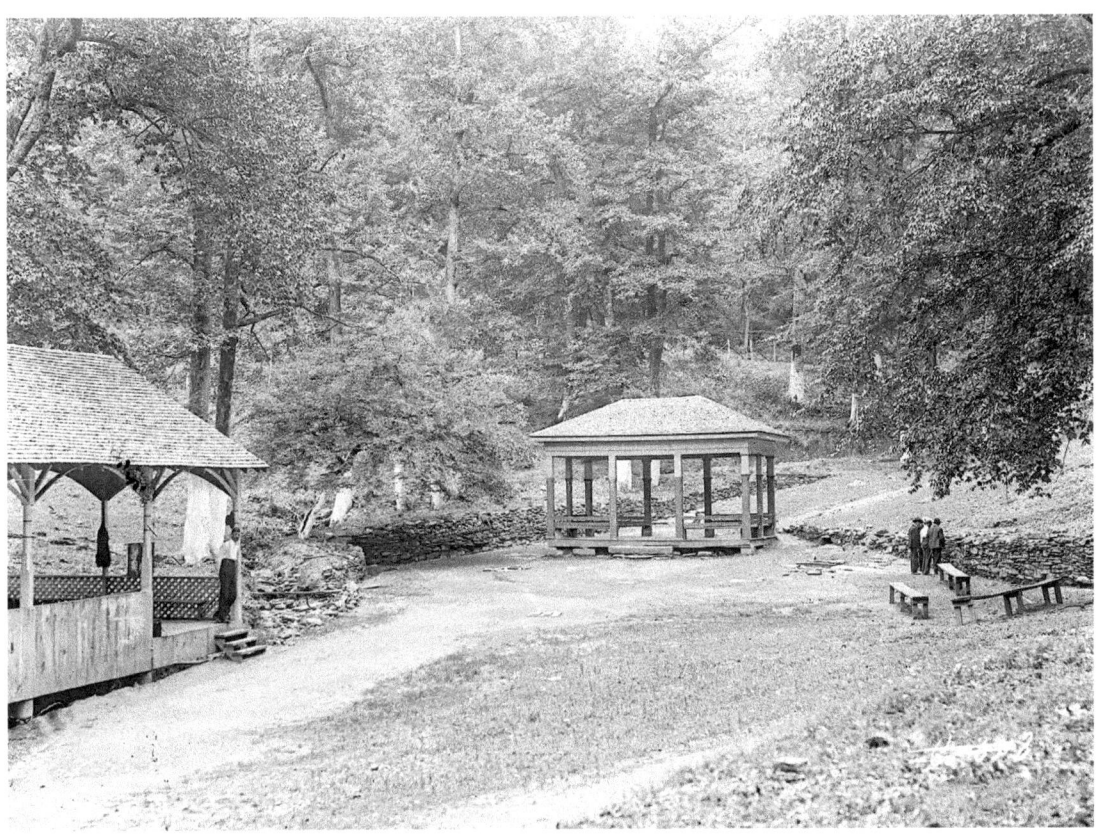

"Pavilion and Springs [1904]," Blount Springs, Blount County, Alabama (Robert Shattuck Hodges, photographer. Eugene Allen Smith Collection, The University of Alabama Libraries Special Collections, *https://archives.lib.ua.edu/repositories/3/resources/1647*).

DeKalb County: Mentone, Alabama White Sulphur Springs

The extreme northeastern corner of Alabama may suggest the most common picture of Southern Appalachia, that of a rugged terrain. Jackson County lies at the border of Southeast Tennessee and northwestern Georgia. Immediately to the county's south is DeKalb County, adjacent to Dade and Walker counties in Georgia. Although a nineteenth-century promoter exulted over Jackson County's "bold, refreshing springs," the county did not experience the growth of watering holes as did DeKalb.[63]

DeKalb County was home to at least two health resorts, differentiated by the clientele they initially sought yet connected by the railroad that passed near them carrying potential visitors. Mentone, eleven miles to the northeast of Fort Payne, founded by a Pennsylvanian, advertised for an English colony to settle near its health-giving springs. Alabama White Sulphur Springs, close to the Georgia border, grew in the tradition of many spring resorts: developed by a local familiar with stories of Native American use of the waters back to Native American use.

In DeKalb County, between the Cumberland Plateau's Sand Mountain ridge to the west and the Lookout Mountain ridge to the east, runs a series of valleys and ridges with colorful names such as Sand Valley, Shinbone Ridge, Dugout Valley, and Big Ridge. Fort Payne, the county seat, lies at an elevation of about 900 feet in the Little Wills Valley between Big Ridge, rising about 300 feet high over the town to its west, and the backdrop of Lookout Mountain to its east. Fort Payne experienced short-lived fame from 1888 to 1893 as one of the region's many boom towns when Vermonter W.P. Rice, "The King of Town Builders," spearheaded northern investment in nearby coal and iron ore mining and logistical operations and in the town's infrastructure, including the construction of the posh DeKalb Hotel for northern capitalists.[64] Nearby, Mentone towered over Fort Payne from its Lookout Mountain perch of 1,770 feet. About twelve miles northeast of Mentone, near the head of Sand Valley, stood the Alabama White Sulphur Springs, roughly at the same elevation as Fort Payne. From the Little Wills Valley northeast through the appropriately named Railroad Valley ran the Alabama Great Southern Railroad, respectively passing near Fort Payne, Mentone, and the Alabama White.[65]

Mentone

Mentone stood on Lookout Mountain, about two miles uphill from the Valley Head depot where passengers disembarked from the Alabama Great Southern Railroad after a twenty-minute train ride from Fort Payne.[66] In 1875, John Mason of Iowa bought 200 acres of land in the Valley Head area after regaining his health there; his son Edward, a surveyor and engineer, subsequently purchased more property, which he divided into sales lots. The tracts attracted Pennsylvania physician Frank (Franklin) Caldwell, who bought property on Lookout Mountain from Edward and built in 1883–1884 the Mentone Springs Hotel (Mineral Springs Hotel). Mentone received its name from Edward's sister, who had read about Mentone, France, whose name loosely translates as "mountain tone," a reference to the perceived musical gurgling of two Lookout Mountain springs, the Mineral Springs and the Beauty Springs.[67]

One interesting Mentone guest, another physician from outside the South, was Irishman John E. Purdon, who in the mid- to late–1880s sought to establish an English immigrant agrarian colony at Mentone.[68] After receiving his medical degree from Dublin University in 1863, Purdon served as a British surgeon general in India and other British colonies before being appointed U.S. Army Staff Assistant-Surgeon at Valley Head.[69] The *Virginia Medical Monthly* editor in 1893 hailed Purdon as a "progressive, active worker in whatever is promotive of the scientific development of medicine," not for his interest in mineral water or the mountain air, but for his involvement in "psychical sciences" such as telepathy.[70] Purdon failed to attract English immigrants to Mentone. He continued, however, to thrive both in his Valley Head medical practice and in his demonstrations of his pulse-measuring sphygmograph to allegedly communicate with the deceased. The *Chicago Tribune* praised him at the 1893 Columbian Exhibition for his "immense aid to the physiological study of mediumship."[71]

In the early 1890s, Caldwell sold the thirty-room resort to a nephew of former

Confederate Major General William W. Loring, Charles Loring of New Orleans, who renamed the property as the "Loring Springs Hotel" and nearly doubled the number of rooms by 1897.[72] The three-story frame Queen Anne building featured two rear ells, seven gables, an octagonal turret at each end, and a single-tiered porch along the front and sides. In 1915, the resort's popularity induced the construction of a nearby two-story hotel annex with about twenty-seven rooms, each with a private bath.[73]

Mentone publicized its convenient railroad location forty miles south of Chattanooga and advertised at various times its "fine bathing, chalybeate waters" or its location "far above malaria and wrapped in a cool mountain air."[74] By the early 1920s, as was common at many resorts, the hotel emphasis had shifted from mineral spring therapeutics to such recreational offerings as boating, swimming, hiking, and fishing.[75]

Guests largely traveled during the 1890s–1910s from Chattanooga, eastern Kentucky, Atlanta, northwestern Georgia, and local Alabama municipalities.[76] Limited room rate data also suggest that Mentone may have attracted a more modest

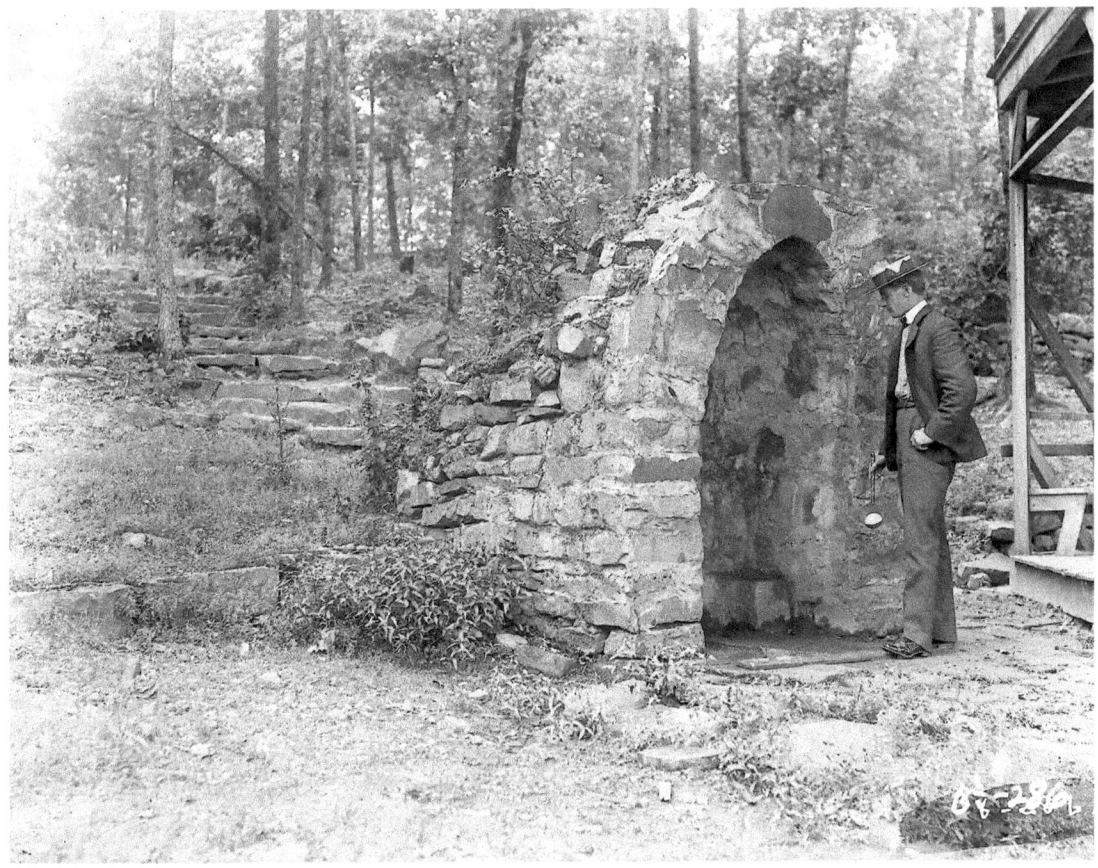

"Spring No. 1 [1905]," Mentone, DeKalb County, Alabama (Robert Shattuck Hodges, photographer. Eugene Allen Smith Collection, The University of Alabama Libraries Special Collections, *https://cdm17336.contentdm.oclc.org/digital/collection/p17336coll1/id/528*).

clientele, perhaps with less funds to travel broadly than guests at Monte Sano, for example, seventy miles to the west, near Huntsville. Monte Sano charged $3 per day in 1894 versus Mentone's monthly rate of only $30 in 1893.[77]

James H. Sulzby, Jr., and Zora Shay Strayhorn, however, imply a geographically more expansive clientele. Sulzby cites Mentone as being "widely known as one of the most healthful and attractive spots in the South." Strayhorn comments that the resort "attracted guests from near and far-away states."[78]

In 1921, the Alabama Baptist Convention began to lease the property each summer until the beginning of the Great Depression in the fall of 1929.[79] The resort subsequently went through a series of owners, with dances and hotel stays continuing through at least the 1920s. In the 1960s, the hotel became a private residence that fell into disrepair.[80] Ray and Sandy Padgett bought it in 1980, began to restore the dilapidated hotel, and successfully nominated it in 1983 for the National Register of Historic Places.[81] They sold the hotel in 1991, and the property saw at least four more owners. Unfortunately, the hotel and the hotel annex, which had been converted into a gallery after the 1960s, burned down in 2014, the 130th anniversary of the resort's founding. The structures have not been rebuilt.[82]

Alabama White Sulphur Springs

Twenty miles northeast of Fort Payne (or about forty-five minutes away if catching a ride on the Alabama Great Southern Railroad's "milk route" in 1895) stood the Sulphur Springs depot, about two miles from the Alabama White Sulphur Springs hotel and its six springs.[83] The six springs, clustered together in an area 200 feet square, were known to Native Americans.[84] Early white settlers developed a nearby academy whose curriculum included lessons about the perceived benefits of the water.[85] Colonel A.B. (Alexander) Hanna, from Rising Fawn in Dade County, Georgia, six miles away, began constructing a hotel and small buildings for family stays around 1871; the unfinished resort partly opened in 1873.[86]

Hanna eponymously called his resort "Hanna Springs" or "Hanna Mineral Springs" and began to entice guests to his three-story, porched hotel through his promotion of the curative powers of the springs and amusements.[87] With the waters' alleged benefits for chronic diseases of the liver, kidneys, bowels, and for other ailments and with the provision of the recreational offerings of a string band, boating, ten pins, and billiards, the resort's gain in popularity prompted an expansion in 1880.[88]

Perhaps as a play to strive for statewide prominence, Hanna also in 1880 rebranded the enlarged resort as the "Alabama White Sulphur Springs."[89] The property now included the addition of luxurious bath-rooms in the main building, larger parlors, and one of the most important improvements, a promenade 800 feet by 12 feet wrapping around the main building. The "grandeur of society," the delightful climate, along with "waters unsurpassed by those of any known mineral springs" were grandly pronounced by the *Vicksburg Herald* as "equal to any watering place in the South."[90]

Throughout the 1920s, the resort management stressed the property's health benefits derived from its water and its rejuvenating mountain air. This emphasis deviated from that of many other Southern Appalachian mineral spring resorts in their mature years, which promoted outdoor activities, dances, and parlor amusements to the near exclusion of the mineral water therapeutics upon which they were founded. One 1878 ad, for example, unabashedly boasted of the Alabama White providing the "best sulphur water and coolest summer resort."[91] About forty-five years later, the resort still underscored its "White Sulphur, Black Sulphur, Epsom, Freestone, and Limestone water," and only secondarily mentioned its "Billiard, Pool, Swimming, Dancing, and Tennis."[92] Seeking to promote the spa's purported healthful altitude in an era in which the bacteria *Salmonella typhi*'s linkage to poor hygiene was not known, the management in 1877 enticed fifty guests to sign a testimonial that typhoid fever was "an impossibility in this salubrious mountain region."[93] An ad three decades later exaggerated the hotel's elevation almost twofold to attract the sickly to the "most healthful mountain resort in the South [at] an eminence 1,700 ft. above sea level insuring [sic] pure, bracing air free from flies and mosquitoes."[94]

Train service provided ease of access to visitors from a broader geography as rail systems expanded. Guests came from Montgomery and other areas of Alabama; the resort's proximity to Tennessee and Georgia also attracted travelers from Chattanooga and Atlanta. Rail transportation also permitted vacationers to visit both Mentone and Alabama White Sulphur Springs on a "local circuit" or to participate in excursions that ran from Birmingham to the resort and then to Lookout Mountain.[95] From the Deep South, train passengers in 1880 traveled "only" twenty hours from Jackson, Mississippi, to reach the Alabama White.[96] Two decades later, a Cincinnati Southern Railway promotional pamphlet featured photographs of the resort in its history of the railroad, whose network now reached from New Orleans to Cincinnati and beyond.[97]

The resort continued from the early 1900s until beginning of the Great Depression. In 1901, the new owner, Dabney Scoville, renamed the hotel as the Lamine Hotel after his wife's first name, but the resort continued to be publicized as the "White Sulphur Springs."[98] In 1927, Fitch commented that ample hotel accommodations were available for those with such afflictions as gastric dyspepsia and skin disorders.[99] The last resort owners, Coca-Cola Bottling Company partner John Thomas Lupton and his wife Elizabeth Lupton of Chattanooga, bought the hotel and land in 1929 and donated it to the Chattanooga YWCA, which used it as a camp that operated through 1953.[100] The resort property was sold again in 1954 for a Christian camp that apparently never materialized as it was put up for auction in 1956.[101] The area around the health resort property today remains surrounded by pasture land and woods.[102]

Monte Sano

The peak of Monte Sano juts more than 1,600 feet above sea level in Madison County on the western edge of the Cumberland Plateau's Jackson County Mountains. Founded in December 1808, Madison County is cradled in the "great bend of the Tennessee" adjacent to Tennessee to the north, Jackson County to the east, and Limestone County to the west. Four miles west of Monte Santo lies Huntsville, originally known as Twickenham when the territorial legislature established it in December 1809. A Huntsville lawyer in 1817 recorded that "[t]he soil is for the most part excellent and admirably adapted to the culture of cotton, corn, wheat and tobacco. Cotton is the staple.... The face of the country is the most beautiful in the world, being in the main a level plain yet affording many mountain prospects and much romantic scenery.... The climate is healthful and in a high degree pleasant. Nowhere do you see more children with ruddy faces."[103]

In 1810, the county's population numbered about 4,700, of which both enslaved and free Blacks composed about a fifth. Fifty years later, Black enslaved laborers had increased by over a factor of fifteen (only 108 "free colored" residents were counted in 1860), accounting for 55 percent of the population in the booming agrarian economy that included oats, corn, and cotton.[104] The county was one of the richest in the state, thanks largely to the "red clay sub-soil and limestone foundation [producing] the highest degree of fertility."[105]

In this antebellum setting, Monte Sano thus appealed to the wealthy planters and other elites of Madison County to escape the lower altitudes' summer heat and afflictions and to connect with nature in a pastoral setting. By 1827, Robert, George, and Dr. Thomas Fearn, three brothers well known in Huntsville public affairs, had established a small community on Monte Santo that was incorporated as the village of Viduta in 1833.[106] The enclave attracted such political notables as the Huntsville Clay family. Clement Comer (C.C.) Clay, Sr., who served as governor and in the U.S. Congress, built a summer home about 1829. His son, politician Clement Claiborne Clay, Jr., followed twenty years later with his cottage, "Cozy Cot," where his family could enjoy the "ice water—pure air—delightful breezes & freed from that cursed ... insect musquitoe [sic]."[107] The Fearns' vision for drawing more visitors (and revenue) was furthered when Robert Fearn became president of the newly incorporated Monte Sano Turnpike Company in 1859.[108] The company built a macadamized road from Huntsville to Monte Sano; by the following year, it had successfully lobbied for legislative authorization to erect a tollgate for passage.[109]

As occurred at many southern resorts during the Civil War, recreational activity ceased. Union General O.M. Mitchel entered Huntsville on April 11, 1862; seized railroad stock; and set up command in the town. Confederate General Phillip Roddey, "Defender of Northern Alabama," countered the Union troops with guerrilla irregulars. Clement Clay, Jr.'s wife, Virginia, recalled that "the courage of our citizens was kept alive by General Roddy [sic], who lay over the crest of Monte Sano. The forays of his men were a perpetual worry to the Federals in the valley. [General Mitchel] razed the houses on 'The Hill' ... and built a stout fort the better to resist the possible attacks from the mountain side by brave General Roddy [sic] and his merry men."[110] A few families refused to abandon Monte Sano when war began. The Union Army, however, burned down the summer colony in 1863 and established a camp at the foot of the mountain.[111]

The resort remained dormant for several years after the Civil War due to lack of funding.[112] By the 1870s, unknown parties had initiated redevelopment on the mountain as the regional press began to comment on Monte Sano as both a place of retreat and refuge. The *Huntsville Advocate* in 1878 announced the presence of several prominent local families on the mountain for the summer. The national cholera epidemic of 1873, which reached as far north as Yankton, Dakota Territory, and the 1879 Memphis yellow fever epidemic brought refugees to Huntsville and Monte Sano where they enjoyed "an occasional picnic on [its] lofty summit."[113]

Another yellow fever epidemic in 1884 precipitated a serious effort to build a hotel on the "Mountain of Health." Michael J. O'Shaughnessy, a New Yorker who came to Huntsville after the Civil War, co-organized and then assumed leadership in 1886 of the North Alabama Improvement Company, backed by both northern capital and Huntsville business interests to further local economic activity. That same year, the company initiated construction on the Hotel Monte Sano.[114]

Newspapers trumpeted the 1887 inaugural season of the Hotel Monte Sano with great fanfare. "The eyes of the world are on North Alabama," gushed one Indiana correspondent about Huntsville and the resort, "a delightful stopping place, easy of access, with views and vistas on either hand that are grandly beautiful."[115] Another observer, in Huntsville for a nephew's wedding, praised the mountain's "exhilarating and bracing effect on the constitution ... [t]he most beautiful scenery ... the panorama of landscape, interspersed with hill and vale ... that is unsurpassed in the

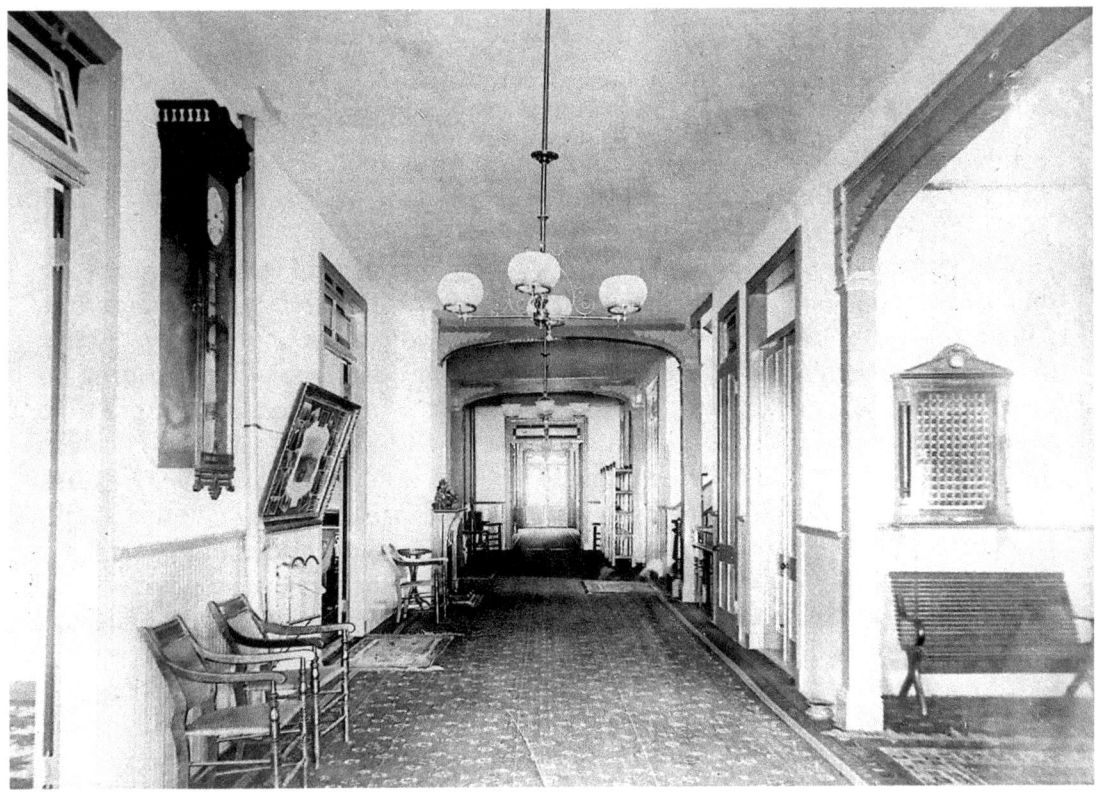

Monte Sano Hotel Lobby (1890), Madison County, Alabama (image courtesy of HMCPL Special Collections, Huntsville-Madison County Public Library, Huntsville, AL).

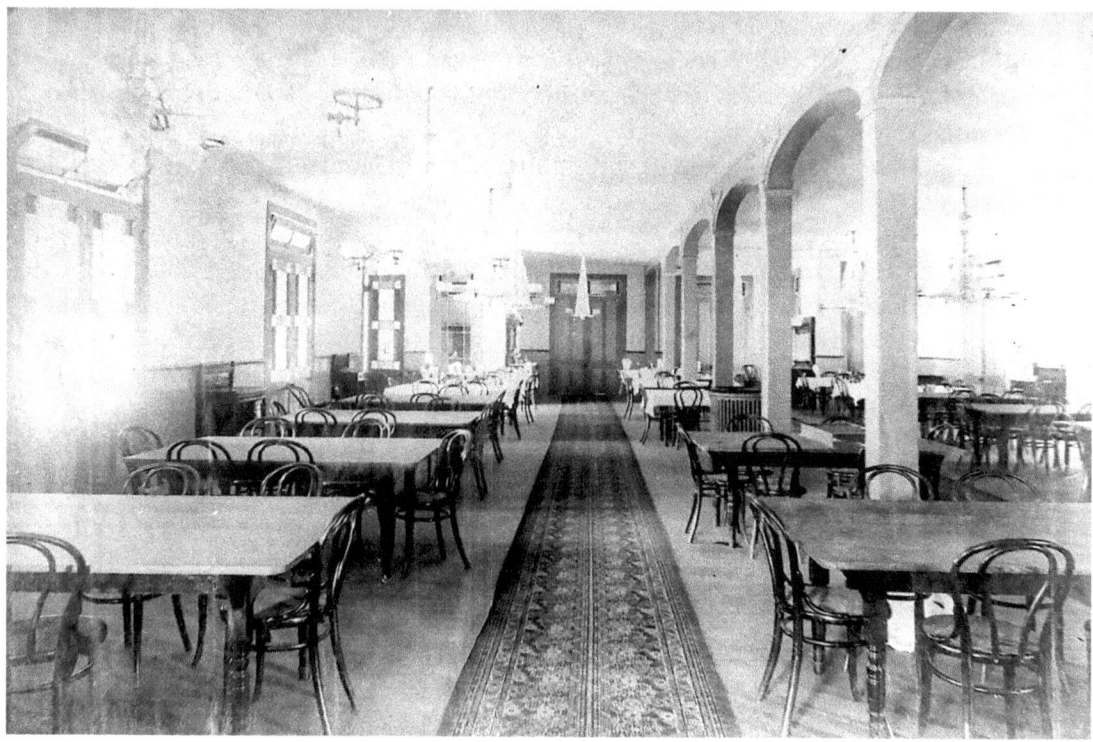

Monte Sano Dining Room (1890), Madison County, Alabama (image courtesy of HMCPL Special Collections, Huntsville-Madison County Public Library, Huntsville, AL).

South." The hotel itself he described as of Queen Anne architectural style with broad galleries surrounding it, with 136 rooms with gas light and steam heat. The hotel's success, he summarized, "has been unparalleled."[116]

Monte Sano's heyday largely occurred from its opening in 1887 through the mid–1890s. The hotel register showed visitors with such surnames as Vanderbilt, Gould, and Astor from the New York City and Newport areas.[117] Probably, though, most guests hailed largely from the Deep South. The correspondent attending his nephew's wedding met the widow of an Alabama Senator and an acquaintance from New Orleans ("more pleased with this climate than he was with the Northwest as a health resort"). The 1890 opening grand ball planning committee included "leading society men" of Louisville, Chattanooga, New Orleans, Memphis and other southern cities.[118] An 1890 newspaper reported that Nashville and Memphis were "perhaps best represented" so far that summer.[119] So many visitors from Memphis came during the first season that a two-story guest cottage with thirty-six rooms built near the hotel was christened the "Memphis Row."[120]

Guests enjoyed the usual fashionable resort amenities: ballroom dancing, billiards, bowling, lawn games, promenades, and excursions around the mountain. One trail, the "Flirtation Walk," according to one wag, was largely "conspicuous by the absence of lovers." Natural formations such as the "Ella Rock" (the four letters mysteriously carved on it), the "Needle's Eye," and the "Earthquake Glen" served as destinations for entertaining excursions. Although mineral waters such as the

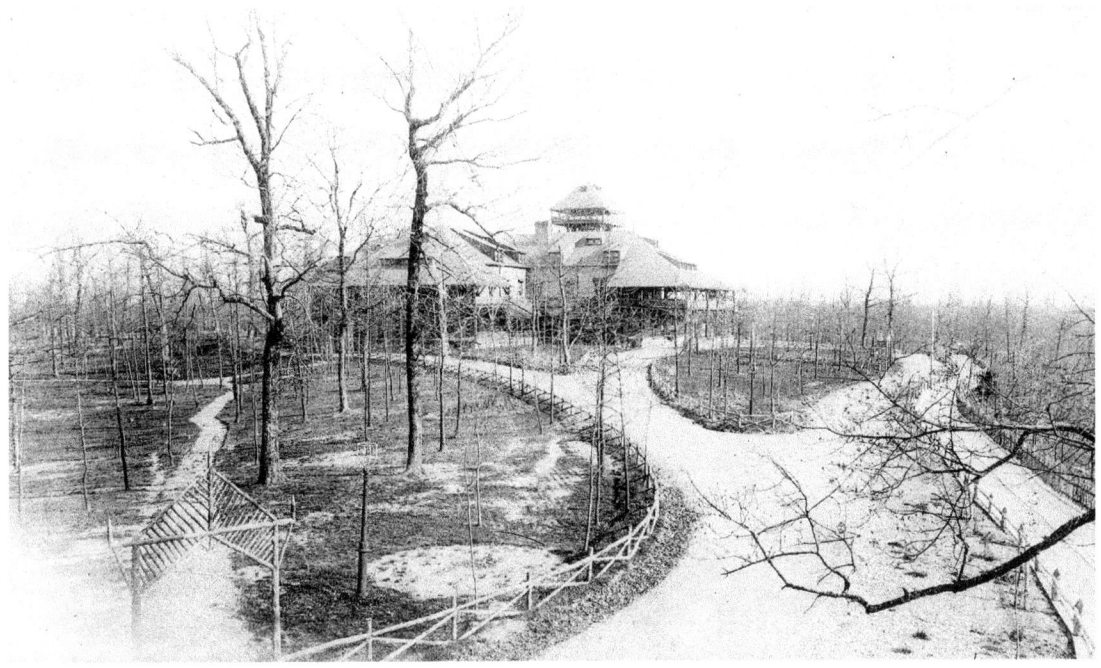

Monte Sano Hotel Exterior [no date], Madison County, Alabama. Ira F. Collins, photographer (image courtesy of HMCPL Special Collections, Huntsville-Madison County Public Library, Huntsville, AL).

Chalybeate Spring, Alum Spring, and Magnesia Spring were noted with markers along paths, they may have served during this period as more as points of amusement or curiosity rather than as stops for purely medicinal purposes as newspapers at that time framed the hotel largely as a destination for pleasure or escape from summer heat and fevers.[121]

In 1892, O'Shaughnessy's North Alabama Improvement Company sold its properties for $5–$6 million to the Northwestern Land Association of Pierre, South Dakota. Included as part of the sale were the Monte Sano Hotel ("lovely surroundings, used as a summer resort"), the Monte Sano Railway, and the turnpike connecting Huntsville with the resort. O'Shaughnessy remained as an association director. Other association board members included R.F. Pettigrew and A.C. Mellette, U.S. senator and governor respectively from South Dakota; several Cedar Rapids, Iowa, capitalists; and Huntsville businessmen. O'Shaughnessy's business connections in the North undoubtedly enticed the midwestern holding company to seek profit south.[122]

Within eight years, however, Monte Sano experienced a downturn in clientele, complicated by transportation and financial problems. Whereas in 1890 the daily rate was $3.50, by 1894, the rate had dropped to $3.00 per day, perhaps due in part to the 1893 depression. The following year, the hotel did not open due to stockholder litigation and a court order to liquidate the eight-mile railroad that ran from Huntsville to the hotel to pay creditors. The hotel reopened in 1897, but financial difficulties permanently shuttered the hotel in 1901.[123]

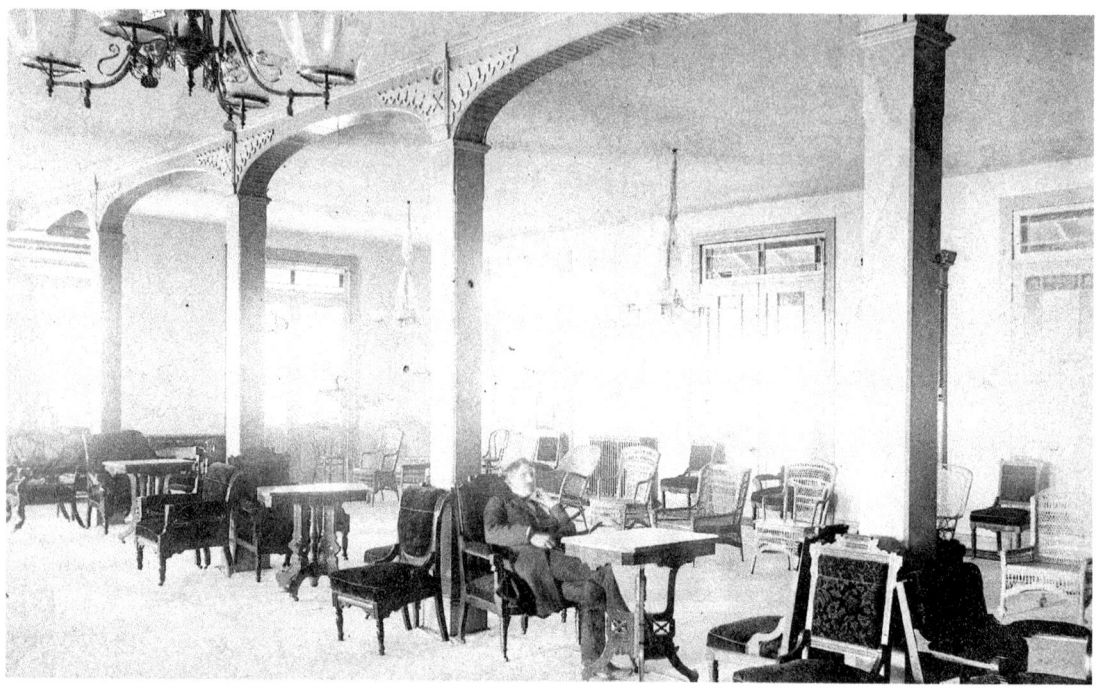

Monte Sano Hotel Parlor [no date], Madison County, Alabama. Photo caption reads, "A corner in the Parlor of Monte Sano Hotel where Concerts, Receptions and Balls were given when this resort was the most popular in all The South" (image courtesy of HMCPL Special Collections, Huntsville-Madison County Public Library, Huntsville, AL).

The daughter of Horace Garth, a former resident of New York then living in Huntsville, purchased the hotel and its twenty-seven acres for $20,000 in 1909 for use as a private home for her father.[124] That same year, the Huntsville, Chattanooga, and Birmingham Railway, Light and Power Company constructed an electric line from Huntsville to Monte Sano, suggesting the continued attractiveness of the mountain for residences.[125] After Horace Garth's death in 1920, the hotel building remained closed until the executors of the Garth estate sold the hotel building in 1944 at a dramatic loss for only $9,000 for salvage and scrap timber. A real estate developer bought the associated land. Only the chimney remains of the hotel itself off the appropriately named "Old Chimney Road." Visitors today seeking a stay on the "Mountain of Health" can do so at nearby Monte Sano State Park.[126]

Talladega County: Chandler Springs, Talladega Springs, and Shocco Springs

The Coosa River courses southwesterly from Rome, Georgia, through northeastern Alabama where the river serves as the western boundary of Talladega County before merging with the Tallapoosa River at Montgomery to form the Alabama River. Within the Coosa River Valley lies most of Talladega County at the southernmost of the Appalachian Valley and Ridge physiographic section. A narrow band of the county's entire eastern side is situated in the Piedmont Upland.[127] Because of these topographical features and combination of igneous and metamorphic geology, Talladega County contains a wide variety of minerals and was home to at least three nineteenth-century mineral spring resorts. Near the Coosa River in northeastern Talladega County stood Shocco (Chocco) Springs at an elevation of about 800 feet, about two miles west of the county seat of Talladega. About thirty-five miles south of Shocco, about a mile from the Coosa River's eastern bank, lay Talladega Springs at an elevation almost half that of Shocco's. About fourteen miles southeast of Shocco, on the western side of the Piedmont Upland in the Talladega Mountain range near the Coosa River tributary of Talladega Creek, stood Chandler Springs at a higher elevation of about 1,200 feet. The three resorts attracted mainly in-state clientele, never seemed to have engaged in rivalry, and were situated in a county riddled with hematite and some exaggerated nineteenth-century claims of the quantity of gold deposits.

The Alabama gold rush followed that of northeastern Georgia's gold discovery. Central Alabama's Chilton County is generally considered the site of the state's inaugural find in the period between 1830 and 1836. Arbacoochee in what is now Cleburne County, adjacent to Talladega County's northeastern border, received a surge in miners; by 1845, it had reputedly become Alabama's largest town. Within five years, however, most of the state's miners, including those in the optimistically named "Goldville" in Tallapoosa County, had left for the promise of California's gold fields.[128]

Opportunistic businessmen and regional newspapers continued for several years to hype Talladega County's potential for and progress in gold mining. Treatises in 1872 and 1888 respectively emphasized that "gold is now being sought" and that gold mines were yielding "decided profit."[129] Newspaper articles published seven years apart extolled Talladega's gold boom.[130] For perspective, for the period 1831–1946, Alabama gold amounted to only 2 percent of all mined southern gold and less than 6 percent of the value of gold extracted from Georgia mines.[131]

Although gold only panned out to a limited extent relative to elsewhere in the Southern Appalachians, Talladega County experienced some success in the iron ore extraction industry during the nineteenth century. The *Atlanta Constitution* in 1887, for example, billed Talladega as the "New Birmingham" for its county's potential to "make a higher grade of iron … than can be made from any other ores" in Alabama.[132] Earlier, from 1836 through 1854, Talladega County experienced a minor boom with the construction of eight forges and one blast furnace processing hematite or "brown ore" mined from deposits about six miles east of Talladega.[133]

Chandler Springs and Talladega Springs— Antebellum Beginnings

Chandler Springs began during Talladega County's early iron ore processing years. Around 1832, Pendleton, South Carolina, native James Chandler moved to the county with his new Georgia bride to capitalize on the land rush in the Coosa Land District for property taken from the Creeks as part of the 1830 Indian Removal

Act.[134] He rediscovered springs Native Americans used, registered deeds for 500 acres including the springs, and sometime before 1839 had built a two-and-one half story hotel with a dance pavilion surrounded by log cottages.[135] The resort, coupled with the several forges located between it and Talladega, likely served as the impetus for a weekly stage stop in place by 1842 at the Mountain Spring post office a few miles away.[136] Because the resort's three springs contained traces of iron from the nearby hematite deposits, they were considered chalybeate, "cold, strong, but pleasant."[137] The water purportedly treated visitors "laboring under nervous diseases, indigestion, and an impure state of the blood."[138]

Chandler Springs' location in the Hillabee (Talladega) mountains rendered it ideal for outdoor excursions. One hardy group from the resort in 1858 took an hour-long horse ride to the base of a nearby peak followed by a tiring hike to the summit, which rewarded the guests with a view of "mountains piled upon mountains, where peaks blended with the azure sky." The group sipped Heidsick (champagne) and enjoyed dinner prepared by "Boney," probably a nickname for an enslaved person or a wage-earning servant, before descending back to the springs, the "delightful place [of] one uninterrupted scene of pleasure."[139]

Talladega Springs stood about thirty miles away from Chandler Springs and like Chandler, was known to Native Americans and rediscovered by a white man, in this case, a Tennessee soldier in 1813 serving under Andrew Jackson in the Creek War.[140] B.W. Bell built a hotel in the 1830s and added double cabins around 1843.[141] In the early 1850s, a thirty-room, one-story hotel with a front porch across its length welcomed travelers.[142] Although Talladega Springs also possessed chalybeate water like Chandler Springs, it was better known for its strong sulphur water that provided the resort's and surrounding community's early name of "Sulphur Springs." By 1845, the resort's then appellation, "Talladega White Sulphur Springs," had simplified to "Talladega Springs."[143]

Talladega Springs' waters, advertised for dropsy (heart failure), rheumatism, and "all other diseases," allegedly cured many but fell short of perceived therapeutic benefit for others.[144] Antebellum mineral spring authority John Bell recognized, for example, northwestern Alabama's Lauderdale County's Bailey Springs' sulphur and chalybeate waters but did not find Talladega's waters worthy of comment.[145] A Talladega Springs community merchant advertised that only "Dr. Spencer's Vegetable Pills" had cured his chronic dyspepsia, sick headaches, and other health complaints despite taking at least eighty boxes of pills from assorted medicinal suppliers; he made no mention of the virtues of the nearby Talladega waters.[146] A Montgomery County planter, pessimistic of the promise of Talladega, drafted his will: "I leave this day for the Talledega [sic] springs. Should I not return, I give my Pintlala plantation to my mother."[147]

Neither Talladega Springs nor Chandler Springs apparently retained a resident physician to advise guests and to attest to the curative power of the springs; perhaps the owners possessed modest capital that prohibited hiring one. An early history of the county's doctors excludes any mention of mineral spring affiliations.[148]

As occurred at other Southern Appalachian mineral spring resorts, both Talladega and Chandler hosted political forums. In 1848, for example, Talladega served as the site for a discussion on Democratic and Whig party differences; the event concluded with an evening ball.[149] By the 1850s, Talladega County, as was the case in the rest of the country, increasingly debated slavery, internal improvements, and states' rights. Some Alabama Whigs, dismayed with the northern Whigs' increased emphasis on abolitionism after the 1854 passage of the Kansas-Nebraska Act, abandoned the Whig Party for the Know Nothing (American) Party, a nativist and anti–Catholic party that advocated for internal state improvements. Democratic attacks on the Know Nothings in the summer of 1855 precipitated some shifts in party allegiance and won over the electorate for the pro-slavery Democratic Party in Alabama. That summer, Chandler Springs hosted a heated Know Nothing political meeting in which the Know Nothing council refused to accept some members' resignation, possibly for those members to align with Democrats; those members met separately and "*resolved* [italics original] themselves out of the order."[150]

The Civil War wrought much devastation and hardship in Talladega County. Rampant inflation prompted one Talladega drug firm to issue over $500,000 in "shinplasters," nearly worthless promissory notes, used throughout eastern Alabama.[151] With able-bodied men in the military, women and children worked the fields, resulting in fewer crops and therefore much agricultural inflation, flour priced, for example, at $50 per barrel locally and the same flour inflated to $100 per barrel in Mobile.[152] In summer 1863, a Talladega County assembly resolved to assist the beats [districts or precincts] destitute of labor to attempt to save the wheat crop. A mere three landowners offered up only six "hands." Perhaps with a tinge of cynicism, the sheriff noted that he "presume[d] many of the planters have contributed to the laudable object contemplated by the resolution without reporting to me" as only Chandler Springs and another beat had publicly asked for assistance. The county sheriff then delegated two workers to assist the Chandler Springs beat.[153]

In July 1864 Rousseau's Raid brought about the destruction of the Talladega railroad depot and the ransacking of property primarily for food, livestock, and feed.[154] Chandler Springs served as a refuge. A Talladega widow charged one of the family's enslaved persons and her 12-year-old son to convey his two sisters and family valuables by wagon to Chandler. Once at Chandler, worried about his mother, the boy hastily rode the fourteen miles back to Talladega late at night, frightened along the way by a blackened pine stump near the road that he thought was a deserter waiting to shoot him. Once home, his mother assured him of the courtesies extended to her by the "Kentucky gentleman," Union Major General Lovell Rousseau, and promptly sent the boy back to Chandler Springs.[155]

Shocco Springs—Postbellum Beginnings

Shocco (Chocco) Springs, like Chandler Springs and Talladega Springs, also was discovered by Native Americans, and its name may reflect Native American origins. The Shocco Springs Conference Center website speculates that "Shocco" may derive from a Native American word meaning "the gathering place."[156] "Shocco" may also have originated from Native American use in North Carolina where another Shocco Springs near Warrenton welcomed fashionable guests.[157] According to a nineteenth-century account, Talladega County Confederate veteran Jarrett Thompson, wounded at both Gettysburg and the Battle of the Wilderness, bought and named the springs after finding relief from chronic health afflictions on the purported advice of Shocco, an elderly Creek medicine man.[158]

Although Shocco Springs received guests by 1874, the resort did not become fully established until 1878.[159] In that year, Thompson opened a new hotel and eight nearby cabins and provided recreational activities to guests.[160] Amusements included a fishpond for the "delightful sport of the ladies and children," a ten-pin alley, bathing, riding, and "good music."[161] The resort also began an annual ice cream festival to coincide with each season's opening and boasted of the availability of ice cream at any time of the day.[162]

Shocco Springs' sulphur, chalybeate, and freestone (non-mineralized) waters were marketed in a variety of ways.[163] To attract summer visitors from humid southern Alabama, Thompson advertised mineral water "spiked in icicles" from stored ice.[164] In 1905, the resort publicized daily delivery of water for twenty-five cents per five gallons, eliminating a reason for locals to trek to the resort.[165] In 1916, the newly formed Shocco Springs Company began to ship the water.[166] In 1919, a regional soft drink, Chero-Cola, later bought by the Coca-Cola Company, was bottled with Shocco Springs water when the normally used Talladega town water became contaminated with *Salmonella typhi* bacteria, the source of typhoid fever.[167] Shocco engaged in commercial water sales as late as 1924.[168]

The Three Resorts: Postbellum Discussion and Aftermath

In the postbellum period, Chandler Springs, Talladega Springs, and Shocco received guests largely from both southern Alabama and the local area. Shocco visitors from one week hailed from Montgomery, Talladega, Selma, and Easonville in Alabama.[169] Chandler Springs received guests from Mobile and hosted the Clay County–Talladega County Democratic state senate convention.[170] Talladega for one week in 1879 reported visitors from Montgomery and Coosa counties.[171]

To accommodate more visitors, Chandler and Talladega expanded and renovated (it is not clear as to whether Shocco enlarged its accommodations). Chandler Springs built several bath houses and ballrooms, added new cabins, and repaired the hotel, which eventually accommodated 150 guests.[172] Talladega Springs also erected new bath houses, provided rental cottages, and enlarged its hotel in 1891 to fifty-two rooms to take advantage of the Louisville & Nashville Railroad's construction of the Alabama Mineral Line providing connections to several Alabama towns.[173]

No apparent competition existed among the three resorts, nor did one health resort consistently garner more accolades than the other two. On the one hand, the local newspaper, *Our Mountain Home*, considered Talladega Springs the most outstanding of the three. On the other hand, a national newspaper directory omitted Talladega Springs but listed Shocco and Chandler as prominent county resorts.[174] Perhaps the only examples of one-upmanship occurred in the claims of escaping from Black Belt and coastal heat. Chandler boasted that "blankets are necessary throughout the summer nights." Talladega Springs emphasized itself as a "retreat from the heat and sickness of the hot." Shocco stressed its "ten tons of thick ice" in winter storage for use in summer drinks.[175]

The twentieth century saw a slow decline in the three properties, Shocco's occurring before the other two. As early as 1895, Shocco Springs pleaded in an ad: "Help to revive the past glory of this excellent resort."[176] In 1911, Shocco began to rent its grounds to the Alabama Baptist Convention for summer use while continuing hotel operations at least into 1926 and hosting dances into the Depression years.[177] During World War II, the hotel and its twenty-five cottages served as defense industry housing. Today, the resort has been reinvigorated as the Shocco Springs Alabama Baptist Conference Center.[178]

Talladega Springs and Chandler Springs no longer exist. In 1907, Talladega rebranded itself "hereafter … not only a health but also a pleasure resort" to attract more visitors.[179] The previous year, the resort's new owner, Anniston's Dr. A.A. Greene, had infused the resort with $5,000 capital to construct a twenty-four room hotel addition, an ice-skating rink, and other improvements, which opened to great fanfare in 1907 with a masque ball.[180] Talladega continued its original health model that year by initiating bottled water shipments and by providing its water on tap at local fountains.[181] The resort closed in 1914 because of travelers motoring elsewhere and because of concerns that the Coosa River's newly built Lay Dam might submerge the grounds. In 1921, Talladega furnishings were auctioned off.[182] Chandler Springs' hotel burned down in 1918. The property served as a CCC camp during the Depression. In 1958, only a few buildings remained, including one cottage the Ed Ponder family remodeled into a private residence.[183]

Valhermoso Springs

In northeastern Morgan County, about twelve miles south of neighboring Madison County's Huntsville, was nestled the health resort of Valhermoso Springs in a "beautiful valley," as the English translation of its Spanish name implies. Towering over Valhermoso's 568-foot elevation about three miles to the east was Brindley Mountain at about 1,322 feet.[184] Although both Morgan County and Madison County compose part of the Cereal Belt described by Riley, Morgan County was less agriculturally developed than Madison in the nineteenth century.[185] Riley focused on Morgan's minerals and rocks, in particular asphalt, coal, limestone, and what he exaggerated as potentially large quantities of gold. The limestone's porosity allowed water with dissolved minerals to flow through it, resulting in the mineral springs found in the county.[186]

Valhermoso Springs' early history is in dispute. Many sources differ about the ownership and the development of the resort until the late 1830s, when all agree that the Manning brothers owned and improved the resort. All concur that a family by the name of Chunn moved to the area from Maryland in the early nineteenth century. Lancelot Chunn, the patriarch, appears to have settled by the mineral springs by the early 1810s. Although some sources state that Robert or James (perhaps Robert James) Manning may have operated a hotel at the site between 1818 and 1823, it appears more likely that prior to his death in 1830, Lancelot gave or sold the property to his son William Ridgely in or before 1826.[187]

The resort history becomes less entangled after 1825. In 1826, William "agree[d]" to lease, for 5 years, to Elizabeth Woods, of Madison County, Alabama, "the Sulpher [sic] and other springs at which the said William R. Chunn now resides such lying and being in the County of Morgan and commonly called and Knowing as Chunns [sic] Springs." The lease also included all household, kitchen, and farming equipment except horses. Yearly rent was established at $700.[188] The following year, per an 1895 newspaper article, William sold the property, purportedly consisting of a hotel and fifty cottages, to James T. Sykes. The article marveled that "in that dangerous time of traveling, and in this then sparsely settled country," that 200–300 travelers annually found their way to Valhermoso Springs to drink the waters.[189] The newspaper account may have exaggerated the numbers, but the comment that the springs attracted a large gathering in the 1820s speaks to the high volume of travel occurring in allegedly remote Southern Appalachia.

In the following decade, according to the 1895 history, Valhermoso hosted at one time as many as 500 guests attracted to the variety of mineral springs. Of Valhermoso's chalybeate, limestone, black sulphur, and white sulphur springs, the white sulphur water gained fame for treating such afflictions as rheumatism, gastrointestinal ailments, and consumption.[190] Its popularity gave rise to another name for the resort, White Sulphur Springs. A post office with that name was established in 1834, indicating high resort traffic, as noted by the 1895 history, but the post office inexplicably closed in 1835.[191]

The property ownership stabilized in 1838 for about four years. The resort proprietor, Joseph Wallace, who had bought the property from Sykes, sold White Sulphur to brothers R.J. (presumably Robert James), P.T., and G.F. Manning.[192] The Manning brothers engaged the former managers of the popular Richmond, Virginia, Bell Tavern as operators.[193] The Mannings improved the resort infrastructure, likely due to the resort's gaining so many patrons that it had become a daily stage stop. They erected a much larger main hotel with three stories and a front colonnade, twenty-five or thirty frame cottages, a new bath house, an icehouse, and a "Bar ... of the first order."[194]

The Mannings miscalculated their potential income from the health resort and mismanaged the funds they did earn. In 1839, they advertised their rates as more moderate than the renovated accommodations would justify to offset rumors that board and lodging prices would increase with the improvements[195] By the next summer, because of "great pressure in monetary matters," perhaps linked to the lingering effects of the Panic of 1837, as well as to their financial incompetence, the brothers reduced their room rates by over 14 percent and slashed dinner prices by a third.[196] Moreover, a few years later, gambling losses added to their financial woes, such that the Mannings declared bankruptcy and the resort was sold at public auction in 1842 to the Bank of Huntsville.[197]

The resort, however, apparently did not fade even as it went into receivership as evidenced by the guests it attracted. Notables included politician William Rufus King and reformer Julia Tutwiler.[198] One guest, Jean Joseph Giers, a native German, lived in Washington, D.C., during the winter and at Valhermoso Springs in the summer. He bought the property in 1855 from the Bank of Huntsville, eventually around 1870 establishing a colony of German and Swiss settlers around Valhermoso.[199] By 1857, resort and community business again necessitated the establishment of a post office, this time known as Valhermoso Springs, with the hotel called the Cedar Hotel after a line of cedars found at a gorge nearby.[200]

Valhermoso was not immune to the sectional tensions preceding the Civil War. Giers, a close friend of Lincoln yet condoned slavery, per Sulzby, invited a Bostonian, William J. Brewster, to teach at the nearby Somerville Academy in 1860.[201] Within a few weeks of Brewster's arrival in the South, a local court summoned him to address the charge of "being an Abolition emissary who had come to incite the slaves to murder and rapine." The Bostonian, after some effort, including thwarting a lynch mob, made his way back to Valhermoso Springs where the Giers family warmly welcomed him for the night. Several local planters armed with guns stood sentry at the home as assailants threatened to burn down the house for harboring an abolitionist. Once safely back in the North, Brewster wrote a graphic, gripping letter to the *New York Tribune* republished in *The Liberator* of his experience with "mob law in Northern Alabama."[202]

In April 1862, Union forces took possession of the Memphis and Charleston Railroad and towns along its wayside, including Decatur and Huntsville.[203] The *Philadelphia Inquirer* in one issue not only covered the Union victories but also, to educate northern readers unfamiliar with northern Alabama, published on the same page a glowing account of Huntsville ("reputed to be the most beautiful of Southern inland cities") and its environs. The *Inquirer* extolled Valhermoso's "beautifully located" white sulphur and chalybeate waters of "considerable resort" and the "remarkably cool and pleasant" sulfur water of the Artesian Wells, a watering place about six miles west of Decatur.[204]

Unlike most southern resorts, Valhermoso was not abandoned during the war. Giers' wife hid Confederate soldiers beneath the hotel eaves when Union troops entered the area.[205] A guest at the resort in 1863 described a Union ambush near Huntsville in which "our little squad behaved gallantly [shooting] a Federal Captain in the face and [killing] his horse." The guest concluded his description with the admonition that "Those on our side, who go over, have more to fear from some of our own people than from the Yankees."[206]

In the postbellum period, the resort continued to attract patronage based on its publicity for its scenery and mineral waters. Valhermoso Springs did not advertise recreational activities; it emphasized its location, the "'Switzerland of the South,' with its cool and bracing atmosphere" where the "temperature is cool and pleasant, and there are no musquitoes [sic]."[207] The mineral waters were advertised in "great abundance" and in "inexhaustible supplies—more heavily impregnated ... than any similar waters in the United States."[208] Physicians, notably from summer fever-stricken New Orleans, avowed that the iconic white sulphur was "equal to any in Virginia."[209]

During the same period, however, Valhermoso Springs began a very gradual decline, as evidenced by a close review of advertisements. Giers in 1869 advertised in the *Huntsville Advocate* for "a partner with some capitol [sic] to aid me in furnishing Valhermoso Springs and take charge of them."[210] In 1869, Valhermoso charged $10 per week; by comparison, Montvale Springs in the Tennessee Smokies commanded over 50 percent more at $16.50 for weekly board.[211] In fact, the Valhermoso rates adjusted via the Consumer Price Index gradually fell after the antebellum period, thus indicating an attempt to attract a fading clientele. The 1839 weekly rate of $10.50, the 1869 weekly rate of $10, and the 1904 weekly rate of $6 normalize in 2022 dollars respectively to $341, $222, and $203.[212] Moreover, the 1895 history noted that the property was neglected: "The buildings and surroundings are badly in need of repair and with the proper management and means could be made the finest health resort property in North Alabama."[213]

The decline in resort maintenance and therefore a decrease in visitors most likely resulted from the lack of owner capital. Giers died in 1880, and his son Ernst operated the resort until at least 1920, attempting to sell or lease the property as late as 1928.[214]

The year 1950 proved to be the final blow to the property. A tornado ripped through the top floor of the hotel, collapsing the porches. Later that year, a fire burned down the remaining hotel structure and swept through most of the cottages.[215] Today, a historical marker on Highway 36 east of Thomas Road stands near the site of the once-thriving resort.[216]

Georgia

Introduction

Images of northern Georgia abound in popular culture. They teeter on stereotypes, thanks to CBS's *The Dukes of Hazzard* moonshine-running family and to James Dickey's *Deliverance*, the chilling tale of ruthless Georgia mountain men torturing Atlanta businessmen on a canoe trip. More realistic of the mountainous region is the *Foxfire Book* series on Southern Appalachian customs and the incorporation of northern Georgia settings into works by native novelists Olive Ann Burns (*Cold Sassy Tree*) and Terry Kay (*To Dance with the White Dog*).

Northern Georgia's Southern Appalachian topography consists of four geologic regions or physiographic provinces: the Cumberland or Appalachian Plateau, the Valley and Ridge, the Piedmont, and the Blue Ridge Mountains.[1] Found within the Appalachian Plateau in the state's northwestern corner are Dade County and Walker County, home to Cloudland Canyon.[2]

On Walker County's eastern border, Catoosa County lies in the Valley and Ridge province that runs southerly to Bartow County and Polk County, the latter on the Alabama state line.[3] The Piedmont cuts an easterly swath from Cherokee County (Bartow's neighbor to the east) through Forsyth, Hall, and Banks counties to the Blue Ridge Mountains.[4] In turn, the Blue Ridge, home to Tallulah Gorge State Park lies in the state's northeastern corner. Counties associated with the Blue Ridge include Lumpkin, Habersham, and Rabun.[5] The nineteenth-century Georgia poet Sidney Lanier captured part of the topography in "The Song of the Chattahoochee": "Out of the hills of Habersham, Down the valleys of Hall, I hurry."[6]

Southern Appalachian Georgia contains many types of minerals and rocks. Alumina, mica, iron, copper, and, most famously, gold near Dahlonega were mined in the nineteenth century. An antebellum physician commented that the northern part of the Piedmont "contains most of the rich mines of gold, copper, &c., with mineral springs in various places."[7] State geologist S.W. McCallie in 1913 described manganese ore near Murray County's Cohutta Springs on the cusp of the Piedmont and Blue Ridge Mountains, mica mining in Lumpkin and Union counties, ochre mining near Bartow County's Rowland Springs, and noted the discovery of garnets in Hall, Lumpkin, Dawson, and Cherokee counties.[8]

Prolific in the Valley and Ridge and present to a lesser extent on the Appalachian Plateau was limestone. *De Bow's Review* in 1858 wondered why Georgia (and

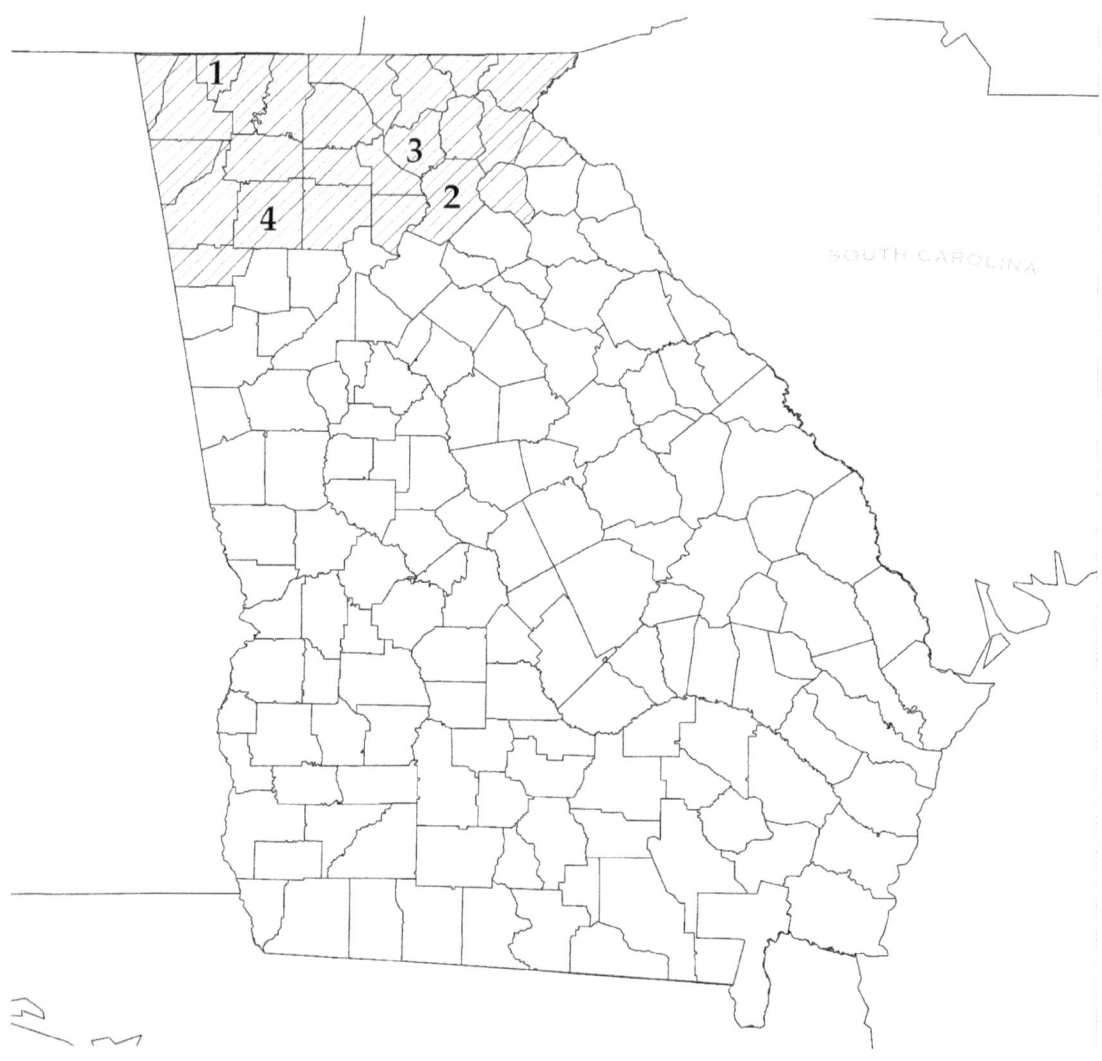

Georgia counties with featured health resorts: (1) Catoosa County, Catoosa Springs; (2) Hall County, Gower's Spring, New Holland Springs and Oconee White Sulphur Springs; (3) Lumpkin County, Porter's Springs; (4) Bartow County, Rowland Springs (Sources: Esri, NOAA, USGS. Cartographer: Sayona Turner, East Tennessee State University).

presumably, the South in general) imported New York cement when "magnesian and argillaceous limestones, of exactly the composition for hydraulic cement … exists in abundance in our limestone country?"[9] Fifty-five years later, McCallie noted limestone's "great economic importance" in Georgia for its use in building materials and as flux in the smelting of ore.[10] An 1857 American Medical Association report described Southern Appalachian Georgia's "large springs, which gush up from beneath the substratum of limestone" but withheld comment on any therapeutic benefit of the resulting mineral-laced waters.[11] Two decades later, however, the Association's Committee of Sanitaria and Mineral Waters listed mineral waters by chemical analysis but explained that patients' benefits were derived in part from the "good effects of change of scene" and a "bracing climate" and not exclusively from the waters' medicinal agents.[12] Among Southern Appalachian Georgia springs the committee listed, therefore demonstrating their curative reputations in a national context, were Catoosa, Oconee White Sulphur, and Gower's Spring.[13]

The most popular antebellum Mountain South Georgia mineral spring resorts dotted northwestern Georgia where the state-owned Western and Atlantic Railroad (the "State Road") provided relative ease of access to Rowland Springs, Catoosa Springs, Gordon Springs, and Cohutta Springs. Murray County's Cohutta Springs, about twenty-four miles from Dalton, may be the oldest resort in northern Georgia; in 1837, it appeared on a proposed federal postal run from Athens to Spring Place.[14] Gordon Springs in modern Whitfield County provided its chalybeate and magnesia waters in a somber setting that prohibited dancing and "all dissipation" so that a "moral and religious public [could] sojourn without being offended."[15] About seven miles from the sobriety of Gordon's, Catoosa Springs stood in lively contrast, known for its chivalrous tournaments and grand balls.[16] Cass (now Barlow) County's John Sharpe Rowland developed Rowland Springs and its elaborate fountains lining promenades. Rowland Springs may have been the most fashionable antebellum Southern Appalachian Georgia resort, rivaled only by Catoosa, and favorably compared to the *crème de la crème* antebellum Georgia resorts outside the Mountain South, Butts County's Indian Springs and Madison County's Madison Springs.[17]

During the Civil War, resorts in northwestern Georgia closed, went on the market, or served as hospitals, given their proximity to such battle sites as Chickamauga and Tunnel Hill. Gordon Springs management sought a buyer to pay in "Confederate Notes or Exchange for Negroes."[18] Catoosa Springs and nearby Cherokee Springs (operated by Catoosa Springs' owner at one time) cared for wounded Confederate soldiers, who benefited from Cherokee's waters.[19]

Thirty years later, a national mineral springs survey reported that while Catoosa had updated its facilities with modern conveniences for up to 600 guests, Gordon Springs and Cohutta Springs were on the decline.[20] Rowland Springs, marked by less capital investment and frequent ownership change, had "not been so extensively patronized," according to the national mineral springs survey's diplomatic wording.[21]

In northeastern Georgia, the lack of antebellum rail infrastructure in the mountains hindered resort development.[22] Nonetheless, the Gainesville area boasted three mineral springs of interest in antebellum times—Gower's Spring, New Holland Springs, and Oconee White Sulphur Springs—that boomed with the introduction of the Atlanta and Richmond Air Line Railway service to Gainesville in 1871. These three health resorts primarily attracted visitors from Atlanta and Savannah and secondarily from central Georgia, who sought a higher and cooler elevation, relief from poorly understood summer fevers, and a cure for almost every physical ailment ever diagnosed. The three resorts and Gainesville hotels vied with Marietta, another stop on the Western and Atlantic Railroad from Atlanta, which boasted that its 1,100-foot elevation allowed visitors to "escap[e] the extreme heat and the malarial influences."[23]

Other resorts opened in northeastern Georgia in the 1870s in the Blue

Ridge. From Gainesville, travelers endured a bouncing hack ride over a winding twenty-eight mile road to Lumpkin County's Porter Springs. Porter gained fame both for its "blend" of iron, sulphur, and other minerals in its water and for its mountain air, purportedly rich with ozone to cure invalids and high enough in elevation to ward off malaria.[24] About thirty miles to the east of Porter Springs stood Habersham County's Mount Airy Hotel, in which the New Holland Springs owner may have invested during the early 1870s.[25] Mount Airy took advantage of its singularity as the highest point on the Air Line Railroad by marketing itself as a hay fever retreat.[26] With its high elevation, Mount Airy also attracted "refugees from the heat and malaria of Memphis, New Orleans, and Savannah."[27]

Visitors to the Blue Ridge occasionally condescended, in some cases unintentionally, to the locals. A New Englander in 1850 commented on the "astounding" ignorance of the populace in her book chapter, "Habits, Pursuits, and Ignorance of the People in the Northern Part of the State" (she placed blame on the state for inadequate public education funding).[28] An impudent female from southern Georgia, on an outing from Porter Springs, denigrated a mountaineer family that her party chanced upon.[29] In the early twentieth century, when do good associations were increasing involvement in rural Appalachian mission work, one longtime northern Georgia resident rebuked a Christian publication that claimed the mountaineers were "living in a state of 'degradation, poverty and ignorance....' These people of the mountains are a very shrewd people, and he 'who shoots one for a fool, wasteth a load.'"[30]

In the spirit of *De Bow's*, southern articles called for Georgians to patronize Southern Appalachian resorts rather than to spend their funds in the North. A Columbus newspaper editorial railed against southerners who migrated like birds to the North annually only to see daughters to be introduced to the "dissipation and frivolity which reign in the saloons of Saratoga" and sons "decoyed to the gaming table": "The money spent in one summer ... would make the watering plaaes [*sic*] of Georgia, equal to any in the Union but, above all, would be kept it here among us."[31] By the eve of the Civil War, a newspaper reiterated the theme: "We have heard much of late about non-intercourse with the North.... Instead of patronizing Newport, Rockaway, Sharon and Saratoga, spend your time and money at home."[32] The refrain continued after the war. Four years after Henry W. Grady's "New South" editorial appeared in the *Atlanta Constitution*, an 1879 Macon newspaper continued the antebellum call as well as implicitly endorsing Grady's manifesto: "no need of going beyond State lines for the most charming entertainment and health-giving powers" of Porter Springs and Catoosa Springs.[33]

The resorts selected for this chapter epitomize a cross-section of Georgia topography and culture. Wealthy plantation owner John Sharpe Rowland worked enslaved laborers to shape his wooded property into a premier antebellum resort near the Valley and Ridge's southern border of Southern Appalachian Georgia. Close to the northern border of the Valley and Ridge with Tennessee stood Catoosa Springs, the self-proclaimed "Saratoga of the South," whose enslaved persons provided an "efficient force of attentive servants."[34] To the southeast of Catoosa, in the Piedmont's Gainesville area, were clustered Gower's Spring, New Holland Springs, and Oconee White Sulphur Springs that thrived after the Civil War. In the Blue Ridge, tucked away on the side of Cedar Mountain, was postbellum Porter Springs, relatively remote and plain in offerings compared to the Gainesville resorts yet a genial gathering place for almost fifty years.

Catoosa Springs

Catoosa County, bordering East Tennessee at the Chattanooga metropolitan area boundary, was carved from Whitfield and Walker counties in northwestern Georgia in 1853, which in turn had been formed earlier from partitions of land stolen from the Cherokee Nation. With the discovery of gold in northeastern Georgia in 1828, whites forced the Cherokee out of their homes into small settlements until the 1830 Indian Removal Act and the 1835 Treaty of New Echota empowered federal soldiers to remove the Cherokee via the Trail of Tears in 1838–39 to the Indian Territory (present-day Oklahoma).[35] Civil War buffs know Catoosa County for its role in the 1862 Great Locomotive Chase, the battles of Chickamauga and Ringgold Gap in 1863, and in the Atlanta Campaign that began in May 1864.

Catoosa County lies in Georgia's Valley and Ridge physiographic province where winding creeks and narrow valleys separate long ridges running in a southwesterly to northeasterly direction. Catoosa Springs stands at an elevation of about 860 feet in a hilly area about one mile southeast of the 1,340-foot peak of the Sand Mountain ridge. In fact, the word "Catoosa" evolved from the Cherokee "gatusi" or "gahdoosi," alluding to either a mound or a small mountain.[36] From the resort, the Catoosa Springs Branch waters eventually reach Chickamauga Creek, which enters Ringgold Gap between Taylor Ridge and the White Oak Mountain ridge near the southern edge of Ringgold. Tunnel Hill and Dalton are southeast of Catoosa Springs in Whitfield County, about seven miles and sixteen miles respectively from Ringgold. The gaps in this area provided a natural route for early white settler migration and for later Civil War Union and Confederate troop movements.[37]

Catoosa County contains many mineral deposits. Scattered throughout Taylor Ridge are so-called "fossil" iron ores, fossil cavities filled with ferric oxide, that by the early 1900s had been "more or less extensively exploited."[38] Calcium carbonate is found in abundance as both limestone and, per a 1906 state agricultural bulletin, as marble "suitable for huge columns ... quarried with ease."[39] Fluorite (calcium fluoride), gypsum (calcium sulfate dihydrate), an Onondaga salt deposit, and alum constitute a few of the mineral sources documented in the county.[40] The leaching of minerals from these and other deposits accounts for the varied chemical content of springs in the county, including Catoosa Springs' fifty-two springs and those of the minor watering hole of Cherokee Springs found within a few miles of Ringgold.[41]

Use of the Catoosa Spring waters predates white settlement. The Cherokee discovered the medicinal value of the waters and attempted as revenge to plug up a dozen of its springs before they were forcibly marched away on the Trail of Tears.[42] Sometime before 1849, an oft-quoted horticulturist in the area, Colonel William Murray, an expert on potato, Catawba grape, and white blackberry cultivation among other edibles, came into possession of the springs, which eponymously became known as "Murray Springs."[43] An 1849 medical journal's list of the top Georgia mineral springs included Murray's waters, whose "very numerous" springs "break out in the bottom of a small stream; and contain *Lime, Sulphur,* and *Iron* [italics original]."[44]

In late summer 1849, Murray sold his springs in two tracts to four Georgians residing over 300 miles away in central Georgia, indicating that the springs' potentiality for profit was known outside northwestern Georgia. Jefferson County's Dr. T.W. Battey and neighboring Richmond County's Major W.H. Battey (relationship to T.W. unknown) and H.H. Hickman bought the tract containing the primary cluster of springs; Macon's Dr. G. McDonald received title to the second tract. The four partners planned to "erect large and commodious houses for public entertainment on the premises" to give the public an opportunity to try the virtues of the spring water.[45] The men rechristened the springs as "Catoosa" (Cotoosa) Springs; when Catoosa County was formed four years later, they savvily influenced the state legislature to name the county after the springs.[46] Murray established another resort at Cherokee Springs where he continued to cultivate orchards and vineyards.[47]

The four owners spent $30,000 (almost $1.2 million in 2022 dollars) to quickly improve the property for the resort's 1850 opening but incurred a few construction obstacles in their haste.[48] The fifty-two springs, clustered in a "basin-like depression" in fewer than two acres, allowed visitors to sip many types of mineral water within a short distance, but the ground's dampness forced the owners to initiate "extensive ditching."[49] The hotel lacked suitable ventilation in all rooms. A visitor at one of the state's preeminent resorts, Warm Springs in west central Georgia's Meriwether County, gloated that while he "slept comfortably last night under sheet and counterpane," his friend at Catoosa Springs climbed up "four pair of stairs, next to the shingles, with a blazing sun pouring upon them…. [H]e had gone a long way to be uncomfortable."[50] Nonetheless, one July visitor rallied in support of the proprietors: "[W]hen everything is completed, [they will provide a] Splendid Establishment … equal to the first class Hotels in its appointments, such as silver forks, napkins, &c."[51]

Lodging consisted of a three-story hotel and one-story house rows behind it.[52] Front steps led up to a verandah enveloping the second level; one energetic stroller recorded that eleven laps around the twenty-foot-wide verandah equaled a mile, implying that the promenade was at least 120 feet long on two sides.[53] The dining room and bar occupied the entire length of the first level; about one half of the next floor accommodated a ballroom.[54] Catoosa Springs provided sixty rooms for its first season, added 100 "spacious and comfortable rooms" for its second season, and expanded yet again for its third season for a total of 500 rooms in both the hotel and in its "Handsome Cottages, with plastered rooms."[55] The Batteys, Hickman, and McDonald announced to "Georgia and to the Southern States" that Catoosa Springs' "accommodations, comforts and luxuries unsurpassed by any Watering place in the United States" rendered Catoosa "the Saratoga of the South."[56]

The abundance of varied mineral springs served as the nexus around Catoosa offerings. A Medical College of Georgia professor in the late 1850s proclaimed the waters "compar[able] to the best watering places in this country or Europe."[57] The spring waters, even those only a few feet apart, typically differed in chemical properties and were each "strongly mineralized."[58] Their popularity was such that the proprietors and guests christened them with such appellations as "All-healing," the "Red Sweet," the "Alum," the "Cosmetic," the "Congress" (after Saratoga's Congress Spring), the "Salze" (salt), and the "Magnesia," the latter two along with the sulphur springs being the most popular, according to one antebellum visitor.[59] Another antebellum guest, well-traveled to prestigious health resorts, snipped that the Congress water was "not exactly as you will get at Saratoga, nor is the White Sulphur such, perhaps, as you will find in Virginia ... nor the Warm Spring such as that in Meriwether County," but he then mellowed to allow that "take them all together and I will be responsible for saying that there is not such another acre of ground in the world."[60]

From the hotel perched on a knoll, guests strolled down to the bath house and to the springs in what originally was an open, undeveloped area. One antebellum guest wished for "more trees, shrubbery and flowers," but a visitor two years earlier had admired the "spreading oaks, beneath which springs up a lively green sward, with avenues stretching through it in all directions."[61]

Eventually, "fancy little" springhouses, each with a marble or wooden basin, enclosed about twenty-four of the springs, each house engraved with the name of the spring fountain.[62] Names included Epsom Salts, Emetic, Coffee, and the odd-sounding "Chautmobousga," allegedly christened one year by the sole Yankee at the resort, which befuddled southern visitors later deciphered as alternate letters of the words "Catoosa" and "Humbug."[63]

For guests perhaps bored of verandah promenades and sipping the myriad waters, Catoosa Springs offered other activities. A popular outdoor event was "flying horses," in which riders on wooden steeds tried to capture suspended rings within reach.[64] Indoor amusements included tenpins, band music, tableaux, dancing, and, of course, the omnipresent flirting.[65]

The zenith of Catoosa Springs activities occurred in late summer at the annual "Grand Tournament and Fancy Ball," which included a chivalrous tournament replete with guests as knights and fair damsels in the tradition of the popular Sir Walter Scott novels.[66] Notables such as former Governor George W. Crawford in 1856 and former Confederate Major General P.M.B. Young in 1872 served as managers for the masquerade balls for which the resort had on hand a wardrobe of "splendid fancy costumes."[67]

By 1860, visitors could travel by railroad from Charleston, Savannah, Augusta, Macon, and Nashville to connect with the State Road (the Western and Atlantic Railroad) either at Chattanooga, twenty-five miles from the springs depot, or at Atlanta, 112 miles distant.[68] One disgruntled passenger from Macon who stayed at the Atlanta Hotel on his way to Catoosa grumped about being "tortured and phlebotomised [sic] by the bed begs" but pardoned the hotel proprietor on account of "his being without a wife to see to the apartments." He left Atlanta the following day at 8:00 a.m., passed through Tunnel Hill ("dark as Egypt") at 3:00 p.m. and arrived at Ramsey's Depot (near Ringgold) at 3:30 p.m. where a waiting Catoosa Springs hack drove him to the resort about two miles away where he appreciatively noted the "clean beds."[69]

With the start of the Civil War, Catoosa modified its tagline to read "The Saratoga of the Confederate States" when it opened for the season of 1861 with J.J. Harman of Catoosa Springs and J.S. Nichols of Savannah as operators.[70] Newspaper pleas for southerners to frequent southern resorts transitioned into satisfied pronouncements like that of the *Savannah Daily Republican*: "For once, the southern people will be forced to a patriotic duty by the necessities of the times, viz: to remain at home in the summer months and spend their surplus earnings among their own people."[71] Indeed, five months after the outbreak of the war, 300 visitors flocked to the resort. Most guests during this time, as the Savannah newspaper noted, were largely "invalids in pursuit of health, and but few of the customary pleasure seekers, whom the state of the country has either detained at home or called to the more stirring [sic] scenes of the battle ground."[72]

Although Catoosa Springs announced its opening for the season of 1862, the health resort suffered misfortunes. In September, a cannonball killed principal resort owner Captain W.H. Battey, organizer of Jefferson County's so-called Battey Guard, at Sharpsburg (Antietam).[73] As skirmishes intensified in the Chattanooga area, Catoosa Springs and nearby Cherokee Springs evolved into Confederate hospitals under the direction of Army of Tennessee surgeon Samuel H. Stout, recognized today for his innovative and efficient mobile hospital units.[74] In February 1863, Nichols auctioned off "all the Hotel Furniture, including Crockery, Cutlery, and Glass Ware," while concurrently Catoosa's mineral springs catalyzed patients' recovery, per one reminiscer in 1871, to allow them to "go forth to do battle for the Lost Cause."[75] Around September 6, on the cusp of the Battle of Chickamauga, the Confederates began to evacuate Cherokee Springs' hospital to Newnan and Catoosa Springs' hospital to Griffin in advance of Union troops, who, according to an *Atlanta Intelligencer* article reprinted in other Georgia newspapers, had pushed Confederate troops back from Catoosa Springs to Tunnel Hill and had burned all railroad bridges between Tunnel Hill and Chattanooga.[76]

In early May 1864, in the beginning days of the Atlanta Campaign, Union forces camped at the deserted Catoosa Springs. A soldier with the 81st Indiana Infantry Regiment, attached to the Army of the Cumberland, described it as "a very pretty place, and at one time, no doubt, done an extensive business ... a large hotel, ten-pin alleys, billiard rooms, and a number of cottages.... But its glory has departed." The soldier and his comrades sampled the Buffalo, the White, the Blue and "several others with high sounding names, but they all looked alike, tasted alike," and "came to the conclusion that they were all alike."[77] A chaplain with the 101st Ohio Infantry wrote anxiously from Catoosa the following day about his fear that just as the resort had served as a Confederate hospital, it would soon house injured Union troops: "[F]or as I write, seated by a tree just in the rear of the regiment, occasional shots are heard on the skirmish line."[78]

The war left Catoosa County scorched, recounted a Ringgold resident: "[E]verything movable or burnable received the attention of one or both armies ... not even a fence rail left within a circuit of five miles around this place."[79] A Wisconsin traveler in northern Georgia observed that the "planters are terribly afraid of confiscation" while the "blacks [sic] would like land of their own." The traveler went on to note that Catoosa Springs's structures, even the lattice work over the springs, "are all in a state of sad dilapidation. Transitory monuments are they all of the departed glory of the chivalry."[80]

Catoosa Springs' popularity ebbed and flowed after the end of the Civil War until in fall 1871, W.C. Hewitt, formerly with Augusta's Globe Hotel, bought the Catoosa Springs property.[81] Hewitt invested about $30,000 ($742,000 in 2022 dollars) to renovate the existing structures, add gaslights, and construct an additional hotel housing a ballroom, billiard room, reading room, and a telegraph office for visiting businessmen "to give orders to … subordinates a thousand miles away."[82] Hewitt initially charged $60 per month, the same as the elite Montvale Springs in the Smokies, but soon lowered his rates to $45 per month "due to the stringency of the times."[83] Business increased as a result: By mid–August, 325 guests occupied the resort, with 700 predicted for the revival of the "fancy ball."[84]

Hewitt also shrewdly advertised Catoosa Springs as providing an "Old Virginia Welcome," a nostalgic nod to the charm and prestige of the Virginia springs but without the need to spend funds to travel long distances. By undercutting the rates of such Virginia springs health resorts as the Sweet Chalybeate (Red Sweet) Springs ($60 per month) or West Virginia's White Sulphur Springs ($80 per month), Hewitt engaged in a business strategy to appeal to potential clientele with less disposable income than the wealthy elite who could afford the Virginia springs. Encouraged by the resulting increased number of visitors, Hewitt invested another $10,000 to improve Catoosa Springs' infrastructure, raising the resort capacity to 600.[85] Although Hewitt's "affable and kind manner" attracted "ladies and gallant gents from all sections of [the] South," one guest in 1874 speculated that visitors should have been about "a thousand … instead of hundreds," implying that Catoosa was continuing to lose its antebellum charm.[86]

Continuing to face financial difficulties with the resort, Hewitt sold Catoosa Springs in fall 1877 to Augusta's H.H. Hickman, who may have been the same Hickman who previously co-owned the resort.[87] Hickman leased the resort to various parties over the next four years, including a Savannah medical physician, W.A. Spence, a "most genial and cultivated gentleman … untiring in his efforts to please" and B.W. Wrenn, agent for the Western and Atlantic Railroad. Wrenn, whose job included coordination of passenger excursions to the resort, assumed a lease in 1879.[88] Considered "one of [Georgia's] most indefatigable, energetic, and enterprising men," Wrenn's property improvements and continuation of fancy balls attracted southern elites such as former Governor Rufus B. Bullock, whose acquittal on embezzlement charges put him "once more at the top of the social wave" per the *Savannah Morning News*, and the family of former Confederate Brigadier General M.A. Stovall.[89] The influx of visitors from Georgia, Alabama, South Carolina, and Tennessee during Wrenn's 1879 season was so great that an overflow crowd at times camped outdoors.[90]

Despite Wrenn's success, Hickman within two years unsuccessfully attempted to sell Catoosa Springs for $25,000 to the state for a "branch of the Lunatic Asylum."[91] In 1881, G.W. Wilson, a transplant to Dalton from Milwaukee, bought the property for $18,000 on behalf of a Dalton business group with the

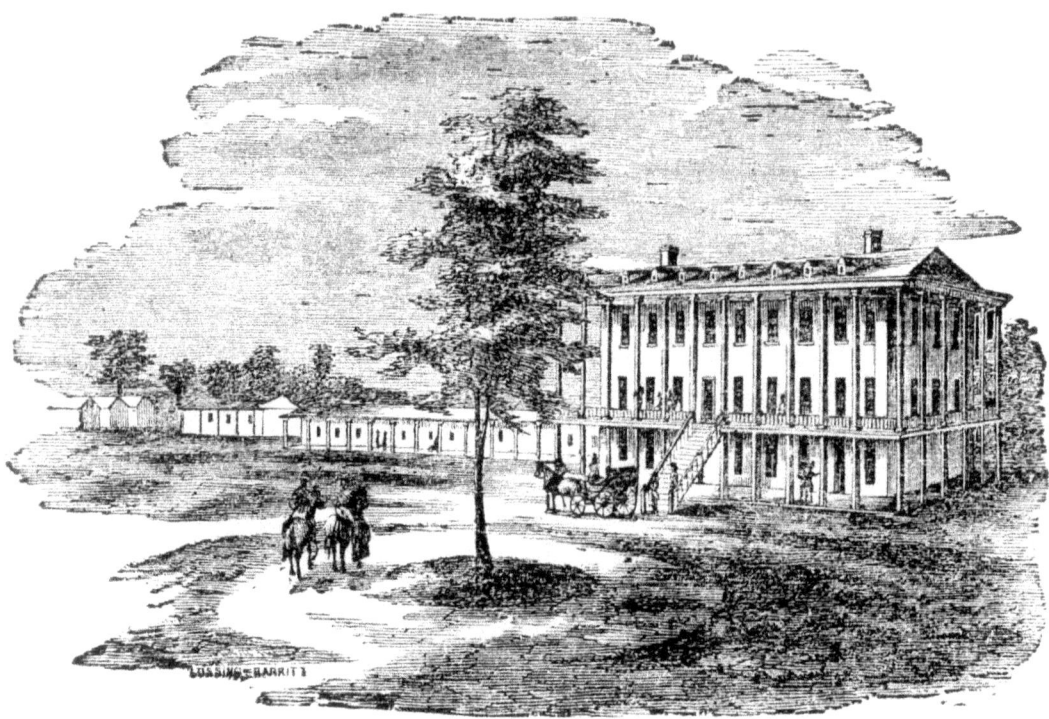

CATOOSA SPRINGS.

"Catoosa Springs [1855]," Catoosa County, Georgia (from the collections of the Catoosa County Historical Society, Tunnel Hill, GA [Image identical to "View of Cotoosa Springs," in George White, *Historical Collections of Georgia* (New York: Pudney & Russell, 1855), 668]).

inspiring vision to "make the springs second to none in the South" through extensive renovations.[92]

The resort operated intermittently for the next four decades but failed to achieve Wilson's objective. It floundered "guestless and tenantless" for part of the 1885 season but entertained 200 guests in June 1887 under the new ownership of a Chattanooga business consortium, which also began to market Catoosa "Buffalo-Epson" water.[93] At least two other groups owned the resort in the 1880s through the early 1900s, a group of Ohio physicians in 1892 and a Savannah group of capitalists in 1901, possibly illustrating the inability of owners with different skillsets to turn a quick profit.[94] After the main hotel burned down in the late 1800s (date unknown), the property attracted fewer guests.[95] In 1903, Brigadier General Theodore A. Baldwin, former commander of the famed Black "Buffalo Soldiers" Tenth Calvary Regiment in Cuba during the Spanish-American War, bought the property to build a new hotel.[96] Baldwin never followed through on his intent, but guests continued to visit the existing hotel even after the U.S. Army in 1904 acquired land for a rifle range that stood only one-half mile from the hotel.[97] In the 1920s, although only a small hotel and a few cottages received guests, Catoosa Springs was still shipping bottled waters from several springs.[98] After Baldwin's death in 1925, at some point (year unknown), Baldwin's daughter Emma and her husband, Brigadier General S.D. Rockenbach, instrumental in the formation of the U.S. Army Tank Corps, used the resort as their private home into the 1930s.[99] Community gatherings occurred at the springs into the 1940s; as of 2009, six of the fifty-two springs continued to flow.[100]

Today, perhaps appropriately, near the location of the now-gone resort that entertained former Confederate officers, saw nearby Civil War skirmishes, and that tended to both Confederate and Union wounded, a military connection still exists. The Tennessee Army National Guard maintains the rifle range for training its members at the federally owned Volunteer Training Site Catoosa (VTS-C).[101]

Gainesville: Gower's Spring, New Holland Springs, Oconee White Sulphur Springs

About fifty miles northeast of Atlanta, Interstate 985 enters the metro area of Gainesville, the county seat of Hall County. Hall County, with Forsyth County to its west and Banks County to its east, forms part of the southern boundary of Campbell's construct for Southern Appalachia. Hall County lies within the Piedmont physiographic province, a broad swath of small hills and narrow valleys running southwesterly to northeasterly across the state, delineated by the fall line to its south and the Valley and Ridge and Blue Ridge physiographic provinces to its north. Gainesville lies at about 1,200 feet elevation, near Lake Lanier.[102]

The Piedmont region constitutes a complicated geology of igneous (e.g., granite), sedimentary (e.g., limestone), and metamorphic (e.g., schist) rock. Over the epochs, many periods of volcanic activity have thrust minerals from deep within the earth towards the surface, resulting in numerous ore deposits throughout the Georgia Piedmont.[103] An antebellum handbook noted that Hall County contained "minerals in great variety," including "gold, lead, ruby, tourmaline, cyanite, and emerald … and a few diamonds."[104] Hall County's Glade Mine, north of Gainesville, for example, was so successful that it advertised in 1835 for fifty enslaved laborers.[105] Marble, iron ore, mica, lead, almandine (an iron alumina garnet), and slate were also extracted in Hall County in the nineteenth and early twentieth century.[106]

Although Hall County contains fewer limestone deposits than other northern Georgia counties, the deposits are sufficiently numerous along with iron ore and other minerals to have yielded many mineral springs. As Gainesville earned fame "for the salubrity of its summer climate" for wealthy Lowcountry planters, its hotels began to publicize area mineral springs as an additional calling card.[107] A new "House of Entertainment" in Gainesville in 1829 for "[p]ersons wishing to spend the summer in the up country" advertised its proximity to the mountains and "several Limestone Springs."[108] Three years later, Gainesville's Planters' Hotel in its praise of Gainesville as "perhaps one of the healthiest places in the State" mentioned that two limestone springs lay near it, "with a good road to each."[109] In fact, at least eighteen springs noted in historical works, most ambiguously named, can be

Gower's Spring

Gower's Spring (Gower Springs) played an early role in Gainesville's social life before E.N. (Ebenezer Norton) Gower built a resort hotel there in 1877. In the 1830s, residents mingled on benches to sip the water from the chalybeate (iron) spring, then called the "Town Spring." A visitor to Gainesville in 1837 observed that the spring seeped from a "low piece of ground, prettily cleared, and there were enough trees left to form an agreeable shade."[111]

In early 1856, Gower, a Maine native who had cofounded South Carolina's Greenville Coach Factory, the largest such enterprise south of the Potomac with annual sales of $80,000 (or about $2.85 million in 2022 dollars) sold his interest in the company and moved his family from Greenville about 100 miles southwest to Gainesville.[112] Gower purchased mineral land leases and around 1857 bought the Gainesville Hotel, "situate[d] on the North-East corner of the public square," which subsequently also became known as "Gower's Hotel."[113] By 1859, Gower became partner in a Gainesville carriage factory; in the following year, he had succeeded so well in his ventures that he claimed personal real estate valued at $26,000.[114]

Little is known about Gower and his family during the Civil War and for the eight years after the war's end. Gower continued to advertise the Gainesville Hotel at least until July 1861; a son in the Georgia Volunteers' Eleventh Regiment died of wounds received at Manassas (Bull Run) in 1862.[115] An 1863 newspaper recorded that Gower was fabricating mule shoes from his iron forge for the Confederacy, promising to sell iron cheaper than prevailing prices.[116]

In 1873, an Atlanta newspaper contributor excitedly described "a spring but recently discovered, and which is about three-quarters of a mile out from Gainesville … known by the name of the Gower Spring," almost certainly the Town Spring, which had evidently fallen into disuse. The chalybeate waters' sweet flavor and healing properties, according to the writer, filled the road to the spring each afternoon "with vehicles and pedestrians of almost every description."[117] Gower, who owned the property, and not one to miss a business opportunity, constructed a hotel that opened in summer 1877.[118]

The two-story, thirty-room frame hotel featured a simple design compared to others in postbellum Southern Appalachia although newspaper contributor Jack Plane, who visited many Georgia resorts, considered it "elegant." The facility had no ornamentation such as fountains, turrets, and porticos; even a dozen years after its completion, it lacked the usual verandahs that encircled more sophisticated resorts.[119]

The building stood on a "high eminence" in an oak forest overlooking the spring and provided a distant view of the Blue Ridge Mountains about 100 miles away.[120] A nearby hill housed the "elegant country" residence of General James Longstreet, Confederate hero turned Republican post-war. From this vicinity, one could view "'Alps peeping over Alps' until they seem to touch the skies."[121]

The main attraction, of course, was the water. Marketed by Gower as the "best chalybeate water in the State," the state analytical chemist endorsed Gower's claim by pronouncing that the spring's twenty chemical constituents produced "one of the best chalybeate waters which I have ever examined."[122] National mineral water authority James K. Crook in the late 1800s recommended the waters for "general debility, digestive orders, and kidney affections."[123] A Macon physician attested to the spring water's efficacy to treat "long exposure to malarial poison."[124] The waters also inspired Gower ads aimed at mothers to "take your babies for the summer," a reference to the alleged benefits of the minerals for teething infants.[125]

Not everyone enthused over Gower's Spring. One guest called it "the queerest summer resort on the face of the earth." The hotel in his view appeared as an "immense, ugly, weather-stained, old frame house, standing solitary and alone on a hillside in a grove of scrubby oaks." About 100 yards downhill from the hotel was "an old shed [which sheltered] the spring in a square pit fifteen feet in diameter and about as deep as a grave." A "big rusty dipper" lay by the side of the spring. The sight reminded him of a "post house for the isolation of smallpox patients." To his bewilderment, Gower's "[held] its own against New Holland, White Sulphur, and all the other elegant and beautiful watering places in this section of the country." Although the resort lacked the usual social amenities such as dancing, games, and music during his stay, he noted that the hotel interior with its "airy" rooms, "clean and comfortable" beds, and "excellent" fare was "perfect." In conclusion, he decided that guests could "devote themselves exclusively to eating and sleeping and doing nothing. [T]heir happiness is that of a stall-fed ox."[126]

Gower began to divest much of the land adjacent to the resort in 1879, perhaps to devote more time to his iron forge enterprise (he listed his occupation as "blacksmith" in the 1880 federal census).[127] In 1880 he placed the hotel with its nearby vineyards and orchards on the market.[128] State and federal politician Allen D. Candler of Gainesville bought much of Gower's property, but whether he also purchased the hotel is unknown.[129] In 1885 Brunswick merchant P.B. (Preston Brooks) Holzendorf bought the hotel with seventy acres for about $4,000.[130]

Holzendorf implemented a series of investments in the health resort to capitalize on the influx of visitors, largely from Georgia and Florida, including Georgia Congressman Henry G. Turner and Florida politician and judge Henry L. Mitchell.[131] In 1886, Holzendorf initiated an expansion of the hotel; by 1893 it boasted 200 rooms.[132] In 1888, Holzendorf added the recreational features that the disgruntled visitor a few years earlier might have appreciated: "a handsome dancing hall, skating rink and ten pin alley."[133]

Visitors wishing to sip the water did not always board at Holzendorf's. General Longstreet's Piedmont Hotel publicized its location a streetcar ride away from the springs.[134] Holzendorf recommended the Hunt House, the Florida Hotel, and the Arlington Hotel for visitors who wanted to lodge in Gainesville, from where they could take the streetcar, which also ran directly from the Air Line Railroad depot to the spring.[135] As a shrewd businessman, Holzendorf conveniently omitted in his hotel recommendations for Gainesville-based travelers that the spring water was provided free "only to guests" staying at his Gower's Springs lodging.[136]

The original Gower's Springs tract lost more land beginning in 1888. Atlanta real estate agents arranged for special excursion fares for potential buyers to visit the sixty-two surveyed lots for summer homes, recognizing that "the best people of Georgia go to Gainesville every summer." As additional draws, sale publicity noted the location as providing both the "best known climate for teething children" and easy accessibility to "superior doctors." Particularly targeted in the campaign were residents of the malaria-prone and humid Georgia coast, the "chance for Savannah people to secure a cottage lot very desirably located."[137]

The health resort suffered a final blow in 1893. A hotel office fire one late October morning destroyed the timbered structure in ninety minutes. Only a few pieces of damaged furniture were salvaged. Total loss was estimated at over $6,000, about $4,000 over Holzendorf's insurance coverage. Holzendorf placed the property, now whittled down to twenty-five acres, on the market.[138]

The next several years saw many failed owners and a foreclosure in 1900 as grand visions of new hotels or an "up-to-date pleasure park" never materialized.[139] One owner, a liveryman, "[fitted the] grounds with two dancing pavilions, tennis court, ten pin alley, and ice cream saloon" with plans to recoup his investment via streetcar and bus fare.[140] The amusements, assuming that they actually opened, did not capture the press's attention as newspaper descriptions of spring activities in later years concentrated on the occasional picnic or afternoon Sunday School class meeting held on the grounds.[141]

In October 1909, W.A. Roper & Company announced a planned forty-one acre "Green Street Circle" acre residential neighborhood that incorporated the spring as part of its envisioned "Maple Park."[142] Gower's Spring remained popular. Clamoring demand for the water resulted in curbside delivery in 1910 (although the state board of health the next year criticized the water as the worst of its local samples); the streetcar route continued until at least 1924, ensuring a "delightful trip in carriage or auto right by the Springs."[143] Today, the likely location of Gower's Spring and its hotel lies between the Green Street Circle and Thompson Bridge Road.[144]

New Holland Springs

Over forty years before Atlanta businessman E.W. (Edmund Weyman) Holland bought the property that became known as the "New Holland Springs," travelers and locals praised the waters of a limestone spring, two miles east of Gainesville on the Clarksville Road, that the Cherokee frequented before their removal during the Trail of Tears.[145] Gainesville's Georgia Hotel and Planters' Hotel in the early 1830s publicized their proximity to the "beautiful and excellent Limestone Springs" and the "good road" to get there.[146] A couple in 1834 on the way from the environs of Athens to North Carolina in search of health stopped to imbibe the waters, which "hourly improved" their health such that the husband heartily recommended the "splendid" spring, convinced "that invalids would be greatly improved [and that] men of health [would become even] better."[147]

A person who regained his health was Augusta businessman Joseph Rivers, a "broken-down invalid," who in 1833 moved with his family to Gainesville where the spring cured his various ills.[148] Rivers, who became a prominent Gainesville merchant, subsequently bought the marshy spring property and transformed it into a "beautiful summer resort" according to his son; a less biased observer in 1887 recalled that the resort in 1849 was an "humble cottage on a hill."[149] Hearing of Rivers' cure, many family friends from the Augusta region began to journey to Gainesville to try the water. As at Gower's Spring, the road to the Limestone Springs, or Rivers' Springs, teemed with traffic, with as many as fifty carriages traveling the Clarksville Road daily to the springs.[150]

The property's ownership is unknown until the early 1870s when, "[i]n his declining years," Holland bought the Limestone Springs and rechristened it as the "New Holland Springs."[151] Born in 1807 in South Carolina's Laurens District, Holland first became a teacher in Alabama and then headed to the gold fields of Georgia where he succeeded in accumulating a "snug fortune" from placer mining near Villa Rica.[152] In 1848, the entrepreneurial Holland moved to the growing railroad center of Atlanta where he built the Holland House, "one of the finest hotels in the city," and partnered with financier Alfred Austell to purchase the Bank of Fulton around 1856 and assisted Austell and others in 1865 to organize the Atlanta National Bank.[153]

In spring 1874, the New Holland Springs opened, replete with a "large new Hotel and several Cottages for families" and promises of a weekly barbecue dinner, "Ten Pins, Billiards, [and] Bath."[154] The resort's initial monthly rate was $35, about midway between the $50 monthly rate of Catoosa, Alabama's Blount Springs, and East Tennessee's Montvale Springs and the $22 monthly rate charged by upper East Tennessee's relatively obscure Easley's Springs near Jonesborough.[155] Holland may have intended that the new resort target a mid-range class of society, or he may have meant to undercut the rates of well-known Southern Appalachian resorts.

Regardless of Holland's pricing strategy objective, his resort quickly brought a following of largely in-state elites, particularly from Atlanta, but also from Savannah and central Georgia, and to a lesser extent from southern Georgia towns such as Americus and Albany.[156] Several former Confederate officers and their families vacationed at New Holland, including General A.R. Lawton, commander of the Georgia troops that captured Fort Pulaski at Savannah, and General Eli Warren.[157] The "central figure in our social life," however, according to a ball attendee, was revered Georgia politician and former secretary of state for the Confederacy Robert Toombs who, along with his "refined and agreeable lady, present[ed] a picture of domestic happiness."[158] The attendee's protracted account of the ball regaled in name-dropping of Georgia elites whose surnames are associated now with Georgia municipalities and counties: Lumpkin, Milledge, Cobb, Jackson, and a "Mrs. Montgomery Cumming, who is universally regarded as one of the 'reigning queens' of Georgia society."[159]

The weekly barbecue meals morphed into more refined offerings to cater to the demands of the sophisticated elites at the resort. Sunday entrée offerings for one sample week in 1885 consisted of baked lake trout with bordelaise sauce, western ham with champagne sauce, fresh beef tongue with pecan sauce, mutton with caper sauce, beef with horse radish, Tennessee beef, loin with apple sauce, barbecued lamb ribs, chicken with French dressing, beef ribs, fried chicken livers, and salmon. While the feasts sated the palates of the wealthy guests, they also provided variety "enough for the worst dyspeptic in the state."[160]

Dyspeptics and others sought the spring water for all matters of affliction over the decades, from sufferers of "Chronic Liver Complaints" in the 1840s to "teething babies" in the 1890s, the latter also treated at Gower's Spring.[161] The water was best known for treating dyspepsia because of its high concentration of carbonic acid that released a steady stream of carbon dioxide bubbles and that precipitated salts such as the carbonates of magnesium, potassium, and calcium, which also acted as antacids.[162] Holland also billed his resort water as a curative for "skin eruptions, private and chronic diseases.... Dropsy [edema] ... Typhoid and other Fevers."[163] The "trace of iron" found in the spring probably inspired Holland to claim that the spring "restores feeble women and children to health."[164] As if knowledge of the all-curing spring alone were insufficient, Holland also advertised a "very fine chalybeate spring" a half a mile away and promoted neighboring resorts such as the Oconee White Sulphur Springs, four miles away.[165]

To reach the mineral waters, guests descended a slope next to the hotel to a "pretty pavilion overshadowing the principal spring."[166] A "boxing" about eighteen feet square and about three feet deep contained the water, which "flow[ed] out into a beautiful rivulet, whose course through the park [was] marked by the ribbon of *bright green grass*, which *fringe[d]* its pebbly way [italics original]."[167] The water flow was estimated at over 1,200 gallons per hour, considerably more than that, for example, of neighboring Lumpkin County's Porter Springs's 800 gallons flow per hour.[168]

A contemporary account described the hotel as surrounded by a cluster of cottages in the "foliage of a magnificent grove."[169] Each cottage was named in honor of southern cities such as Augusta, Chattanooga, and Atlanta, and housed renters from the corresponding town.[170] While little is known about the hotel architecture, the resort was spacious: It could accommodate 275–300 guests; the dining room could seat 300.[171]

From the hotel, a gravel path led to the Atlanta and Richmond Air Line Railway depot only 300 yards away.[172] During the season of 1875, one daily train, two hours each way, ran between Atlanta and New Holland Springs. Passengers bound for Oconee White Sulphur could also disembark at the Air Line Railway depot and take a hack to Oconee White Sulphur to save an extra two-mile buggy ride from Gainesville.[173] By 1886, trains ran three times daily from Atlanta to New Holland's depot where resort visitors could also board a train to travel ten miles northeast to Lula to transfer to Athens on the Northeastern Railroad of Georgia or to continue on to Toccoa.[174] In addition, the Gainesville Street Railway Company began in 1875 to convey Gainesville visitors by horse- or mule-drawn carriage to both Gower's Spring and to New Holland.[175]

Recreational offerings easily surpassed the little to none provided at Gower's Spring. Within five years of its opening, New Holland by 1879 offered band and orchestra music, dancing ("Ball Room, forty by eighty"), two ten-pin alleys, swings, croquet, and a "Bathing Pool, forty by sixty feet."[176] Also advertised throughout the years were the "Promenades in a Natural Grove, cool breezes, and pleasant nights" at an elevation considered "one of the highest in the South," publicized anywhere from 1,500 feet above sea level to an exaggerated 2,000 feet in altitude, intended to entice clients.[177]

Misleading altitudes aside, steamy hot weather sent Atlantans to New Holland Springs. During one heat wave, an Atlanta correspondent for a Savannah newspaper reported that "some twenty of our leading families put out for New Holland Springs for the heated term, which place will be Atlanta's summer resort." Several weeks later, the same newspaper again lamented the high temperatures: "[T]here has been a perfect rush to New Holland Springs by our Atlanta families.… It is the nearest refuge from heat and dust."[178]

New Holland provided refuge to a greater danger than the discomfort and unpleasantness of summer heat: yellow fever. In 1876, Savannah experienced a yellow fever epidemic that killed more than 1,000 citizens in two weeks, leading to a mass exodus from the city.[179] Georgia newspapers carried daily reports of municipalities' yellow fever mortalities; at the same time, Savannah physicians were overwhelmed by the epidemic, several "broken down" and almost all "worn down by over exertion."[180] Atlanta hotels teemed with travelers either escaping the epidemic or heading to the Georgia coast but paralyzed by apprehension as to whether to proceed to Savannah. When General A.R. Lawton and his family reached Atlanta by train from Savannah on their way to New Holland Springs, crowds besieged him for news: "'He *will* give us the truth' [italics original]."[181] New Holland and other northern Georgia resorts hosted refugees throughout the September epidemic; while many guests were preparing to return home for the autumn, the Savannahians stayed because they "scarcely [knew] what to do."[182] When three Savannahians in Gainesville came down with yellow fever, the health authorities determined that they contracted it in Savannah, not in the higher Piedmont elevation, which therefore did not "excite any alarm."[183]

After Holland's death in December 1885, the resort began an uneven decline.[184] Holland's daughter-in-law, Kate B. Holland inherited the resort but in early 1887 found herself in a legal sparring match with the resort lessee over renewal of the lease that Holland had executed.[185] After a successful lawsuit, Kate's husband Ed, who by this time was partner in Atlanta's Pemberton Chemical Company, later the Coca-Cola Company, spent several thousand dollars in resort improvements.[186] The couple in 1890 sold the resort with its 600 acres to the Georgia Development Company, which also bought the nearby Oconee White Sulphur Springs property. The firm planned to pave a 130-foot-wide avenue from Gainesville to the two resorts that included a "dummy line" (rail line) and to construct a new hotel at New Holland.[187] The next year saw the proprietor of Gainesville's Arlington Hotel lease New Holland; his ads did not mention road improvements.[188]

The resort limped along for a few more years. In 1898, the press raised hope that a new hotel might replace the "old" structure, but no source consulted indicated that happened.[189] A syndicate of "eastern and western capitalists" bought the property in late 1899 but failed to deliver on its promise to spend at least $100,000 on improvements.[190]

In March 1900, any envisioned revival of New Holland Springs ended. The

South Carolina–based Pacolet Manufacturing Company purchased the resort property to build a large cotton mill with employment anticipated around 1,400 workers.[191] The next year, the company constructed a granite and marble basin around the spring, which on one Sunday alone attracted "hundreds of people." As late as 1906, a national medical directory listed it in its tabulation of mineral springs. Today, Milliken & Company owns and operates the mill in the unincorporated community of New Holland.[192]

Oconee White Sulphur Springs

In the early 1800s, two frontiersmen hunting game near the Oconee River supposedly passed by a pungent sulfur spring about four miles northeast of a limestone spring, site of the future New Holland Springs.[193] The spring evidently lay forgotten for almost four decades until advertisements for establishments such as Gainesville's Mansion House announced in 1841 the "recently discovered White Sulphur Spring" a few miles from the hotel.[194] In December of that year, the state legislature passed an act listing six Gainesville citizens as trustees for the incorporated White Sulphur Springs, including eminent surgeon Richard Banks, for whom Banks County was named after upon its founding in 1858, and L.A. (Lemuel Austin) McAfee (McAffee).[195]

McAfee, a North Carolina native, moved to Hall County sometime before 1840, at which time he lived next to Joseph Rivers and two households away from Banks.[196] He served as a justice of Hall County Inferior Court and as a charter member, along with Banks, of the short-lived Gainesville Railroad Company that aspired to connect the Atlanta area to Gainesville.[197] Perhaps aligned with his interest in the curative powers of mineral waters, McAfee also was Gainesville agent for a Mississippi physician's "Vegetable Liver Medicine, Purifying Pills, and Vegetable Tonic," advertised reassuringly "that they will not *kill* any one [italics original]."[198]

By 1843, McAfee had assumed sole proprietorship of the mineral springs resort and "extended his buildings, so as to enable him to accommodate his guests with that comfort, which he flatters himself, will be satisfactory."[199] Within three years, however, he advertised the sale of the sulphur springs because of his "not being able to improve the Springs in a deserving manner," recounting that "hundreds [had] received its benefits."[200]

McAfee found no buyers for the resort for the next several years. Despite his objective to sell, he patiently continued to cater solicitously to guests. A contemporary handbook called him "a gentleman eminently qualified to take charge of a watering establishment."[201] A visitor in 1850 agreed with that assessment: McAfee "is one of the most obliging and attentive of obliging and attentive landlords."[202]

Before the season of 1851, McAfee sold the resort to Ewsiel (Ensil) Pace, a tavern keeper with property valued at $8,000 in Oglethorpe County, who began hotel improvements.[203] Within the next four years, Pace constructed a new two-story hotel, with the second floor for guests and the ground story for a "capacious ball room."[204] A visitor from Athens in 1855 noted the same troubling situation that a guest in 1850 had observed: The resort housed only a few boarders despite Pace's tavern experience and his provision of the new building and offering of outdoor activities such as hunting and fishing and, of course, visits to the mineral springs.[205]

An explanation for the low attendance may be attributed to the location of the sulphur springs downhill from the hotel. Jack Plane wrote that "the water is so far from the hotel invalids could not walk to the springs" and was the most difficult of all the Gainesville springs to access.[206] The topography partially explains the low attendance: The hotel stood on "a steep hill" above the springs, "nestling under the side of this giant hill," at least one hundred yards away from the hotel.[207] In fact, the resort may not have achieved its greatest popularity until the 1919 season, after mineral spring accessibility had improved, when "hundreds of people … enjoyed the pleasures of the hotel," an anomaly as most mineral spring resorts began to fade in the early 1900s.[208]

Guests whose mobility allowed them to reach the mineral water detected it "at some yards distance by the sulphurious odour."[209] The sulphur properties allegedly treated dyspepsia, dropsy, rheumatism, and dermal afflictions. As an antebellum foreshadowing to modern office stress, an 1855 article promised that the water would treat "a loss of appetite … and general debility from too close confinement to business."[210]

Little is known about the resort from 1860 through 1869. A post office opened at White Sulphur Springs in July 1860, demonstrating the resort's success in attracting lodgers (Pace's $14,000 estate value recorded that year attests to the resort's prosperity). Pace in 1861 owned sixteen enslaved people, who may have labored at the resort.[211] Even in June 1861, three months into the Civil War, E.N. Gower, then proprietor of the Gainesville Hotel, in a promotion of his hotel also publicized the "excellent hotel at the Sulphur Springs, with ample accommodations for visitors to the Springs." Both hotels charged the same, $25 monthly or $1 per day, indicating that neither establishment commanded a more exclusive price than the other.[212]

The completion of the Air Line Railroad from Atlanta to Gainesville in 1871 saw a renaissance of the White Sulphur Springs. In 1869, local press had clamored for a "railroad and telegraph" to make Gainesville the "Saratoga of the South" to invigorate, among other area mineral springs, the "formerly much celebrated" "sulphur spring of superior quality."[213] In 1871, with the advent of the railroad, Samuel R. McCamy reopened the resort, which one enthusiastic guest recommended for its "excellent water, romantic scenery, and above all, the boundless continuity of shade."[214]

Within two years, McCamy was dead. In early January 1875, the executor sale included 400 acres of largely forested land, the thirty-two room hotel, its adjacent cabins, and an additional ten acres "now grown up" adjacent to the springs.[215]

Although rumors began to spread in spring 1877 that a new hotel accommodating up to 500 visitors would be built at the resort, now occasionally called "Oconee White Sulphur" due to its proximity to the Oconee River a few miles away, the resort languished.[216] A new hotel was built in spring 1878, which attracted 130 guests one week that summer, including stays that summer by Toombs and former Confederate officer and state politician James B. Mathews (who died there), but its occupancy rate never reached the envisioned (probably exaggerated) 500.[217]

Oconee White Sulphur saw another rebirth around 1879 under Ferdinand Phinizy, grandson of Italian immigrants to Philadelphia who eventually settled in central Georgia's Oglethorpe County. After Phinizy's graduation in 1838 from the University of Georgia, he pursued railroad construction and cotton trading, among other business ventures. Phinizy acquired the White Sulphur Springs as payment for a debt and immediately hired an architect to improve the property and a Charleston hotelier to manage the resort.[218] As a result, one traveler in 1880 who made the rounds of Gower's, New Holland, and White Sulphur pronounced the latter as "*the place* [italics original]" to visit in the Gainesville area, calling it "most beautifully improved." Indeed, according to the traveler, he had seen no place since he "left Virginia to which an invalid might go with such certainty of recovering health."[219] Another guest, perhaps relieved to relax at the end of a grueling eleven-hour journey from Columbus, Georgia, gushed over Phinizy as "a prince of a man" who had "crown[ed] his family name with one of the most beautiful and attractive places in the south."[220]

Phinizy's improved hotel stood on a hilltop with "sixteen cottages on either hand, stylishly painted, plastered, and carpeted with matting."[221] The cottages with their "spring beds, bureaux ... and ample ventilation" surpassed even those of West Virginia's Greenbrier according to one discriminating guest. Just as New Holland's cottages were named after Georgia cities, so were some of Oconee White Sulphur's christened with well-known Georgia surnames such as Toombs and Cobb or with the state names of Georgia and Mississippi. The two-story hotel contained "bright, spacious, and airy" rooms with "spacious" verandahs hugging the exterior.[222] Amusements included billiards, bowling alley, "fine drives," and grand evening balls.[223] Phinizy enlarged the lodging to house around 300 guests, built a church on the grounds, and improved the property to such an extent that his expenditures were estimated in 1900 to have been about $30,000–$35,000, about five times the value of Gower's Springs when it burnt down in 1893.[224]

In 1890, the Georgia Development Company bought the resort from Phinizy's several sons and son-in-law, A.W. Calhoun, a renowned ophthalmologist whose father established the forerunner of today's Emory University School of Medicine.[225] Just as the Georgia Development Company lost the New Holland property, so did it forfeit the Oconee White Sulphur: the Phinizy sons and Calhoun once again received ownership.[226] Lacking time to tend to the property, the Phinizy sons and Calhoun sold the resort with no asking price; the winning bid was only $4,800. Within a week, the new owners put the property back on the market to sell or to rent, perhaps to "flip" it to make a handsome profit.[227]

The resort continued for the next three decades primarily under J.W. Oglesby, head of a southern Georgia railroad, who bought it in 1905, with plans to vastly improve the property, ultimately spending about a million dollars.[228] By summer 1907, he had renovated the hotel rooms with mahogany, oak, brass, and iron decorative features; built a graveled road to the spring pavilion; installed porcelain-lined tubs in a bath house supplied with heated sulphur spring water; and had added the "largest pool and billiard room of any hotel in north Georgia." Oglesby's *pièce de resistance* was his design of a sixty-foot-long semicircular "perfectly grooved" white oak porch that doubled as an outdoor ballroom. A ribbed roof fanned out from one sole support post to protect the porch, "perhaps the largest of its kind in the state."[229]

Oglesby suffered a severe setback in the 1929 stock market crash and closed the resort. In January 1933, the hotel burned down; the local fire department saved fourteen cottages. As of 2009, Cathryn Smith and her sister whose grandparents had worked at the hotel and sold dairy products and produce to the resort owned the property.[230]

These three Gainesville-area resorts share characteristics that speak to their socioeconomic interconnectivity to areas outside Southern Appalachia. First, they welcomed primarily families from Atlanta and Savannah to enjoy cooler temperatures and secondarily those from other communities such as Columbus and Athens to mingle with Georgia politicians and former Confederate officers. Guests from outside Southern Appalachian Hall County might spend their funds at all three as they made the rounds. Second, the three health resorts began as undeveloped antebellum watering holes, only to fall into disuse for several decades each, before being rediscovered and developed by a series of well-heeled entrepreneurs originally from outside Hall County with various business foci. These businessmen included Maine native Gower and his stagecoach manufactory expertise, Holland and his banking acumen, and Phinizy's and Oglesby's railroad management talents among other enterprise skills. These businessmen were not absentee landlords but engaged in the resorts, spending much outside capital on them as well as contributing to the local economy via their other businesses, particularly Gower's Gainesville hotel operation and carriage factory. The three resorts by their provision of services and the contribution of the owners via their capital expenditures exemplify Southern Appalachia's Hall County's linkage to areas outside North Georgia.

Porter's Springs

On a sunny spring day in 1878, a young woman climbed to a ridge overlooking Dahlonega, Georgia, to admire the vista: "The mountains run farther away, hill behind hill, hill beyond hill, stretching on and on. You see where the ridge seems to break abruptly, ending in a graceful curve? That is Cedar mountain, at whose base lie the celebrated Porter's springs. Those two peaks whose summits alone you can see are Blood and Slaughter mountains. The scene is beautiful."[231]

These undulating rugged ridges lie mainly in northeastern Georgia's Blue Ridge Mountains' Chattahoochee National Forest. Dahlonega, the county seat of Lumpkin County, about nine miles south of Porter's Springs and about twenty miles north of Gainesville, may be best known in historical circles for its affiliation with the 1829 Georgia gold rush and subsequent removal of the Cherokee from their lands. Outdoor enthusiasts identify the town with the Appalachian Trail (A.T.) because of Dahlonega's proximity to Amicalola Falls State Park where many "thru hikers" use an approach trail to connect with the A.T.'s southernmost trailhead at Springer Mountain; much of Robert Redford's 2015 film based on Bill Bryson's book, *A Walk in the Woods*, took place in the state park. Blood Mountain, about fifteen miles north of Porter's Springs in Union County, with an elevation of 4,461 feet, is the highest point of the A.T. in Georgia.[232]

The steep terrain of Lumpkin County and other parts of northeastern Georgia derives from the thrusting of plates that formed the Appalachians. The Blue Ridge province in Georgia consists of several so-called thrust sheets, including the Dahlonega gold belt along the Chattahoochee fault.[233] The presence of gold near Dahlonega resulted from the push of rocks containing gold ore from deep within the earth into contact with hot water that dissolved the gold, which precipitated out at the surface. The same geological process explains the presence of gold in regions such as California's Sierra Nevada or Colorado's San Juan mountains.

Native Americans as early as 1528 recounted tales to Spanish explorers of the fabled gold-ore rich land of "Apalachen," now determined to be in the vicinity of the headwaters of the Chattahoochee. Hernando de Soto in 1540 sought to locate the gold after hearing of its presence in an area that correlates to northern Georgia. Possibly, his men or other Spanish expeditions explored or worked the land in the Nacoochee Valley about twenty-five miles east of Blood Mountain.[234]

The major rediscovery of gold occurred in 1828–1829 when miners began to migrate from North Carolina goldfields into northeastern Georgia. Although various authorities give credit to at least five men, including two enslaved persons, the front runner for discovering gold in Georgia may be John Witheroods (Witherow) of North Carolina, who uncovered a three-ounce nugget in Habersham County's Duke's Creek in 1828.[235]

The ensuing gold rush saw Georgia's removal of the Cherokees from their lands and the subsequent initiation of the 1832 Land Lottery for the former Cherokee property. With the influx of several thousand miners into the northeastern Georgia mountains, gold-mining villages quickly formed, including Licklog, which was rechristened "Dahlonega," and in 1833 became the county seat of Lumpkin County, named after Governor Wilson Lumpkin, a fierce supporter of Cherokee eviction.[236]

The miners and lot owners in northeastern Georgia in general were white southern males although the gold rush also attracted large numbers of western Europeans who mined as laborers or who provided engineering expertise before scattering to Texas or California in the next fifteen years. Interestingly, a small number of white females and a larger group of Blacks, some freemen but mainly enslaved persons, labored as miners.[237] John C. Calhoun, for instance, worked twenty enslaved laborers in his mine south of Dahlonega. A relative of Ferdinand Phinizy, the postbellum owner of Gainesville's Oconee White Sulphur Springs, brought enslaved persons annually from Augusta to work in the gold mines.[238]

The 1849 California gold rush precipitated the decline of the Georgia gold mining industry and the bustling trade centers that had been built around them.[239] By the late 1860s, Dahlonega appeared as a "a very old looking town [with] some indication of life and trade."[240]

In 1868, Dawson County Methodist minister Joseph McKee on a walking excursion in neighboring Lumpkin County found at the foot of Cedar Mountain a brush-covered mineral spring bordered by rocks forming a makeshift culvert. According to tradition, probably first documented with McKee's discovery, the

Cherokees drank from the spring because of its quarter-mile proximity to Stone Pile Gap where allegedly lies buried the Cherokee princess Trahlyta, whose rejected suitor promised Trahlyta on her deathbed to bury her near a magic spring of youth.[241]

McKee communicated his finding to the landowner, Basil S. Porter, who decided to develop the property, infrequently known as Bethesda Springs or Cedar Mountain Springs in its early years but more popularly known as Porter's (Porter) Springs.[242] By summer 1869, a visitor observed at least sixteen dwellings clustered about the springs and over one hundred sojourners of "all ages and sizes."[243]

The Lumpkin County springs attracted much attention because of the water's blend of iron, sulphur, magnesia, and other minerals. The springs purportedly cured "kidney affections, dyspepsia, rheumatism, neuralgia, old sores, [and] diseases of the skin."[244] In Gainesville, about thirty miles south of Porter's Springs, the town's *Air Line Eagle* in an article republished in the Macon press exulted over the region's great excitement over the springs, which "will doubtless prove a blessing to the hundreds of the afflicted." The article cautioned that "delicate females" might experience "almost intoxication," such were the "exhilarating effects" of the water.[245] One traveler who had made the rounds of four Virginia mineral springs provided the supreme compliment: Porter's waters were "equal, if not superior, to any of them."[246]

Accordingly, the first five years following McKee's 1868 rediscovery of the Cherokee waters prompted much construction activity to provide hotel accommodations and better road access. In 1869, John Woody built a hotel located west of the springs on "Radical Hill," so called because of the Republican lot owners and lessees there. The property teemed with campers and cabin guests. One visitor commented that several hundred would congregate at the springs if sufficient lodging were available.[247] Before the season of 1873, James M. Harris built an addition to his hotel, the second one at the springs, to accommodate yet more visitors.[248] To facilitate transportation, the *Atlanta Daily Sun* reported, the state legislature in 1872 authorized $1,500 to make Porter's Springs, "claimed to be of superior mineral and healing qualities," "accessible to people generally" by constructing public roads from the health resort via Blairsville, county seat of Union County to the north of Lumpkin County, to the North Carolina border, a distance roughly of 35–40 miles.[249]

In 1874, the resort came under the management of H.P. (Henry Pattillo) Farrow for a tenure that lasted until Farrow's death in 1907. Farrow, a South Carolina resident before his move to Cartersville, Georgia, in 1856, was a former slaveowner who served as superintendent of the Confederacy's niter and mining bureau in Georgia and in parts of Alabama and South Carolina. After the war, he served as attorney general in Georgia's Reconstruction government in Atlanta for four years and then resigned to accept President Grant's appointment as U.S. District Attorney for Georgia's northern and southern districts for eight years. While serving in this last position, Farrow in October 1874 signed a lease with Porter, having sojourned previously at the resort to treat, according to tradition, a lingering Civil War injury.[250]

Farrow's resort was located about a quarter mile uphill on Cedar Mountain from the springs. In 1888, about 150 guests could occupy the two-story, frame hotel connected by an elevated causeway to the dining room and the ball room a considerable distance away; by 1895, the lodging could accommodate about 300.[251] Farrow provided many of the amenities expected at nineteenth-century resorts: a ten-pin alley, billiards, and spring-fed bath rooms, "free to guests of Porter Springs Hotel, and open to none others."[252] For those interested in musical entertainment and dancing, Porter's offered a brass band and an orchestra, which Farrow proudly advertised as the "only watering place in Georgia" to provide both. A walk from the hotel led to the pavilion-covered springs, a swimming pool, and to a dozen bath rooms.[253] For those who enjoyed fishing or found simple pleasure in watching fish, Farrow built two fish ponds in front of the hotel, one stocked with carp and the other with trout; one writer penned, "It is a treat to go to those ponds and watch the fish playing in the pure, clear water and have them to come up and feed from your hand."[254]

Farrow was an unsuspecting trends-setter of today's "farm to table" movement that advocates locally sourced food, grass-fed cows, and free-range hens. He served local trout as a staple, a "luxury to many."[255] One ad, for instance, rhapsodized of the "delicious butter" and "[p]ure milk at every meal from ten Jerseys that drink pure water and graze on clover" and of chickens "fat and healthy from never having been cooped up."[256] One satisfied boarder wrote in the *Barnesville Gazette* in 1895 that Porter's table was "unsurpassed" by that of any summer resort; he savored "some of the finest peaches at Porter Springs I ever had in my life, grown by Alfred Harrington, one of Porter's formerly enslaved workers."[257]

Although guests may have extolled the table fare, it was much simpler than, for example, Gainesville's New Holland Springs' Sunday dinner spread of a dozen entrees. In fact, Farrow did not invest the same level of capital into any of his resort offerings as did his fellow proprietors of Gainesville's New Holland Springs, Oconee White Sulphur Springs, and Gower's Spring. One visitor in 1883, for example, opined of Porter's: "The buildings are not fine but are comfortable."[258] Fourteen years later, two guests still described the structures as "plain and neat."[259] Even an 1888 Gainesville promotional brochure given to flowery exaggeration described Porter Springs' lodging as of the "cheap order, but comfortable."[260]

Accordingly, Farrow's early rates remained lower than those of Gainesville area hotels. In 1875, New Holland Springs charged a monthly $40 for a single person and $70 for a married couple; Porter's Springs charged a flat $25 per month.[261] A year later, General Longstreet's Piedmont Hotel in Gainesville charged $40 per month contrasted to Porter's $30 monthly rate (in 1878, the same lessee ran both the Piedmont and Porter's and shrewdly offered a "one house" rate of $30 for guests wishing to divide their time between these two establishments).[262] Although no rivalry evidently existed among the Gainesville resorts, some Gainesville establishments discouraged travel to Porter's, perhaps to keep tourist dollars in their coffers, possibly providing another partial explanation for Porter's relatively low prices. One satisfied coastal Georgia guest at Porter Springs, for example, expressed dismay at the Gainesville populace's dismissive attitude towards the resort: "Not one good word could be heard about the Springs … 'hot place,' 'lonesome,' 'dreadful roads,' 'nothing to see.'"[263]

Farrow also may have offered lower rates to offset the expense and inconvenience of reaching his resort. Traveling to Porter Springs from Gainesville, the latter easily reached from Atlanta via the Air Line Railroad beginning in 1871, required money and stamina to withstand rough terrain. In 1873, for example, visitors who traveled to Gainesville might ride the mail hack to Dahlonega for $2.50 one way and then pay another dollar for coach fare from Dahlonega to Porter's, a one-day trip whose expense exceeded three times the cost of one night's lodging and two meals at Porter's (one dollar).[264] If guests took a stage with no stops between Gainesville and Porter's Springs, the coach drive required seven hours to cover the jarring twenty-eight miles to the resort, preferably during daylight.[265] One group that toured the Ivey gold mine near Dahlonega in 1883 frantically hurried back to Porter Springs as the sun was setting on unfamiliar "mountain roads, with perpendicular walls on one side and fifty-foot ravines on the other.... [T]he last mile of the way was the roughest and the darkest, for it lay right over Rock-pile Gap in the mountain."[266] One observer dryly understated that Porter's Springs did not attract as many visitors as New Holland because of the former's "not being directly on the railroad."[267]

Why, despite the plainness of the hotel and difficult travel, did the resort attract hundreds of guests over the years, including several southern notables? Well-known visitors included Georgia Secretary of State Nathan C. Barnett, former Confederate vice president Alexander H. Stephens, and former Confederate General James Longstreet on his second honeymoon.[268]

In fact, the lure of Porter's lay in its medical attributes: the mineral water and the high elevation, billed by Porter's at 3,000 feet (roughly the height of Cedar Mountain, not the elevation of the hotel).[269] McKee wrote in *The Methodist Advocate* in 1870 of several who had been cured at the springs, including a gentleman from neighboring White County, afflicted with dropsy (edema), who measured at least ten feet in circumference around his waist and left the springs four weeks later with his coat now large enough to button around both his brother and him. Another North Georgian, according to McKee, was covered with "the leprosy," which disappeared after three weeks' use of the water, leaving his skin as "natural as that of a child."[270] A resident physician, a surprising attribute for such a modest resort, consulted with invalids over several seasons.[271] In 1884, an Atlanta doctor who had bought interest in the property unsuccessfully attempted to create a sanitarium in the cool mountain air.[272] In addition, in an era of misinformation around malaria transmission, an *Atlanta Constitution* article reprinted in other Georgia newspapers admonished readers: "People living within the malarial region would do well to spend a month or two at Porter Springs each summer and get the malarial poison out of them."[273] Ozone, thought to be plentiful in the mountain air, with "stimulating" "electro-negative" properties, enabled invalids to "climb the heights [of nearby peaks] with an ease astonishing to themselves and to their friends at home."[274]

The mountains near Porter Springs lured guests for day or overnight expeditions. Visitors climbed to the top of Stone Pile in front of the hotel where the flat top afforded a "entrancing view of the mountains and valleys."[275] Those more adventuresome engaged a local guide to reach the top of Cedar Mountain. One young lady commented on the trip to and from the top of Cedar Mountain's spur: "When the road got very steep and the horses seemed to be having a hard pull, [the young guide] would give vigorous pushes from behind." On the way down, when "the brakes did not seem sufficient, he would jump on the spokes of the wheel and hold the vehicle back by main force."[276] Only the very intrepid rode to the peak of Blood Mountain, either spending the night at the home of a mountaineer or making the round trip within the same day. A horseback rider wrote of the steep and rough terrain to the top of Blood Mountain that made for "pretty dangerous traveling"; once at the top, he felt rewarded by the "grandest view imaginable."[277]

As visitors to Porter's Springs trekked northerly into the Blue Ridge, some wrote of the mountaineers almost as often as they did of the natural scenery about them. Porter guests typically hailed from coastal and central Georgia, some perhaps not having previously engaged with mountain residents. Although most guests expressed no overt prejudice against mountaineers (one traveler, for example, in 1869 called out the "kind mountain people"), some depicted them in a manner reminiscent of the title of Will Wallace Harney's seminal 1873 magazine article, "A Strange Land and a Peculiar People," as if they were Mountain South isolates.[278] One visitor observed that "[t]he natives are a stout, healthy, robust class" "not very highly educated and care but little for the outside world. [It is] certainly very interesting to go among the mountaineers of North Georgia and see them and watch their habits, manners and customs. It is well worth the while and expense."[279] In a similar fashion, another Porter's guest classified his fellow citizens in the Blue Ridge as "a hardy race," one that was "friendly and hospitable to an extreme." He then clarified his view of them as a group disjunct to his own by relegating them to another stratum of Georgia society: The "free swinging walk" of the mountaineers "is in marked contrast to the shuffling gait of their prototype, the low country 'cracker.'"[280] A female from Thomasville, located at the Florida border, however, did not refer to South Georgians as "crackers": She reserved the slur for the "genuine 'Georgia cracker[s]' [who] live along this road to Porter Springs in all their pristine originality." She wrote disdainfully of one mountaineer's oldest daughter, "Our mountain Sue," who wore a "blue plaid homespun dress and evidently considered her costume for an August day complete without shoes of any kind." The Thomasville woman criticized the family's housekeeping ("cleanliness was not one of the virtues"); the family's small cabin ("served them as both kitchen and dining room"); and the cabin's draftiness, caused in part by a gap by the fireplace ("quite large enough for me to crawl through, were I disposed to take the trouble"). Her scorn, however, dissolved into perhaps inadvertent envy upon leaving the family: "Something not less beautiful than [the mountains and a rose vine at the door] existed in that home. It was the spirit of contentment."[281] Possibly, the writers of these commentaries recorded their true impressions of the mountaineers. It is also conceivable that one or more, especially the Thomasville author, may have slanted or embellished their accounts to appeal to the same readership that Harney, Mary Noailles Murfree, and other local color writers attracted with their descriptions of a fictitious isolated Southern Appalachia.

At the turn of the twentieth century, Porter Springs continued to attract guests. For the season of 1899, over 450 visitors came, with many others turned away in the hot months of July and August.[282] The branding of Porter Springs as "Queen of the

Mountains" appeared widely during this period in ads as if the resort's longevity, especially under Farrow's long tenure (twenty-five seasons in 1899), had earned it this royal sobriquet.[283]

According to Joseph Whitner, Farrow's great-grandson, the hotel began to decline after the death of H.P. in 1907.[284] The hotel closed for the season of 1922; however, a full house was anticipated for 1925.[285] The resort operated as "Trahlyta Lodge" in the late 1920s under the proprietorship of two of Farrow's granddaughters, after which the Porter family used the property as a private summer home and as a site for community functions for many years.[286] In 1960, the Porter Springs Land Company advertised an auction for a tract of 1,400 acres that included the hotel site. As of 2009, McKee's direct descendant, George David, owned the undeveloped hotel property.[287]

Rowland Springs

Along the Interstate 75 corridor between Atlanta and Chattanooga in northwestern Georgia lies Bartow County, flanked by Floyd County to the west, Gordon County to the north, and partially by Cobb and Paulding counties to the south. Bartow County along with its neighboring counties of Polk to its southwest and Cherokee to its east delineates part of the southern boundary of Campbell's Southern Appalachia.

Most of Bartow County is situated in Georgia's Valley and Ridge geological province; about 10–25 percent lies in the Piedmont province in the county's southeastern area.[288] The rolling plateau of the Valley and Ridge's Coosa Valley section in western Bartow County rises only slightly in elevation from west to east, from Mullinax Mountain (1,100 feet) to Sproull Mountain (1,200 feet), about five miles west of the county seat of Cartersville; the eastern hilly part of the county includes the county's highest point, Pine Log Mountain at over 2,000 feet. The Etowah River, a popular paddling trail, flows westerly past the Etowah Indian Mounds, about three miles south of Cartersville, dipping to the county's low elevation of about 600 feet at the Bartow—Floyd county line.[289] The county's Cartersville Fault, at the intersection of the Piedmont and Valley and Ridge physiographic provinces, has provided the county's mining industry with a wealth of iron and manganese ores, bauxite, and other minerals to extract from the sedimentary and metamorphic layers.[290]

In 1832, the state legislature carved the county out of Cherokee County, naming it in honor of Lewis Cass, President Andrew Jackson's Secretary of War. Once the Civil War began, a Cass County state legislator denounced Cass, who had resigned as President James Buchanan's Secretary of State over Buchanan's indecisiveness over secession, as "inimical to the South" and introduced a bill enacted in late 1861 to change the county name to "Bartow" to memorialize Georgia native Colonel Francis Bartow, killed at the First Battle of Manassas (Bull Run).[291]

Migration to Cass County from eastern states in the 1830s partially occurred from participation in the 1832 land-lot and gold-lot state lottery held to distribute former Cherokee land.[292] In addition, many South Carolinians settled in Cass

County for the cooler summers and fertile farmland; transplanted Virginians grew tobacco in the "Little Virginia" colony along the Cass—Cherokee counties border.[293]

One new arrival to Cass County in 1839 was North Carolinian John Sharpe Rowland who as a 15-year-old moved with his family to South Carolina's Greenville District in 1810. He served in the War of 1812, then held appointed government positions in the Pendleton and Spartanburg districts before purchasing an initial 320 acres in the Etowah River Valley that he later expanded into 1,300 acres. Rowland moved his log cabin from the valley into the cooler elevation of the surrounding hills and transformed it over the next few years into the magnificent plantation manor, "Etowah Valley," which one antebellum writer designated as "one of the most handsomely improved places in the State."[294]

Rowland developed his wooded acreage into a thriving plantation that included fruit orchards, a vineyard, livestock and crops such as wheat, corn, and cotton.[295] To maintain such a large agrarian enterprise, Rowland relied largely on enslaved laborers, who also had built Etowah Valley "from the stonework of the foundation to the balustrade upon the roof."[296] In 1840, he owned fifty-four enslaved persons, making him the largest slaveowner in the county (his brother-in-law John W. Lewis ranked third with forty enslaved people).[297] By the time of Rowland's death in 1863, he owned at least 125 enslaved persons valued at $82,000 "specie value" ($246,500 "Confederate value"), thus indicating the expansion of his prosperity in two decades, gained largely through the labor of his enslaved workers, making him one of the wealthiest Southern Appalachian planters.[298]

In the early 1840s (antebellum sources disagree as to the exact year), Rowland bought another 2,100 acres in the area and subsequently built a resort around a series of mineral springs previously used by Native Americans, about ten miles from his Etowah Valley home and about six or seven miles from Cartersville, a depot for the "State Road" (the state-owned Western and Atlantic Railroad).[299] One prolific newspaper writer, the "Rambler," predicted in 1846 that the "new establishment … being near the Railroad, bids fair to become a place of considerable resort."[300] Although Rowland had not yet finished construction, that same year sojourners from Savannah 300 miles away were imbibing the resort's chalybeate (iron-containing) waters.[301]

During the next two years, Rowland continued to upgrade transportation and resort infrastructure, demonstrating both his wealth and the resort's growing popularity. In 1847, Rowland initiated a run of two six-passenger carriages from the railroad depot to the springs so that large parties arriving at Cartersville at noon could be conveyed to the resort in time for dinner.[302] In 1848, Rowland enlarged the existing house, built an additional sixteen-room structure, and repaired cabins and constructed additional ones.[303]

To make the grounds attractive for the fashionably ill, Rowland engaged in careful engineering and landscaping. He laid a mile-long pipe from the base of a neighboring mountain as an aqueduct to the front of the hotel where it generated water for a central fountain topped with a statue of Hygeia holding a bowl from which the water gushed fifty-five feet high and installed additional pipework to feed fountains located along shady paths surrounding the hotel.[304] Of the over twenty springs within a few hundred yards of the resort, he connected paths from the main hotel to a popular freestone spring and the upper and lower springs, covering the upper chalybeate spring with a pavilion roof an impressive thirty-six by twenty-four feet. Lastly, at the lower spring, he constructed a four-room bathing house.[305]

Taking the waters in such a thoughtfully orchestrated setting of fountains and promenade pathways appears to have constituted more of a social activity rather than one of medicinal therapy. Although antebellum publicity sought guests seeking health or pleasure, advertisements and visitor testimonials concentrated on the latter.[306] One guest, for example, briefly noted the chalybeate water's beneficial effects on several Savannah visitors before rhapsodizing at length about the comforts found at the resort, from Rowland's "courteous attention [to] the good order of the house, the promptness of the servants [likely enslaved workers], [and] the neatness of the rooms."[307]

Guests compared the mineral waters with those found at prestigious Georgia resorts located outside the Mountain South, not for the springs' therapeutic virtue, but for their taste, just as oenophiles might discuss subtle differences among Merlots. One commentator praised Rowland's waters: "The freestone water is hard to beat any where [sic], and decidedly the coolest (without ice) we have tasted during the summer. As to the mineral or Chalybeate spring, it is nothing like as strong as the Madison Springs, nor does it seem as strong as that of the Meriwether Springs. It may be a shade or two weaker, but it is more pleasant to the taste."[308] Another guest, however, scoffed at Rowland's: "[As] far as the mineral properties of the springs, their location, &c. are concerned, the place is, in my humble opinion, a perfect humbug. [Rowland's chalybeate waters] have not one fifth the strength of the Madison or other Chalybeate waters I have tasted."[309]

Rowland made a major coup in the Georgia antebellum resort management business when he hired Sterling Lanier, future owner of Tennessee's Montvale Springs, to operate Rowland Springs for the season of 1848. Lanier hailed from Macon where he had managed the Floyd House, which, according to Judge Richard H. Clark, he had shaped into a "first-class hotel, with a reputation as such from New York to New Orleans."[310] Publicity for Rowland's that year beckoned Lanier's past clientele "for whose accommodation he has made very extensive preparations."[311] One visitor emphasized that Rowland "has done more than all [the improvements by engaging] Sterling Lanier, Esq., of Macon, favorably known to the traveling world, and Georgians especially ... to contribute to the comfort of guests."[312]

When Rowland reassumed Lanier's responsibilities for the season of 1849, one newspaper lauded him as an "extremely courteous and obliging gentleman [who] deserves infinite credit, for the efforts which he has made to accommodate those who seek comfort or pleasure."[313] In an article widely reprinted from the *Charleston Mercury*, for instance, Rowland's organization of a fancy ball in 1849 captivated southern readers with its dazzling account of guests costumed as European nobility, peasants, mythological creatures, and military figures.[314]

Daily activities compared favorably to those offered at other fashionable antebellum resorts. Guests took morning and evening strolls to the springs, bowled in the ten-pin alley, danced at night, listened to parlor music, and gathered for convivial conversation after meals.[315] Courting constituted a most favorable pastime among the numerous younger visitors; one observer wrote that "nine-tenths of the company is composed of maidens who have 'come out,' at least to 'see and be seen,' and 'trim gallants full of courtship and of state.'"[316]

Resort life, under Rowland, was mannered and wholesome, if also invigorating. On Sundays, the guests conducted themselves piously in the hotel parlor at services conducted by visiting ministers. Rowland forbade card playing; one correspondent wrote that he had "heard complaints of him only on that score."[317] A school master in his advertisement for an adjacent boarding academy, which educated Rowland's sons, consoled potentially concerned parents that "*above all* [italics original] it is remote from the evil influence of grog-shops, card tables, and other vices with which youth are now so industrially and fatally baited."[318]

For nearby excursions, guests visited the Cooper & Stroup iron works and flour mills on the Etowah River and the local saltpetre cave. Local newspapers boasted of these manufactories as much as they did of the northern Georgia natural scenery. The *Albany Patriot*, for example, called out the iron works and the salt-petre cave, which "together with the good [hotel] fare ... the pure blue limestone water, and the urbanity of the inhabitants will make Cassville [ten miles from Rowland Springs] a desirable summer residence for anyone seeking health or amusement."[319]

Visitors to Rowland's traveled largely from central Georgia, Charleston, and Savannah, and occasionally from Alabama and Mississippi. Rowland's for some served as a stop on a grand tour, not as prestigious as that associated with the Virginia springs, but fashionable just the same for those with sufficient time and income. Charlestonians and Savannahians might travel by rail to Atlanta where they might spend the night before continuing on the Western and Atlantic Railroad to the Cartersville depot to engage a hack to Rowland's.[320] One energetic group, the senior class of the La Grange Female Institute, went by railroad in 1851 from La Grange, Georgia, on the Alabama border, through Atlanta to Chattanooga where they climbed Lookout Mountain and visited its environs. From Chattanooga, they traveled about twenty-five miles south to Georgia's Catoosa Springs for two days and then journeyed to Rowland Springs where they enjoyed "promenading its velvet tossed walks." The next day, they visited the Cooper & Stroup iron works, "one of the grand developements [sic] of the resources of Georgia we should all be proud of" before continuing to La Grange.[321]

Rowland Springs could accommodate about 600 visitors in its heyday before the Civil War.[322] An 1847 visitor estimated guests during his stay at 225.[323] Three years later, the season of 1850 left one observer dizzy attempting to bean-count: "We have even a larger company here than when I last wrote: as fast as one party leaves, another arrives, and it is one continual coming and going, not in parties of two or three, but of 25 or 30."[324]

Elites included an array of Georgia politicians hosted by Rowland, "among the cleverest of all clever democrats [sic]," according to one writer.[325] Democrat George W. Towns and Whig Duncan L. Clinch met there during the 1847 gubernatorial campaign. Democratic Congressman Thomas C. Hackett was rapidly regaining his health there in the summer of 1850.[326] The Rambler reported the next year that retired U.S. senator and former Governor George Troup was staying at the

Springs ("his health is not so good as when I last met him") and praised him for his states' rights views: "He would have had no compromises by which we lost all and the North gained all."[327] Contrary to the Rambler's report, however, another guest remarked that "very little is said of politics here. Indeed I have not heard the subject mentioned more than once or twice."[328]

Georgia Governor Joseph Brown and his family sojourned in 1860 in a house furnished by Rowland at the resort. Brown, preoccupied by health concerns and evidently unsatisfied with his brief convalescence at central Georgia's Indian Springs the year before, believed that Rowland Springs' high altitude and spring water would benefit him and transacted both government and private business affairs during his stay.[329]

Brown knew Rowland well. In 1851 Rowland had retained Brown to defend him successfully in a lawsuit in which the plaintiffs, a widow and her son-in-law, attempted to gain possession of the resort property via altered documents.[330] In addition, in 1858, Brown hired John W. Lewis, Rowland's brother-in-law, as the Western and Atlantic Railroad superintendent.[331] Lewis's frustration with Brown's micro-management of the rail (Brown had a lifelong fascination with railroads) led to his surprised resignation in the middle of Brown's 1861 gubernatorial campaign. Largely due to their friendship and kindred political views, Brown immediately appointed Rowland to replace Lewis.[332]

Consumed by railroad management responsibilities and the organization of local Confederate companies of soldiers (the Rowlander Highlanders were named in his honor), Rowland put the resort and slave cabins on the market in late summer 1863, publicizing the resort as suitable for war refugees.[333] Rowland, however, died of a sudden illness in mid–September 1863 before he could sell the property. His obituary omitted mention of the resort; rather, it somewhat cryptically alluded to Rowland's "[devotion] to his agricultural interests and private affairs." In more detail, the obituary lauded him as "warmly attached to the South, the land of his birth, and to its institutions" and praised him as a "kind and careful and benignant master."[334]

Rowland Springs apparently closed during the Civil War (no source consulted provides direct confirmation) and began a gradual decline after the war, marked by frequent changes in owners and fewer guests than during its halcyon antebellum days. A doctor and his Atlanta partners were preparing to take charge of the resort in 1870; by 1873, however, the resort was "being put in good condition" by Colonel William L. Rowland, one of Rowland's sons.[335] The next year, a former Atlantan, M.G. Dobbins, bought the resort and spent $10,000 for the addition of a dance hall and two buildings and other improvements. Because of the scarcity of money, according to one writer, who possibly was alluding to the lingering impacts of the Panic of 1873, Rowland's attracted few visitors in 1875, mainly from Georgia and Florida.[336] In 1878, Dr. U.O. Robertson, in vogue with a national hygienic movement that espoused various electrical and water-based therapies, advertised the Rowland Springs Hygienic Institute, apparently located near the mineral springs, firmly declaring it "not a summer resort for the gay and fashionable world."[337] Within a year, however, he had relocated his practice to Atlanta because of the inaccessibility of Rowland Springs for potential patients.[338]

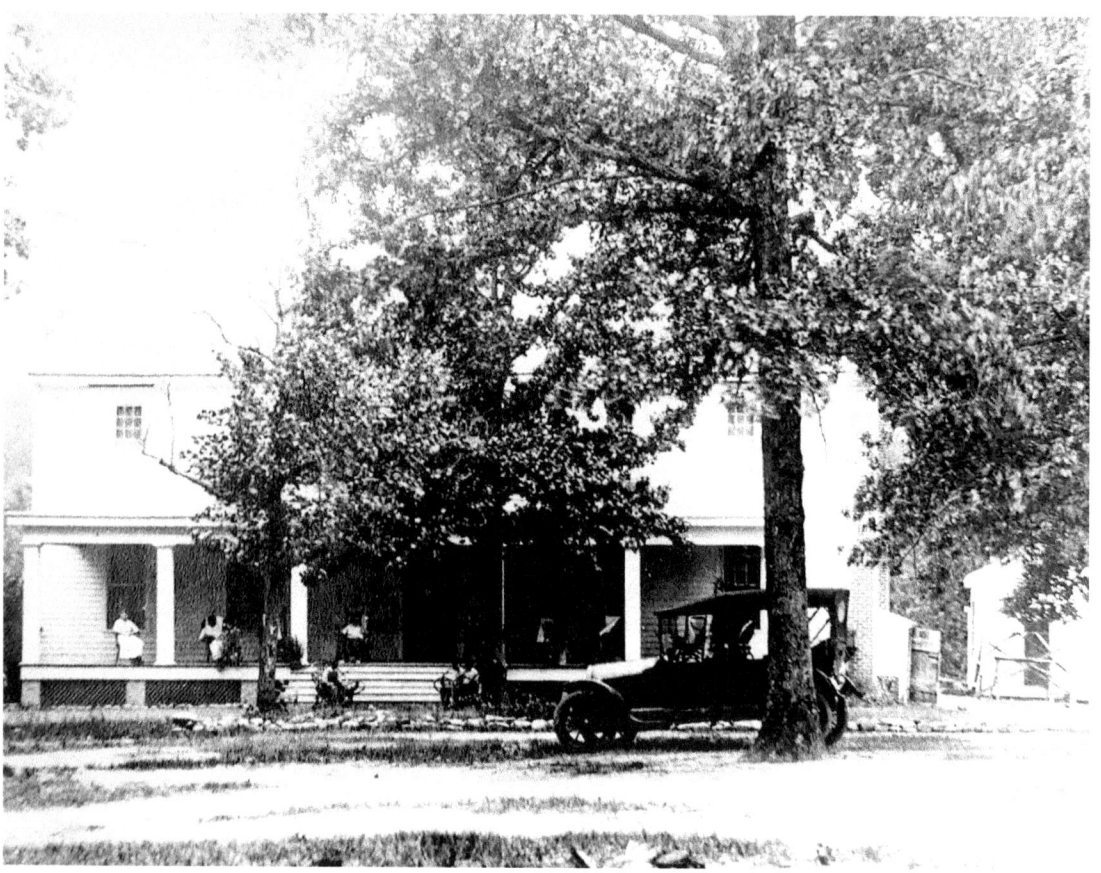

Rowland Springs [1910s?], Bartow County, Georgia (courtesy of the Bartow History Museum, Cartersville, GA).

Rowland Springs' postbellum decline may be attributed to several interrelated causes. First, as Robertson noted, the expansion of railroad service to other popular destinations rendered Rowland's relatively inaccessible. Second, the Civil War left many in Bartow County in financial ruin, and persistent drought over several years inhibited economic recovery.[339] Third, perhaps the absence of knowledgeable enslaved workers, potentially a lower cost to the resort than that of hiring free laborers unfamiliar with the property's operations, may have posed an obstacle. Fourth, the death of Rowland, a strong hands-on proprietor (not an absentee landlord), left a vacuum in resort management.

In 1907, Dobbins and the co-owners of the Rowland property answered the plea of an Atlanta newspaper to provide a summer place in the country for a group of children from the Sheltering Arms Orphanage in Atlanta. Publicity covering the orphans' stays at the resort described Rowland Springs as an "old summer hotel" and "one of the relics of antebellum days ... with many fine springs."[340]

Only locals visited the resort grounds in the next decade, as almost all buildings were in ruins, until Robert and Rebecca Donahoo invested in the property in 1917, initiating a bottling operation and entertaining largely Georgians and Floridians.[341]

The hotel during the Donahoos' ownership was a three-story, wooden-frame structure with double chimneys on each side, with a grand sixty-foot-long interior hall separating double parlors and a spacious dining room. Guests also stayed in three tenant houses converted to cottages.[342]

The resort closed for good in 1925 when the Donahoos sold the property to a Florida real estate broker, who failed to develop it.[343] As a death knell, a tornado demolished the former Donahoo hotel in 1948.[344] An historical marker now commemorates the site of one of Georgia's most fashionable antebellum health resorts, owned and largely managed by a wealthy Mountain South plantation owner, a resort not isolated in the Etowah River Valley but linked with southern elite guests outside Appalachian Georgia.[345]

Kentucky

Introduction

The region of eastern Kentucky may evoke distinctly different historical images, ranging from Daniel Boone's eighteenth-century expeditions to the 1930s "Bloody Harlan" skirmishes to today's "KFC" originating from Harland Sander's Corbin café's fried chicken. Probably more obscure is the history of several health resorts located in the Cumberland Plateau's Eastern Kentucky Coal Field (Coalfields) physiographic province, Kentucky's contribution to Campbell's Southern Appalachia.[1] These health resorts largely stood near the western escarpment of the plateau, not the Coal Field's eastern mountain ridges, with the notable exception of Bell County's Cedar Creek Springs, now part of Pine Mountain State Park, in southeastern Kentucky.[2] The weathered sandstone gorges and cliffs along the escarpment hindered travel to several of the Southern Appalachian health resorts; the northern Bluegrass Region to the west of the Coal Field contained the most popular antebellum Kentucky resorts such as Graham Springs and Olympian Springs.[3]

J. Winston Coleman, Jr., the foremost twentieth-century scholar on Kentucky watering places, observed that most mineral spring resorts reached their zenith before the Civil War.[4] Earlier, mineral springs authority James K. Crook had noted in the 1890s that Kentucky springs "are not enjoying the high measure of popular esteem which they once possessed" and described only four Southern Appalachian resorts among the 15 he covered for the state.[5] Even in the antebellum period, the venerable *Appletons'* travel guide gave just passing mention to one Southern Appalachian Kentucky health resort, Esculapia Springs.[6] The resulting lack of documentation on Southern Appalachian Kentucky health resorts resulted in my selection of five resorts in the region based on the quantity of available information to piece together narratives: Estill County's Estill Springs, Lewis County's Esculapia and Glen (Glenn) Springs, and Pulaski County's Rockcastle and Sublimity Springs.

All five resorts began in the antebellum period: Estill Springs, Esculapia, and Glen Springs in the 1810s followed by Rockcastle around 1835 and Sublimity about 1854. Estill Springs was first owned by Green Clay, a distant relative of Henry Clay, and then by his son Brutus, which may have helped cement ties in the 1820s–1840s with visitors who personally knew or wanted to mingle with members of the prominent Clay aristocracy of Kentucky. Esculapia was developed by a real estate magnate, M.T.C. Gould, whose business transactions may have attracted some of his clientele

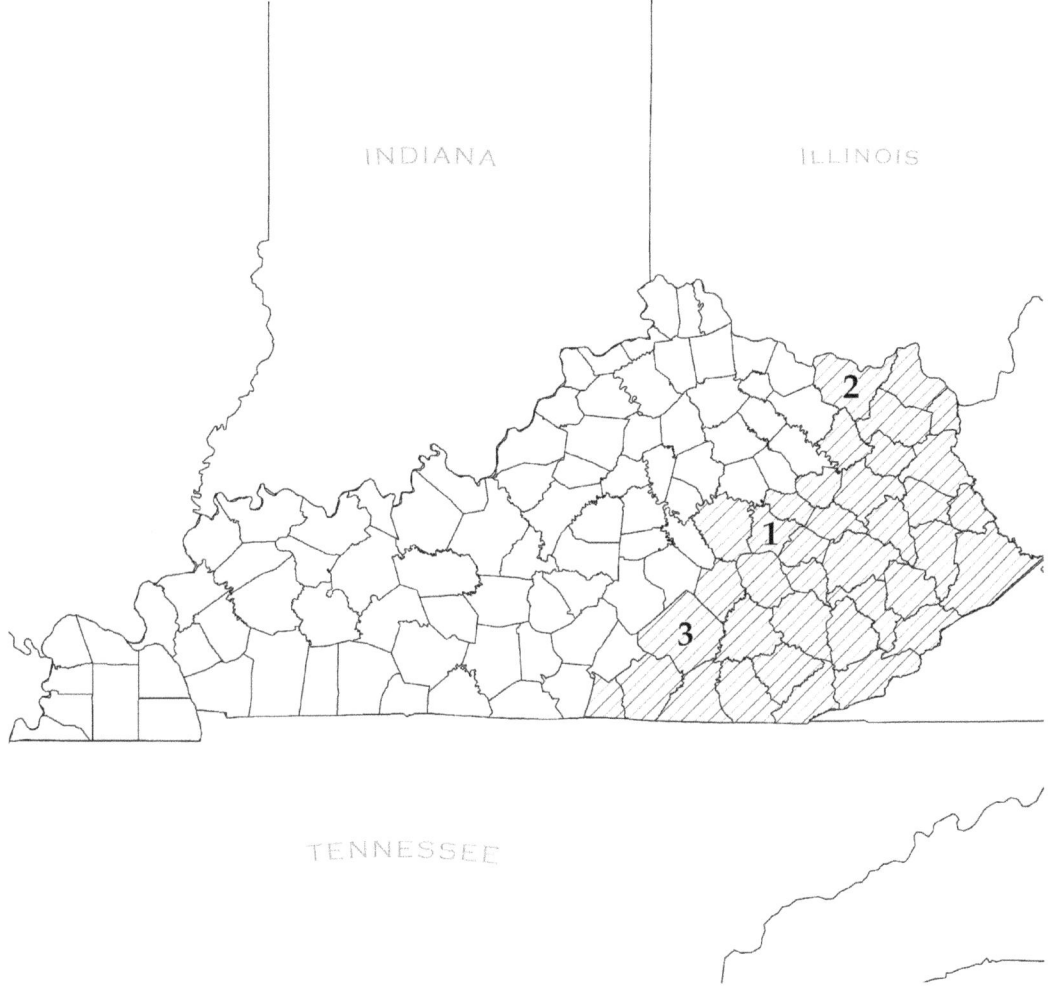

Kentucky counties with featured health resorts: (1) Estill County, Estill Springs; (2) Lewis County, Esculapia Springs and Glen Springs; (3) Pulaski County, Rockcastle Springs and Sublimity Springs (Sources: Esri, NOAA, USGS. Cartographer: Sayona Turner, East Tennessee State University).

to the resort. Perhaps this affinity of the Estill and Esculapia clientele for the resort owners, who also lavishly invested in the resorts, swelled the ranks of visitors to the point that they rivaled the most popular Blue Grass regional resorts.[7] Rockcastle and Sublimity Springs were much more remote due to their location along a gorge of the Rockcastle River. By the 1850s, Rockcastle, however, vied with Esculapia and Estill Springs as one of the most popular Kentucky resorts in the Mississippi and Ohio River valleys.[8]

Most Kentucky resorts, including those in the Eastern Coal Fields, closed during the Civil War.[9] The Southern Appalachian resorts discussed in this chapter reopened afterwards, with various degrees of popularity. On the one hand, the fashionable Esculapia, after experiencing a cholera outbreak in 1850, faded for the next decade and, after the war, regained only a regional patronage. On the other hand,

Rockcastle Springs received fewer guests than Esculapia or Estill in the antebellum era but welcomed the likes of former Confederate generals and Kentucky governors in the postbellum period. Likewise, Glen Springs, overshadowed by Esculapia before the Civil War, attracted a wider geographic range of visitors after the construction of the railroad through Vanceburg in the late 1880s and after management invested in its infrastructure.

The demise of the resorts began in the late 1800s due to weather events, fires, or sale of the non-lucrative properties as potential visitors went elsewhere in automobiles or on the expanded railroad network in the country. The Rockcastle Springs' main section burned down in 1900; Esculapia's hotel, in 1912. Ice floes and flooding of the Rockcastle River destroyed several of Sublimity Springs' structures before 1882. Glen Springs found new life as an academic institution but burned down in 1918.

Three interesting topics for further research result from the relative proximity of the resorts to the Ohio River. First, why did southern planters with their families and retinues of slaves traveling by steamer often bypass the Ohio River port towns of Maysville or Vanceburg, relatively close to some of Kentucky's Southern Appalachian resorts, to disembark farther upstream at Wyandotte, Virginia, to then endure an arduous coach ride to the White Sulphur Springs, almost 200 miles to the southeast? To answer this question in part, it must be noted that the White Sulphur, despite its mountainous location, prevailed among all southern watering holes as the locus for the country's social and political elite. Henry Clay, for example, probably accrued more days at the White Sulphur in his unofficial role as host for part of each season than he did while sojourning at his father-in-law Thomas Hart's Olympian Springs in Kentucky's Bath County or at Green Clay's Estill Springs.[10] Perhaps southern agrarians who wished to socialize with the likes of Clay and to be seen by others mingling with the national elite gladly undertook the journey to the White Sulphur and other Virginia springs.

A second question arises from the nature of interactions of antebellum resort clientele hailing from both sides of the Ohio River. How did antebellum visitors from Mississippi, Louisiana, and Memphis mingle at Esculapia, for example, with guests from Pittsburgh and other northern cities? Were the issues of slavery and states' rights *verboten*, or did the guests largely segregate into like-minded groups?

Third, as a corollary question to the above, what was the general sociopolitical nature of the northern visitors? Were they abolitionists in theory (not practice), supporters of attempts to broker national compromises between the admission of slave and free states to the Union, and / or passive recipients of the services provided by the resort owners' "servants?" Estill Springs' owner Green Clay, for example, was the largest slaveowner in Kentucky at one point, and his son Brutus owned over 40 slaves in 1860. Esculapia Springs' M.T.C. Gould employed over ten white laborers but also held three enslaved adults in 1850.[11] Visitors from the north could scarcely have been ignorant of the role of enslaved persons at the mineral spring resorts.

These three topics are beyond the scope of this chapter but appear to be a fascinating area for further investigation. Accessing diaries, letters, and other sources of the antebellum period related to the resorts might yield an enhanced understanding of Southern Appalachian watering holes in a border state such as Kentucky.

Lewis County: Esculapia and Glen Springs

Kentucky's Lewis County lies in the northeastern corner of the state, demarcating a northern boundary for Campbell's definition of Southern Appalachia. The county is surrounded in a clockwise direction by the Ohio River to the north, Greenup and Carter counties to the east, Rowan County to the south, Fleming County to the southwest, and Mason County to the west. Its topography rises from the rolling Outer Bluegrass physiographic province in the west to the hilly Eastern Coal Fields elsewhere in the county, with elevations in the valleys at about 520 to 540 feet. Vanceburg, the county seat, for example, lies at an elevation of 525 feet on the banks of the Ohio River. Farther inland, Tollesboro, about 35 miles to the southwest, stands at 816 feet. Esculapia (Eskalapia) Mountain, slightly less than four miles to the southeast of Tollesboro, rises to about 1,200 feet.[12]

Before its formation in 1808, Lewis County was well known for a salt lick located at the head of the aptly named Salt Lick Creek. Native Americans, largely Shawnees, staked out the lick for buffalo and deer. Early explorers traveled by it on their way to the Cabin Creek War Road that led farther into Bluegrass country. The French knew of the salt lick as early as 1762; Daniel Boone camped at the head of Salt Lick Creek near Esculapia Mountain in 1776. Later, Vanceburg developed in part as a landing point for those traveling to the nearby Ohio Salt Works established in 1794.[13]

Through the Salt Lick Creek valley's limestone and shale seeped several magnesia, sulphur, and chalybeate springs. The springs near the headwaters of the Big Salt Lick Creek at the bottom of Esculapia Mountain became the basis for the health resorts of Esculapia Springs and Glen (Glenn) Springs, about one mile from each other, and about 12 miles south of Vanceburg.[14] Kirk's Springs, contemporaneous with Esculapia and Glen, lay about six to eight miles to the southwest, near the community of Burtonville, but remained largely undeveloped.[15] This chapter will explore the histories of Esculapia and Glen, both dating back to the antebellum period. Esculapia rose to fashionable prominence before 1850 as a convenient resort for steamboat passengers disembarking at Vanceburg. Glen, however, came into its element, perhaps surpassing the opulence of Esculapia, with the completion of railroad service through Lewis County in 1888.

Esculapia and Glen Springs' origins date back to at least the late 1810s when they were known by other names. In 1822, English immigrant John Powling received a license to operate a tavern at White Sulphur Springs, an early name for Esculapia Springs, and built several crude structures around the springs. By 1826, Peter January received the tavern license from William O. Powling (relation to John Powling unclear) as John Powling had moved to Maysville.[16] Possibly a few years before John Powling began the White Sulphur Springs tavern, native Kentuckian James McCormick founded McCormick's Springs, as Glen Springs was originally called: In 1819, he was already associated with the springs when he was appointed overseer for a mountain road in the area.[17]

Both resorts flourished during the next three decades although less information is available for McCormick's Springs, implying that it attracted less public interest than White Sulphur. By the early 1850s, however, McCormick's Springs was thriving to such an extent that It served as a post office and generated profit for McCormick.[18] McCormick in 1850, for instance, reported to the census taker that he owned real estate valued at $4,000 ($155,000 in 2022 dollars); in addition, as a landowner, he likely supplied his hotel table from the 200 improved acres of his total 800 acres.[19] As another example of his prosperity, his household in 1850 included five men, largely in farming occupations (the census taker recorded "hotel" in the margin of the household record by their names). One of the males was Ohioan Simpson Grant, brother to Ulysses S. (Hiram Ulysses) Grant; their father in 1847 owned a tan yard near Esculapia Springs.[20]

Two households away from McCormick in 1850 lived M.T.C. (Marcus Tullius Cicero) Gould. Gould was a regional real estate agent and well-known stenographer who authored several treatises on the art of shorthand.[21] In 1845, he bought Carter's Springs, as White Sulphur Springs was then known, from owner R.G. (Robert G.) Carter.[22] The following year, Gould and two others changed the resort name to Esculapia Springs, incorporated the Esculapia Mineral Spring Company (or Esculapia Springs Company) around 1846 or 1849 with capital of $50,000, and through the late 1840s retained professional hoteliers to manage the health resort.[23] To provide, in part, easier access to the watering holes, Gould, McCormick, and others attempted unsuccessfully to procure resources to construct a turnpike from Maysville to Vanceburg via Esculapia.[24]

Gould accordingly listed his occupation as "Hotel Keeper" in the 1850 population census and estimated his real estate at a value more than triple than that of McCormick's ($15,000). His household included several laborers who likely worked at Esculapia along with his three adult enslaved persons, the latter a rarity in a county where slaves comprised less than 5 percent of the population.[25]

Esculapia Springs reached its zenith from 1840 through 1850.[26] An 1854 gazetteer in its description on Lewis County singled out the resort (excluding McCormick's), describing it as "a fashionable watering place."[27] During the first half of the decade, the property consisted of a two-story white frame hotel flanked by a cottage row on both sides. In 1846, Gould enlarged the hotel and built 20–30 additional cottages to double the capacity from 100 to 200 guests. Gould also constructed additional bathing houses and landscape features such as labyrinths and arbors.[28] Shady paths led to the white sulphur spring ("equally efficacious" to the White Sulphur Springs of Virginia) and to a chalybeate fountain about 300 yards away (used to treat "most of the chronic disturbances of the female system").[29] Outdoor activities included fishing, fox and deer hunts, a pistol gallery, and "gymnastic and kalisthinic [sic] apparatus … for the invigoration of the body." A typical day included an early morning walk to the sulphur spring for a shower bath, breakfast followed by a "segar," scandal-free conversation with ladies or gentlemen, dinner, lounging around the property, visiting the chalybeate fountain, supper, more conversation, and evening dancing.[30]

Esculapia guests in the antebellum era appear to have mainly hailed from the Deep South and the Ohio River Valley. A Louisiana planter planning to return in 1845 to Esculapia inquired about the availability of five cottages "on the upper range, west end" for three couples, three unmarried ladies, two single gentlemen, seven children, and five servants (likely enslaved persons).[31] Other Deep South visitors from Mississippi, Arkansas, and Memphis intermingled with northern guests from Pittsburgh, Ohio, and Wheeling.[32]

Several notables visited Esculapia Springs for medicinal purposes and also most likely for social activities, if their health allowed. Newport, Kentucky's founder, General James Taylor, a connoisseur of Saratoga and the Virginia springs, testified that the white sulphur water aided his digestion.[33] Benjamin Harrison, born near the Ohio River banks, sought the watering hole to improve his health decades before his presidency.[34]

Deep South elites' travel to Esculapia partially mimicked the journeys of those from the Delta who sojourned at western Virginia's White Sulphur Springs. Planters went by steamboat up the Mississippi through the Ohio River where they might disembark at Vanceburg to ride by stage to Esculapia within two or three hours. Regional residents traveled by daily packets from Cincinnati, Maysville, and Portsmouth to dock at Vanceburg or Maysville where they could board a coach to ride directly to Esculapia.[35]

Gould lamented the lack of "good roads and carriages" to attract more from the "lower country"; he unsuccessfully lobbied the state legislature for turnpike funding several times.[36] To compensate for the apparently uncomfortable stage ride, he boasted that Esculapia was "[more] near the Ohio river than any other watering place" even though many southern families obviously continued past the Kentucky ports to disembark at Wyandotte, about 170 miles from the premier watering hole, White Sulphur Springs in western Virginia.[37]

The sophistication and gaiety of Esculapia Springs greatly diminished after 1850. Throughout the 1840s and 1850s, the region around Maysville suffered cholera outbreaks.[38] In 1849, a massive cholera epidemic killed 8,000 residents of Cincinnati and precipitated the postponement of the Ohio Constitutional Convention of 1850–1851.[39] Typical of the day, those in areas stricken by cholera fled elsewhere, including to Esculapia Springs. In 1850, cholera struck at the health resort, resulting in the death of at least two persons within four days. Guests vied for transportation away from Esculapia, paying premium stagecoach fares to head to Maysville.[40] Gould himself contracted cholera while leaving on horseback but survived. The resort's reputation faltered for the next several years although it hosted such Kentucky luminaries as future U.S. Senator Archibald Dixon in 1851. Buildings were not maintained, and fire destroyed the hotel in 1860.[41]

Any effects of the Civil War on Glen Springs and Esculapia Springs in Lewis County, where residents were "intensively devoted to the Union cause," are not known, but both resorts received guests in the postbellum era.[42] Esculapia Springs received more publicity than Glen Springs in the first two decades following the war, a sign of its relative popularity at the time.

Esculapia, despite the taint of the cholera epidemic, rebounded under the ownership of Greenup County's William F. Jones from around 1867, when he acquired the property, to November 1886, when he sold his interest.[43] Within three years of his purchase, Jones had prospered to the point that he claimed real estate worth $12,000 (about $278,000 in 2022 dollars) and personal estate of $3,535.[44] He built a hotel served by sulphur water piped from the springs and connected the house by telephone to Vanceburg.[45] He eschewed the use of alcohol at the resort, advertising no bar-room, no wines, and no liquors.[46] The prohibition of alcohol probably changed soon after May 1886, when Jones incorporated the Esculapia Springs (Hotel) Company with several other regional businessmen, including wholesale and retail liquor dealer A.R. Mullins who became company president.[47] Jones sold his interest in November of that year because he intended to move west.[48]

The Esculapia Springs Company remodeled the hotel and improved the grounds.[49] In addition to the usual amusements, including grand masquerade balls, the company offered hot and cold sulphur baths and cuisine prepared by French cooks.[50] As evidence of the growing popularity of Esculapia, the number of visitors in the third week of July 1886 doubled from 100 to 200 the same week five years later.[51]

The years 1892, 1893, and 1905 brought about misfortune and scandal to Esculapia Springs. An attempt failed in spring 1892 to establish a Keely institute at Esculapia to treat alcoholism, indicating the loss of potential revenue.[52] In September 1892, resort manager Charles Beach lost almost all possessions in a devasting hotel fire with loss valued at $20,000; after receiving a 25-year lease from the hotel syndicate to rebuild, Beach determined to "surpass Glenn Springs in the way of grandeur and beauty."[53] The opening of the new Esculapia hotel in July 1893, however, was tarnished by lawsuits and counter lawsuits between Mullins and Beach earlier that year over shared profits and liquor payments allegedly due to Mullins.[54] Beach evidently won the litigation: He replaced Mullins as the syndicate president, and his attorneys in the lawsuits, prominent Kentucky politicians and Newport law partners R.W. Nelson and George Washington, Jr., became syndicate directors.[55] In 1905, Beach, by then a physician as well as proprietor, killed the local mail carrier allegedly for trespassing. The press sensationally reported on the incident until the doctor's eventual acquittal in October 1906.[56]

Glen Springs began to vie with Esculapia Springs for visitors after the Chesapeake & Ohio (C&O) Railroad, operating the Maysville and Big Sandy Railroad, came to Lewis County in June 1888, bisecting Vanceburg.[57] Carriages met the dwindling number of steamboat and packet arrivals and the increasing frequency of trains at Vanceburg to convey guests over an "unusually fine" road that passed through farming country and old growth forests to reach the Glen Springs hotel.[58]

Improved transportation alone cannot account for the escalating demand for Glen Springs that caused Beach to vow to outcompete Glen when rebuilding the Esculapia Springs hotel in 1893. The Glen Springs owner, tobacconist I.N. (Isaac Nash) Walker and members of his family operated the health resort from around 1889 until about 1912, providing friendly management (guests "feel perfectly at home") and steady maintenance and improvement of the property.[59]

Walker spent lavishly on Glen Springs. In 1890, he expended almost $100,000 in improvements to accommodate 300 guests.[60] Within five years, he had enlarged the dining room to 131 feet; added new parlors, one of which contained a prized white onyx mantel costing $1,000; and increased capacity to hold 500 visitors.[61] The three-story white-frame main hotel was surrounded by wrap-around, sixteen-foot-wide verandahs on the first and second floors and was topped by a tower positioned between two front gables. Walker's addition of a one and a half story wing stood perpendicular to the main building.[62] A shady fern-lined path led to a cluster of springs, including sulphur, alum, iron, and alkaline waters.[63] An artificial lake for bathing and boating was constructed nearby.[64]

Despite the assumed rivalry between Glen Springs and Esculapia, guests visited both resorts, staying at one or the other at different times and strolling between them, perhaps to take in a dance at "The Glen."[65] A Maysville family, for instance, boarded at Esculapia in 1886 and at Glen in 1892, perhaps an implication of nothing more than a change of resort venue or perhaps a reflection of Glen's vaulted reputation in the 1890s.[66] In addition, religious services and social activities at the Ruggles campground near Burtonsville, about eight miles west of Glen Springs, appealed to both health resorts' visitors.[67] Likewise, Ruggles attendees and locals visited Glen and Esculapia for the day.[68]

The health benefits of the water, the lack of mosquitos, the "pure mountain air," and "escape [from] the heat and discomfort of the city" attracted Esculapia and Glen guests in the postbellum period.[69] At Glen, a Cincinnati man recovered from 15 years of chronic dyspepsia, and his wife regained 35 pounds during a two-month stay.[70] Regional newspapers reported that Esculapia guests returned home "much refreshed" and with health "fully restored."[71]

Postbellum guests at both watering holes included ministers, judges, professors, and businessmen and families from such Ohio River Valley towns as Portsmouth or Covington. Esculapia in the early 1880s also advertised outside the region in large cities such as Memphis, Nashville, and Indianapolis but appears to have drawn more regional elites a decade later based on newspaper society columns. Glen Springs in the early 1890s, however, hosted travelers from New York, New Orleans, Indianapolis, and Washington, D.C., perhaps indicating wider popularity of Glen's appeal.[72]

The 1910s saw fires severely damage both resorts. In 1910, Beach sold Esculapia to John and Will Hamrick of Tolesboro (Tollesboro); the hotel burned down in 1912.[73] A Baptist concern bought Glen Springs in fall 1916 or early 1917 to convert it into an educational academy after it was sold to settle an estate. Unfortunately, a kitchen fire in February 1918 at Glen Springs College destroyed the campus's three-story main building; only one of the 50 occupants was injured.[74]

These two bygone resorts ebbed and flowed as epidemics, transportation, and ownership affected their fortunes. A cholera epidemic blemished Esculapia's reputation in the antebellum era. In the postbellum era, both resorts prospered, Glen perhaps more so than Esculapia owing to the coming of the railroad and a proprietor with deep pockets to invest in the property. Today, a Kentucky Historical Society marker commemorates Esculapia Springs.[75] Glen Springs lives on as the name of a small farming community at the crossroads of Salt Lick Road (State Highway 989) and Toller Branch Road.

Estill Springs

The Kentucky River meanders through Estill County, located on the western edge of the Eastern Coal Fields physiographic region in eastern Kentucky, about 40

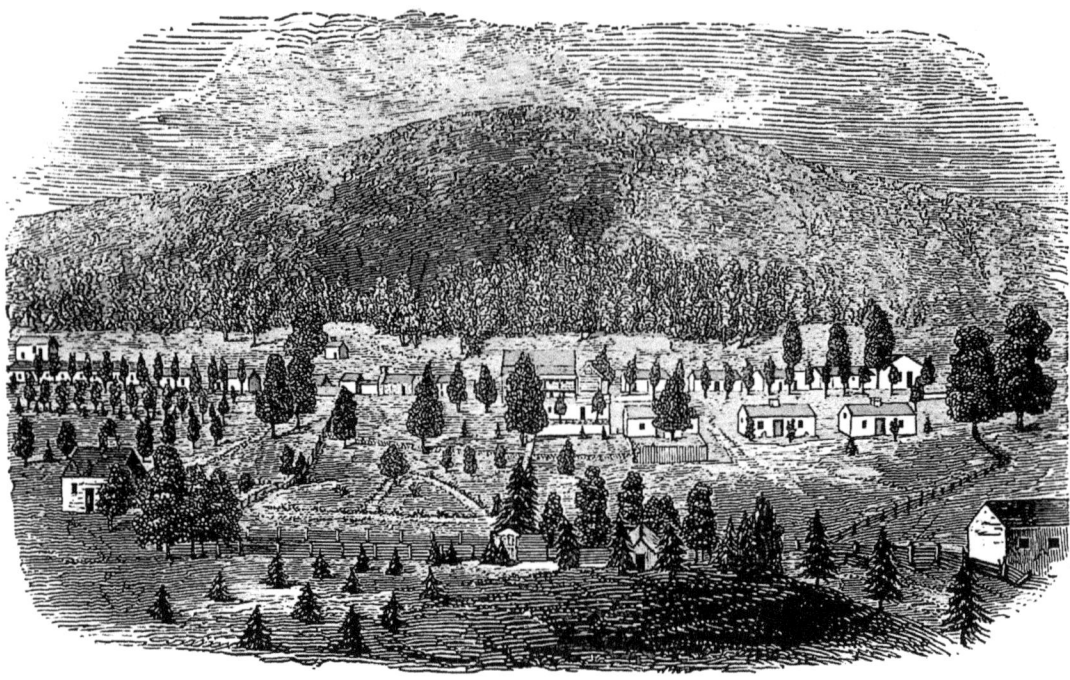

Esculapia Springs, Lewis County, Kentucky [~1847]. Lewis Collins, *Historical Sketches of Kentucky: History of Kentucky* (Maysville, KY: Lewis Collins; Cincinnati: J.A. & U.P. James, 1847), *Revised, Enlarged Three-Fold, and Brought Down to the Year 1874 by His Son, Richard H. Collins*, vol. 2 (Covington, KY: Collins & Co., 1874; reprint, Louisville: John P. Morton & Co., 1924), 465 (image courtesy of the University Archives & Special Collections, Lincoln Memorial University, Harrogate, Tennessee).

miles southeast of Lexington.[76] In the deep-cut river valley lies the county seat of Irvine at an elevation of about 585 feet in the shadows of Henry Mountain (1,247 feet high) and Sweet Lick Knob (1,160 feet high).[77] At the base of Sweet Lick Knob is a cluster of mineral springs that gave rise in the early 1800s to the county's most prominent business, the fashionable resort of Sweet Springs, later called Estill Springs, which endured for 120 years.[78]

The use of the Sweet Springs can be traced to Native Americans, followed by eighteenth-century white explorers. Native Americans used the springs as a resting place along a prong of the Warriors' Path; the Shawnees also established a camp there at some point.[79] Early white visitors included Daniel Boone's 1769 hunting party, which established a base at Station Camp, about ten miles from the springs, and the 1773 McAfee party, which stayed at "some sweet springs in a white oak flat of a mountain."[80]

The sweet springs became the property of Green Clay in the early 1800s, about the time of Estill County's formation in 1808.[81] Clay, distant kin to Henry Clay and father of Cassius M. Clay, born in 1810, was a wealthy slaveowner and largest land owner in the county.[82] Clay constructed some rough cabins around the springs.[83] By 1814, the so-called "Sweet Springs at Estill Courthouse" was firmly established as a

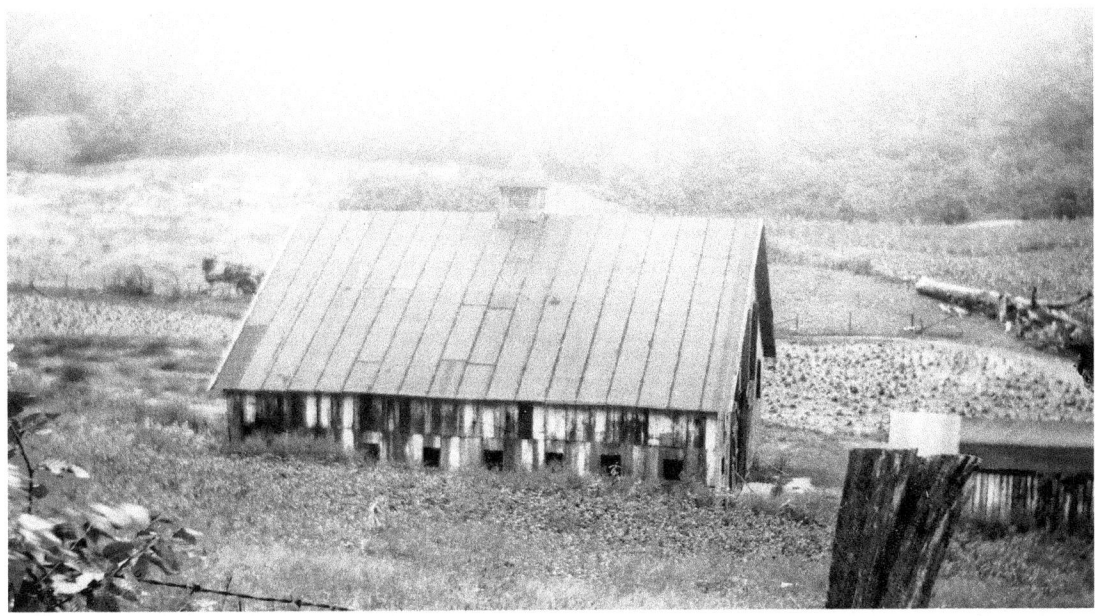

"This barn is the only building that remains on the site of Esculapia Springs [1920s]" (Warren Kellar Frederick, photographer. Warren Kellar Frederick Collection, ULPA 1980_029_888a, University of Louisville Photographic Archives-Archives & Special Collections, University of Louisville, *https://digital.library.louisville.edu/concern/images/ulpa_1980_029_888a?locale=en*).

mineral springs resort, with "fifteen rooms wel [sic] furnished, with a fire place in each," within a half mile of the courthouse.[84]

Upon Green Clay's death in 1826, his son Brutus became owner, followed by at least three other owners, until William Chiles and his son John bought the resort about 1846. John sold his interest to his father, who then managed the resort with another son, Henry.[85]

William, a native of Virginia, constructed on the cabin sites a large hotel, which he rechristened as "Estill Springs."[86] The main hotel with its wrap-around verandahs conveyed a sense of grandeur: The second-floor dining room, measured at 3,000 square feet and adjacent to six bedrooms, was upstairs from three large first-floor parlors. Chiles also built a two-story addition with 28 more bedrooms and two other one-story row buildings, one building called "Ashland Row," after Chiles' friend Henry Clay's home. Two-room cottages were also erected by Chiles.[87] By 1850, due to his improvements, Chiles estimated the property value at $20,000 ($773,000 in 2022 dollars).[88]

Chiles also improved the grounds: planting shrubs, pruning the large oaks, and, of course, providing easy access to the springs.[89] The white sulphur Sweet Springs flowed near a gum tree that by 1874 had so encircled it that the tree was undergoing petrification from the mineral deposits.[90] Two red sulphur and a black sulphur springs were close by. A path led about a quarter of a mile away to a fifth spring, that of chalybeate water, in a shaded gorge.[91]

The waters were prized for various attributes. The Sweet Springs, as the name implies, was sought for its pleasant taste, considered "quite as good" by one antebellum visitor as that of Lewis County's fashionable Esculapia Springs at the Ohio border.[92] The chalybeate, containing iron, was used to treat pulmonary diseases.[93] A peculiarity of the springs was the rapid precipitation of the mineral content. Therefore, those seeking the water had to drink it soon after taking it from the springs.[94]

Sources consulted indicate that visitors perhaps emphasized Estill's recreational activities over its water's medicinal benefits. Dancing to a "superior band of music" occurred every evening, occasionally in the form of a grand masquerade or a fancy ball, at which young women vied for men's attention in elaborate dresses described as "rich pink silk with two deep flounces of white lace" and head dresses of rose buds and leaves.[95] The massive oaks provided shade for rounds of Boston, whist, and backgammon, played by gentlemen guests such as Henry Clay.[96] Bowling, long promenades, plays, and a well-used "proposition log," used even in the 1890s for love-struck guests to discuss matrimony, comprised other social activities.[97]

Like several other antebellum Southern Appalachian resorts, men gathered to discuss topics of the day such as philosophy, politics, and economics, perhaps while nursing a whisky from the "competent and obliging bar-keepers."[98] In addition to Henry Clay, fellow Kentucky Whigs who engaged in discourse at the springs included state and federal politicians such as John J. Crittenden, Robert Letcher, Daniel Breck, William Owsley, and John C. Breckinridge.[99] A mass Whig meeting at Estill Springs in 1852 touting party presidential candidate Winfield Scott prompted one newspaper to extol the "people in the mountains" for their participation in "one of the most enthusiastic and soul-stirring [Whig gatherings] ever held in that section of the country."[100]

Antebellum visitors came not only from the likes of central Kentucky and Lexington but also from the Deep South and states north of the Ohio River. In a typical season of 2,000 guests, visitors from Illinois mingled with those from Louisiana and Mississippi. With overflow crowds, male guests often slept in halls, in the ballroom, or even outside just as men did at the Virginia springs at the peak of their season.[101]

The popularity of Estill Springs may have resulted in part by good transportation. Travelers at the Louisville depot rode the Louisville & Frankfurt Railroad to Lexington for five hours, then took a stage to Richmond, where they then engaged a transfer stage to the resort via the Richmond and Irvine Turnpike.[102] The macadamization of the turnpike by 1858 ensured a road "in good order" that "can be traveled over in safety."[103]

Upon Chiles' death in 1856, Sidney M. Barnes bought the property and continued to operate the resort (although he unsuccessfully attempted to sell it) until the advent of the Civil War.[104] During the first year of the war, Barnes transformed the property into a Union training camp (Estill County supplied about 1,000 Union and 150 Confederate soldiers during the conflict) for the Eighth Kentucky Infantry Regiment, which later became the first Union unit to crest Lookout Mountain, Tennessee, during that battle in 1863.[105] Confederate Brigadier General John Hunt Morgan briefly occupied the resort that same year, allowing his men to ransack the property.[106]

The postbellum period saw several owners and periods of litigation. Following the end of the Civil War, Barnes moved to Somerset, having lost the resort when his brother, to whom he had entrusted his financial affairs during the war, suddenly died, leaving legal entanglements.[107] In 1888, a syndicate headed by W.H. Lilly bought the resort, then under a property dispute in court, for $9,200, two weeks after it had sold for $11,500.[108] The Estill Springs Company managed the property, largely with J.M. Thomas, a future Democratic state senator, at the helm for the next many years, apparently even in 1890 when a Louisville syndicate, Coleman-Bush Investment Company, purchased the resort for $30,000 and owned it for an unspecified period of time.[109]

The shifting ownership, however, did not affect patronage. Postbellum visitors included former Confederate Brigadier General and U.S. Senator Jonathan S. Williams, former Union Colonel J.H. Holloway, whiskey distiller and Frankfort politician E.H. Taylor, Jr., and former Arkansas Governor James Phillip Eagle.[110] Alice Lloyd, the educator from Boston who began a school in Knott County now bearing her name, accompanied her students to the resort for a weekend outing in 1894.[111] Estill Springs also hosted a variety of railroad excursions organized to benefit organizations such as the Y.M.C.A. and the Knights of Pythias.[112]

Postbellum guests enjoyed a range of activities over the decades. In the 1870s, croquet, ten pins, rowing on the river, and visits to the springs constituted some offerings.[113] By 1900, visitors could play tennis, enjoy a round of golf, pedal on a bicycle track, and relax after a sporting day in a steamy sulphur bath in a genuine porcelain-lined tub.[114]

The springs maintained their staying power through the late nineteenth century. Ads from this period boasted of the "Finest White Sulphur and Chalybeate Water in the World."[115] To assist the steady flow of visitors seeking the water in this era, management constructed a new path and a rustic summer house over the popular chalybeate spring.[116] Visitors taking the waters were complimented, as in antebellum times, of appearing "fat and stout" at their weight gains.[117] A minister in 1888 went to Estill to recuperate from an illness; ten years later, a Lexington newspaper man stayed at the resort to convalesce.[118] The baths also greatly benefited U.S. Senator Joseph Clay Stiles Blackburn, an Estill regular; however, his and Thomas's political allegiance to fellow Democrat William Jennings Bryan evidently failed to entice the Great Commoner to carry through on an invitation extended by Thomas to visit the springs.[119]

In 1911, a court ordered the property sold again to satisfy a complicated legal ownership quagmire that involved the Lilly and Thomas families.[120] The resort, subsequently under the ownership of Labe Riddell and family members, continued until fire consumed the main hotel building and most of the cottages in 1924. Today, a private home stands at the site of the hotel.[121]

The legacy of Estill Springs perhaps lies in attributes traditionally associated with the better known Virginia springs. The resort attracted guests from both the Deep South and neighboring states from the antebellum period through the early 1900s. Politicians and elite gathered there to discourse on issues of the day, to sip the waters, and to engage in a myriad of social activities. Estill Springs ranks as one of the more fashionable resorts in Southern Appalachia for the whole of the nineteenth century.

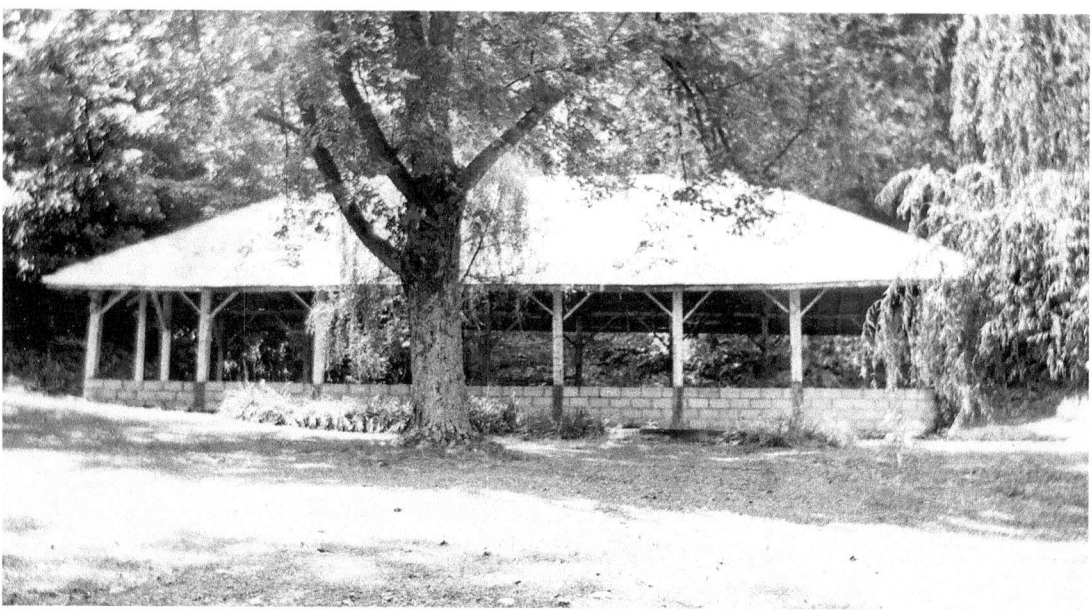

"Estill Springs at Irvine, Estill Co. KY [1920s]" (Warren Kellar Frederick, photographer. Warren Kellar Frederick Collection, ULPA 1980_029_868a, University of Louisville Photographic Archives-Archives & Special Collections, University of Louisville, *https://digital.library.louisville.edu/concern/images/ulpa_1980_029_868a?locale=en*).

Pulaski County: Rockcastle Springs and Sublimity Springs

Through towering sandstone and limestone bluffs of the Cumberland Plateau of southeastern Kentucky, the Rockcastle River meanders south from the edge of Jackson County, defining the border between Pulaski and Laurel counties on its way to flow into the Cumberland River. Part of the Rockcastle River through Pulaski and Laurel counties rushes through a rugged, boulder-filled gorge called the Narrows, an experienced whitewater paddler's paradise of Class IV rapids.[122] About a mile from the Narrows on the river's north bank in Pulaski County, the health resort of Sublimity Springs stood in the shadows of Bee Rock, an impressive 300 feet wide and 100 feet high.[123] Seven miles downstream from Sublimity, on the same side of the Rockcastle River gorge, lay the Rockcastle Springs hotel.[124]

The histories of the two resorts are intertwined for several reasons beyond their proximity to each other. According to one tradition, Sublimity existed for several years before the development of Rockcastle Springs, giving rise to a local belief that the phrase "Old Rockcastle" actually referenced Sublimity Springs. Other sources state that both names applied to a single resort. Some residents during the postbellum period maintained that the same proprietor, Josephus Campbell, operated or owned both resorts for long periods. This chapter will attempt to clarify some confusion. At the same time, however, the stories of the two resorts will, for now, remain incomplete due to the paucity of verifiable data to eliminate all ambiguity surrounding their chronologies.

Information on Rockcastle Springs in the antebellum period is sketchy in sources consulted. In 1835, Rockcastle Springs most likely first opened for guests.[125] Early ownership and appearance of the resort are unknown. In 1853, C.C. Carson (no information available) was proprietor; the next year, J. Campbell (most likely Josephus Campbell) replaced Carson as proprietor.[126] No sources consulted provide information if these gentlemen owned the resort or leased it from another party (most likely, they were lessees). In 1860 and in early 1861, Pulaski County's Whittington Lear apparently owned Rockcastle Springs; his proprietor was F.C. McLean of Fayette County.[127]

Information is more available, however, for Sublimity Springs in the antebellum period. In February 1853, Dr. C.C. (Christopher Columbus) Graham bought 1,500 acres in the vicinity of Sublimity Springs and began purchasing additional tracts.[128] Graham, a wealthy physician, may have been anticipating the sale of his fashionable Graham Springs health resort at Harrodsburg, Kentucky, located about 80 miles to the northwest of the Rockcastle and Sublimity springs area.[129] In fact, three months later, in May 1853, he sold his wildly popular resort known as the "Saratoga of the West" to the U.S. government for $100,000 (almost $4 million in 2022 dollars) for use as an asylum for elderly and invalid soldiers.[130]

A year later found Graham developing the area at Bee Rock, which tradition says he named "Sublimity Springs" for its awe-inspiring wilderness of monumental cliffsides pierced by the cascading river.[131] That year, for example, he successfully petitioned the state to incorporate a company to improve the navigation of the Rockcastle River.[132] He also constructed a sawmill and grist mill at Bee Rock, followed by his erection of a hotel near the mineral spring and a three-room, batten structure that served both as a kitchen and as slave quarters.[133]

The hotel was not a crude rustic lodge hunkered under a cliff but a two-story structure with a grand foyer dividing the building into two sections, each with five guest rooms on both floors and a dining room on the first level. The requisite verandah fronted the Rockcastle River.[134] Union troops in 1862 described the hotel as "large and commodious" and as "a large building covering the two sides of a square."[135]

Sublimity Springs proprietors under Graham included J. (Josephus) Campbell from at least 1858 through 1860 and Montrose Graham, C.C. Graham's son and a member of Campbell's household in 1860.[136] Both served in 1860 as state-appointed judges for the newly incorporated town of Sublimity's first election of trustees, the town beginning "10 poles above the ferry."[137] Campbell left his proprietorship by 1870 to work as a lawyer in Pulaski County's Somerset.[138]

Other information about Campbell is debatable. A 1954 newspaper article speculates that "Ceph" Campbell (Josephus was also known as "Seaf") may have operated Sublimity Springs before going to Rockcastle.[139] Josephus's obituary in 1885 states that "for the past thirty years [he was] an important fixture at Rock Castle Springs and owner of Sublimity in its palmy days."[140] Discounting the incorrect ownership statement in the 1885 obituary and from reviewing fragmentary information on Campbell, it seems likely that he served as proprietor at Rockcastle Springs around 1854 and at Sublimity, under Graham, from at least 1858 through 1860 and then frequented Rockcastle Springs once he had established himself as an attorney in Somerset.

Montrose Graham was considered eccentric, due in part to an unconventional lifestyle that included walking great distances and shunning society for the solitude of nature.[141] Perhaps then his father wisely hired him as a proprietor of a resort in the wilderness of the river gorge. At some point in the postbellum era, he moved to the vicinity of Rockcastle Springs, where he led hunting trips and served as a boatman and guide to guests.[142]

Little is known about visitors to either Rockcastle Springs or to Sublimity Springs during the antebellum period. In view of Graham's 25 years of ownership of the exclusive Graham Springs, perhaps his new resort attracted guests because of his "brand recognition" or because of their relationships formed at Harrodsburg with Graham, a "genial host" providing "gracious hospitality," according to Coleman.[143] A Union soldier from Ohio wrote that the Sublimity Springs hotel was "used in the summer time as the quarters for the fashionable frequenters," implying that its clientele did not consist solely of the sickly.[144] Clark comments that both resorts "played an active role in Kentucky society" in the antebellum period, attracting local elites and visitors from the lower South for the waters and as refuge from malaria and yellow fever.[145]

As might be expected, transportation to the two resorts in the antebellum period was somewhat difficult compared to such mineral spring resorts as Nicholas County's Blue Lick Springs located in the gently rolling hills of Kentucky's Bluegrass Region physiographic province. Graham in the late 1850s spearheaded a move to obtain a state-funded road to Sublimity Springs from both Pulaski and Laurel counties.[146] No bridge was apparently included in the appropriation; travelers from the Laurel County side, more accessible than from the Pulaski County side, crossed the river by ferry. To reach the ferry, guests might travel via stage from Crab Orchard to London in Laurel County, where they transferred coaches to then journey along a mountain ridge road before making a cautious descent to the Rockcastle River.[147]

Although the remote location of the resorts may suggest that they served as places of refugee for families and men who did not want to serve in the military during the Civil War, they stood in the path of troop movements. Consequently, Rockcastle Springs closed and did not reopen until the end of the war.[148] Sublimity Springs may have received a few guests in summer 1861; a Union soldier recorded in February 1862 that the "gentleman [unspecified] who keeps the hotel at present" was "driven from London [where he was staying] by the rebels and robbed of almost everything he owned."[149]

The Union soldier was part of the 16th Ohio Regiment on the move from the January 1862 Battle of Mill Springs to Cumberland Gap with the intent to flush out Confederate troops there. Heavy rains forced the troops to stay at Sublimity Springs two days, enough time to record their observations of the "nearly deserted" Sublimity Springs.[150] The ferry, a "rickety old boat," conveyed their cannons and gunnery across the river to the Laurel County road, "so steep and muddy that it took from 12 to 16 horses to draw a cannon up the hill."[151] Despite the downpour, one soldier admired the "tall pines shooting straight up one hundred and twenty-five feet" and the "huge rocks forty feet above the ground covered with beautiful moss."[152] Another wrote that the locale was a "magnificent place—a valley hemmed in with mountains you can scarcely describe."[153]

The inhabitants they saw on their march through the region appear to have been both objects of pity and curiosity. Two Union soldiers commented on the residents' poverty: "[S]oil is as poor as desolation, and the people are poorer if possible. They look as though they could hardly keep soul and body together."[154] They also remarked on the locals' insularity and lack of education: "In their houses you can see no books or papers. None of them ever saw a cannon or a railroad."[155] Whether or not the local residents interacted with the resort proprietors or guests apart from a Sunday School Graham established is not known.[156]

After the end of the Civil War, both resorts reopened. More information for Rockcastle Springs can be found for its postbellum history, in part because F.J. Campbell, the Rockcastle Springs proprietor for many years, also edited the Stanford newspaper that conveniently published resort news. Less is known about Sublimity Springs in this era.

Sublimity Springs saw at least two ownership changes following the Civil War. C.C. Graham began to sell his acreage along the Rockcastle River as early as February 1865 while retaining as Sublimity Springs coproprietors his son Montrose and C.C. Jackson, son of a local judge.[157] Sometime before 1875, Jackson bought the resort from Graham (or from another intermediate party) and then resold it to his brother-in-law Christopher Pitman.[158] Pitman in 1874 added new furniture and 20 "well ventilated" rooms, presumably for clientele to experience the cool mountain breezes.[159]

The status of Rockcastle Springs for the five years after the Civil War is not recorded. In 1870, Burnside, Anderson & Co., a local business engaged in livestock sales and perhaps in other commerce, owned Rockcastle Springs.[160] The company publicized the health resort as both "Rockcastle Springs" and "Old Rockcastle Springs," the latter perhaps a throwback to its antebellum days but certainly not a pseudonym for Sublimity Springs as some sources content.[161] Burnside and Anderson apparently experienced such good business that by the 1871 season they had constructed "new and commodious buildings" and "thoroughly repaired the old."[162] As part of the dissolution of their partnership, they sold the resort in 1874 to T.C. Everett of Montana Territory, formerly of Louisville.[163] Until the early 1880s when Rockcastle Springs came under the control of the Rockcastle Springs Company, little information can be located on the resort. Rockcastle Springs Company's partners included J.S. Hughes and F.J. (Francis Josephus) Campbell, perhaps a nephew of the J. (Josephus) Campbell who most likely served as proprietor briefly at both Sublimity Springs and Rockcastle Springs in the antebellum period.[164]

F.J. Campbell continued to improve the property and to enhance recreational offerings. The resort, fronting the river, consisted of either two or three two-story buildings with verandahs across the front.[165] A somewhat stylized illustration for an 1885 ad shows one building with a central tower and two other buildings with turrets at their four corners; a photograph, however, more realistically depicts two two-story structures with verandahs facing each other on each level.[166] Outdoor recreational activities expanded greatly from the simple hunting and fishing advertised in 1854 to include walks along mountain paths, strenuous hikes to the Narrows, river bathing, barge or boat excursions, and rowing in the 1870s and later.[167] Indoor activities in the postbellum era included fancy dress balls, germans, cornet band performances, and billiards.[168] The director of Stanford's Gold and Silver Band, which performed regularly at the resort, recorded a list of typical daily activities: guests awakening to brass band music at 7:00 a.m.; rowing or rambling after breakfast; listening to music at a grotto at 9:30 a.m.; lunch; napping; bathing or swimming at 4:00 p.m.; a river concert at 5:00 p.m.; and dancing at 8:30 p.m.[169]

Although the band director omitted from his list the ritual of taking the waters, the springs' health benefits and mountain gorge location attracted the sickly, who consulted the Rockcastle Springs resident physician. The high sodium sulfate, calcium carbonate, and iron carbonate of the springs purportedly treated such ills as chronic dyspepsia, nervous prostration, uterine affections and "all depraved conditions of the blood."[170] In addition, the "pure air and equable temperature, as well as the isolation from the thoroughfares of travel," allegedly relieved catarrh, asthma, and hay fever, and provided a safe retreat from summer epidemics and the "ills of hot weather."[171]

The resort's "isolation from the thoroughfares of travel" in the Rockcastle River gorge continued in the postbellum period as no railroad stopped nearby. By 1882, visitors could travel by railroad from Louisville to London and then take a coach for the 16 miles to Rockcastle Springs.[172] One traveler in 1888 wrote that the mountain ridge road was sufficiently improved to be considered as "good as the best pike" and that the stage driver knew how to handle his passengers with humor as he drove his coach down the same steep road that the Union troops had grumbled about climbing up with their cannon.[173]

Rockcastle Springs' isolation did not, in fact, deter postbellum visitors, whose ranks swelled the resort grounds anywhere from 100 to 200 in July.[174] They largely hailed from central and eastern Kentucky, Cincinnati, Indiana, and to a lesser extent from points farther south.[175] Notables included former Confederate General George B. Crittenden; E.T. Sturgeon, captain of the famous racing steamboat *Eclipse*; Soule Smith; and Kentucky Governor William Bradley's family.[176] A commentator wrote that the refined guests were from "some of the most wealthy and distinguished families of the State."[177] Exclusiveness, however, apparently was absent; the same observer described Rockcastle Springs as a "pleasant, cultivated family" while another guest described the clientele as a "whole happy family."[178]

The resort saw ownership change hands at least three times from the turn of the century until its closing a decade later. In 1897, F.J. Campbell became the sole proprietor of the resort, having been a partner in the Rockcastle Springs Company for 18 years.[179] Within two years, Campbell sold the resort to Thomas Morgan and H. Hummell and moved to Somerset where he bought and served as editor of the *Somerset Journal*.[180] In 1900, the resort's principal portion burned down; Danville attorney and real estate agent L.F. Hubble bought the property the following year.[181] It is unclear if Hubble rebuilt any of the damaged part of the hotel complex, but newspapers continued to report on activities at Rockcastle Springs through 1913, including a lady's stay of six weeks in that year.[182] No further information is available on the resort although Hubble continued to own the property until his death in 1922.[183]

The demise of Sublimity Springs resulted not from a hotel fire but from damage caused by the Rockcastle River. Either ice floes in the winter of 1877–1878 or flooding sometime before September 1882 destroyed the mills and a section of the hotel.[184] Apparently the structures were not rebuilt. In 1912, Hubble as real estate agent for perhaps the Pitman family sold the "old Sublimity Springs" property, so-called by at least two newspapers.[185]

President Franklin D. Roosevelt's administration purchased the land encompassing both resort properties as part of the Cumberland National Forest (now the Daniel Boone National Forest).[186] In 1936, the Civilian Conservation Corps built a suspension bridge across the Rockcastle River where the mill stood at Bee Rock. Today, that area is the Bee Rock Campground.[187] As for Rockcastle Springs, only a few foundation stones may remain scattered near the river.[188]

North Carolina

Introduction

Western North Carolina has been known as the "Land of the Sky" for almost 150 years, ever since the publication of Frances Tiernan's 1875 serialized novel of the same name.[1] Names of communities such as Little Switzerland, Loafers Glory, Swiss, Spruce Pine, Balsam Grove, Sapphire, and Micaville also provide clues as to the natural beauty, the flora, and minerals associated with the mountainous region. Just as the Land of the Sky has welcomed tourists and sightseers since the antebellum period, its mineral springs and near pollen-free high elevations also attracted those in search of improved health.

No doubt the antebellum western North Carolina resorts most recognizable today are Madison County's Warm Springs, now known as Hot Springs, and Buncombe County's Sulphur Springs, in the vicinity of the modern west Asheville area of Malvern Hills. Both thrived as fashionable resorts after the completion of the Buncombe Turnpike from Greeneville, Tennessee, through Asheville, to Greenville, South Carolina, in 1827.[2]

Because much has been written about Warm Springs and Sulphur Springs, especially in regard to their prominence in the development of Asheville regional tourism, a history of each will not be provided.[3] This chapter instead will focus on seven less well documented resorts: Haywood White Sulphur Springs, the Eagles Nest, Healing Springs, Shatley Springs, Piedmont Springs, Connelly Springs, and Glen Alpine Springs. For many of these resorts, their health attributes attracted patrons as much as or more than their recreational or sightseeing activities, in which guests could readily indulge during stays at other area hotels or resorts.

By contrast, several western North Carolina destinations pivoted in the antebellum period from providing a recuperative ambiance to attracting tourists or those in search of social activities. As early as 1839, for example, Warm Springs' clientele had shifted from health-seeking to pleasure-seeking: the British traveler James Silk Buckingham wrote that only half of the roughly 50 guests were invalids during his stay that year at Warm Springs.[4] Sulphur Springs in 1840 publicized its "thoroughly refitted" stables and "pleasure grounds."[5] Furthermore, Richard D. Starnes observes that Asheville in 1850 attracted about 500 health seekers but that the majority of visitors constituted sightseers or travelers from their second residences in the mountains.[6] Burke County's Piedmont Springs, on the other hand, one of the health

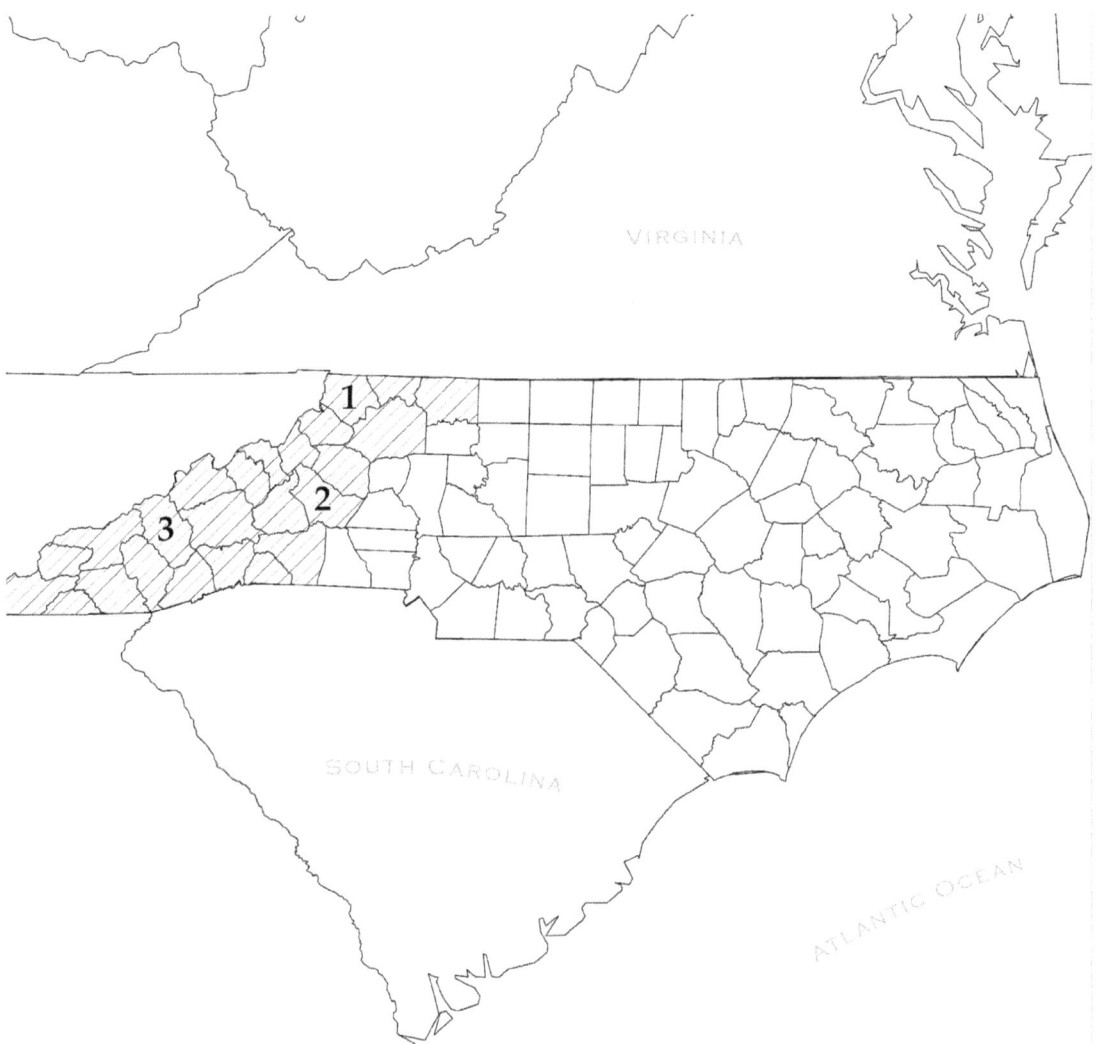

North Carolina counties with featured health resorts: (1) Ashe County, Healing (Thompson's) Springs and Shatley Springs; (2) Burke County, Piedmont Springs, Glen Alpine Springs and Connelly Springs; (3) Haywood County, Haywood White Sulphur Springs and Eagles Nest (Sources: Esri, NOAA, USGS. Cartographer: Sayona Turner, East Tennessee State University).

resorts researched for this chapter, drew "many broken-down and almost wasted invalids" in addition to the slave-owning "gentry of the lower Yadkin and Catawba ... with a full retinue of servants."[7]

In the postbellum era, many health resorts in North Carolina, including several researched for this chapter, benefited from the railroad boom, especially the continued construction of the Western North Carolina Railroad after the Civil War (an 84-mile stretch had been completed from Salisbury to within four miles of Morganton in 1858).[8] Rail not only carried livestock, tobacco, lumber, textiles, and brick but also tourists, seekers of health, and permanent residents.[9] In Asheville alone, population increased by 900 percent and property values quadrupled in the two decades after the railroad came through in 1880.[10] The most famous visitor to put down roots was George W. Vanderbilt, who built his prominent residence Biltmore in the late 1800s after his second trip to Asheville.[11] In the Waynesville area, Haywood White Sulphur Springs and the Eagles Nest hay fever resort gained visitors from the rail expansion through Waynesville in 1882.[12] Extension of the Murphy branch of the railroad through Jackson County's Balsam Gap in 1883, the highest railroad stop east of the Rockies and seven miles west of Waynesville, encouraged the construction of the Balsam Inn, originally a "rough and uncouth" one-story structure housing invalids to gain strength from the balsam-scented air and mineral springs and for sightseers from Waynesville and Asheville.[13] Farther to the east, Burke County's Connelly Springs and Glen Alpine Springs attracted visitors due to these resorts' accessibility to the Western North Carolina Railroad, including the elite who traveled by private car.

Other railroad lines in the region inspired visions for health resorts. The East Tennessee and Western North Carolina Railroad, which carried magnetite iron ore from General John T. Wilder's forge in Cranberry, North Carolina, to Johnson City, Tennessee, passed through Avery County's Elk Park, a modest timber and tanbark hub for the railroad. Carter County, Tennessee, physician Abraham Jobe, who lived in Elk Park in the 1880s, speculated on development possibilities: "Elk Park is also becoming a great summer resort, and with a little capital invested, could be made one of the most popular watering places in the South. The mineral water on the Taylor place is unsurpassed."[14] About 100 miles to the south, the passage of the Asheville and Spartanburg Railroad through Henderson County helped lay the groundwork for the creation of the Skyland Springs resort, which boasted of its 48 mineral springs and its main hotel's 75-yard distance from the passenger station.[15]

In contrast, health resorts in northwestern North Carolina at the Virginia border were less accessible by rail than were resorts elsewhere in western North Carolina. Virginia railroads provided access to Ashe County's Thompson's Bromine-Arsenic Springs and Surry County's Mount Airy White Sulphur Springs but required coach or wagon rides of over 20 miles from the Virginia depot communities of Glade Springs and Stuart respectively in the 1870s–1880s.[16] In addition, Mount Airy White Sulphur Springs advised guests coming from the south to allow 12 hours for the journey from the Winston, North Carolina, depot stop 41 miles away.[17] These relatively isolated resorts, especially Thompson's, tended to bring in visitors more intent on imbibing the water than in engaging in social activities, easily found in resorts closer to rail depots in the days before automobiles and good roads.[18]

In contrast to an Asheville visitor's comment in the 1870s that the town was a "mecca for consumptives," many western North Carolina health resorts, as well as Asheville, Waynesville, and Highlands hotels denied consumptives entry by the late nineteenth century to concentrate on the lucrative tourist trade.[19] Starnes points out that resort and hotel owners sought to convey the image that their properties were not catering to the sickly but were providing leisure activities for travelers.[20] As one Ashevillean noted: "The tourist business paid better than the tuberculosis patients did."[21] Although a few tubercular patients may have sought the Balsam Gap air because of a belief that both the area's balsam fragrance and its higher elevation than Waynesville's conferred therapeutic benefit, the dilapidated Balsam Inn in 1906, even before the erection of its new hotel in 1908, barred consumptives.[22] Haywood County's Eagles Nest, the Haywood White Sulphur Springs, and Burke County's Connelly Springs also advertised "no consumptives." Indeed, after the federal government ended its lease of Haywood White Sulphur Springs as a sanitarium for tubercular soldiers in 1918, the resort quickly tried to recapture the public's interest by publicizing its "thoroughly renovated and remodeled" hotel and "[e]very variety amusement: golf, tennis, fishing, swimming, riding, orchestra, and dancing."[23]

The seven health retreats explored in this chapter lie in three counties widely dispersed across western North Carolina: Ashe County at the Tennessee and Virginia border; Burke County about 70 miles south of Ashe on the cusp of Southern Appalachia and the Piedmont; and lofty Haywood County about 85 miles to the southeast of Burke, touching the Qualla Boundary and the Great Smoky Mountains National Park. Despite the different county geographies, two themes, as mentioned in this book's introduction, the role of enslaved and free Blacks at health resorts and the local (as opposed to northern) ownership of health resorts, connect these resorts in addition to their shared health objective.

First, one or more of the researched health resorts in each of the three counties revealed that its proprietors either held enslaved Black persons or rented them from other slaveholders. Although they lived in the Blue Ridge Mountain region, the proprietors and the lessees did not need to travel to the Lowcountry to gain easy access to slaves. Drovers or slave traders marched slaves in coffles, for example, through Catawba County, adjacent to Burke County; whites also could buy slaves advertised for sale in the Morganton environs.[24] Burke County's Piedmont Springs antebellum owner held a few enslaved persons and may have hired slaves from a Morganton physician / hotel owner to work at Piedmont Springs. Ashe County's Healing Springs (Thompson's Bromine-Arsenic Springs) was started in the late 1880s by a Washington County, Virginia, hotel keeper who owned eight slaves in 1860.[25] Both the owners of Burke County's Glen Alpine Springs and Haywood County's Haywood White Sulphur Springs (both hotels opened in 1878) came from or married into families comprising two of the largest slave-holding clans in western North Carolina, the Loves and the Waltons.

Following the Civil War, Blacks living near the resorts found employment at them in subservient roles. Blacks served as waiters at the Haywood White Sulphur Springs and, when not waiting tables, also performed as minstrels.[26] A young Black man employed at the Eagles Nest as a wood hauler died when a horse crushed him.[27]

Second, six of the seven resorts described in this chapter were under southern ownership in their later years. In line with conventional thought of postbellum northern investment domination in the region, C. Brenden Martin highlights Warm Springs as one of the few remaining southern-held Blue Ridge Mountain resorts when the Western North Carolina Railroad came through in 1881 but notes that northerners eventually bought it.[28] Four of the seven health resorts in this chapter, however, stayed exclusively in southern hands. Of the three remaining health resorts, Glen Alpine eventually was bought by a northern Christian denomination (not a business concern); Piedmont Springs and Shatley Springs each reverted to regional ownership after failed northern capitalist ventures.[29]

The health resorts described in this chapter illuminate health and social activities in western North Carolina, from the antebellum Piedmont Springs to today's Shatley Springs. They stand apart from the hostelries that sought to appeal to strictly tourists or sightseers in the "Land of the Sky."

Ashe County: Healing Springs and Shatley Springs

Healing Springs

In 1998, President Bill Clinton and Vice President Al Gore stood along the banks of the New River in rugged Ashe County, North Carolina, greeted by a crowd of several thousand who watched them dedicate the body of water as an American Heritage River.[30] The New River, ironically one of the world's oldest rivers despite the name, begins as the North Fork New River and the South Fork New River from springs in Watauga County, Ashe County's neighbor to its southwest. The forks converge to form part of Ashe's northeastern boundary with the northwestern tip of Alleghany County, North Carolina. The New River then flows into neighboring Grayson County, Virginia, and eventually joins with the Gauley River in West Virginia to form the Kanawha River.[31] Along the South Fork, near the community of Crumpler lay the postbellum mineral resort of Thompson's Bromine-Arsenic Springs, known in modern times as Healing Springs, at an elevation of about 2,600 feet. Less than four miles south of Healing Springs and about 11 miles north of the 4,683-foot-tall Mount Jefferson, stands Shatley Springs, renowned for its country family-style restaurant as well as for its radium spring.

In July 1885, a young boy, Willie Barker, discovered a bromine-arsenic spring when searching for water for his father working in a nearby field. Not only did Eli Barker, the father, proclaim that it was the best water he had ever drunk, but both he and Willie noticed that poison oak sores on their hands almost completely healed in the next few days after splashing the water on them. As word spread, Willie recounted that "everybody got to using the water and it has cured a power of folks.... Sometimes 300 come here in one day."[32]

One of the invalids who camped by the water was Saltville, Virginia, native Hiram V. Thompson. Since at least 1860, Thompson had operated a boarding house and seasonal hotel near the Virginia and Tennessee Railroad in Glade Springs, Virginia, about fifty-five miles northwest of Crumpler.[33] By September 1885, Thompson had purchased 28 acres that included the springs for about $5,000 ($157,000 in 2022 dollars).[34] In the three months between the springs' discovery and Thompson's acquisition, the water had purportedly cured ulcers, palsy, tetter (pustular patches), indigestion, and kidney disease among other ailments.[35]

Shortly after his acquisition, Thompson initiated a campaign to raise $25,000 to organize a stock company to transform his "Bethesda Healing Springs" into a health resort comparable to Arkansas's Eureka Springs in the Ozarks, which at the time was attracting thousands.³⁶ As a savvy marketing move the following summer, he fended off a rival with a similar name, Bethesda Healing Water, by changing the name of his springs to "Thompson['s] Bromine and Arsenic Springs," also subsequently referred to in the press as the Bromine Arsenic Healing Spring, Thompson Springs, All-Healing Springs, and Healing Springs.³⁷

In 1887, the stock company decided to lure guests (and increase profits) by erecting a two-story frame hotel, with a 120-foot-long front verandah, to accommodate seventy-five visitors.³⁸ An early visitor described the lodging house as having a "rough, temporary appearance but … thoroughly comfortable now and clean."³⁹ The food he found "unexceptional" but surprising that "in such remote a place a bill of fare can be presented and so delightfully prepared."⁴⁰ He excused the rather unremarkable hostelry by his admission that "shipping the water is the main business of this place."⁴¹

Shipping the water indeed constituted the focus of the health resort, which never advertised any recreational activities such as croquet or ten pins. The shipping business model expanded after March 1887, when Thompson sold the spring for $4,000 to a Saltville, Virginia, four-person venture firm, led by industrialist George W. Palmer, who had begun a bottling operation next to the spring.⁴²

The spring lay in what one 1887 visitor described as a "ravine, scarcely wide enough to accommodate the public road and creek, hotel and other buildings."⁴³ Another writer fifty-two years later related that the spring "was situated in more or less a canyon," with a copper vein running on one side and a magnetite vein on the other.⁴⁴ In the narrow ravine, the bottling enterprise carefully installed a marble lining around the spring basin and sheltered the water with a pavilion.⁴⁵ The company then diverted the spring's flow, calculated at about sixty gallons per hour, into a pipeline capped by a funnel that filled six glass half-gallon bottles simultaneously, keeping workers busy exchanging out the full jugs for empty containers.⁴⁶ Employees loaded the full bottles onto wagons for transport about thirty-five miles northwest to the East Tennessee, Virginia & Georgia Railway depot at Seven Mile Ford, Virginia, between Glade Springs and Marion, Virginia, or a few miles farther to the Marion train depot.⁴⁷ As an illustration of the growing popularity of the water, in February 1887, seven wagons in one day carried water from the bottling house to the railroad depot; by April, thirteen four-horse wagons were required to meet demand.⁴⁸ By 1889, about fifty wagons daily hauled the water, an average that was sustained between 1888 and 1898.⁴⁹

Drugstores and distributors mainly in the South but also in Canada and Europe ordered or inquired about the water during the resort's early days. A Richmond dealer advertised that two of the city's drug firms had purchased $2,000 worth ($4.65 for a dozen half gallons or 40 cents per bottle) of the "recognized panacea for so many of the ills of suffering humanity."⁵⁰ An Atlanta broker acknowledged the impatience of its customers in Columbus, Georgia, and Kansas and promised to ship 500 cases per week and to "put on a night force" if "the demand continues to increase rapidly."⁵¹ An unidentified European firm purportedly ordered 9,000 cases.⁵²

Perhaps the publications that most influenced sales were two newspaper articles, the fall 1887 *New York World's* "Another Pool of Siloam" and the *New York Sun's* January 1888 provocative "Eager for Its Healing Waters: North Carolina Mountaineers

Wrought Up Over a Mineral Spring." The articles, propagating Southern Appalachian stereotypes, were widely reprinted in other newspapers and fascinated readers as far south as Florida in their embellished tales of Thompson the invalid brandishing his rifle at mountaineers fortified with moonshine attempting to use his spring. The *New York World* correspondent depicted locals who traveled to the "pizen" (poison) spring as "fat old women, bandy-legged men and artless mountain maidens dangling their shanks in the healing water."[53] The *New York Sun* reporter described his interchange with an "old man" weighed down with "[p]oultry, ginseng, and two pigs" and carting a barrel that the reporter mistook for moonshine. The mountaineer explained that the barrel contained a valuable commodity, water that he had hauled more than forty miles from the spring to sell: "I b'lieves the furder I gits from ole Thompson's pison spring the wusser they is arter it."[54] Both articles testified to the rampant popularity of the water—more than 6,000 "vessels" (half gallons) filled in a month—and to its phenomenal powers, such as "draw[ing] out by the roots" a cancerous tumor.[55]

Water sales consequently increased throughout the South and catapulted the springs into the ranks of esteemed mineral waters. Savannah druggists gave Thompson's water top billing in ads, above the waters of Virginia's Buffalo Lithia and Carlsbad Sprudel.[56] Charlotte dealers promoted it along with Apollinaris, South Carolina's Glenn Springs, Congress, and Hunyadi Janos waters for their discriminating clientele.[57] Caught up in the excitement (and for its own potential profit as a railway in southwest Virginia), the Norfolk and Western Railroad touted the water's "many cures" and "[T]housands of testimonials and letters from sufferers," but the railroad cautioned that the "demand by drug stores and dealers and by individuals is greater than the supply."[58] So widespread was public interest in the therapeutic power of the water that an Atlanta newspaper relayed the rumor that the U.S. Congress might purchase the spring for the "purpose of offering a free panacea to the thousands of invalids in this broad land of ours."[59]

Because of the Thompson water's fame, area entrepreneurs capitalized on bottling the water from other bromine-arsenic springs in Ashe County. R.E.L. (Robert E. Lee) Plummer, a noted Ashe County educator, sold the aptly named "Plummer Bromine Arsenic Water" over a wide area, including the Richmond market, from a spring about a half mile away from Thompson's spring.[60] Bristol, Tennessee, tobacco capitalist, A.D. (Abram) Reynolds, older brother to R.J. Reynolds, established a bottling operation near Lansing, about ten miles west of Crumpler.[61] Headquartered in Bristol, Reynold's enterprise marketed "Ashley's Bromine and Arsenic Water," a "Boon to Women" for their complexions and also a remedy for "Rheumatism, Syphilis, Erysipelas [a dermal infection], Old Sores [and] Chronic Sore Eyes."[62] Like Plummer's and Thompson's, Ashley's spring water was heavily sold in cities such as Roanoke or Richmond, easily reached by rail.[63] Its popularity was such that Reynolds contemplated, but never followed through, building a pipeline from the springs to Bristol, fifty miles away, to keep up with demand.[64]

Palmer, who had bought Thompson's share of the Thompson Bromine-Arsenic Springs enterprise in May 1888 for $25,000, threw down the gauntlet at his increased competition. Thompson's challenged the medical profession to "report any of the following cases they fail to cure with [Thompson's] wonderful water"; the published list of over two dozen illnesses included malaria, nausea, and "exhausted vitality."[65] Thompson's further warned the public "against newly-sprung (but OLD Springs) Bromine-Arsenic Waters, claiming same analysis or similar!"[66] The company's distribution network of druggists ran notices of gratitude to the "numerous other Bromine Arsenic Springs ... [that] delight in making comparisons with the Thompson Spring. We thank them for their help in making the ORIGINAL and DESERVEDLY-POPULAR water still better known [capitals original]."[67]

Visitors who chose to visit the springs rather than ordering bottled water were largely regional. A Raleigh visitor commented in 1889 that the springs were "difficult to reach but we found people there from Texas."[68] Prominent Johnson City, Tennessee, businessman H.H. Stratton returned from the springs with several bottles and gave one to the local newspaper editor, perhaps as a gift or to curry publicity for the water.[69] Ashe County as a whole mainly connected with markets via the turnpike built in 1887 that detoured by Thompson's to head north to the railroad near Marion, Virginia. Most visitors, therefore, especially the very ill, probably traveled from Marion as opposed to traversing more exhausting terrain and rough paths from, for example, neighboring Johnson County, Tennessee. Ashe County, in fact, and neighboring Watauga and Alleghany counties, became known as the state's "Lost Provinces" because they developed trading routes mainly with Virginia and secondarily with other regions in North Carolina.[70]

The resort changed ownership many times after the early 1900s. In 1910, Palmer's daughter, Helen Palmer Wiley, sold the property to an Abingdon syndicate for $10,000.[71] The syndicate expanded the hotel to one hundred rooms and built several cottages to replace or to supplement those built in 1889 out of bottle crate planks.[72] Lou Dora Plummer Porter of Wyoming, the sister of R.E.L. Plummer, purchased the resort in 1938 and made improvements.[73] In the late 1940s, Dr. and Mrs. Robert L. Dickson acquired the property and operated the hotel until it burned down in 1962.[74] Today, the property is on the National Register of Historic Places, and the renovated cottages known as "The Cabins at Healing Springs" are available for rental.[75]

Shatley Springs

Shatley Springs originated similarly to Healing Springs: the discovery of a spring that cured a dermatological affliction and then attracted hundreds to its waters. In summer 1890, while walking through his farm property, Martin Shatley paused to wash his face and hands from a spring at the source of Long Shoals Creek, a small tributary of the North Fork of the New River. Within a few hours, the water had begun to heal the painful sores and pustules that had routinely afflicted him to the point that he was not able to open his eyes for days at a time.[76]

Word spread of Shatley's cure. Much like Thompson's Springs in its early years, visitors camped around the springs in the absence of a hotel.[77] Sometime before 1923, for reasons unclear, Shatley sold his Ashe County property, retaining title to the springs and moved to a peach farm a few miles outside of North Wilkesboro, about thirty-five miles southeast of Shatley Springs.[78]

Several attempts were made to develop the property after Shatley sold it. In

1923, Charlotte businessman W.C. Phillips took the tract under option to "build a fine resort hotel and perhaps a new resort town" to take advantage of improvements in the Ashe County roads system.[79] Phillips did not succeed, and in 1925, Shatley joined with North Wilkesboro businessman E.E. Eller and a few others to form the Shatley Springs Hotel Company with a capital investment of $100,000.[80] By February 1926, engineering surveys that divided the acreage into lots had finished but developer interest fell short.[81]

In June 1926, however, what might have been considered a routine chemical analysis of the water sparked intense business interest in the spring, which almost caused the property to be developed into a motion picture backlot. Dr. Henry Froehling, of the Richmond engineering firm of Froehling and Robertson, determined that the water contained not only many of the trace minerals analyzed in Healing Springs water but also radium, a "very valuable" quality.[82] At the time, some considered radium to be a cure-all for ailments. In an age when deleterious effects of radioactivity were little understood, patients might sip a Revigator (radium dissolved in water), wash with Radisavon Radium Soap, or bathe in Radio-Sulpho Brew to allegedly cure cancer.[83] Not all products marketed as "radium" contained the element: for example, analysis of Radio-Sulpho Brew by the Colorado State Board of Health revealed that it consisted of mainly Epsom salts. The marketing of "radium" or "radioactive" claims was sure to draw a large customer base.[84]

The spring's most spectacular curative trait, however, according to Froehling, was its extremely low level of sediment, only forty-one parts of solids per million parts of water.[85] The purity of the Shatley water, in Froehling's judgment, rather than its mineral content, provided its therapeutic value: The water was able to absorb all foreign substances.[86] In actuality, although labs or medical environments may use pure water or distilled water as a solvent in various formulations, the medical profession does not typically use distilled water alone to treat dermal conditions.

As a result of Froehling's analytical conclusions, the Radium Springs Distributing Company was organized about 1927 to sell the water, now rechristened as "Shatley Radium Springs" or simply "Radium Springs."[87] Billed as the "Purest Water in America!" with the tagline "Radium is the most wonderful curative agent known to science," the spring water was advertised to treat cancer, rheumatism, a variety of dermal conditions, and stomach diseases such as gastric ulcers and "Gastric Catarrh" (chronic gastritis).[88]

Concurrently, the Radium Springs Corporation of America organized with a two million-dollar capitalization to develop 1,200 acres, including the spring tract, into a resort with a fifty-room sanitorium, clubhouse, auditorium, bath houses, a golf course, tennis courts, and a movie studio.[89] Among officers and backers were former New York Supreme Court Chief Justice Charles J. Guy, New York City black diamond merchant Arthur S. Bandler, and North Carolinians W.A. McNeill (the springs proprietor), E.E. Eller, and Thomas Dixon, Jr., best known for his controversial book *The Clansman* that D.W. Griffith adapted into his 1915 blockbuster *The Birth of a Nation*. The Radium Springs Corporation contracted with the Southern Producing Corporation to produce films at the resort, the first one to be based on Dixon's book *Facing South*.[90]

By August 1927, for unknown reasons, the grand vision of the Radium Springs Corporation ended in a trustee's sale.[91] The property ownership for the next few years is unclear. By 1930, W.A. (Alonzo) McNeill was president of the Shatley Springs Company that distributed Shatley's Spring Water (no mention of radium). Other officers were S.C. Harper, J.C. Grimes, and J.B. Williams. The company in late spring of that year erected eleven new cottages and remodeled others, expanded the tearoom's eating capacity to forty people, and walled the spring with marble slabs.[92]

Over the next three decades, J.B. "Bid" Williams was the primary owner although Grimes and Harper were co-partners in at least 1939; C.L. Collins of Marion, Virginia, also provided continuity by serving as proprietor for at least a decade during this period as well.[93] A shift in management occurred in 1958 when Lee McMillan bought the resort and engaged his parents, Frank and Goldie, to operate it as he was then serving in the U.S. Navy.[94]

The McMillans' country-style cooking and the free spring water have attracted thousands in the years since. In 1967, for example, the *Charlotte Observer* noted that over 10,000 meals were served between each May and October, featuring southern specialties such as "pan fried chicken, country cured ham, mashed potatoes, red eye and cream gravy."[95] Almost thirty-five years later, Noah Adams of NPR's *All Things Considered* wrote that Shatley Springs' family-style dining, with its overflowing platters, is where "You have to remember to sit up straight and take slow breaths."[96]

Visitors staying at the Shatley Springs cottages during the 1930s and the 1940s mainly hailed from North Carolina towns such as Elkin (fifty miles to the southeast), Lenoir, North Wilkesboro, and Sands (thirty miles to the southwest) and occasionally traveled from surrounding states.[97] The dark red dining hall hosted various groups such as North Carolina university alumni chapters, press associations, civic groups, and in more recent years, bus tours for dinner.[98]

The water continues to be a draw. From the 1970s to the 2010s, visitors from states as distant as New York, Oklahoma, Michigan, and Pennsylvania traveled to the resort exclusively to fill up their jugs with the free water.[99] One Philadelphia resident told Lee McMillan that she had taken the spring water back to her terminally ill sister, who then recovered from cancer.[100] Unlike many mineral spring resorts where recreational activities eclipsed the allure of the water over time, Shatley Springs has continually attracted a clientele to its springs for the promise of good health.

Burke County: Piedmont Springs, Glen Alpine Springs, and Connelly Springs

The 1974 Watergate hearings introduced Americans to a folksy lawyer, North Carolina Senator Samuel J. Ervin, Jr., who chaired the Senate Select Committee to Investigate Campaign Practices. Ervin's pithy observations—"Divine Right of kings went out with the American Revolution and doesn't belong to White House aides"—won him a national following, including coverage in *Rolling Stone*.[101] Ervin, with jocular hyperbole, claimed that "humorists lived in all areas of North Carolina, but they were undoubtedly more numerous and gifted in my home county of Burke than elsewhere."[102]

Few outside of Ervin's constituency may have heard of Burke County, but many may recognize a few of the natural wonders in it and neighboring counties. In Avery County, to the northwest of Burke County, the Linville River originates on the high slopes of Grandfather Mountain (5,496 feet). From there, it descends southerly into Burke County to course for a dozen miles through the Pisgah National Forest's 2,000-foot-deep Linville Wilderness Gorge, as defined by the Linville thrust fault. Along the way, the Linville River cascades as a series of two falls; trails climbing above the Linville Falls basin offer spectacular overlooks.[103] The Linville Mountain ridge on the west side of the gorge defines the boundary between Burke and McDowell counties; Jonas Ridge runs on the east. Other local peaks, ranging from about 3,900 feet to about 4,100 feet, include Table Rock Mountain, Hawksbill, and Cranberry Knob.[104] The Linville River eventually meets up with the Catawba River at the Lake James reservoir that straddles Burke and McDowell. About fifteen miles south of Morganton, the county seat of Burke, lies the South Mountain ridge, with elevations up to about 3,000 feet.

The other counties bordering Burke are Rutherford to the southwest, Cleveland to the south, Lincoln and Catawba to the southeast, and Caldwell to the northeast. Cleveland, Lincoln, and Catawba lie outside Campbell's definition of Southern Appalachia. Burke, therefore, is on the cusp of Southern Appalachia, reflecting the descending terrain from northwest to southeast. The designation makes intuitive sense if one considers central North Carolina topography. Catawba County's Hickory lies twenty-five miles east of Morganton at an elevation 300 feet lower than Morganton's 1,200 feet. Other locales east of Hickory in Catawba County lie another 100 to 200 feet lower than Hickory, thus considerably less in altitude than the peaks of Burke.[105]

The complex geology of the Blue Ridge in Burke County, largely quartzite and metamorphosed sedimentary and igneous rocks, has yielded such minerals and rocks as brown hematite (brown iron ore), mica, monazite (a phosphate mineral of rare earth metals), gold, garnet, diamond, silver, aquamarine, zircon, and tetradymite (telluric bismuth, a sulfur-containing mineral). Groundwater seepage therefore contains a variety of mineral salts. The abundance of mineral-laced water led to the nineteenth-century development of three prominent Burke County mineral spring resorts: Piedmont Springs, Glen Alpine Springs, and Connelly Springs.[106]

The American Revolution provided names for both Burke County and Morganton. Burke, originally part of western Rowan County and divided into five more counties between 1790 and 1911, received its name in 1777 from Thomas Burke, who was then serving in the Continental Congress.[107] In 1782, the state legislature formed the Morgan Judicial District, named after Brigadier General Daniel W. Morgan of Saratoga and Cowpens fame. The district created a commission a few years later to select a county courthouse site. Consequently, the commission bought a tract of land known as the "Alder Springs" to lay out the town of Morgan (later Morganton).[108]

The largely Scots-Irish, English, and German immigrants who settled in Burke County began a budding textile industry. By 1810, the 542 looms in the county were producing 77,000 yards of cloth. Other early industries included whiskey and brandy distilling, leather tanning, and iron-ore mining.[109] More alluring than any of these industries, however, was the promise of wealth associated with gold mining.

In 1828, gold discovered at Brindle Creek near the South Mountains triggered a gold rush. According to one tradition, "Brindle and wife" panned the first gold in Burke County and sold the flakes to Morganton merchant Thomas Walton, father of the future builder of the county's Glen Alpine Springs health resort, Colonel Thomas George Walton. The latter recalled that Mrs. Brindle, evidently a strong-willed matron, refused to accept her husband's agreement to sell the mine until a potential buyer offered her a red cashmere shawl, at which point she assented.[110] The gold rush resulted in such a stampede of elites from Virginia and other parts of North Carolina that one local wrote: "The fact that numbers of [North Carolina's] most intelligent, wealthy, and enterprizing [sic] citizens from the eastern and middle counties … are withdrawing their slaves entirely from the cultivation of cotton and tobacco, and removing them to the deposit mines in this county … proves conclusively the importance [the mines] are destined to assume."[111] By 1833, about 5,000 enslaved persons toiled in Burke County gold mines.[112] Although mining activity began to diminish in the next few years as miners left for the northeastern Georgia mines or as the elites redeployed their slaves for agricultural field work or for railroad building, various mining forays continued in the county until about 1920.[113]

Piedmont Springs

Despite the downturn in Burke County gold-mining operations after 1835, the lust for gold continued to excite regional newspaper readers. In 1847, a correspondent for a Raleigh newspaper opined: "The 'Shuffler mine,' in Burke county [sic], on Upper Creek, promises to be extremely rich. This mine is just in its infancy; no excavations to any extent having been made…. I found here gold, silver, lead and copper ore; and the whole vein is skirted by a strong 'Talc' formation." The writer continued: "At the base of this mountain [Brown Mountain] there are two mineral springs; one is sulphur and the other chalybeate [iron-containing]."[114]

That same year, James C. (E.) Estes (Estis), the lessee of the Brown Mountain springs property, decided to build a hotel to open the following summer.[115] Whether or not he intended to capitalize on travelers prospecting for land and mineral rights in the area cannot be determined; but, as so many health resort owners boasted, he grandly pronounced the Piedmont Sulphur and Chalybeate Springs as a watering hole where "invalids, as well as those seeking pleasure, may find a Summer residence, calculated to restore the last energies of the Physical Constitution and gratify the most fastidious."[116]

Within four years, fueled by increasing sectional views, a Raleigh editorialist complained about fellow southerners who would "spend the money which has been obtained from the labor of the negro [sic] among those [in the North] who do everything to destroy the industrial capital of which the negro [sic] forms the chief item." To the contrary, he continued, "the attractions that can be worth any thing [sic] to the invalid or the votary of pleasure, are to found at Deaver's and the Warm Springs in Buncombe and at the Piedmont in Burke."[117] In just a few years, therefore, Estes had shaped Piedmont Springs into a resort sufficiently fashionable to be favorably compared to the *crème de la crème* of western North Carolina watering holes.

Estes held a few enslaved people, a six-year-old male in 1850 and a 22-year-old female in 1860; therefore, any slave labor at Piedmont Springs most probably had to be hired from other slaveowners.[118] One slaveowner with whom Estes had a business relationship was physician John Michael Happoldt, owner of Morganton's Mountain Hotel and inventor of Dr. Michael's Pills, marketed as a cure for chills and fevers.[119] Whether Happoldt hired out any of his slaves to Estes cannot be ascertained, but Estes did savvily recommend to travelers stopping at the Mountain Hotel to leverage Happoldt's medical expertise about the springs' "curative effect and application to certain forms of disease."[120]

Piedmont Springs, "surpassed by none for their health giving [sic] properties," purportedly treated a variety of ailments.[121] One antebellum ad carefully distinguished between the two springs: it specifically recommended the sulphur water for "liver and skin diseases" and the chalybeate (iron) water for "all enemic [anemic] and debilitated conditions of the system."[122] Other antebellum notices emphasized the springs' benefit for a host of digestive afflictions: "Dyspepsia, disorders of the stomach, bowels, liver and kidneys—in rheumatism and many of the forms of nervous diseases."[123] Even in the late nineteenth century, Piedmont Springs continued to advertise its water for "enemic" illnesses and "female diseases" (probably related to anemia). Publicity during this period, however, included treatment for "scrofulous" (tubercular) illnesses, perhaps a marketing move made in response to Asheville's increasing number of sanatoriums.[124]

Piedmont Springs boasted of its accessibility over "good roads," whether from Morganton, sixteen miles away, or from Wilkesboro, fifty miles away. A morning or afternoon ride from Morganton via a twice-weekly hack conveyed guests to the "large Boarding House with spacious and ample accommodations."[125]

Piedmont Springs in reality remained relatively remote despite continued road building and improvements. In 1857, the North Carolina General Assembly, for example, authorized the Morganton and Cranberry Turnpike Company, in which Estes served as a commissioner, to construct a public road from Morganton via Piedmont Springs to the Cranberry Forge, forty-two miles to the northeast.[126] Two years later, future Tennessee State Geologist and North Carolina native Henry E. Colton, however, lamented that the Piedmont Springs' "somewhat out-of-the-way location has kept them from being much resorted to; but the beauty of the scenery around, and the health-restoring properties of the waters, certainly demand for them more attention."[127]

Another antebellum traveler on his way to Table Rock Mountain described the journey from Morganton to Piedmont Springs as one with "some tedious windings over [the mountains that] descended into a narrow alley and pursued … along the banks of a beautiful stream [Upper Creek]" to reach Piedmont Springs. He "enjoy[ed] a refreshing night's sleep" at the hotel and continued the next day to Table Rock, enduring a "narrow and difficult path, sometimes ascending some lofty peak and then descending into a narrow valley, jutted in by the almost perpendicular sides of the contiguous mountains."[128] Ironically, the rugged scenery that attracted some visitors to Piedmont Springs for mountain exploration also deterred others from journeying to the resort.

Piedmont Springs did not close during the Civil War. Whether Estes continued to have a role in the resort after 1860 is unknown as two other proprietors, John W. McElrath and "Capt. E. Barton," appeared respectively in advertisements for 1862 and 1864, hired by the newly formed Piedmont Springs Company, led by E.C. Lindsey.[129] Although the 1863 season opened two weeks later than normal, in July, due to difficulty in engaging a proprietor, the health resort during most of the war publicized its "quiet home to families and persons in pursuit of health and recreation" and, as late as 1862, was improving the property.[130] The Western North Carolina Railroad, despite construction stoppages during the war, was still publicized by the resort as conveying passengers from Salisbury to near Morganton three times weekly as of early summer 1864.[131]

Fighting came close to the resort in summer 1864. From Morristown, Tennessee, Colonel George W. Kirk led Union troops in mid–June, largely consisting of disenchanted Confederate deserters, Unionists, and Cherokees, to the Confederate Camp Vance, about six miles below Morganton. There, in late June, the Union soldiers destroyed several railcars, the depot, and other structures at the Western North Carolina Railroad terminus. About two to three miles away from Piedmont Springs, additional skirmishes occurred. Kirk's Raiders captured 279 Confederate troops and thirty-two Blacks and made their way northwest to Mitchell County's Yellow Mountain where they successfully thwarted the pursuing Confederates on the steep, rough terrain.[132] A Salisbury newspaper cautioned secessionists: "Col. Kirk, the commander of the raiding party, conducted his retreat with admiring skill.… We have now seen that the tories of the border counties and of East Tennessee can inflict serious damage upon us."[133]

Piedmont Springs quickly reassured the public that "[n]o danger from raiders" existed: "The whole surrounding country has been rendered secure. Even the deserters, who formerly sheltered in the mountains, have been swept out."[134] Its seclusion in the mountains acted as a potential drawing card as the resort championed that its "romantic scenery, pure water, and remoteness from danger is perhaps unsurpassed by any place in the Southern Confederacy."[135] A Union raid that December, however, resulted in about $20,000 damage to the resort property. In addition, the "tories" took two wagons, all moveable property, and several slaves, who later escaped back to Piedmont Springs.[136]

The number of visitors who stayed at the resort during the war is not known. With the economy in shambles and the confederate currency's rampant inflation, most southerners lacked disposable income to visit the resort. As an illustration of the hyperinflation, the monthly rate for summer 1862 was $30. By summer 1863, the rate had climbed to $90 and by June 1864 had skyrocketed to an exorbitant $13 daily charge, with a required stay of one month, or a total of $390.[137] More research is needed to determine the type of currency or currencies in use in Burke County during each of these periods and the approximate values to one another, but Piedmont Springs almost certainly experienced a downturn in clientele during the war.

Piedmont Springs reopened in June 1873, at the beginning of a decade of North

Carolina transportation improvements aimed in part to open the western part of the state to tourism.[138] The state legislature approved a road from Morganton via Piedmont Springs and Linville Falls to the Toe River in Mitchell County. The press praised the road, not only as an outlet for Mitchell County goods, but also as a means to provide visitor access to Linville Falls, Table Rock, and Roan Mountain.[139] In 1879, some Morganton citizens began to push for a turnpike to be built from Morganton via Piedmont Springs to Roan Mountain's Cloudland Hotel, a new resort for hay fever sufferers and recreation seekers, that a Raleigh newspaper accurately predicted would be "one of our great watering places."[140] Predicting an increasing clientele, the Piedmont Springs proprietor Gabriel Pearcy, who had lived in Estes' household in 1860 and therefore may have been a longstanding employee, paid for a two-mile-long road to connect with the so-called Mitchell turnpike.[141] Concurrently, the Western North Carolina Railroad completed the Swannanoa Tunnel in 1879 and then laid rail to five miles north of Asheville by the following summer.[142]

It remains uncertain that Piedmont's visitor numbers in the 1880s increased with the improved transportation infrastructure. Those who did visit the health resort continued to come primarily for the springs and secondarily for leisure activities. Ads emphasized the "Waters Blue and white Sulphur, Chalybeate, and the most sparkling freestone" for use "especially in female diseases."[143] The curative powers of the water, however, sometimes fell short: a Union County government official and a young Charlotte girl both died within weeks of each other in 1883 after sojourning at Piedmont Springs to recover their health.[144] Visitors seeking recreation found limited options such as dancing, fishing, horseback riding, and creekside strolls.[145] A visitor describing a festive dance at the hotel lamented that "It is a pity that Piedmont is no better known and more largely patronized."[146]

The increased numbers of roads and rail lines that theoretically afforded better access to Piedmont Springs therefore also took some tourists and health-seekers away from Burke County. Local boosters asserted that "one can go by rail to Morganton, and twenty miles beyond, and with not more fatigue than is enjoyable, [to] be in the very heart of the mountains."[147] Yet an observer noted that "[t]he near approach of the railroads to Asheville and Warm Springs seems to have crowded out" Piedmont Springs and other watering holes and that Asheville "is well filled."[148] Demonstrative of the popularity of Asheville-area watering holes, Deaver's Sulphur Springs around 1887 often commanded a daily rate 50 percent more than that of Piedmont Springs.[149]

In 1883, in response to reports the previous year of gold at the resort property, the Louisville Gold Mining Company offered $7,000 to Pearcy for the Piedmont Springs' buildings and twenty-four acres, but the deal never materialized (little to no gold was apparently mined at the resort site).[150] A few years later, the Piedmont Lumber, Ranch, & Mining Company, a group of northern capitalists represented by Captain R.H. Blake, bought the property from Pearcy for $6,000.[151] The firm, which owned upwards of 40,000 acres by 1887, stocked streams with trout, devised plans to breed deer, initiated an iron-ore mining operation at Linville Mountain, and bought ewes and corn from locals for a sheep ranch on its property.[152]

Piedmont Springs experienced financial instability beginning in 1888. In

August of that year, the Piedmont Lumber, Ranch, & Mining Company began construction on a new hotel valued at about $30,000 (about $952,000 in 2022 dollars).[153] It is not clear if the hotel was completed: the press did not cover building progress nor any grand reopening. The local newspaper reported in December 1890 that Piedmont Springs was closed to the public but wistfully hoped that the completion of the Southern and Western Railroad from Shelby to Cranberry would allow the springs to "more than eclipse their antebellum reputation, which was of the best."[154] Local families such as the Crites, Piercys, Beans, and Pritchards owned the hotel property after 1888 but lacked the capital resources of investment syndicates to make major improvements. Moreover, northern timber interests began buying land tracts around the hotel.[155]

In 1892, a torrential rain hit Burke County. At Piedmont Springs, water flooded offices in the yard and washed away the dining room foundations.[156] The damage was repaired and the hotel reopened: an 1895 medical article, praising the Piedmont water as "not unlike the White Sulphur of Virginia," described the resort as a "long, rambling hotel, venerable in service, offer[ing] attractions of quiet and rest."[157]

By the turn of the twentieth century, the hotel continued to receive visitors. Irene Margaret Crites, daughter of Solomon Vance Crites, the proprietor from around 1890 through 1904, recalled that the hotel was always full of people.[158] Within the next few years, however, the resort apparently catered largely to a local crowd although proprietors continued to lease the property.[159]

In 1916, the so-called Great Flood ravaged western North Carolina, destroying all Burke County bridges over the Catawba River, washing away much of the turnpike near Piedmont Springs, causing millions of dollars of damage in Asheville, and claiming several lives.[160] Esther Pritchard remembered that she and her husband, the last to occupy the hotel, escaped to a nearby hill where they lived for three days off a gallon of milk, coffee, and a jar of blackberries that they collected in their haste.[161] The hotel incurred much damage and was not rebuilt.[162] Today, Piedmont Springs lies within the Pisgah National Forest near the intersection of Mortimer Road and N.C. Highway 181.[163]

Glen Alpine Springs

The history of Glen Alpines Springs, built in 1878 near the South Mountains, begins with Colonel Thomas George Walton, the memoirist of the early gold-mining days of Burke County and leader of the Confederate Burke County Home Guard that fought against Kirk at Camp Vance.[164] Moulton Avery, who married into the Walton family, "discovered" the springs in the antebellum period (the Cherokees may or may not have used the waters) and built a summer cottage there.[165] Walton, a former slaveowner and a wealthy landowner with an estate valued at $39,000 (over $1.4 million in 2022 dollars), headed the Glen Alpine Springs Company, incorporated in 1870 "for establishing a first class watering place in the salubrious and healthy mountains of Burke county [sic]."[166] By 1872, at least a dozen crude cabins stood near the springs, which had attracted about sixty persons the year before.[167] A visitor during that period grandly declared that no place, with the exception of the White Sulphur

Springs in Virginia, "combines so much that is desirable for the invalid, and attractive to the lover of the sublime and beautiful in nature."[168]

Glen Alpine Springs held its grand opening ball in July 1878. The honorary and floor managers included Congressman A.M. Waddell and several businessmen and lawyers from Charlotte, Statesville, Hickory, and Morganton, thus indicating Walton's network outside Burke County.[169] The *Charlotte Observer* billed the hotel as "large and elegant," even though it was still incomplete by September.[170] The final three-story building with a central tower did indeed include extraordinary dimensions: seventeen-foot-high ceilings in most of the fifty guest rooms of 360 square feet each, a roof promenade extending 115 feet, and overall accommodations for 200.[171] Walton's investment resulted in the most ambitious effort undertaken of any of Burke County's mineral springs resorts.[172]

Early advertisements and visitor narratives largely focused on three elements: the hotel architecture, the mountainous ambiance, and social amenities. Walton and his son-in-law John H. Pearson, the proprietor, published a promotional notice throughout the summer of 1879, largely in the Raleigh press, in which an illustration of the hotel occupied over half of the ad.[173] The prominence of the hotel sketch relative to the text suggested visual evidence that the hotel anecdotally was the largest frame building in North Carolina.[174] In the Raleigh ad and in other publicity, Walton and Pearson emphasized the "large, well ventilated" rooms fed by the mountain breezes and "Spacious Verandahs and Terrace" that were designed "with a view to the greatest convenience of the guests."[175]

The natural beauty of Glen Alpine's surroundings captivated guests. One Raleigh visitor, sitting by his hotel window, wrote that he was "watching the white mists unfold themselves and roll slowly off the mountains"; the cool mountain air made it "hard to realize that this is the same earth as it was last Saturday [in Raleigh] when the rampant mercury rose over 100° and the air was like a breath of a Sirocco."[176] A guest from the North Carolina coast marveled that "the view from Glen Alpine heights, Monte Crusis and Raven's Cliff [respectively three-quarters and one and a half miles from the hotel] is so extensive and sublime, that description can scarcely give the faintest conception of the reality."[177] As a Charlotte ad for the resort boldly summed up: "The surrounding scenery is unsurpassed in the Southern Alleghanies."[178]

Social amenities constituted a major facet of Glen Alpine Springs' culture. Unlike Piedmont Springs, which publicized its quiet environs, Glen Alpine routinely hosted a "gay crowd that throngs the corridors of the hotel" and where "pool, billiards, euchre, and dancing hold full sway every day."[179] The Raleigh guest who wrote of the mountain view from his window embraced the "peals of merry laughter from the young folks in the large hall where we gather in the mornings and dance in the evenings ... mirthful voices mingled with the rolling balls [in the ten pin alley] ... a hilarious party shouting and laughing over the noisy and disreputable game of *grab* [italics original]."[180] Ads for the season's opening ball promised an "excellent band" and a "large crowd" (over 200 attended the 1878 function, with dancing until 4:00 a.m.).[181] Important to the resort's amenities were foods shipped from New York to supplement local "tender mountain beef and mutton" [and] the "delicious fruits for which the South Mountains are celebrated."[182] For 1879 Walton and Pearson engaged "one of the most experienced pastry cooks in the South" to bolster their claim that "the cuisine is superior."[183] A guest described a tea in the "supper-room," which preceded a gala as a "busy interesting scene ... the merry laughing crowd; the sparkling silver and glass; the hurrying waiters, balancing with skillful hand their trays high above their heads...."[184]

Resort ads and visitor narratives for the resort's first few years largely minimized the therapeutic uses of the springs' waters relative to the pharmaceutical ads and medical journals that touted the water. The lowermost text of an 1878 resort ad, almost overshadowed by the hotel building drawing, merely advised that the water would be sold "by all the leading Druggists in the state."[185] At least one enterprising druggist, however, catapulted the water into the same league as Saratoga and European springs by publicizing it prominently with Congress, Empire, Vichy, and Apollinaris mineral waters.[186] Moreover, an 1880 American Medical Association committee report summarizing medicinal mineral springs singled out Glen Alpine water with about fifty other springs (including Red Sulphur, one of the famous antebellum Virginia springs) as "chemically indifferent ... but which still possess peculiarities which may give them some medicinal value."[187]

By 1890, the resort, now managed by C.S. Smith for Walton, had begun to reassert the "wonderful curative properties of its water and salubrious climate," presenting a testimonial by a Raleigh minister and normal school principal, who certified that taking the waters for his "general run down condition ... very feeble, with dispepsia [and] kidney troubles" had "strengthened him and fitted him to return to work."[188] Various accounts favorably compared the five mineral springs at Glen Alpine with England's Turnbridge Wells and Virginia's Buffalo Lithia water 200 miles to the northeast, Glen Alpine's being "of such exceeding lightness that one may drink to surfeiting without experiencing ill effects."[189] In 1897, Smith was still publicizing four "excellent" springs (lithia, sulphur, alum and iron) "whose efficacy have been proven in many extreme cases of disease."[190]

Unlike many Southern Appalachian resorts in their twilight years, Glen Alpine Springs sustained its appeal to regional elite throughout its existence until it closed in the late 1890s. In the early 1880s, U.S. Senator Matthew Butler of South Carolina engaged rooms for the summer; North Carolina's U.S. Senator M.W. Ransom's family vacationed there; and Colonel George W. Stanton, erstwhile Radical Republican candidate for state office, traveled to the springs where his wife had taken ill.[191] Several years later, Eugene Morehead, Durham banker and industrialist and son of Governor John M. Morehead, convalesced at the resort for several weeks: "The water makes everything agree with me.... I sleep like a pig in a pen, day and night."[192] In 1890, Morganton native William S. Pearson, who served as U.S. consul in Italy and engaged in other public and private sector activities, stayed several days to regain his health.[193] Other state notables who signed the guest register included Governor Zebulon Vance and tobacco industrialist Benjamin Duke. As a local newspaper proudly summed up: "[Glen Alpine Springs's] patronage is largely recruited from the *elite* [italics original] of this and other Southern States."[194]

Glen Alpine patrons typically arrived at the resort by hack from the Western

North Carolina Railroad's Morganton depot, twelve to fifteen miles away, or from its Glen Alpine station, seven or eight miles distant.[195] If they stopped at Morganton, they could arrange for "any kind of conveyance they wish" from the Hunt House (formerly the Walton House, owned by Walton and his brother, W.M.).[196] The extremely wealthy, such as railroad baron Jay Gould, who stayed at Glen Alpine, perhaps as a wayside during a trip to Asheville to meet with George W. Vanderbilt and other capitalists, traveled by private rail car.[197]

As the southern network of railroads increased, the Richmond and Danville, as well as the Atlantic Coast Line, offered special excursion fares to Glen Alpine Springs from such hubs as Charlotte, Concord, and Wilmington, North Carolina.[198] With the expansion of the rail system, travel guides such as *Appletons'* developed; the 1896 edition included Glen Alpine Springs, advising the Mountain Hotel for Morganton, from which travelers could leave for the resort.[199]

In 1900, the resort was put on the market.[200] Glen Alpine Springs had been closed for a few years by then: auctions had been held in 1898 and 1899 to sell the property, including "household and kitchen furniture" and an undivided tract "with a three-story hotel building, cottages, barns … containing 300 acres."[201] In 1901, J.W. Taylor leased the property for that summer only; the next year, Marguerite G. Grant of New York and the Reverend Dalzell Schoonmaker of New Jersey leased the resort tract with an option to buy for use as a Presbyterian mission school.[202] The Northern Presbyterian Mission Board operated a school with Schoonmaker as principal until 1911.[203] Schoonmaker bought the property outright in 1912 and sold it in 1918 to Clifton Pearson, an agent for others who planned to construct a new hotel.[204] The property was eventually abandoned; the dilapidated hotel burned down in 1934.[205]

Connelly Springs

The third major health resort in Burke County, Connelly Springs, may be considered a hybrid of Piedmont Springs and Glen Alpine Springs: it appealed throughout its operation to both those who sought the therapeutic waters and to those who were part of an elite business and political element of eastern North Carolina society. Unique of the three resorts, however, was its very accessible location to travelers: it stood less than a half mile away from the Western North Carolina Railroad.

In January 1865, as North Carolina was bracing for possible invasion by General William T. Sherman after his victorious march from Atlanta to Savannah, Elizabeth Connelly (Conley) placed a Salisbury newspaper ad advising "refugees, or others wishing a comfortable home" at her "plantation and tenements" to contact her son, W.W., for rental terms.[206] Elizabeth had been a widow for a decade. Her late husband, Captain William Lewis Connelly, had led a state militia in 1838 to round up Cherokees for the infamous "Trail of Tears" forced march and then built a stagecoach waystation about midway between Salisbury and Asheville, which evolved into the small village of Happy Home.[207] Being of limited means as suggested by the ad, Elizabeth performed many household chores herself. Around 1871, when doing laundry, she rediscovered a mineral spring that Cherokees purportedly had used: yarn or clothes that she washed in a side branch of only that spring (several springs stood on her property) accumulated a mysterious yellowish-brown stain.[208] Testing revealed a high content of iron bicarbonate in the spring's water; subsequently, many persons in the region began to travel to the spring.[209]

The spring continued to attract seekers of health for the next decade. By the early 1880s, one of Elizabeth's daughters, Charity Louisiana Connelly Goode, and her husband, D.P. (David Parham) Goode, operated a boarding house near the springs that they expanded in 1883 to meet demand, particularly from the Salisbury area.[210] One Salisbury resident, Thomas J. Merony, "broken down in health," drank the spring water to regain his "stout and strong" vigor, and convinced his brother, Philip J., to make an offer with him on the springs to then develop into a health resort near Icard Station, Happy Home's rail depot.[211] The Meronys subsequently bought almost four acres of land that contained the spring from W.W. and an additional five-eighths acre from Goode and Emma Connelly, a sister to W.W. and Charity Louisiana.[212]

The Meronys' hotel opened in June 1886 to much favorable publicity. A Salisbury newspaper trumpeted that "Connelly Spring at Icard Station is looming up as one of the conspicuous watering places and pleasure resorts in Western North Carolina. The medicinal character of the water has been shown to be of great value."[213] Several newspaper articles took great pains to detail the grand size of the wooden structure. Measurements varied for the length, ranging from 110 to 120 feet; the central tower height, up to seventy-five feet high; and the number of rooms, estimated at thirty-seven to fifty.[214] The verandah on the first and second stories—an important feature for sheltered promenades—measured 200 feet long, adding "so greatly to the comfort of the pleasure-seeker or invalid."[215]

In appearance, the Connelly Springs hotel resembled the Glen Alpine hotel: both structures contained a central turret or tower flanked by two two-story wings with dormer windows on the top or third level. The Glen Alpine hotel, designed by an English architect, appeared more ornate in design (e.g., a rooftop verandah) than did the Connelly Springs hotel, designed by a local architect and featuring simple spindled balustrades.[216]

The Connelly Springs hotel interior emphasized spaciousness and engineering advances. The hotel showcased its dining room table—100 feet long—that could seat one hundred guests comfortably. Hallways were advertised as ten feet wide, perhaps to impart the concept of good ventilation in the mountain setting. With an eye on the numerous kitchen fires common in the era, the Meronys installed iron cladding on the kitchen walls and ceiling in hopes of rendering it fireproof.[217] Pipes conveyed water from a South Mountain spring to a holding tank at the top of the hotel tower with a 25,000 gallon capacity. Directly below the tank was a parlor with windows overlooking the Blue Ridge peaks in all directions.[218]

Connelly Springs provided a variety of recreational activities. A building near the mineral spring housed a "magnificent ball room, a ten pin alley, billard and pool tables, [and] bath rooms[,] etc., all kept in first class repair for the convenience and comfort of the guests of the hotel."[219] Guests, as at Piedmont Springs and Glen Alpine Springs, might hike, fish, or secure horses, "sure-footed and gentle … for rides or drives up the mountains…."[220]

The careful landscaping and terracing of the resort's grounds and the voluminous publicity given to the water's attributes indicate that the spring was the resort's main attraction. The Meronys painstakingly drained the ground around the mineral spring—avoiding the other springs, all freestone, that seeped on the property—to concentrate the iron bicarbonate salts. In addition, they encased the spring with a marble basin and enclosed both by a pagoda.[221] Guests strolled "a few steps" down a shady slope from either the hotel or the health resort's "neat and attractive cottages" along a path to the pagoda. There, they might sip the "health-restoring beverage" on benches around the pavilion and inhale the "health laden breezes."[222]

Connelly Springs' extensive publicity around its therapeutic water extended throughout its history and generally minimized or omitted mention of the resort's recreational aspects. Early ads shouted the heading "Invalid's Home!" to broadcast the water's use for "Bright's Disease [acute kidney inflammation], Gravel [kidney stones], Gout, and other depraved diseases of the dependent upon Uric Acid Diathesis."[223] Ads from 1887 through 1912 continually emphasized the spring water's curative power: an 1887 ad touted the use of the iron-containing water for conditions as varied as dyspepsia and "all diseases peculiar to women," and a 1912 notice recommended the spring for "nervousness, a run down system, and all blood diseases."[224]

Relieved patrons touted the waters, equating weight gain with robust health. William Smithdeal, a Salisburian who led the Connelly Springs Company that bought the health retreat from the Melronys, marveled that he had "gained six pounds in eight days … my digestion greatly improved."[225] A husband from Wilson, North Carolina, expressed delight that his formerly invalid wife after fifteen days of drinking the water had "walked four measured miles and gained six or eight pounds."[226]

Connelly Springs water was compared favorably to well-known springs. Following Glen Alpine's lead, Connelly Springs proclaimed its water "equal to the celebrated Buffalo Lithia Springs of Virginia."[227] One guest, familiar with the health resorts in northeastern Virginia, opined that Connelly Springs provided "a most palatable water resembling much the celebrated Chalybeate of Virginia, the Rawby Springs."[228] As late as 1924, the press compared the water with that of European watering places, and Fitch in 1927 briefly discussed its "diuretic and slight tonic properties."[229]

Connelly Springs initiated mineral water sales within its first five years: in 1889, the resort began periodic shipments to a Londoner who had taken the waters earlier in the year for chronic kidney issues while conducting business in Salisbury.[230] Passenger trains stopping at Connelly Springs picked up water for shipping "all over the country" for about a dime per gallon in the early 1900s (about $3.43 in 2022 dollars).[231] From 1913 through 1917, Connelly Springs stands out as one of only fifteen North Carolina health resorts and one of two in Southern Appalachian North Carolina to continually market its water.[232] Although no source consulted lists international sales apart from those originating in London, the span of Connelly Springs water shipments for over two decades offsets its somewhat exaggerated claim that "hundreds of people at home and abroad in unsolicited testimonials attest its efficacy."[233]

The health resort also drew upon its elevation as a health benefit, linking the perceived efficaciousness of both mountain air and inability of mosquitos to populate at higher, less humid altitudes. In 1900, the resort's Savannah newspaper advertisements emphasized to coastal Georgia readers its "magnificent mountains 1,200 feet above sea.... No malaria."[234] Again, in 1916, it publicized its lack of mosquitoes, presumably absent at its altitude, to a South Carolina newspaper audience.[235] Interestingly, unlike the Asheville area sanitariums, Connelly Springs remonstrated in the 1910s against potentially contagious, tubercular clientele: "No consumptives taken."[236]

By billing itself as "the only Mineral Springs directly on the railroad in Western North Carolina," Connelly Springs aimed to attract patrons with easy access to rail, particularly from eastern North Carolina cities such as Salisbury, Raleigh, Greensboro, and Charlotte.[237] Nearby Rutherford College, founded by a Methodist minister, recommended the Connelly Springs hotel for its visitors, including those attending religious gatherings on its campus (implying that the resort provided a healthy, perhaps non-alcohol ambiance).[238]

In common with Glen Alpine Springs, a smaller number of Connelly Springs guests traveled regularly from many southern states such as Louisiana, Florida, and Alabama and reconnected each year as what one visitor termed, "a great big family."[239] Even into the 1910s, as good roads and rail were opening up venues in other parts of the country, Connelly Springs prospered. One week in June 1910, for example, saw the arrival of travelers from points as diverse as Massachusetts, New York, Richmond, Mississippi, New Orleans, and Bristol, Tennessee.[240] The son of the last owner, Jeff Davis, an adult when his father bought the hotel in 1913, remembered that the hotel remained full during the summer, especially from Charlotte and Statesville visitors, who stayed one to two months.[241]

The political and business elite who travelled to Connelly Springs included North Carolina Governors A.M. Scales and T.J. Jarvis; Charlotte banker and Spartanburg and Atlantic Railroad President Rufus Yancey McAden, who came for health reasons; and Judge Thomas Ruffin, Jr.[242] According to tradition, George W. Vanderbilt visited by private rail car to Connelly Springs and tried unsuccessfully to purchase nearby Hoosier's Knob (now known as "The Knob").[243]

In 1890, a Salisbury-based syndicate purchased the Connelly Springs property from the Merony brothers for $11,000, with a newspaper reporting that the "ever popular place has even outgrown the excellent management of the Merony's [sic]."[244] The newly formed Connelly Springs Company had such a successful season with overflowing crowds that it embarked on a twenty-room hotel addition that it completed in time for the next spring.[245]

A decade later, despite seemingly good resort attendance and the railroad's construction of an additional track at the depot, the Connelly Springs Company defaulted on its mortgage payments for unclear reasons.[246] The hotel continued for the season of 1900 under the proprietorship of B.B. Abernethy; J.F. Battle bought the furnishings in May 1902 to sell at an auction in Morganton, and Horace W. Connelly purchased the property itself that year.[247] Connelly operated the Connelly Mineral Springs Company until his death in 1905, after which Henry Vanstory bought the property. Vanstory continued to ship the water "all over the country" and promised clientele "reasonable rates" to enjoy "[a]ll amusements" and to cure their "run down system[s]."[248]

In 1913 the health resort underwent major improvements. In that year, Jeff (William Jefferson) Davis, an experienced hotelier in the region, bought Connelly Springs, modernized it with electric lights, and undertook other renovations.[249] In 1927, Fitch's mineral waters guide described the hotel as a "commodious building equipped with modern conveniences … [the] spring well improved and enclosed in a marble basin. The water is clear and sparkling but has a metallic taste due to the iron." Illustrative of the cachet that the hotel continued to carry, the handbook continued: "Many of the best families of the section sojourn there for several weeks during the summer season."[250] When Davis died in 1930, his widow Eunice continued the hotel's operation for a period. After her death in 1941, the hotel was dismantled and the lumber shipped to Winston-Salem to repurpose in construction of a school.[251]

Haywood County: Haywood White Sulphur Springs and Eagles Nest

Among the undulating Smoky, Balsam, and Plott Balsam mountain ridges in rugged southwestern North Carolina lies Haywood County at a mean elevation of 3,600 feet, the highest average altitude of any county in the eastern United States.[252] The northern part of the county is home to the Great Smoky Mountains National Park's Cataloochee Valley, a picturesque cove nestled in the shadows of mountains over 6,000 feet tall, including Mount Guyot, on the Tennessee and North Carolina border.[253] Other notable peaks in the county, which claims over 200 named mountains, include Waterrock Knob (6,292 feet) and Cold Mountain (6,030 feet), the setting for Charles Frazier's National Book Award-winning novel of the same name.[254]

Haywood is also bordered by Madison and Buncombe counties to the northeast, Transylvania County to the south, and Jackson and Swain counties to the southwest in a region that today is known for its tourism and "halfbacks," northern retirees who moved to the Deep South and now have resettled in or established second homes in the Southern Appalachians. The county seat of Waynesville, however, has received visitors since the nineteenth century, rivaling Asheville's tourist trade in the late 1800s. Travelers during that era journeyed to Waynesville's nearby resorts of Haywood White Sulphur Springs and Eagles Nest to seek the "health and ozone of the mountains" and to flee from the periodic yellow fever epidemics of the Deep South.[255]

Haywood White Sulphur Springs

Around 1845 or 1846, an elderly enslaved person, "Uncle Jerry," was digging a ditch on the property of his owner, Colonel Robert (James Robert) Love, when he struck a stream of what he thought was water contaminated with milk sickness due to its odd color and smell, but which Love correctly identified as a sulphur spring.[256] Love cleared the area around the spring, which subsequently attracted regional attention. In 1849, a traveler from the Raleigh area wrote of Waynesville's "healthy and beautiful" location "with a fine mountain view" and singled out the "excellent Sulphur Spring about a mile from the Court House."[257] A year later, a writer opined that the "White Sulphur, in Haywood, will become a place of very great resort, if only the gentlemanly proprietor can be prevailed on to open his house to the public."[258]

Love was one of Haywood County's wealthiest landowners, with personal estate valued at $50,000 in 1850 (about $1.9 million in 2022 dollars).[259] He was also the county's largest slaveowner for over a decade, holding 85 enslaved persons in 1850, about 20 percent of the county's 418 slaves, and about 56 in 1860, around 18 percent of the county's 313 slaves.[260]

James Robert had gained much of his wealth through his father, Colonel Robert (Robert Gustavus Adolphus) Love, at one point one of the wealthiest men in North Carolina, who owned 758,000 acres of land sweeping across Buncombe County through Swain County.[261] Robert G. left a noted legacy in both western North Carolina and upper East Tennessee: He fought under General Anthony Wayne in the American Revolution, naming the Haywood County seat after his commander; helped to defeat John Sevier's attempt to form the independent State of Franklin out of North Carolina; and famously beat Andrew Jackson on a horse track about a mile from the site of the Unaka Springs resort near modern Erwin (the section of Tennessee Route 36 near the race track site is known today as the Jackson Love Highway).[262]

James Robert's youngest daughter, Maria, in 1871 married a Tennessean, W.W. (William Williams) Stringfield, a Confederate veteran who later served in a variety of appointed and elected positions, including as an Assistant Doorkeeper in the U.S. House of Representatives, as a North Carolina state senator, and as the head of Confederate veteran associations.[263] By the late 1870s, the Stringfields were living on Maria's family's property (Union Colonel George W. Kirk's troops had destroyed Robert L.'s home in March 1865).[264] In 1878, according to various sources, the Stringfields either opened their private home or another building as the Haywood White Sulphur Springs Hotel.[265]

The couple did not undertake such a venture due to dire financial conditions. In addition to Maria's moneyed background, W.W. had accumulated $4,000 (about $92,500 in 2022 dollars) as an upper East Tennessee merchant before their marriage.[266] Most likely, they recognized that the ongoing westward expansion of the Western North Carolina Railroad would further open their region to industry, especially timbering, and to tourism in the cool mountain climes. Even in the antebellum period, Maria's father James Robert wanted to bring a railroad through the town and had willed to his children sites next to the land he had donated for a depot,[267] Accordingly, within four months of the resort's opening, Stringfield published an opinion piece referencing "The great health resort of the South. By all means push forward the broad guage [sic] full fledge Railroad [sic], and let the iron horse arouse the now latent energy in our people."[268]

The resort proved popular even though the Murphy Branch of the Western North Carolina Railroad did not reach Waynesville until 1882, forcing travelers in the first five years to arrive via a daily stage from Asheville.[269] Although Stringfield only offered limited accommodations the first season, within five years, he had enlarged the three-story frame structure so many times, extending its length to at least 150 feet, that a commentator described it as a "large farmhouse, remodeled and added to it until its original proportions and design are lost."[270] To further meet the demand for accommodations, Stringfield constructed a line of cottages accommodating 100 guests, which stood along a gravel path leading from the sulphur spring uphill to the enlarged hotel that could receive 150 visitors.[271]

Calamity in the way of a fire, with racist overtones as to its origin, struck in August 1885. The hotel burned down at a loss estimated at $30,000 ($942,000 in 2019 dollars).[272] The 200 guests, including North Carolina Governor A.M. Scales and his family, escaped unharmed.[273] While a few accounts attributed the blaze to a kitchen stove, one newspaper narrative blamed a "colored servant" for vowing vengeance against the hotel manager, J.S.C. Timberlake, who had struck him between the eyes with a hammer for a "little difficulty" a few days before the fire.[274] Timberlake's alleged violent behavior, analogous to that of an antebellum overseer, not only went unpunished but appeared tacitly justified as no recrimination appeared in the press for his violence. The definitive cause of the fire remained unknown.

The resort stayed open, however, as the unscathed cottages continued to receive guests through November.[275] Eleven months later, a new hotel opened in July 1886 on the site of its predecessor.[276] The new main structure was made of brick, again boasted three stories, and publicized its "verandahs 12 feet wide and 250 feet long.... Everything new, bright and clean."[277] Its sixty-two rooms accommodated about 250 guests, with the cottages generally reserved for families and invalids.[278] From the hotel, surrounded by large shade trees, a path led directly to the sulphur spring about 100 yards away while other trails, including the popular Lovers' Walk near Richland Creek, wandered around the property's 25 acres.[279]

As was typical of mineral spring resorts, a protective pavilion stood over the spring.[280] A stone basin estimated at 14–24 inches deep and about 18 inches in diameter surrounded the spring itself.[281] Pavilion seats surrounded the basin where Waynesville visitors not lodging at the resort could imbibe all they wished for a small fee (five cents in 1902) or purchase the water by the gallon.[282] An attendant in the early 1900s served the water; one young man, who had an eye on the female employee during his stay, frequented the spring so much that he claimed to have gained fifteen pounds in two months to become a "new man with a new lease on life" (no information available on any outcome of his infatuation).[283]

Two other springs, both chalybeate (iron-containing), were discovered respectively in the late 1870s and in 1893.[284] Although mineral water authority William Edward Fitch in 1927 favored the chalybeate water to that of the "celebrated steel spring at Pyrmont, Germany" due to the former's much higher iron concentration and recommended the white sulphur water for "chronic fuctional disturbances of the gastrointestinal tract," the resort itself inexplicably did not advertise the medical attributes of its waters in newspapers or the availability of a resident physician.[285] Rather, Haywood ads in vague terms referenced the resort's "finest and purest white sulphur," its "health giving springs," and its water's "wonderful reputation" without specifying afflictions treated or providing testimonials from cured clientele. Even though Haywood White Sulphur did contract with physicians—one even owned the resort at one point—only one testimonial, that of a physician cured of Bright's Disease from drinking the water, was found in hundreds of newspapers browsed.[286]

Most likely, the imbibing of the spring water constituted largely a social, not a therapeutic, activity for Waynesville visitors, who typically came to the "Land of the Sky" for mountain scenery and cool summer weather. Accordingly, an 1892 Haywood White Sulphur ad emphasized the resort's "cool and invigorating" climate.[287] Two newspaper ads in 1895 respectively publicized the resort's devotion to the "comfort and entertainment of guests" and its self-branding as "Truly the Switzerland of America."[288] Even an 1894 notice directly mentioning the water put it in context of its location: "The lowest temperature and highest elevation of any known Sulphur Springs in the world."[289]

Guests therefore indulged in a variety of activities apart from the springs, many of them instead focused on the outdoors. In addition to the typical mineral spring resort offerings of lawn tennis, croquet, and bowling, the hotel arranged or publicized excursions to natural attractions within fifty miles.[290] Local excursions included carriage rides up the Junaluska Mountain Road (site of the Eagles Nest resort) to admire the view, trout fishing at Cataloochee, journeying to Mount Clingman (Kuwohi), and riding horseback near Richland Creek to the base of Old Bald mountain.[291] The hotel also hosted an occasional Cherokee ball game for guests, most of whom had never encountered Native Americans. As one excited observer recorded, the ball game was played by "real live Cherokee Indians ... their faces painted ... they look savage and aboriginal to the last degree."[292]

Indoor events included dancing with orchestral music and the occasional formal ball.[293] The 1889 gala attracted 200 guests, many from Asheville, who enjoyed an elegant supper and a performance by Swiss bell ringers before the dance.[294] At the 1891 "fancy dress ball," many men assumed the roles of phantoms while women masqueraded in costumes as varied as nuns or red poppy flowers.[295] Prohibited at the dances was alcohol; not only was Waynesville a dry community but Stringfield was formerly Grand Worthy Patriarch of the Sons of Temperance of Tennessee.[296]

Summer visitors crowded Waynesville in the late 1800s. The town's four hotels and the Haywood White Sulphur resort were continually full. According to a local minister, "almost every family in the place have [sic] to surrender their extra rooms to prevent turning away summer visitors."[297] Accordingly, in the early 1890s, the Haywood White Sulphur constructed a two-story annex of thirty rooms.[298] Within a few years, however, the press reported that the popular resort was again overflowing with visitors.[299]

Guests visited from largely the South although a few attendees at the 1891 fancy dress ball traveled from New York City, Rhode Island, and Nebraska.[300] Visitors from the Deep South might take a train, as one Alabamian did, to Chattanooga for the night and then travel the next day to Morristown, Tennessee, to board a Richmond & Danville train to Asheville, and then transfer to the Western North Carolina Railroad to reach Waynesville.[301] So many Alabamians frequented the resort that one letter writer noted that "It looked like Selma at the springs one day."[302]

Notables visiting the resort included Woodrow and Ellen Louise Wilson and General Thomas "Stonewall" Jackson's widow, Anna, who was feted at a Confederate veteran and Daughters of the Confederacy reception.[303] As one writer put it, "Some of the best people from all over the South gather there, quiet, cultured, refined people, and that is what makes the Hayward [sic] White Sulphur a popular resort."[304]

The quietude of Haywood White Sulphur was spoiled early one Wednesday in August 1898. The Black head waiter and 15 Black waiters left the resort immediately before breakfast to protest their wages.[305] The proprietors scurried to find sufficient staff to serve breakfast; in addition, they telegraphed Asheville to locate waiters and placed an ad for assistance in an Asheville newspaper promising "good wages."[306] The Black waiters, however, had told their Asheville counterparts in advance not to respond.[307]

No further information in sources consulted can be found on the resolution of the walkout.[308] However, the work stoppage, undertaken in a hotel built on land owned by a prominent slave-holding family and which catered in large part to southern sympathizers, perhaps reflects a bold empowerment in an era in which many Blacks still worked in servitude for whites. In addition, the year 1898 is notable for North Carolina race relations in at least two aspects. The successful Democratic gubernatorial candidate, Charles Brantley Aycock, lobbied that year throughout the state, including Waynesville, for a disfranchisement amendment, and Democratic white elite supremacists overthrew Wilmington's legitimate Republican biracial city government and burned a Black newspaper office in November 1898.[309] Whether the waiter walkout was part of a larger movement to protest increasing Black inequality in the state cannot easily be ascertained but is worthy of further research.

The resort changed hands several times and subsequently underwent various renovations with new proprietors. The most extravagant remodeling occurred in the 1899–1900 period when the new owner, the southwestern Georgia lumber and logging railway firm of Alford & Sloan, thoroughly renovated the resort: ordering "new furniture of the latest pattern," building a new forty to fifty room annex on a nearby hill, erecting a dancing pavilion, and overhauling or adding lawn tennis, ball grounds, and a golf link.[310] As an Asheville newspaper reported, the owners are "men of means and will spare no pains to have this resort a first-class one."[311]

The resort under C.A. Alford and B.J. Sloan, later managed by Sloan and his son, continued to welcome largely southern guests, including Florida Governor Park Trammel.[312] In addition, Haywood White Sulphur hosted state groups as diverse as the Masons, the Gastonia Pythian Drum Corps who paraded from the train depot to the hotel for the corps' annual banquet, newspaper press conventions, and pharmacy students undergoing their state board examination (not known is if the latter de-stressed at the spring bathing house following the test).[313] Tourism in the 1910s was booming so much in western North Carolina that many resorts remained open past the traditional closing of early September; Haywood White Sulphur elected to receive visitors until early November in 1913.[314]

The resort most likely would have continued in popularity if not for World War I. Whereas one visitor in June 1916 wrote that the hotel was a "delightful spot, with fine sulphur water," by the following May, B.J. Sloan had offered the resort to the federal government to house captured German crews of civilian merchant ships, an option the government later turned down in favor of using Hot Springs' Mountain View Hotel as an internment camp.[315] In March 1918, however, the U.S. government leased the hotel as a temporary hospital for tubercular soldiers until the completion of a permanent hospital at Azalea near Asheville in December 1918.[316]

The end of the war saw a short-lived revival of the mineral spring resort. In 1919, Sloan and his son reopened Haywood White Sulphur after fumigating its buildings and ensuring that "every room [was] repainted and repapered or kalsomined" to reassure guests anxious about tuberculosis.[317] Once again, the state newspaper press association met there; while acknowledging the previous use of the property for veterans, the press reporter exclaimed that "It would be hard to imagine a more delightful place to hold a convention."[318]

Within two years, however, the federal government leased the property again. The government closed a vocational training program at Johnson City, Tennessee's National Soldiers Home for veterans recovered from injuries and transported the student veterans by train to Haywood White Sulphur where they continued their trade education.[319] In addition, the government moved equipment to Haywood from the former Chick Springs, South Carolina, resort, which had also been employed as a vocational school.[320] The school at Haywood White Sulphur lasted two years; the government closed it in November 1924.[321]

Whether the Sloans reopened the hotel for a short period after the government ended its lease is not clear. The hotel, however, closed permanently in 1927; a former Waynesville mayor reminiscing about the town's history commented in 1928 that the hotel was now "deserted and desolate."[322] The hotel was demolished around 1940 or 1941.[323] Sloan family members operated a summer guest house, Blink Bonnie, on the site of the Haywood White Sulphur Hotel for a few years.[324] In 1971, the Sloan family donated the last remaining structure on the property, the spring house pavilion, to Waynesville.[325] The Sulphur Springs Park of about one acre stands today on Timothy Lane as a tribute to the grand southern resort.[326]

Eagles Nest

S.C. (Samuel Clement) Satterthwaite (Satterthwait), born around 1848 or 1849 in New Jersey, moved with his family to Aiken, South Carolina, as a teen. There, he began a family but lost his wife and his five-year-old daughter to unknown causes within two years of each other by 1881.[327] According to tradition, he visited the Haywood White Sulphur Springs in 1879 where he met his future wife, Hester Smathers of Turnpike, Buncombe County, a modest resort with a chalybeate spring.[328] Smathers was one of thirteen children whose parents descended from prominent pioneer families and was sister to George Henry Smathers, Waynesville mayor, state politician and land title legal expert, who cleared the Eastern Band of Cherokee Indians' title to the Qualla Indian Boundary in southwestern North Carolina.[329] The couple married in November 1881, a few months after the death of Satterthwaite's daughter, lived several years in Aiken, South Carolina, and then moved to Waynesville in 1890 where Satterthwaite opened a lumberyard.[330]

Perhaps due to the increase in Haywood County tourism brought by the expansion of the Western North Carolina Railroad in the late 1800s, Satterthwaite decided early in his family's move to Waynesville to build a hotel at the summit of the 5,066-foot-tall Junaluska Mountain (now known as North Eaglenest Mountain), about five miles northwest of Waynesville.[331] Over the next three years, Satterthwaite purchased four tracts of land on Junaluska Mountain, three of them with his brother-in-law, George Henry Smathers, and contracted around 1893 with largely a local Cherokee labor force to construct a road in five years from the mountain's base, in the rear of the White Sulphur Springs hotel, to its summit.[332]

According to contemporary accounts, the road was a masterpiece of construction, finished within the stipulated five years for a cost estimated at $5,000 to $6,000 or about $1,000 per mile.[333] The road consisted of a series of tight switchbacks, with about a 500 foot elevation gain per mile, roughly a 9.5 percent grade.[334] The Cherokee workmanship was such that when the road required resurfacing in subsequent decades, only two slight grade changes were required.[335]

The view from the Junaluska summit was outstanding. The North Carolina Press Association, meeting at the Haywood White Sulphur in 1898, traveled the newly constructed Junaluska Mountain road. One attendee wrote that from the top, "one can see into four states, some twenty counties; one can see the Blue Ridge, the Alleghany, the Smoky Mountains, Black Mountain, Mount Pisgah and the Nantahala or Valley River mountains."[336] Another newspaper editor offered that "[t]he view was truly magnificent and beyond description. As one looked out upon Nature's grand panorama of sky and mountain and valley and forest he stood enchanted by the ... beauty and grandeur...."[337]

With the completion of the road, hotel construction on the summit began the following year, and the Eagles Nest (Eagle's Nest) resort opened in June 1900.[338] The imposing hotel jutted out from the steep summit; one could stand on the resort's porch and drop a stone 200–300 feet before it hit the mountain slope.[339] Built largely from timber cleared from the road construction and from the mountain top, the majestic three-story hotel stood on a foundation made from the mountain's fieldstone; despite the hotel's high prominence on the mountain, no newspaper researched mentioned it ever being struck by lightning.[340]

The Eagles Nest followed the architectural style of many fashionable nineteenth-century health resorts but incorporated details to highlight its altitude. On the first floor were game rooms, ladies and gentlemen parlors or bathrooms, a dining room that sat one hundred or more guests, and a large lobby with a huge stone fireplace used even in summer months at that high elevation.[341] At least thirty bedrooms with ample windows to admire the scenery stood on the second and third levels; mid-roof, an observation platform similar to a widow's walk was perched between two large stone chimneys.[342] Visitors could sip cold mountain water (temperature ranging from 44 to 47 degrees) that a mechanical ram pumped up to the hotel from a nearby spring. To maximize views for guests to espy Waynesville 2,000 feet below and to permit healthy mountain air promenades, a wide verandah wrapped around half of the hotel; visitors often strolled after dining the thirty laps needed to complete a mile.[343] As the Tampa newspaper society editor Louise Frances

Dodge wrote for her readers about the "pretty hotel" looking over "cultivated valleys and forest-covered mountains": "The place is ideal! Just enough of the comforts of civilization and not too much!"[344]

The resort proved popular from the start. Over 1,000 visitors stayed at the hotel in 1903, its third season of operation.[345] Within a few years, Satterthwaite added ten rooms and eventually erected tents for overflow guests (and presumably for those who desired a more rugged experience while still near the hotel amenities).[346]

The Eagles Nest attracted a spectrum of largely southern visitors, from those who visited for a few hours from their hotels in Waynesville or Asheville to those who resided in the cool breezes at the Eagles Nest from June until the first killing frost.[347] A Tampa visitor from a Waynesville boarding house contrasted the "nice and cool" mountain weather to that of Florida's and admired the "one continuous stretch of mountains as far as the eye can see.... I was up on Junaluska mountain a few days ago. You get the most beautiful view from there."[348] An Eagles Nest guest from Birmingham described the "numbers of long and short surries [from Waynesville] loaded with passengers, all seeking the mountain top" where they might observe, from the hotel's tall platform called the "Point," the villages of Dellwood and Hazelwood and the Great Smoky and Nantahala mountain ranges.[349] Dodge in her 1903 visit recorded hotel guests from South Carolina, Alabama, Texas, Georgia, Florida, Tennessee, Louisiana, and Mississippi either enjoying the view from the verandah or huddled inside before the evening fire.[350]

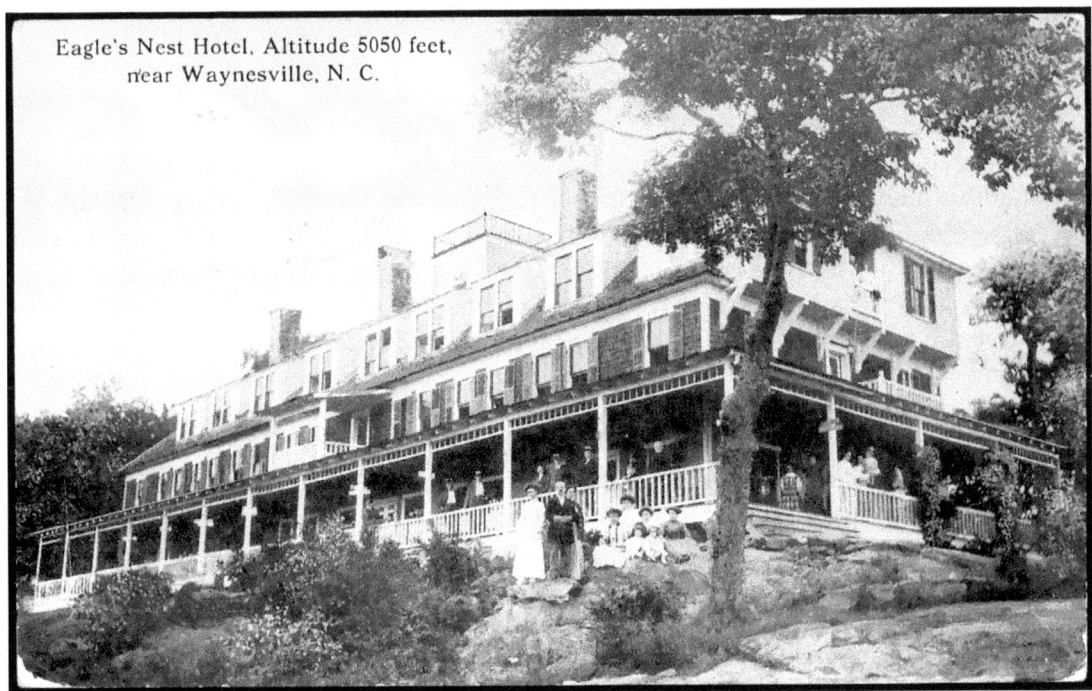

"Eagle's Nest Hotel. Altitude 5050 feet. Near Waynesville, N.C. [1907–1915]" (Postcard image from Buncombe County Special Collections, Pack Memorial Public Library, Asheville, NC. ID: AB118).

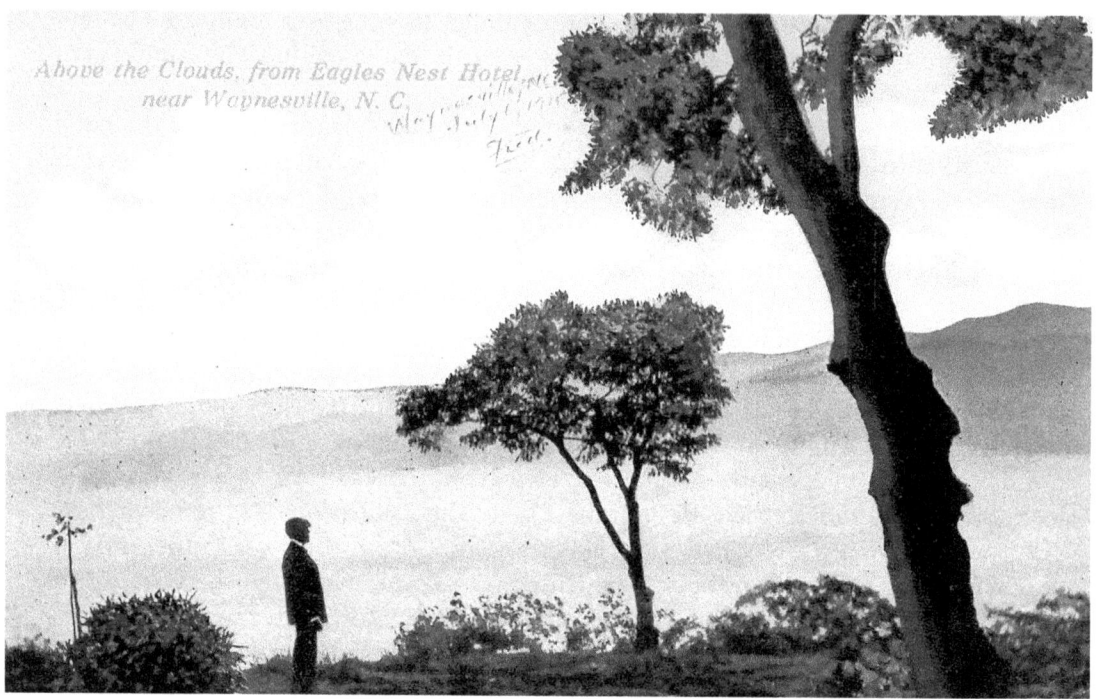

"Above the Clouds, from Eagles Nest Hotel, near Waynesville, N.C. [1915]" (Postcard image from Buncombe County Special Collections, Pack Memorial Public Library, Asheville, NC. ID: AD580).

Other guests were those with sufficient discretionary income who spent the summers making the rounds of early twentieth-century vacation spots (and homes of benevolent friends). An Augusta mother and two children left the Eagles Nest after two months to spend an additional two months in Chattanooga before heading home.[351] A Florida minister and his wife visited the Eagles Nest, traveled northeast to Johnson City, Tennessee, and then returned southwest to Hendersonville, North Carolina, to recreate.[352] An intricate itinerary was devised by a wealthy matron who traveled from Selma, Alabama, in the heat of July to Pensacola and then to the cool climes of Asheville, Waynesville and the Eagles Nest, and on to Washington, D.C., and New York City where she returned to the south via steamer to Savannah in September.[353]

The "Sneezers," however, constituted a major segment of the Eagles Nest's guests. Just as Roan Mountain's Cloudland Hotel one hundred miles to the northeast on the Tennessee—North Carolina border at 6,285 feet advertised its absence of hay fever, so did the Junaluska Mountain resort at 1,200 feet lower in elevation proclaim its "Ideal conditions to build up mind and body. Immunity from Hay fever."[354] Although the *Journal of the American Medical Association* disputed the popular notion that altitude alone protected against hay fever unless the elevation exceeded 6,000 feet, it endorsed the Eagles Nest for providing "complete temporary relief."[355] Accordingly, an Asheville resident reported that he "had seen the most violent cases almost instantly relieved at Junaluska."[356] A regional newspaper reported

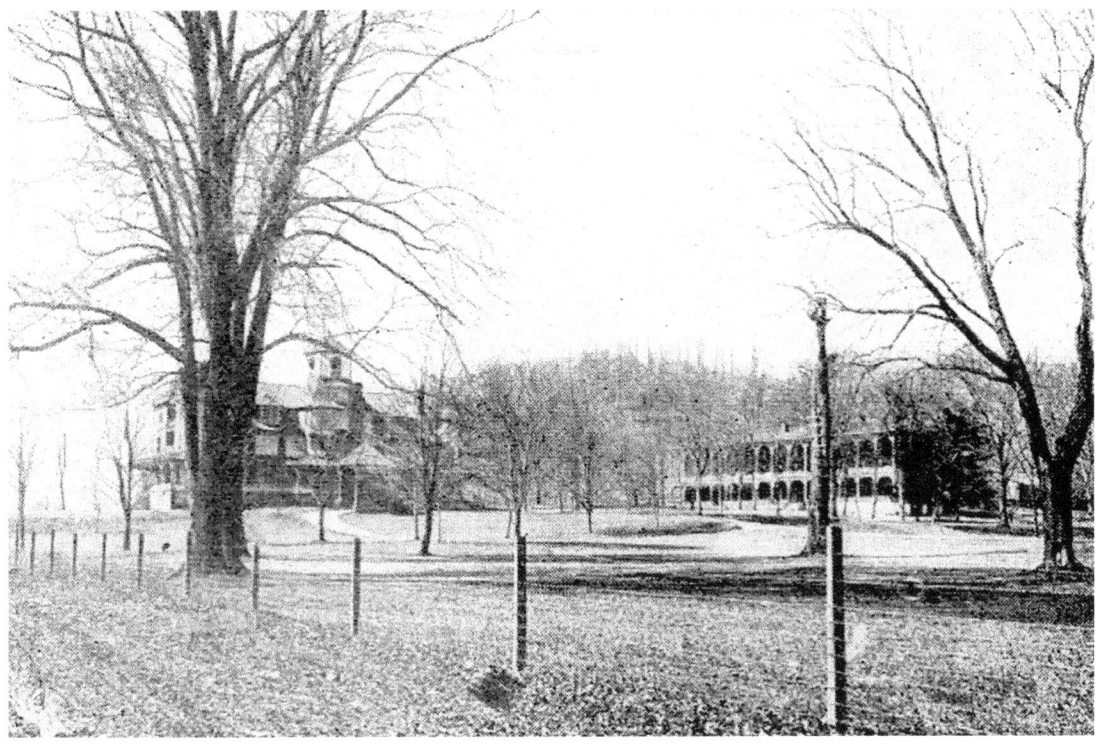

"Haywood White Sulphur Springs [1900–1910]" (Image from Buncombe County Special Collections, Pack Memorial Public Library, Asheville, NC. ID: M939-5).

that "sufferers are immediately relieved on Junaluska's top, and so they go up there, whether the house is ready [open for the season] or not" to explain why the Eagles Nest opened earlier than most mountain resorts.[357]

One newspaper journalist described the average hay fever sufferer who eventually found relief on Junaluska as looking like a "joke" to those ignorant of the affliction.[358] To the journalist, sufferers appeared to have "extremely bad colds.... [T]hey go about with tearful eyes to an accompaniment of sneezes. Rag-weed is to them as red flannel to a bull."[359] Perhaps as a sign of sympathy or hospitality to provide the sufferers and other guests, especially those recovering from acute diseases, with tranquility, Eagles Nest ads promised, in perhaps an unintended comparative juxtaposition, "No consumptives or annoyance from mosquitoes, flies, fleas or unruly children. No hay fever."[360]

National hay fever groups assessed the Eagles Nest for pollen irritants. The U.S. Hay Fever Association withdrew the resort from consideration to host an annual meeting after ranking it lower than New Hampshire's White Mountain health resorts; the North Carolina press then accused the association of being "New England in sentiment altogether."[361] The American Hay Fever Association's hundreds of so-called "Sneezers," however, convened there after determining that all hay fever sufferers who had visited the Eagles Nest the season before had remained symptom-free during their sojourns.[362] The large convention drew the attention of the Southern Railway, the successor to the Western North Carolina Railroad, which

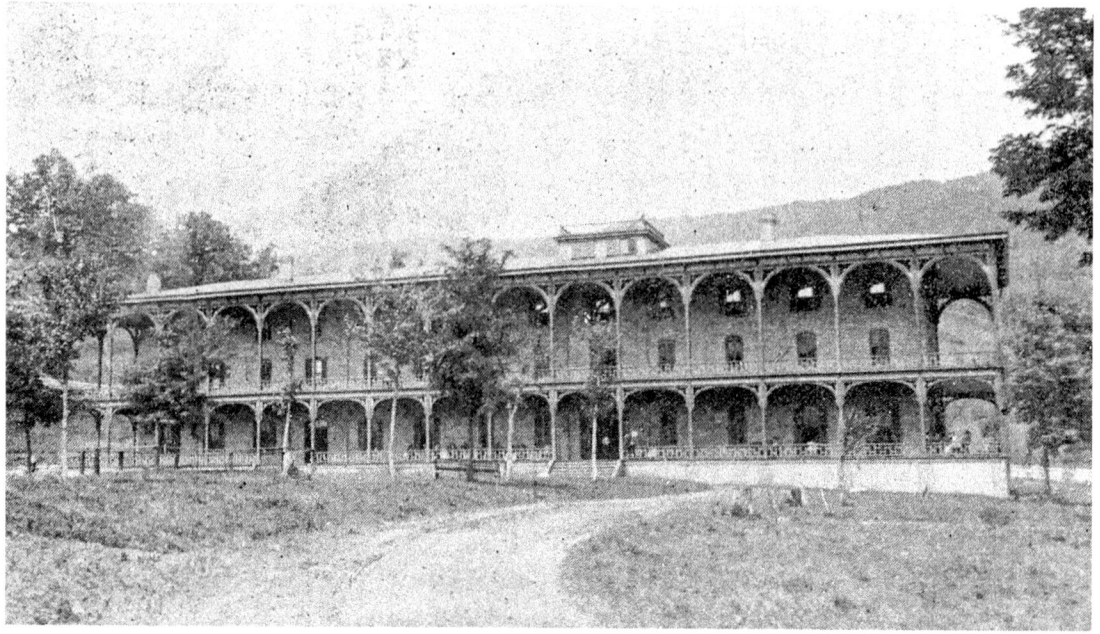

"The Haywood White Sulphur Springs Hotel, Waynesville" (*Health Resorts of the South* [Boston: George H. Chapin, 1892], 303. Buncombe County Special Collections, Pack Memorial Public Library, Asheville, NC).

contemplated publicizing the Eagles Nest to hay fever sufferers who had been traveling to the White Mountains and the Michigan lakeshore resorts after the demise of Roan Mountain's Cloudland Hotel in the early 1910s.[363] Even into the 1940s, the Hay Fever Prevention Association endorsed the Eagles Nest location for its pollen-free air; it stood out along with Glen Ayre, North Carolina, a hamlet on the Roan Mountain slopes, among a list of locales recommended for hay fever sufferers that was largely centered in New York, Vermont, New Hampshire, and Maine.[364]

Less than three years after the successful American Hay Fever Association convention, however, the Eagles Nest burned down in a fire of unknown origin. In April 1918, Waynesville residents noticed plumes of smoke rising from the hotel's upper rooms and roof. By the time S.C. Satterthwaite's son and son-in-law could motor up the steep road to the hotel, the fire had destroyed everything; the loss was estimated at $50,000 with insurance for $20,000.[365] Letters and telegrams poured into Waynesville from past guests, many of whom had been coming to the Eagles Nest for over a decade, who bemoaned the loss and encouraged the Satterthwaites to build anew.[366]

The Satterthwaites did not rebuild and sold the property and road over the decades. The road was rebranded as a toll road, the "Scenic Eagle's Nest Road," which operated from 1937 to 1941.[367] Various parties established hostelries and camps bearing the "Eagles Nest" moniker, one inn advertising itself in 1925 as the "NEW Eagle's Nest Hotel" for hay fever sufferers.[368] In the late 1950s–early 1960s, three Florida realtors built a new road and developed an 800-acre tract on Junaluska's slopes.[369] As of 2018, the Eagles Nest hotel site was in private hands.[370]

South Carolina

Introduction

The state of South Carolina conjures a variety of impressions and memories for those who have visited or lived in the Palmetto State. Charleston, founded in 1670 by English colonists, may suggest the Rainbow Row of homes along the Battery, Fort Sumter, Boone Hall Plantation, or the annual Spoleto Festival USA. South of Charleston are Lowcountry barrier islands such as Hilton Head Island and St. Helena Island, the latter known as the site of the Penn Center, one of the first free schools in the U.S. for emancipated slaves and where Martin Luther King, Jr., led Southern Christian Conference Leadership retreats. North of Charleston is the Pee Dee River region, home to the Darlington Raceway and the "Grand Strand" coast. Columbia, the state capital, and the counties of Newberry and Lancaster constitute a few of the geopolitical entities in the Midlands. To the Midlands' northwest lies the Upstate region, also known as the Upcountry. This region includes the Piedmont and the Blue Ridge Mountains along the North Carolina border. In the Upstate, one can root for Clemson or Furman University sports teams, buy a peach from a road stand along the Cherokee Foothills Scenic Highway, or climb to the top of Pinnacle Mountain in Table Rock State Park.[1] The Upstate also is home to South Carolina's four counties that fall into Southern Appalachia: Oconee, Pickens, Greenville and Spartanburg.

Health resorts in northwestern South Carolina developed, apart from the lure of mineral waters, as reactions to two major initiatives: Lowcountry planters seeking cooler climes and the building of intra-state railroads. Although Charleston itself was largely unaffected by malaria due to its salty marshes, it was susceptible to yellow fever and, of course, to the hot humid weather that ran from late spring through late summer.[2] Originally, Lowcountry planters around Charleston visited Sullivan's Island for relief while planters situated south of Charleston established second residences at other seaside resorts, for example, Eding's Bay for Edisto Island planters.[3] About 1800, Lowcountry planters began traveling to the northern parts of the state during the "sickly season," which usually lasted from May through the first hard frost, generally in November.[4] Greenville erected its first hotel for summer visitors around 1815. Spartanburg began developing as a resort area in the 1830s.[5] The more mountainous counties of Oconee and Pickens received Charlestonians largely in the postbellum period when the Atlanta and Charlotte Air Line Railway (also known

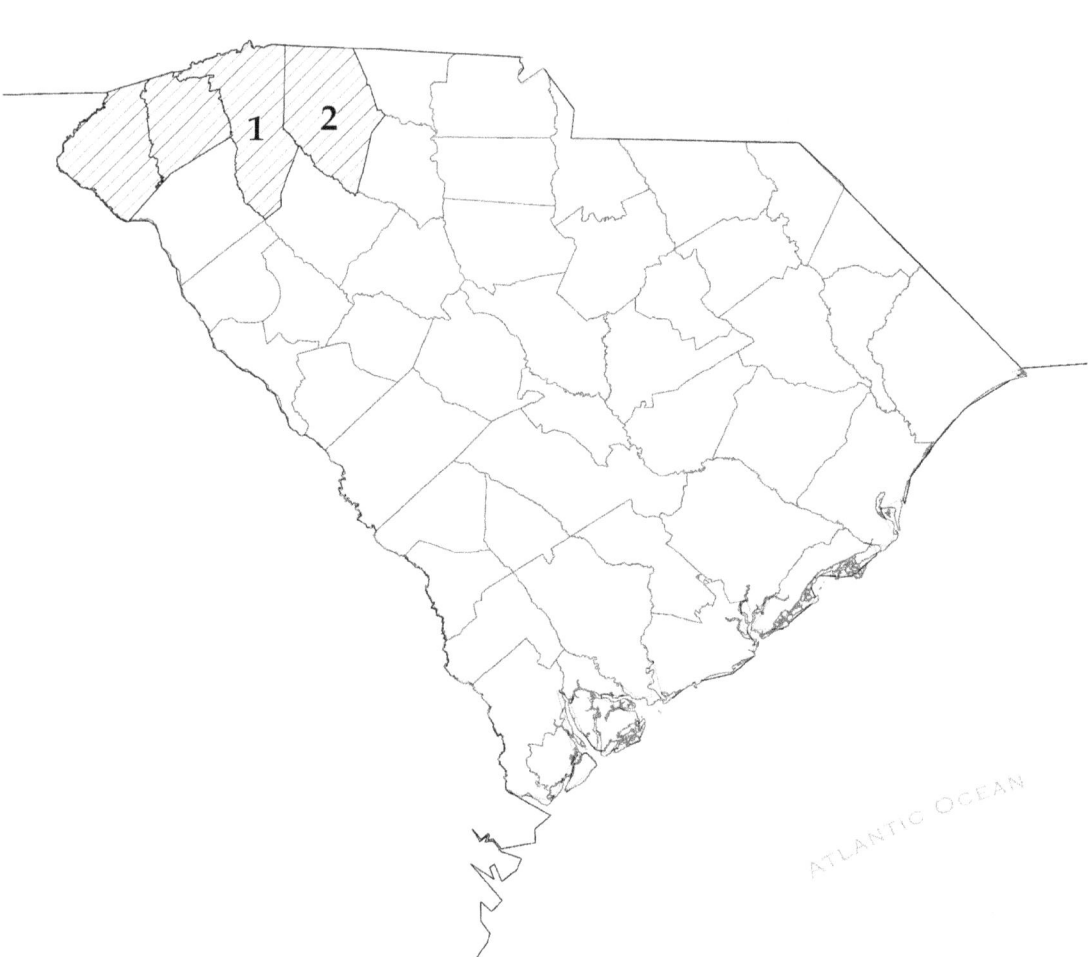

South Carolina counties with featured health resorts: (1) Greenville County, Chick Springs; (2) Spartanburg County, Glenn Springs (Sources: Esri, NOAA, USGS. Cartographer: Sayona Turner, East Tennessee State University).

by many other names due to mergers) began stopping in Seneca; in addition, the much shorter (and uncompleted) Blue Ridge Railroad ran from Anderson to Walhalla.[6] Although most of the Southern Appalachian health resorts of South Carolina were found in Spartanburg County, Greenville claimed the fashionable Chick Springs resort and Oconee and Pickens were home to a few short-lived and less publicized mineral springs establishments.

Oconee County was formed in 1868 from the division of the Pickens District into Oconee and Pickens counties, but its county seat of Walhalla dates back to 1850 when the German Colonization Society conceived of the "beautiful garden of immortal heroes" of Norse mythology.[7] Walhalla and Seneca, about nine miles to the southeast, developed regional reputations as resorts along the Piedmont Air Line

Railroad (Atlanta and Richmond Air Line Railroad) due to their elevation ("malaria is unknown") and dry air to "strengthen those troubled with throat or lung affections."[8] In keeping with the county's name—Oconee can roughly be translated from the Cherokee as "place of the springs"—the Keowee Hotel in Seneca publicized a chalybeate springs from which "[s]everal wonderful cures have been reported."[9] About a mile from Walhalla was West Union's Blue Ridge Mineral Springs that opened in 1903 to capitalize in part on rail passengers connecting from Anderson on the Blue Ridge Railroad, a planned line through Georgia's Rabun Gap to Knoxville that terminated at Walhalla due to insufficient funding and corruption.[10]

J.C. Shockley built the Blue Ridge Mineral Springs Hotel behind a lumber company that fronted the railroad. Although ads noted the health resort's "three fine springs," the ads mainly accentuated the hotel's location in the "Land of the Sky and Sapphire Country" as the chief drawing card.[11] After the lumber company moved to a different location ("the Keller place"), M.E. Ruthrauff and his wife, who had leased the property from Shockley in 1905, planned to landscape the front grounds, add walks and flowers to the grove surrounding the springs, build a tennis court and to offer "other out-door amusements."[12]

The season of 1905 appears to have been a success for the Ruthrauffs. One week in August saw the arrival of over sixty guests, largely from Anderson and Columbia (the Ruthrauffs' hometown) and to a lesser extent from Atlanta, Pine Mountain, and Toccoa in Georgia. A few visitors also registered from Alabama, St. Louis, Cincinnati, and Texas. Because husbands often registered families under only their surnames, it cannot be determined how many guests from outside South Carolina were tourists versus drummers (salesmen) or other businessmen.[13]

By 1907, the resort consisted of a hotel with thirty-two rooms and six cottages over twelve acres. That spring, Shockley auctioned off the property, including furnishings.[14] W.C. Woods owned and managed the property in 1909; the Stuckes (perhaps two sisters) managed the hotel in 1911. Today, the hotel as well as the nearby railroad depot no longer stand.[15]

Pickens County is home to Sassafras Mountain, the state's highest peak (3,560 feet), and to Table Rock State Park, built by the Civilian Conservation Corps in the late 1930s to provide access to one of the state's premier geological formations. While the northern part of the county is mountainous, the southern area evolves into rolling hills. John C. Calhoun resided in the southern area at his plantation, Fort Hill, which became the foundation for Clemson University after the death in 1888 of Thomas Clemson, the widower of Anna Maria, Calhoun's daughter.[16] With the building of the Atlanta and Charlotte Air Line Railroad through the county in the early 1870s, small communities such as Easley and Liberty grew along its route.[17]

One Pickens County mineral spring resort that most likely benefited from the railroad was Ambler Springs. Known until the late 1870s as Griffin's Springs, the resort began appearing in the local press a few years after rail had reached Pickens County.[18] Although little documentation survives about the resort, the physician James K. Crook, one of the foremost mineral water authorities of the late nineteenth century, highlighted Ambler Springs in a 1906 medical journal as one of South Carolina's "most important localities now in use."[19] Ambler's two springs lay about a mile from the "small" resort hotel, the Ambler House, which itself stood about six or seven miles north of Pickens Court House.[20] The springs' dissolved salts—largely calcium carbonate (an antacid), sodium carbonate, magnesium carbonate (Epsom salts), and potassium sulphate—attracted those afflicted by dyspepsia and "skin affections of the eczematous class."[21] The resort supplied its water commercially in the late 1800s but had stopped bottling production by 1911.[22] Guests in the late nineteenth and early twentieth centuries largely visited from two ends of the state: many from Greenville, about 20 miles away, but the majority from Charleston to escape the city's summer heat and humidity. Other guests seeking cooler temperatures hailed from Florida and the Lowcountry's Edisto. Less frequently, visitors arrived from the Midlands' Edgefield and Newberry and from other Upstate counties such as Laurens and Anderson. Quite a few guests over the years consisted of families and young single ladies accompanied by their mothers or presumedly female chaperones.[23] Visitors often spent two weeks or more during the summer and enjoyed outdoor activities such as picnics and excursions in the mountains to Table Rock, Caesars Head, and North Carolina.[24]

In Greenville County, visitors frequented the Caesars Head resort and the elite Chick Springs. Caesars Head, perhaps named for a granitic gneiss outcropping, is preserved as a state park today and known for its spectacular vistas from its 3,208-foot peak.[25] In the mid–1850s, Colonel Benjamin Hagood of the Pickens District purchased 500 acres and in 1860 built a hotel near the summit that could be reached by the Jones Gap Road from Greenville to Asheville.[26] Although the hotel publicized in the postbellum period its elevation for treating "all diseases of the Throat and Lungs.... Hay Fever and Malarial Affections" and its mineral spring "possessing fine tonic and alterative qualities," it was much more widely known as a recreative place for antebellum Lowcountry planters or as a sight-seeing destination rather than as a health resort.[27]

Greenville County's Chick Springs rivaled neighboring Spartanburg County's Glenn Springs throughout the decades. Visitors to each contrasted the hotel, company, and water. Such a guest in 1852 wrote that the Chick "accommodations are tolerably good, although inferior to Glenn's" and that resorts such as Chick's become "dull to those who have no special object in view."[28] Two Newberry residents visiting Chick, for example, miserably complained of being "cribbed, cabined, and confined" in their small cottage and consoled themselves that they would soon travel to Glenn Springs to drink its curative water, "not surpassed by any other in the whole country, for Liver Complaints, Dyspepsia, Neuralgia, Cutaneous Diseases, etc."[29] Glenn Springs hosted a lively clientele, including many state office-holders such as the governor, during the summer. One guest in 1844, thinking of the heated presidential campaign around the annexation of the pro-slavery Republic of Texas, penned that the 400–500 persons that he encountered at Glenn Springs enabled him to "[converse] with gentlemen from various quarters of the State upon the interesting and in some places exciting topics, which are now being agitated before the people."[30] At Chick Springs, on the other hand, an antebellum patron complained of the lack of stimulating conversation among the many card-playing guests.[31]

In addition to Glenn Springs, Spartanburg County contained several other watering holes exclusive of those found in adjacent Cherokee County, which was carved out of Spartanburg, Union, and Laurens counties in 1897 (Limestone Springs, a venerable antebellum resort and today the site of Limestone College, lies in Cherokee County, outside of Southern Appalachia).[32] These health resorts, supplying largely chalybeate and sulphur mineral waters, included Cherokee, Pacolet, Garrett, and White Stone Lithia Springs.[33]

Antebellum travelers made the rounds of some of these springs in the old Spartanburg District, notably Cherokee, Glenn, and Limestone, just as they traveled between Chick and Glenn. One writer in 1839 made the inevitable comparison between the Spartanburg springs and the Virginia springs by penning that "we are beginning to rival Virginia in watering places, and that the time has come when we may claim the favorable consideration of the whole South for our own State." Cherokee Springs, he declared, was "equal in purity and efficacy to the celebrated red sulphur of Virginia … highly curative for many diseases, particularly those arising from impurities, or a phlogi-tic [sic] state of the blood."[34]

The accommodations at Cherokee Springs, about eight miles north of Spartanburg, were "very fair for a small company" in 1839 but had expanded fourteen years later when Fielding Cantrell, a large landowner and owner of eleven enslaved people, purchased the property and erected a twenty-room hotel with a four-column portico.[35] In 1856, the hotel advertised its "sweet and airy bed-rooms and piazzas to both stories the entire length of the building" for those desiring fresh air and porches for promenades. The springs, "known all over the State for their valuable medical properties," bubbled out of a hand-hewn rock basin to reduce the water's temperature; in addition, plunge baths and a shower were attached to the springs.[36] Cherokee Springs, which catered to Lowcountry planters, nonetheless was not as fashionable as Chick Springs, whose demand allowed it to charge a monthly rate of $25, a quarter more than that of Cherokee's $20 monthly rate.[37]

Cherokee remained open for the first few years of the Civil War. In 1862, a guest described hotel dances; ads that same year encouraged "our low country friends" to experience the springs, "unsurpassed by any for health and comfort." Meanwhile, Cantrell listed the resort for sale.[38]

From 1869 through 1872, Methodist minister Robert C. Oliver, who embraced the Holiness movement then taking root in the state, owned the resort as a way to earn income for his charitable work.[39] Following the Methodist and Holiness stance against alcohol, gambling and other perceived vices, Oliver and his physician neighbor Dr. Joseph Wofford, who managed the resort, banned drinking, cards, and dancing. They offered "Gymnastics," however, presumably as a healthy alternative. Oliver also built a church in the vicinity.[40]

Over the next decades, the resort changed hands several times; the usual gaieties resumed upon Oliver's sale in 1872 to a former Confederate officer and Citadel professor from Columbia.[41] In 1906, John Humphreys took ownership and resold the property the following year to the Cherokee Springs Hotel Company, a group of a dozen local men. Controversy erupted around the sale as regional newspapers reported that the company of white businessmen had allegedly bought the property for $3,000 less than the sales price that would have been offered to Booker T.

Washington, who had visited the state several times with a particular interest in educational institutions, and who supposedly had plans to convert the health resort into a school.[42] Washington had no designs on the resort; the resort most likely sold for less due to rail construction that was planned to skirt Cherokee Springs by a good mile and a half as opposed to racism.[43] In 1959, the hotel was disassembled, and the construction of a state road piled dirt into the octagonal pool at the springs. Today, the resort of Cherokee Springs no longer exists in the small unincorporated community of its namesake.[44]

Pacolet Springs, about nine miles east of Spartanburg on the west side of the Pacolet River near Moyer Drive, likely began as the Spartanburg area's earliest watering hole.[45] Phillip Freneau, often called the "Poet of the American Revolution," visited the springs and penned in "The Invalid": "Resolved, he left the cool sea-breeze In Pacolet Springs to drown disease."[46]

A decade later, the *Columbian Herald* publicized the sale of 4,574 acres including "Pacolet Springs and Valuable Iron Works" located near the Pacolet River and Lawson's Fork Creek.[47] Governor John Drayton in 1802 wrote that the springs "are said to be of much virtue in rheumatic, cutaneous, and some other complaints."[48] By 1855, Colonel Robert Coleman Poole, a slaveowner, public official, and owner of Spartanburg's elite Mansion House hotel, was operating a hotel for 40 to 60 guests; the springs consequently also became known as Poole's Springs.[49] Perhaps due in part to the Panic of 1857, Poole lost the property through a state bank sale that year (his son took over the operations of the Mansion House) but evidently his family regained title.[50] Like Cherokee Springs, Pacolet Springs provided no amusements or recreational activities during its existence; the sickly and those families desiring a quiet ambiance therefore constituted most of its guests.[51] A massive flood in 1903 heavily damaged the hotel, swept away former slave cabins, and dumped mud into the mineral spring. The Poole family tore down the hotel and never rebuilt the resort.[52]

About one and a half miles away from the Spartanburg Court House, Garrett Springs began as Thomson's Springs in 1848 when J. Waddy Thomson discovered a chalybeate springs on his farm that promptly found favor with locals as "improv[ing] our health, to a considerable degree."[53] By 1874, G.P. Garrett owned the springs—Thomson had died in 1868—and offered an "ice cream garden," boat riding on Lawson's Fork, croquet, and picnics. A minor scandal erupted when rumors swirled that the resort was offering lager beer, not just its usual lemonade, and on Sundays to boot.[54]

By 1885, Garrett Springs was one of three South Carolina establishments bottling its water for sale; the other two were the more famous Chick Springs and Glenn Springs.[55] Garrett further expanded his mineral springs operations in 1890 by opening a fountain in Spartanburg from water pumped from the springs via his family's patented hydraulic motor. The ensuing interest piqued local media to speculate if other resorts such as Glenn Springs or Union's West Springs might employ the technology to boost the local economies.[56] Garrett, a resourceful entrepreneur, at the same time operated a bookstore, an ice cream parlor (no doubt based on his successful ice cream garden at the springs), and an office for shipping his water at $4 per crate across the country, guaranteed "you will feel [like] a new *person* [italics original]."[57]

Textile magnate J.P. Stevens and local businessman J.T. Harris bought the resort property and began in 1906 to develop it into a new resort, Rock[y] Cliff Lithia Springs, naturally claiming the water to be superior to all others in the region, and to be shipped by the newly formed Rock Cliff Lithia Water Company. Stevens devised plans to install a dance pavilion and a large swimming pool.[58]

In 1910, Rock Cliff Park opened on the old springs resort site. It boasted a Ferris wheel, a merry-go-round, and a stomach-churning feature, the "ocean wave," which dipped its occupants while turning. In addition to the swimming pool and dance pavilion, boating and bowling were also offered. The park, which stood near Spartanburg's Heywood Avenue, is gone today.[59]

J.T. Harris, Stevens' business partner, previously had developed Laurens County's financially successful Harris Lithia Springs health resort. Harris Lithia Springs not only guaranteed a cure for cancer but also gloated that "Persons ... given up by the best medical skill of the country as incurable, but after a short stay at the Springs are entirely cured."[60] In 1901, having sold the Laurens health resort, Harris partnered with local investors to purchase Spartanburg County's Irby Springs, a relatively unimproved watering hole for picnics and outdoor activities located a few miles from the Rich Hill depot.[61]

Harris's new resort opened for the summer of 1902 as White Stone Lithia Springs, named for the color of the top of the rocks where the mineral water flowed.[62] To demonstrate its rank among the exclusive resorts of the region, the hotel publicized its grand dimensions: "800 feet of piazza" for its 350 guests to enjoy the fresh air, the dining room ("40 by 80" feet) for 200, and the ball room ("40 by 100" feet) with "286 incandescent lights grouped most artistically in the ceiling." The hotel, with at least 109 rooms, contained a rotunda around which the second and third floors circled to provide a view for "hundreds of spectators."[63] To further its prestige, the resort branded itself as "the largest brick Hotel in the Carolinas or in Georgia" and billed its water as "The Lightest Mineral Water Known," "a marvel among Springs."[64]

The immodestly worded ads about the mineral water claimed some truth: the White Stone Lithia Water garnered first honors at the 1904 Louisiana Purchase Exposition in St. Louis and won prizes at other fairs as well.[65] Just as Chick Springs and Glenn Springs marketed their ginger ales made from their mineral waters, so did White Stone. The health resort, however, taking a creative cue from the spring water's carbonation, pitched its White Stone Lithia Ale as retaining its gasses "after remaining open 48 hours, while most Ginger Ale on the market will not retain theirs [for] 48 seconds."[66] The resort also offered plain water and carbonated water for shipping.[67]

In common with the investors who rebuilt large hotels at Chick Springs and Glenn Springs in the late 1800s through early 1900s, Harris also perceived the potential of income from hosting large conventions. In 1903, White Stone hosted the state press association. The following year, 300 members of the Mystic Shriners of the Carolinas met at the resort.[68]

In August 1904, Harris sold the resort and its 187 acres for about $100,000 (more than $3 million in 2022 dollars) to the Savannah wholesale grocer Dougan & Sheftall and to Solomon Sheftall, also from Savannah. Harris, however, at a cost of $50,000, received a ten-year exclusivity to the mineral waters shipping business.[69] Unfortunately, for Dougan & Sheftall, a kitchen fire a mere two years later destroyed the brick hotel, which was only partially insured for the estimated loss of $30,000.[70] Harris bought the property again in 1908; by 1911, E.A. Dugan of Savannah had purchased it from the holding bank as a family home. The U.S. Army bought the property as part of a larger land purchase for the building of Camp Croft Military Center during World War II. Today, the mineral springs land lies within Croft State Park.[71]

The Southern Appalachian resorts in South Carolina in the antebellum era discussed in this chapter are broadly characterized by their hosting of fire-eating, pro-slavery secessionist guests.[72] Although Greenville County Unionists beat Nullifiers for state legislature seats in 1830 and 1832 and carried the district for a Unionist who lost to a Nullifier in the 1834 Congressional race, the state as a whole was squarely in the nullification camp against tariffs, considered an economic drain on the cotton economy.[73] Chick Springs and Glenn Springs played host to politicians and planters who espoused rabid secessionist views. To use a modern phrase, the resorts served as "echo chambers" where the fire-eaters could influence and shape ideologies.

Interestingly, John C. Calhoun, one of the most infamous of the South Carolina fire-eaters, may not have frequented these resorts although his wife convalesced for a period at Glenn Springs. On a trip from Washington, D.C., back to his cherished Fort Hill in 1846, he did, however, visit the Salt Sulphur Springs and White Sulphur Springs in modern West Virginia where he joined his wife and daughter for several days. The family then meandered through southwest Virginia's Wytheville and Abingdon, and then rested at Warm Springs (now Hot Springs), North Carolina, before crossing over the mountains into South Carolina.[74] Most likely, he frequented the Virginia springs more than the resorts in his home state as he could consort with his "equals" of the nation's elite at the Virginia springs; furthermore, Chick and Glenn Springs did not come into their own until after his death in 1850.

The Unionist views of much of the Upcountry did not presume a pro-abolitionist stance: one could be pro-slavery and pro–Union. Therefore, whether Unionist or Nullifier, the Southern Appalachian South Carolina antebellum resort owners and managers often owned enslaved persons or leased them from local owners as cooks, maids, porters, or servants.[75] Alfred Taylor, who in 1859 served as Chick Springs' manager and later became part-owner, came from a family that owned 15 slaves.[76] It is not unreasonable to assume that a few of the enslaved persons may have worked at the resort. Owners of Cherokee, Chick, and Glenn Springs held enslaved persons who may have assisted in property improvements as well as in providing services for guests.

The Upcountry resorts largely remained open during at least part of the Civil War due to lack of fighting until Union Major General George Stoneman's spring 1865 raid into South Carolina. For the majority of the war years, the resorts provided an "attractive refuge" for those from areas experiencing warfare.[77] After Union forces captured Beaufort following the Battle of Port Royal Sound in November 1861, Glenn Springs became a second home to refugees from the Beaufort area.[78] Cherokee

Springs advertised in the Charleston newspapers until at least 1863.[79] Although it is not known whether Chick Springs was open during the first year of the war, its hotel burnt down in 1862.

A different threat forced residents in the Deep South to evacuate their homes in the postbellum period: yellow fever. Memphis suffered severe outbreaks in 1878 and 1879, prompting the Tennessee State Board of Health to direct residents to "quietly remove your families to places of safety."[80] The poorly understood fever—some physicians claimed that newsprint and mail harbored its "germs"—caused some areas to bar entry. A Nashville commentator wrote that the "fear of yellow fever is so intense in character that Memphians are often peremptorily and abruptly invited out of houses even by old friends until now the refugee says he is from anywhere else but Memphis."[81] Accordingly, during the 1888 Jacksonville, Florida, yellow fever outbreak, some South Carolina communities barred entry to refugees and heeded the South Carolina State Board of Health warning during an 1898 epidemic that no elevation in the state was immune.[82] Although the Southern Appalachian resorts in the state, however, do not appear to have admitted refugees, the reason may lie with their geographies rather than with governmental mandates or recommendations. Those families traveling from Memphis, New Orleans, Mississippi, and other points west of the Appalachians tended to head toward East Tennessee, North Carolina, or parts of northern Georgia. A Pickens County resident traveling in Georgia in 1879 commented that the "great influx of excursionists and refugees from yellow fever … give Atlanta quite a lively appearance."[83] An Anderson, South Carolina, newspaper reported that families from Jackson, Mississippi, had escaped to the Great Smoky Mountains in North Carolina where hotels and boarding houses had "thrown their doors open to yellow fever refugees." The same newspaper described travel to Walhalla from that part of the Smokies as "very difficult" as it required hacks and wagons through the mountains in the absence of rail.[84] For many of the wealthy families fleeing yellow fever on the Atlantic coast, the resorts in Southern Appalachian South Carolina were bypassed in favor of the more posh and traditional enclaves around Hendersonville in North Carolina.[85] In addition, the federal government arranged for trains to take refugees to western North Carolina.[86]

Chick Springs and Glenn Springs will be examined more closely in the pages to follow. They exemplify antebellum resorts in Southern Appalachia that transitioned from watering holes frequented by politicians and Lowcountry planters to twentieth-century hotels hosting professional associations and business conventions. Over decades of multiple management, the owners generally understood their hotels' key claim to fame: the sulphur and chalybeate mineral waters. From providing facilities that allowed patrons to ease the "itch" in the early days to shipping carbonated ginger ales in the 1900s, the proprietors enabled the resorts' success for nearly a century each.

Chick Springs

Greenville County forms a rough rectangular shape, about twenty miles wide and sixty miles long, in northwestern South Carolina.[87] The county stretches from the North Carolina border to Anderson County to its southwest, Laurens County to its southeast, and meets Abbeville County to the south at a four-county corner shared with Laurens and Anderson. The Southern Appalachian counties of Pickens and Spartanburg lie directly to its west and east respectively. Named for Revolutionary General Nathaniel Greene in 1786 (the last "e" was dropped), Greenville County is home to Furman University and Bob Jones University and birthplace of personalities as varied as the late blues singer Josh "Pinewood Tom" White, civil rights activist Jesse Jackson, and actor Bo Hopkins.[88]

Greenville, the county seat, stands at an elevation of about 960 feet, lower than neighboring North Carolina's Hendersonville's 2,000-foot altitude just forty miles away, but obviously higher than that of the Lowcountry's Charleston. In the early 1800s, Greenville became both a destination and a stopping point for Lowcountry planters seeking cooler climes in the mountains. Its first resort hotel received guests in 1815, and its popularity as a summer resort increased in subsequent decades. Around 1840, James Silk Buckingham, the British author and traveler, wrote about Greenville: "The healthiness and coolness of the atmosphere has gradually drawn persons here for a short summer's sojourn…. [E]very year more and more country villas are built by wealthy people from the low-country; while visitors stop here in great numbers on their way up to the Springs of North Carolina and Virginia; and still more on their return from the mountains to the coast."[89]

In 1825, physician Burrell (or Burwell) Chick moved from Newberry about seventy miles to the northwest to Greenville County. While on a deer hunt in the county in 1838, Chick's Native American guides described to him a mineral spring—Lick Springs—that cured dermatological sores. Intrigued, Chick paid for a chemical analysis of the water, purchased the spring and surrounding area, and then built a hotel that opened in 1842.[90] Chick Springs quickly became popular, competing with more established North Carolina resorts for clientele. Just three years later, a traveler staying in Greenville attested to this fact: "Greenville has been dull during the past week. The amount of traveling through this place seems to have diminished…. [T]hose that do come here are soon attracted to 'Buncombe,' to the 'Warm Springs,'—the 'Chick Springs' twelve miles from the village…."[91]

Upon Chick's death in 1847, his two sons, Reuben S. and Pettus W., bought the property for $3,000 (about $110,000 in 2022 dollars).[92] To accommodate increasing crowds and their desire for recreation, the Chick brothers in 1851 built an addition to the hotel and advertised a "Billiard Table and Ten Pin Alley."[93] As additional evidence of the growth of the health resort and the summer homes around it, a post office was established there by the same year.[94]

Travelers making the rounds of health resorts compared their stays at Chick Springs to other resorts just as online travel forums today might debate the merits of one cruise line to another. For example, one writer penned that Chick rooms were much more "pleasant" than those at Glenn Springs in neighboring Spartanburg County, but that the fare was lacking ("aged and rancid butter" among other deficiencies). Furthermore, the writer also flippantly opined that the free use of the billiards table and ten pin alley was justified because otherwise it "would certainly require handsome pay to induce a good player to approach either of them."[95]

Turning somber, the same writer observed that the chief amusement at Chick Springs lay in "poking fun at an uncouth rustic, Gabe," who evidently was Black.[96] In defense, the slave-owning Chick brothers published a racist rejoinder that the writer had in the past "sung negro [sic] songs and said negro [sic] sayings [for] amusement"; why did he not "join in exclaiming 'hurrah for Gabe,' and the like, then sing dandy Jim, and finish by 'jumping about, turning about, and dancing *Jim Crow* [italics original].'"[97] The writer's jabs at the resort additionally precipitated an indignant defense of the Chick brothers' "excellent attention" in the form of a resolution signed by such outraged guests as planter Drury Scurry, a Newberry County slaveowner, and Charles L. Miot, former owner of Charleston's Planter Hotel.[98]

A few years later, a visitor suffering from a bout of ennui bemoaned the lack of intellectual stimulation at the resort. This visitor, while complimenting the Chicks on providing "everything delightful to the taste of an epicure" (evidently, the butter had improved), complained of fellow guests "little given to reading or anything else calculated to improve the mind." In his judgment, "the water would have a greater and more beneficial effect, were they to drink more of it—take more exercise—and do less dram-drinking and card playing" and engage in reading—if the Chicks were to pay for more than a single newspaper and two books on the shelf.[99]

The water's attributes from a sulphur spring of "sulfates of soda and magnesia" and one or two chalybeate (iron-containing) springs also drew unfavorable comments by some water sophisticates. One guest scoffed that the water was not "so strong, neither so cold and pleasant as the water of the Hanging Rock Spring" in his home county of Lancaster, about 120 miles to the east.[100] Another party left after only two days, finding lodging "as anything else than healthy" and hearing that "a week's use of the waters at [North Carolina's] Deaver's Sulphur Springs was worth a month at Chick's."[101]

The wealthy Chicks parsimoniously elected not to invest capital in the hotel's upkeep or to expand recreation beyond the ten-pin alley and billiards table. In 1857, the Chick brothers sold the resort to two Lowcountry residents, John T. Henery and Franklin Talbird, in partnership with J. Bursey. The new owners vowed to "spare no efforts to make the SPRINGS [capitals original] all that can be desired, whether to the invalid seeking health, or those in quest of pleasure" but assured anxious old-timers that the genial Chick brothers would be in residence "to see their many friends there."[102]

One anonymous antebellum traveler described the improved resort as "commodious": the hotel and surrounding cabins accommodated about 150–200 visitors.[103] The hotel lobby was sufficiently spacious to accommodate Masses for Greenville-area Catholics.[104] The ballroom and parlor likewise were large enough, not only for dances, but for both Protestant ministers and Catholic priests to conduct services there as well.[105]

From the front porch running the length of the two-story hotel, guests peered down a thinly wooded hill to espy the covered spring house about a quarter mile away.[106] A Catholic priest who spent much time at Chick Springs to conduct Mass as part of his diocesan assignment to the Greenville area, wrote that "the invalids were the smallest number among the guests" who "sipped the cold and sparkling liquid bubbling up in silvery sparkles from the generous heart of rock...."[107] Most visitors, in his view, were the "gay and youthful in quest of pleasure or matrimonial alliances."[108]

The number of antebellum guests varied greatly from season to season but appears to have gradually increased to the eve of the Civil War. The 1852 season saw only about twenty-five or thirty guests most of the time, indicating about 20 percent occupancy.[109] One guest estimated about 150 guests in the hot month of August in 1854, but a newspaper reported around sixty or seventy a month later in the cooler September weather.[110] Alfred Taylor, resort proprietor in 1860, recalled in an 1886 interview that the average number of guests for the 1860 season averaged about 500–600.[111]

Antebellum visitors hailed from a number of southern locales, the residents of which overwhelmingly favored such southern "causes" as states' rights and the continuance of slavery. These included a variety of Lowcountry planters from the Charleston and Savannah areas, residents from Lancaster and Newberry in the Midlands, and southern travelers in general making the rounds of the Upstate and North Carolina springs. Foremost were South Carolinians, hostile to northern interests. Governor John Laurence Manning, philosophically a cooperationist but pragmatically a states' right advocate, attended a ball held in his honor at the resort.[112] Secessionist orator and future Confederate officer William King Easley of Pickens County and Greenville lawyer and States' Rights Party candidate William Choice were fellow guests of a writer who penned in the Greenville newspaper: "This watering place should be liberally patronized by the Southern people.... When will the floodtide of travel by our Southern people through the Northern States cease?"[113] Congressman Laurence Massillon Keitt railed against the Know Nothings as a threat to southern interests.[114] Perhaps ironically, considering the fire-eater secessionists who patronized Chick Springs, John Belton O'Neall, Justice of Appeals at Law, rendered from Chick Springs in 1849 a ruling that forced the Spartanburg County sheriff to release from jail a free man of color.[115] The year before, he had published *Negro Law of the Carolinas* to try to guarantee legal protection for enslaved persons.[116]

Chick Springs in the antebellum period attracted regional elites but not the higher echelon who could afford a lengthy stay at Southern Appalachia's Montvale Springs in the Tennessee Smokies. Guests at Montvale generally paid twice as much as Chick visitors. In the 1852–1853 period, for example, Chick charged $1 per day and $6 per week compared to Montvale's $2 daily and $12 weekly rates.[117] Perhaps competition with other Piedmont or North Carolina resorts or Chick's lack of opulence forced Chick Springs management to maintain relatively low rates. Transportation did not pose undue hardship that might have factored into low room and board: state roads through Greenville such as the Saluda Gap Road or those developed by Lowcountry planters and by mountain drovers herding livestock to South Carolina markets were well traveled.[118]

The resort remained open after the start of the Civil War. Its extensive advertisements in the Midlands and Lowcountry newspapers in 1861 and 1862 gave no hint as to national conflict. It continued to publicize its attentive staff and fine food and announced an extensive renovation.[119] It did cease operations, however, not due to the war, but due to a chimney fire that destroyed the hotel in November 1862.[120]

The property never regained its antebellum reputation as a gathering place for regional elites after the end of the Civil War. As Huff notes, many Lowcountry residents began to bypass the Greenville area as a summer retreat for western North Carolina.[121] Furthermore, in the case of Chick Springs, the lack of a hotel for several seasons following the 1862 fire undoubtedly disincentivized many former visitors who had no desire to stay in the resort's spartan cabins.

A second hotel did not materialize until over 15 years later. Burwell's two sons, who had regained title to the resort in 1868, did not rebuild: guests stayed in the cabins and a boarding house although the press speculated in 1870 that W.R.B. Farr, the owner of the boarding house, and the Chicks intended to build a new hotel.[122] A writer a few years later lamented that if the famously frugal Reuben Chick were to be induced "to invest a few of his dollars" to provide "suitable buildings for the accommodation of visitors, Chick Springs [could] again be made famous as a summer resort, as it was in days past."[123] Several years after Reuben's death in 1876, Atlanta attorney George Westmoreland bought the property and constructed a modest hotel with cottages and a lake for "boating and bathing."[124] Twenty-seven years later, Westmoreland sold the property to a group of investors, led by J.A. Bull, a Greenville grocer, who had formed the Chick Springs Company, a stock company worth about $100,000 to erect a new hotel and to start a water-bottling business.[125]

This third hotel apparently was constructed near Westmoreland's buildings, contained about a hundred rooms, according to one local's estimate, and accommodated over 4,000 guests for the 1905 season.[126] Capitalizing on the resort's relatively cool mountain air in the summer, three of the ballroom's sides opened onto porches, and ads promised "large and airy" bedrooms, each with outside windows.[127] The three-story hotel contained "elegant sanitary arrangements" (each room had an attached bath), electric lights and bells, and waterworks.[128] The publicity for the 1907 season was more low key: it offered a few pedestrian details about kitchen improvements (the hotel company owned a farm and dairy) and a "modern laundry" to be "operated by skilled workers."[129]

Vastly increased from Reuben and Pettus's simple billiards and ten pin alley were the resort activities provided in the early twentieth century. In addition to pool and bowling, recreation included tennis, trap shooting, "Donkeys for the children [and] sand beds for their play," and bathing, swimming, and boating in the lake.[130] Special events were held: surprise watermelon parties in the evening, dances festooned by decorations such as Nile green crepe paper with wild bamboo, and sacred Sunday concerts that featured soloists such as South Carolina Governor Martin F. Ansel.[131] As one self-serving ad phrased it, manager J.A. Bull and his assistant "never tire in their work for the pleasure and comfort of their guests."[132]

The years 1907 and 1908 were calamitous for the resort. In December 1907, fire once again destroyed the main hotel at a loss estimated at $30,000 (about $964,000 in 2022 dollars).[133] A smaller hotel costing $50,000 opened in 1908 with 64 rooms; ads proudly promoted the rooms' "felt mattresses, best springs, and iron beds."[134]

In September, a flood burst the dam at the lake and flooded what had been Chick Springs' thriving bottle works business. The water sales recovered; by the next year, Bull was once again taking orders for "Chick Water."[135]

During the early 1900s, Chick Springs emphasized the attributes of its mineral water and mountain air just as much as it publicized its recreational activities. Muddling science via creative advertising, the resort beckoned potential guests from the Deep South to let the water and "the pure mountain air drive that miserable old malaria out of your system."[136] In addition, the health resort implored mothers to bring their "sick and delicate" youngsters to try the water for "stomach trouble" and the ambiguously-worded "children's diseases."[137] Bull recommended a gallon of water daily for adults and promised a money-back guarantee for its "curative powers in Stomach and Liver diseases, etc., and for remarkable increase in bodily weight."[138] One woman who gladly forfeited her money as a result of the guarantee wrote that she was "a mere skeleton" who drank the water from her hotel bed for six weeks before regaining strength to visit the spring house; after three months, she was "strong and rosy and could eat anything." As Bull cheerfully pronounced, "Good health is four-fifths of everything."[139]

By 1913, investors eyed the financial potential of the resort as a convention center in addition to marketing its attributes of "Health, rest, good company, a pleasant place and three good meals a day."[140] The Chick Springs Company, reorganized by Greenville investors (but excluding Bull) and C. Brewster Chapman of New York and Asheville, built a new hotel, the fifth in the resort's history, on the site of the original hotel in summer 1914, at a cost estimated up to $100,000.[141]

The new hotel and its landscaped grounds eclipsed the previous resorts. Designed with "red brick pilasters, with panels of pebble dash," the three-story structure boasted a 300-foot-long verandah running the length of its facade. Additional verandahs lined two sides of the ballroom, which housed stage equipment at one end for large meetings. Above the ballroom lay a dining room with glass doors on opposite walls that each led to a tiled terrace for dining *al fresco*. Three stairways and an elevator conveyed guests to any of a hundred rooms, each with a private bath. Catering to men, the hotel provided a barber shop, pool room, and card rooms. The architects, perhaps mindful of previous hotel fires, installed a Grinnell sprinkler system. The former hotel was renovated into an annex for guests; together with the new hotel, the two buildings accommodated about 350 guests. The Chick Springs Company landscaped around the now enlarged lake (the dam having been repaired) and beautified a park around the spring house. One regional newspaper gushed: "Hereto upper South Carolina has been without an up-to-date resort. Now the Piedmont section of the state will have a resort second to none."[142]

Visitors to Chick Springs from the late 1880s on, essentially the time period of Westmoreland's small hotel through the 1914 grand conference resort, largely came from within the state, especially from the Greenville, Spartanburg, Newberry, and Columbia areas. Georgians, particularly those from the Atlanta and Macon areas as well as Augusta and Waynesboro closer to the South Carolina state line, also traveled to Chick Springs. Relatively fewer traveled from the Lowcountry as contrasted to the antebellum period. A 1914 article boasted that guests "representing every state in the South" registered at the resort, including several from northern Virginia, Jacksonville, and New Orleans.[143]

Many postbellum guests traveled to Chick Springs on trains because of their accessibility. Two of South Carolina's three major postbellum railroads, the Seaboard Air Line and the Southern Railway, provided stops near or at Chick Springs.[144] In the early 1870s, a writer commenting on the economic importance of rail to Spartanburg described vistas along the Atlanta and Charlotte Air Line Railroad track to Greenville: "Carver's Mills in sight, then Benson's Mills on Tiger, Crawfordsville Factory being four miles below … then on by Chick's Springs to Greenville."[145] By 1895, the Air Line had been merged into the extensive track network of the Southern Railway, which heavily advertised its "low summer rates" from Atlanta for destinations as varied as Bar Harbor, Chicago, and Taylors, a depot about a mile away from Chick Springs.[146] A competitor railroad, the Seaboard Air Line, also emphasized its many connections and stops, including Chick Springs. In the 1910s, it publicized that it passed "immediately in front of the hotel and [made] good connections at Spartanburg" with "The Scenic Line" (the Carolina, Clinchfield & Ohio Railway) for "other mountain resorts in North Carolina and Tennessee," such as upper East Tennessee's Unaka Springs.[147]

In addition to rail lines, an electric trolley line stopped by Chick Springs beginning in 1914. The Interurban Street Railway, also known as the Piedmont Northern Electric Line, ran eighteen trains daily between Greenville and Spartanburg as part of an extension of the Anderson Traction Company.[148] Weekend rates for a round trip on the electric rail to reach Chick Springs ranged from two dollars (leaving Greenwood) to sixty-five cents (leaving Piedmont).[149]

In 1907, a year before the Model T's introduction made cars more affordable to the middle class, some regional elites throttled their Oldsmobile or Cadillac roadsters to Chick Springs. A newspaper article that year recapping the "regular Friday hop" commented that "quite a number [came] over in automobiles from Anderson and Belton" about 40 miles away.[150] Others motored to Chick Springs from farther away, making the rounds of resorts just as antebellum travelers did of the Virginia springs. An Athens, Georgia, couple, for example, spent the night at Chick Springs on a weekend trip to Asheville.[151] Barrett Phinizy, most likely the son of Ferdinand, who had owned Georgia's Oconee White Sulphur Springs resort, and his wife traveled from Atlanta to Chick Springs to meet his wife's aunt, who had previously sojourned at Tennessee's Tate Spring.[152] A Hendersonville, North Carolina, newspaper invited its "numerous visiting friends" to visit Chick Springs at the behest of a Chick Springs Company employee who had been in Hendersonville to woo potential guests.[153] As one newspaper proudly noted:

> "In front of the Chick Springs hotel runs the Nationay [sic] highway [sic], the great thoroughfare for motorists.... One can motor from Columbia to Chick Springs in seven hours without speeding.... There should be in South Carolina at least one resort which, in a social way, would be distinctive of the state.... The enlarged and renewed Chick Springs of today has everything that is required to obtain and hold popularity among the best classes of people who patronize summer resorts."[154]

Several organizations embraced the newspaper's pronouncement. Groups as diverse as the South Carolina Pharmaceutical Association, the Summer Southern

States' Checkers Tournament, the South Carolina Short Hand Writers' Association, and—naturally—the South Carolina Press Association convened annual meetings at the resort in the 1910s.[155] The press association called the hotel a "gem" that "surpassed all the promises" made to entice the group to meet there.[156]

In the same decade, Chick Springs introduced a product to capitalize on its mineral water: ginger ale. Made from "Pure, Sparkling, Health-Giving Chick Springs Water and Pure Jamica [sic] Ginger Root," Chick Springs Ginger Ale promised to be "Nature's Remedy for Man's Stomach and Kidneys." Perhaps acknowledging both the trending interest in health food—W.K. Kellogg had formed the Battle Creek Toasted Corn Flake Company in 1906—and the increasing stress of harried businessmen, Chick Springs Ginger Ale vowed that "you will sleep better and wake up feeling brighter." Druggists across the region sold the concoction; Chick Springs also delivered the drink by wagon in the Greenville area.[157]

Unfortunately, despite the resort's ginger ale business and its income from hosting extravagant balls, professional associations, and private hotel guests, Chick Springs defaulted on its mortgage interest payment due in January 1916.[158] In March 1916, the Chick Springs Company entered receivership through action taken by Chapman representing the bondholders' interest, and the property was sold at auction for $48,000 in early April to Jesse R. Boyd, attorney for the bondholders.[159] Chapman then deeded four-fifths interest of it to Bull and three others in exchange for over 1,400 acres in upper Greenville County that he planned to developed.[160] Even though the local press speculated that the resort would function as usual, several associations quickly changed the venue of their annual meetings to other South Carolina locations, thus increasing the indebtedness of Chick Springs.[161]

Chick Springs management announced arrangements in May for a "first-class orchestra" to open the season and promised weekly dances (fifty cents for "young men" who were not registered guests). Options to use the grounds as a military academy, however, began to circulate by the end of the month.[162] Although "hundreds of people" "handsomely gowned" listened to music and dined from "imported articles and from the well-tilled gardens" of the Chick Springs hotel one Sunday in July 1916, the resort by that fall had transitioned into a military institute.[163]

The Chick Springs Military Academy advertised both its objective, "to develop its students into frank, manly, Christian gentlemen," and its location's health attributes, "1200 feet above sea level at a famous health resort" and "celebrated mineral water."[164] The school fielded a football team its first year, added thirteen new students after the Christmas holidays in 1916, but then sustained a $25,000 loss when the second hotel, used as an annex for classrooms, burned down in October 1917.[165] In January 1918, the school announced a suspension of classes for the term and never reopened.[166]

Chick Springs never regained its status as a fashionable resort. Dr. B.B. Steedly rented the hotel as a sanitarium and for overflow patients from his Spartanburg hospital after the demise of the military academy.[167] The U.S. Veterans Bureau leased the property beginning in 1922 for development as a training center for disabled World War I soldiers, with plans for the hotel to serve as the dormitory and for a new building to be constructed as a trades school by the Steedly Sanitarium, the

Chick Springs Water Company, and the leasing companies.[168] After the Chick Springs Water Company declared bankruptcy during the Great Depression, Bull bought some of the former resort property, including the spring, at auction. The eventual buyer of the hotel building itself, however, demolished the structure and sold the property to a local physician, who built a house on the hotel site. By 1972, only a swimming pool remained at the former hotel grounds.[169] In the mid–2000s, interested citizens organized the Chick Springs Historical Society with the objective to preserve the spring house and environs as a park, an endeavor that persists today.[170]

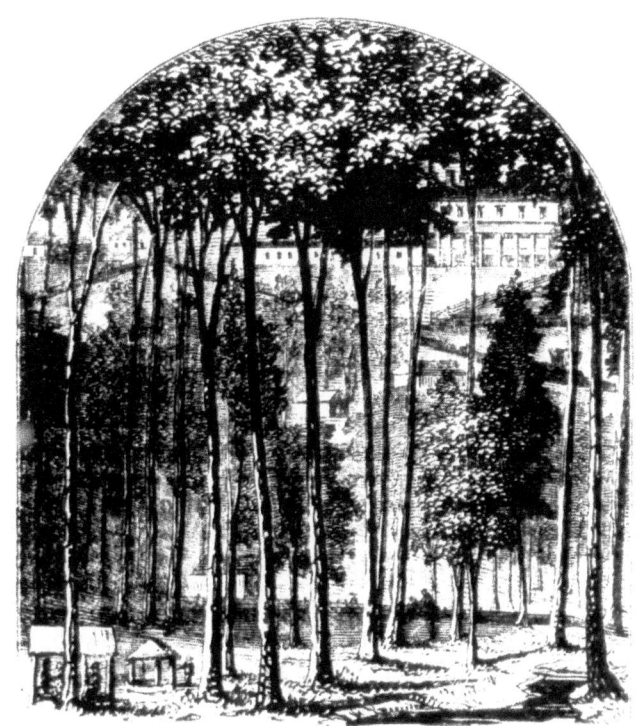

CHICK'S SPRINGS.

Chick Springs, South Carolina. John Warner Barber and Henry Howe, *Our Whole Country*, vol. 1 (Cincinnati: George F. Tuttle and Henry M'Cauley, 1861), 723 (courtesy of the East Tennessee State University Medical Library).

Glenn Springs

In northwestern South Carolina lies Spartanburg County, the largest in square miles of the state's four counties that fall into Southern Appalachia. Spartanburg County is bordered by Cherokee County to its east, Union County to its southeast, Laurens County to its southwest, Greenville County to its west, and North Carolina's Polk and Rutherford counties to its northwest and north respectively. Elevation gradually falls from its northwestern corner, at a high point of almost 1,500 feet on the slope of Bird Mountain, straddling its border with Greenville County, to around 290 feet in the south.[171] The county seat of Spartanburg, for example, stands at an elevation of roughly 800 feet, contrasted with Greenville's 920 foot elevation about thirty-two miles to the west and Columbus's 1,100 foot elevation about thirty miles to the northwest in Polk County. Those who have traveled on Interstate 26E from Hendersonville, North Carolina, to Spartanburg have experienced the highway's winding descent that provides a panoramic expanse of the rolling Piedmont to the southeast.

Named for the Spartan Regiment, a local Revolutionary War militia, Spartanburg County in the 1750s saw its first white settlers, predominantly German, Scot-Irish, and English, who passed through the Shenandoah Valley from Pennsylvania, Virginia, and Maryland.[172] Robert Mills, in his 1826 *Statistics of South*

Carolina, noted the Spartanburg area's cultivation of "all kinds of grains" (e.g., rye, wheat, corn) and the processing of cotton, which grew best in the southern and eastern parts of the region.[173]

Mills also emphasized the Spartanburg region's abundance of limestone ("furnishes very beautiful granular marble") and of pyrite ("will be of great value to the state ... [its sulphur] essential to the manufacture of gunpowder"). Springs in this region therefore contain a variety of carbonate and sulfur salts from the limestone rock (calcium carbonate) and the mineral pyrite (iron sulfide). The lure of these springs' "purest water" coupled with the "temperate, pleasant, and healthy" climate, according to Mills, attracted Lowcountry planters by the early 1800s.[174]

About eleven miles south of the village of Spartanburg, Mills noted, a sulfur spring seeped in a marshy area near Story's Creek.[175] According to one tradition, a boy in search of strayed livestock fell into mud at the spring. A few days later, a skin disease from which he was suffering disappeared; subsequently, the spring quickly gained fame for its curative powers.[176] Another tradition, however, holds that Revolutionary War soldiers discovered that the springs cured the annoying "itch."[177] Regardless of the origin of the recognition of the springs' therapeutic action, by the early 1800s, locals suffering from scabies, sores, or other dermatological distresses dug holes in the "Sulphur Spring" or "Powder Marsh" (aptly named because of its gunpowder odor) to bathe in the soothing waters.[178]

The early antebellum period saw a succession of owners of the spring. By 1815, James B. Means had purchased the tract and had constructed a two-story structure to accommodate health-seekers.[179] About a decade later, John B. Glenn of Union County brought his ailing wife to the spring where her health greatly improved, eventually to the point that "the good wife presented her lord with a son."[180] In 1827, Glenn bought the springs property, about 723 acres, and built another inn and several cabins.[181] Union County physician Maurice A. Moore co-organized the Glenn Springs Company that then purchased the burgeoning resort from Glenn. The company opened a grand three-and one-half-story wood frame hotel in 1838, with three two-story wings. The dining, drawing, and ball rooms each commanded fifty feet in length, decorated with fine furniture bought in New York.[182] In addition, the company landscaped a small portion of the 1,031 acres, leaving most undeveloped and about 200 acres cultivated for crops.[183] By 1839, a post office was established in the vicinity, an example of the influx of visitors and the growth of a small community around the springs.[184]

Unfortunately, the Glenn Springs Company defaulted on payment to Glenn and to a lending bank; a writ of *fieri facias* was served and the property sold at a sheriff's auction in January 1842. Proceeds from the auction were to repay Glenn and the financing bank an initial sum of $5,000 cash up front and $6,000 annually between them until the mortgage was paid, an amount well in excess of $300,000 today.[185]

The expensive venture was perhaps adversely affected by the Panic of 1837, which lasted well into the 1840s.[186] Cotton prices in the state, for example, dropped from eighteen cents in February 1837 to eight cents by May 1837.[187] In addition, the years 1836–1837 witnessed a record cotton crop in the United States, leading to falling prices as British demand declined in the face of Indian cotton exports.[188] Perhaps a combination of overly generous bank loans to the Glenn Springs Company coupled with a decrease in Lowcountry planter discretionary income during the depression caused the new resort to fail.

John C. Zimmerman and William C. Camp joined Glenn as co-owners of the resort after the sale. Camp, a surveyor of modest means, lived near Glenn Springs.[189] Zimmerman, by contrast, married into a prominent Orangeburg family, moved in 1830 from St. Matthews north to the Spartanburg area where he purchased a farm, also near Glenn Springs. Eventually, he became both the largest landowner in Spartanburg County, owning thousands of acres, and the county's largest slaveowner, holding by 1850 almost one hundred enslaved persons to till his land.[190] Zimmerman cofounded a "good Male and Female School" at Glenn Springs, hiring a Methodist minister to teach the girls and retaining a "prominent educator" for the male students, whose parents saw the school as a preparatory academy for their sons to then enter the state college.[191]

For the season of 1842, the three owners hired a "Mr. and Mrs. [William] Murray" to assist "in the comforts" of patrons wishing to try the waters used by "[h]undreds snatched from a premature grave by their healing efficiency." To earn capital, Glenn, Zimmerman, and Camp partitioned the property into lots for buyers to build summer cottages or permanent homes near the springs.[192]

In 1844, Zimmerman obtained exclusive title to the property.[193] Over the next several years, Zimmerman improved the hotel and its offerings. By 1852, he had employed a "water-cure" or hydropathic physician to oversee the treatment of up to one hundred invalids by the use of cold water compresses or bathing therapy as an alternative or supplement to patrons simply imbibing the pungent sulfur water.[194] For such a large enterprise, Zimmerman deployed several of his enslaved persons from his plantation to the resort to maintain the hotel and cabins, serve the meals, and generally cater to desires of the Lowcountry planter families.[195]

In August 1853, Zimmerman, a devout Episcopalian, sold the resort for $15,000 (about $586,000 in 2022 dollars) to the Episcopal Church with the stipulation that his family and owners of nearby lots purchased from him be able to retain access the springs.[196] The denomination turned the resort into a young ladies' academy.[197] Two Episcopal priests, Thomas S. Arthur and J.D. McCullough, served as administrators of the school, whose former hotel buildings had "been thoroughly repaired and fitted up … to make [them] in every respect, such a home as parents would desire for their daughters."[198] The Glenn Springs Female Institute opened with a faculty of six in February 1854; the following year, however, the academy moved to a former boys' school campus in Spartanburg. Arthur sold the property, which subsequently changed ownership at least three times before the Civil War.[199]

By the eve of the Civil War, Glenn Springs had reached its antebellum zenith in terms of numbers of guests and in terms of provision of activities. The hotel, cottages, and nearby private homes, for example, accommodated 1,000 visitors at one time in 1860.[200] One guest, Samuel Burges, employed as a fee collector for a Charleston newspaper, noted that his first evening's entertainment included an informal tableau. Also enjoyed during this era were billiards, ten pins, and cards.[201] Taking the waters was a morning activity, a social occasion for the healthy and a therapeutic session for the sickly. If they were physically able, guests walked downhill about 300 yards along a winding trail across rustic bridges that led to the springs in a cool and shady ravine.[202]

An 1855 issue of the *Charleston Medical Journal and Review* featured the waters in a laudatory article written by none other than one of the former co-owners of the resort, the physician Maurice A. Moore. Despite his obvious conflict of interest as author, Moore may have genuinely believed in the curative power of the waters although his claims stretch modern credibility.[203] Most of the "success stories" he recounted involved patients with symptoms of jaundice and nausea manifested in "total derangement of the liver," "bilious cholic," and dyspepsia. Moore also claimed to have resolved with the water such female issues as painful menstruation, abnormal discharge, and urinary incontinence. The good doctor also attested that he observed the relapse or cure of diseases as wildly unrelated as epilepsy and gonorrhea.[204]

A common theme emphasized in the healing of the patients was weight gain. One female weighing 94 pounds came to the hotel on a bed; in less than a month, her "catamenial derangement" ceased, and in two months, she left Glenn Springs, having gained about two-thirds of her initial weight, a whopping 62 pounds. A male over the course of two long stays at the springs stopped his incessant vomiting, and his weight gradually rose from 110 pounds to 190 pounds. Cured, "he emigrated to the west."[205]

Invalids included enslaved as well as free laborers. Peter, "a servant belonging to Mr. Mims," arrived at the springs in 1839. The large hotel crowd forced the proprietor to put him in "a very small house" where he received water by his bed for two weeks before walking to the springs on his own. Peter so improved in health that Glenn Springs hired him as an ostler from his owner. "Old aunt Sally, a negro [sic] woman aged 75 years" "was hauled to the springs" because of "bloody urine"; the water effected a natural cure.[206]

Others in search of good health came to Glenn Springs, according to Moore, after allegedly exhausting the offerings of the most prestigious, fashionable mineral springs establishments. The Glenn Springs water restored the health of a New Yorker who had tried "time and again all the watering places at the North and in Virginia." Suffering from blood in his urine, a Georgian from Augusta visited "all the watering places in the Southern country" and chanced upon Glenn Springs on his way to the Virginia springs; with his symptom resolved in two weeks, he elected to remain at the resort for the remainder of the season. While one matron had made the rounds of "Saratoga, Ballston and all the Virginia Springs," she only found relief at Glenn.[207] These examples indicate that Glenn Springs often catered to a wealthy, well-connected clientele, those who possessed the financial means to travel for months and whose social networks most likely included those who had awareness of the major spas' attributes.

South Carolina elites who enjoyed the resort's fashionable conviviality and waters during the antebellum period included Mrs. John C. Calhoun ("health is rapidly improving"); Chancellor William Harper, lead author of the Ordinance of Nullification (he died three months after his health rallied at the springs); U.S.

Senator William C. Preston; and Governor Whitemarsh B. Seabrook.[208] Congressman Preston S. Brooks, notorious for his caning of Senator Charles Sumner in 1856, maintained a summer home near Glenn Springs. Fellow Fire-Eater Congressman Laurence Keitt, an accomplice of Brooks in Sumner's beating, frequented Glenn Springs when in the South Carolina mountains; in August 1855, for example, he met 50 or 60 people at the resort and attended two balls over the course of two days.[209] Brewster points out that Glenn Springs served as a "sort of summer capital for the Palmetto State" because the governor was constitutionally forbidden to leave the state during his term of office. Therefore, dozens of South Carolina politicians, jurists, and lawyers debated governmental affairs, jockeyed for position and status, and recreated at Glenn Springs.[210]

Depending on the decade, antebellum travelers used stagecoach, rail, or a combination of both to reach the resort. Before the extension of rail to the Upstate or Piedmont in the 1850s, Lowcountry travelers could take a stagecoach that ran semiweekly from Columbia directly to Glenn Springs.[211] In 1853, Zimmerman as proprietor advertised transportation to the springs via a four-horse coach from the head of the Laurens rail about 28 miles southeast of Glenn Springs or the same from Chester about 45 miles to the west of the resort.[212]

The coming of the rail, in particular, the Spartanburg and Union Railroad, connected Spartanburg with Union, Columbia, and Charleston and opened additional and more direct routes for potential travelers to Glenn Springs.[213] In 1847, the South Carolina General Assembly designated a special fund to aid in state railroad construction; the subsequent year saw the passage of acts to amend the charters of the Spartanburg and Union Rail Road Company and to incorporate the Laurens Rail Road Company.[214] In addition, Zimmerman and Moore lobbied as members of the Glenn Springs delegation to the 1849 Union Rail Road Convention.[215] The funding and lobbying resulted in the 1854 completion of a line from Laurens to Newberry and the 1859 completion of the Spartanburg and Union Railroad.[216]

The resort remained open during the first few years of the Civil War, attracting invalids and Lowcountry residents as usual during the summer of 1861. The Charleston press throughout that summer advised that travelers could reach Glenn Springs via stages run in connection with the Spartanburg and Union Railroad.[217] A prominent Laurens lawyer in feeble health, for example, rested at the health resort until his death there in July 1861.[218]

As the war intensified, however, and as railroad track was damaged or destroyed, potential customers found it difficult to reach the resort. Subsequently, the number of guests plummeted, and social activities diminished. In June 1863, the daughter of a planter living nearby recorded that "Mr. Anderson [W.G. Anderson, the proprietor] opened the hotel at Glenn Springs Saturday at $3.00 per day. He has three or four boarders." About two weeks later, during what normally would be the zenith of the resort season, she noted that the number of guests had risen to only about twelve. With no lively social scene to entice her, she went on to write, "I know very little about the place now for I very seldom ever visit...."[219]

Immediately after the war in 1866, Anderson, still the proprietor, advertised Glenn Springs extensively in the Charleston press. Anderson advertised rates as

$2.50 per day or $65 per month, about the same as Tennessee's premiere antebellum Montvale Springs resort, perhaps indicating that Glenn Springs required less infrastructure improvement than Montvale, which may have served at one point as a makeshift infirmary during the war.[220] Anderson, however, dropped his monthly rate to a more affordable $40 in 1869 to lure more guests in a region devastated by the war.[221]

Nonetheless, business languished in 1869. A newspaper commentator on the region's upcoming summer travels noted that "Glenn's Springs are sometimes mentioned, but they do not advertise; and we hear but little about that place, which enjoys a capital old reputation for its medicinal virtues."[222] A guest in one of the resort cabins wrote rather tongue-in-cheek that the resort was as "dull as ditch water," with one amusement being "catching fleas … of the largest and liveliest kind." Although he jokingly complained that the "big lack [for cabin guests] was 'cold 'vittles'" because the cabins lacked large utensils to cook enough to serve both dinner and cold lunch leftovers, he also yearned for the spring to "once more be the place it was in former days." From his perspective, the foremost reasons as to the lack of visitors were "the depressed condition of the country, the scarcity of money in the south, and the unfavorable seasons, not the place or lack of virtue in the water."[223]

Consequently, a sheriff's sale that summer resulted in two-thirds interest in the property "real and personal" being sold for $4,210.[224] In December, the remaining one third, consisting of about 350 acres, including the hotel buildings and the spring, was sold via bankruptcy proceedings to a partnership, Smith & Fowler, for $1,401.[225]

W.D. Fowler operated the hotel for the next four years. For the season of 1870, he put the buildings through a "thorough repair" that "comfortably accommodated" 400 guests, promising that the hotel would "not be kept as it was a season or two in the past."[226] He advertised for meat and pastry cooks and for a "first-class barber and hairdresser" and brokered an agreement with Spartanburg's Harvey House such that a guest paying a month's rent at one could stay for two weeks at the other.[227]

Fowler evidently failed in his attempt to adequately improve Glenn Springs, because in 1874 Gorman & Calnan of the Columbia Hotel assumed proprietorship and swore their intent to "restore this famous Summer resort to its former glory."[228] Although "nearly all of the rooms [were] engaged" in mid–July 1875 and the services of a resident physician employed that same summer, one guest commented that the health resort lacked "all luxuries of a first class city hotel."[229]

The year 1876 began the health resort's renaissance when physician John Wells Simpson and C.M. Miller assumed ownership. The following year, Simpson's son, J. (John) Wistar (or Wister), a Harvard University law school graduate, joined his father as co-proprietor.[230] When Dr. Simpson died in 1881, his share of the property went to J. Wistar and his brother William Dunlap, then chief justice of the South Carolina Supreme Court.[231]

"Simpson & Simpson," as the partnership was known, ran Glenn Springs over a span of almost thirty years, pulling in largely J. Wistar's sons to manage various aspects such as the hotel and transportation.[232] During that time, the Simpsons greatly improved the property. They landscaped a park of about one hundred acres and added an octagonal open-air pavilion at the springs.[233] In addition, they supplemented the hotel's 60 rooms by constructing more cottages (two-story frame dwellings with front porches), including a prototype "double cottage," along the two cottage rows that flanked the expansive lawn in front of the hotel, for a total of at least ten cottages.[234] Around 1889, the Simpsons spent almost $100,000 to improve the resort. A Kentucky newspaper, mentioning several parties traveling from Maysville to the opening gala, approvingly noted the "very large" ballroom of "exquisite design, without doubt the finest at any resort west of famous White Sulphur."[235] By 1897, the hotel could accommodate 500 guests; it consisted of four joined sections, all but one with three stories, with verandahs running the length of the first two floors of the three-story sections.[236] A couple of years later, the Simpsons again renovated the resort, calling it a "new hotel" with "all modern improvements and conveniences," but inexplicably not providing further detail.[237]

The Simpsons, of course, provided ample recreational activities within and around the improved health resort. Reading novels and newspapers, discussing the social and political events of the day, and—as one writer delicately put it—engaging in "amatory sentiment" represented a few of the more sedentary options.[238] Postbellum guests now less frequently dressed up as knights or ladies of the court to participate in the popular mock jousting tournaments of decades earlier that had attracted hundreds; visitors now amused themselves with a shooting gallery, tennis court, and a "double Track Ten-pin Alley."[239]

Just as in the antebellum period, the medicinal use of the mineral springs remained an important feature of Glenn Springs. Patrons could make use of bathing rooms, consult with the resident physician or osteopath for the season, and engage in the all-important early morning ritual of strolling down the curving paths to take the water.[240] By 1880, Simpson & Simpson was shipping quarts of water across the South from the bottling house next to the springs; the business grew such that in late 1886, Paul Simpson, son of J. Wistar, began managing the newly-established Spartanburg branch office.[241] Although a physician reported to the state board of health in 1881 that Glenn Springs water was not a cure-all as had been largely indicated in the antebellum medical literature (e.g., "may not be used with any hopeful results for good in tuberculosis"), he did aver that it could be successfully used "in all functional derangements of the digestive, uterine, renal, and nervous systems."[242] Forty-five years later, state physicians still endorsed the water for alimentary tract disorders, diarrhea, dysentery, and hemorrhoids.[243]

In the early 1900s, the Simpsons created more options for Glenn Springs water. Perhaps to obscure the sulphur water's "bitter, saline taste" from the general public or perhaps to capitalize on the nation's increasing appetite for "healthy" soft drinks, the resort began to market Glenn Springs Ginger Ale, a "Delightful Beverage, Invigorating, Healthful."[244] About the same time, Glenn Springs began offering both "still" (non-carbonated) and carbonated mineral water that "[c]ures diseases of the Liver, Kidneys, Stomach, and Skin."[245] Glenn Springs bottled water proved so successful that at least one Pepsi-Cola office served as an agent.[246]

The rebuilding of South Carolina rail and the addition of new lines in the 1860s and 1870s eased travel to Glenn Springs. In the mid–1870s, the Spartanburg & Union

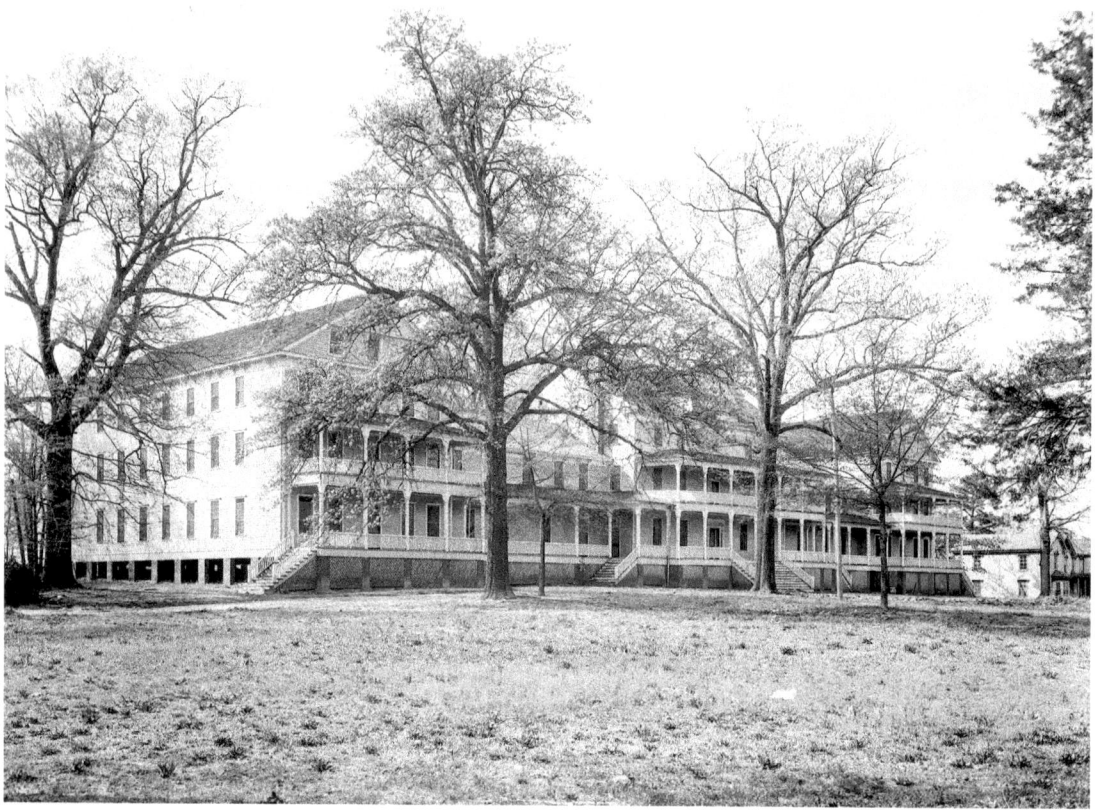

"Glenn Springs Hotel [1926]," Spartanburg County, South Carolina. Alfred Willis, photographer (from the collections of the Spartanburg County Public Libraries, *https://cdm17281.contentdm.oclc.org/digital/collection/shjw/id/250%20Spartanburg%20Public%20Library%201926*).

ran three weekly "downward" trains from Spartanburg to Alston and three weekly "upward" trains that operated in the opposite direction.[247] Spartanburg gained more rail traffic via the completion of both the Atlanta & Richmond Air-Line Railroad in 1873, which passed through Spartanburg, and the Spartanburg & Asheville Railroad in 1879. The various railroads passing through Spartanburg allowed passengers traveling across the South to disembark at the Spartanburg depot and avail themselves of a daily hack to the Glenn Springs.[248] When the Glenn Springs Railroad was completed in 1894, resort guests could then travel to Roebuck from Spartanburg to the north or from Union in the south, jump on the Glen Springs line, and then disembark within 300 yards of the hotel.[249]

Guests in the late nineteenth through the early twentieth century at either Glenn Springs or nearby boarding houses came largely from within the state, notably towns within one hundred miles, although some hailed from other southern states.[250] A visitor in 1890 wrote that out-of-state guests had traveled mainly from North Carolina, Georgia, and Arkansas and that every South Carolina county save one had been represented at the resort that season; in-state guests included a former governor and a variety of judges and military officers.[251] The majority of guests, however, were not the fashionable elite as in the antebellum period but representative of a growing middle class.[252]

The resort began a decline after the Simpsons' December 1905 sale of 55 acres, consisting of the hotel and bottling works, to a syndicate of Spartanburg businessmen, including several textile mill presidents, who planned to invest around $200,000 to improve the resort.[253] The syndicate did not, however, spend lavishly on the property or on its operation. Although the syndicate built an electric plant and installed ceiling fans in central hotel locations, one visitor in 1907 complained that the management did not turn the fans on until after seven in the evening to save money. The same visitor also noted that "very little attention is given to the grounds, and the walk ways to the springs are washed in gullies." He concluded that the 300 guests during his week's stay came with the exclusive aim to drink "probably the best mineral water in the state ... regardless of accommodations."[254] Although the resort hosted several state professional associations in the next few years, by 1927 a writer described it only as a "modest resort hostelry."[255] During Prohibition, Glenn Springs probably evolved into a "speak easy" for the sale and consumption of alcohol. After its condemnation in the 1930s, fire destroyed it in summer 1941.[256] Today the former resort grounds lie within the Glenn Springs Historic District of the National Register of Historic Places.[257]

Tennessee

Introduction

Two iconic images linked with Tennessee are Elvis and Dolly, superstars whom most readers recognize without the need for last names. Although Elvis Presley lived within the splendid grounds of Graceland in Memphis, Dolly Parton grew up some 400 miles to the east, in the rural Smoky Mountains that inspired such hits as "My Tennessee Mountain Home" and "Coat of Many Colors." Many who have never traveled to the Volunteer State might assume that the Smokies "is all there is" to East Tennessee. They might be surprised to learn that East Tennessee, one of the state's three "Grand Divisions," named with Middle Tennessee and West Tennessee in the state constitution as early as 1834, contains three distinct physiographic provinces.[1]

The Unaka Mountains, which include the Great Smokies, form Tennessee's border with North Carolina.[2] The Unakas include Carter County's Roan High Knob (6,285 feet), Unicoi County's Big Bald Mountain (5,516 feet), and Sevier County's Kuwohi (formerly named as Clingmans Dome) (6,643 feet), the highest point in Tennessee. The mountains slope down to the Valley and Ridge Province where long narrow ridges and valleys run northeast to southwest. The valleys' river systems that drain into the Tennessee River, the Ohio River's largest tributary, provided fertile bottomland for cotton, tobacco, and corn in years past. Today, the Tennessee Valley Authority (TVA, established by federal legislation in 1933) regulates many of the rivers in this region via dams for flood control and hydroelectric power generation. To the west of the Valley and Ridge province rises the tableland of the Cumberland Plateau, with an average elevation of 1,800 feet, that stretches southwesterly into Alabama.

Middle Tennessee, as defined in the state constitution, contains counties that Campbell includes in his definition of Southern Appalachia. Examples include Franklin, Warren, and Grundy counties near Alabama and Pickett and Fentress counties near Kentucky.[3] Southern Appalachian Tennessee therefore consists of all East Tennessee and several Cumberland Plateau counties.

Southern Appalachian Tennessee, with its three distinct topographies, contained dozens of local and regional watering holes frequented throughout the nineteenth and early twentieth centuries. J.B. Killebrew, state agricultural commissioner, noted in 1874 that "Tennessee may challenge comparison with any portion of the United States in the number, variety, excellence, and medicinal value of its mineral

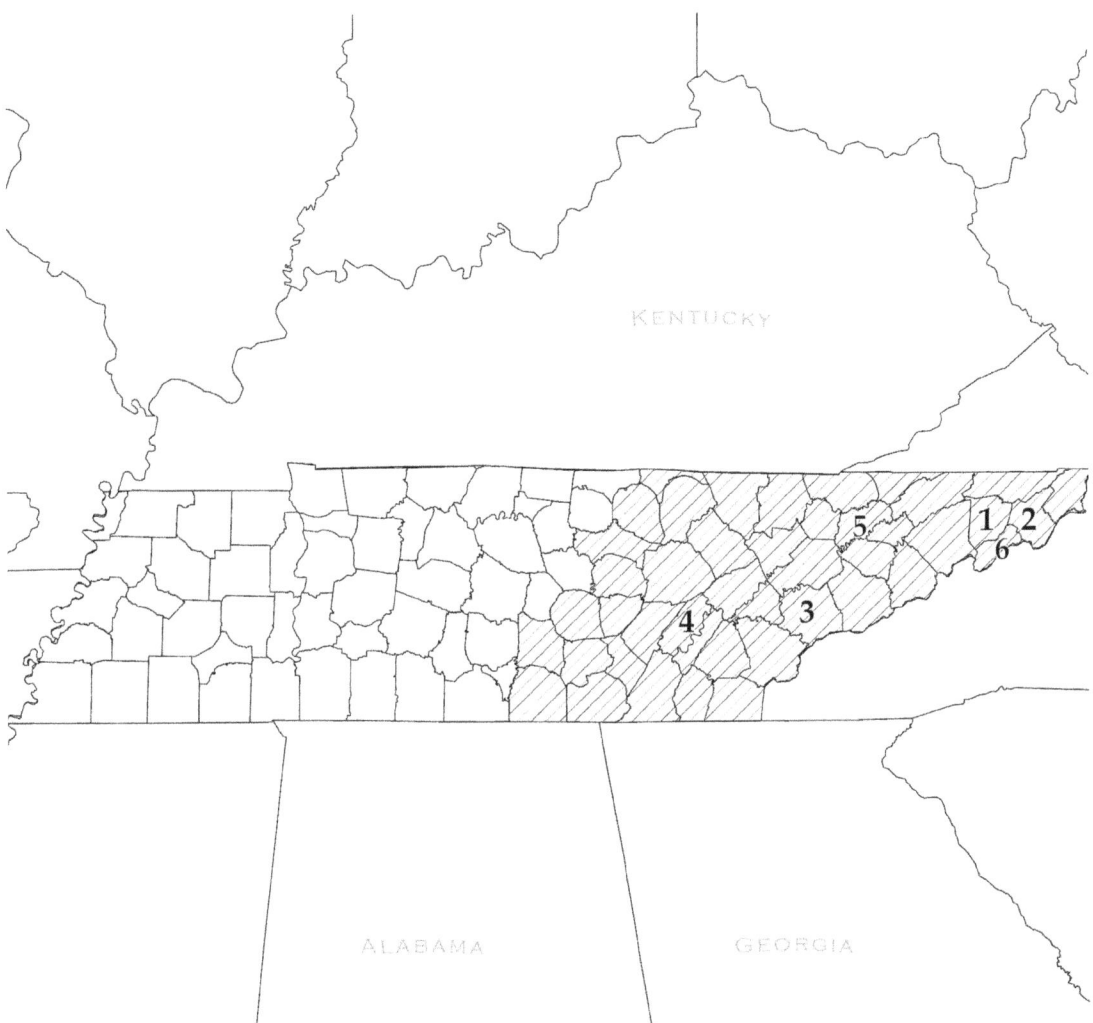

Tennessee counties with featured health resorts: (1) Washington County, Austin's Springs; (2) Carter County, Cloudland Hotel; (3) Blount County, Montvale Springs; (4) Rhea County, Rhea Springs; (5) Grainger County, Tate Spring; (6) Unicoi County, Unaka Springs (Sources: Esri, NOAA, USGS. Cartographer: Sayona Turner, East Tennessee State University).

waters. They occur upon the lofty peaks of the Unakas, and break out in groups from the bases of the long ridges of the Eastern Valley. The Cumberland Table Land is crowned with sparkling chalybeate springs."[4]

Grundy County's Beersheba Springs on the Cumberland Plateau rivaled Blount County's Montvale Springs in the Smokies as a fashionable, sophisticated antebellum mineral springs resort. A crude hotel and a few ramshackle cabins clustered at Beersheba Springs attracted largely locals beginning about 1839 until the mid–1850s when J. John Armfield, a slave trader with ties to Louisiana, bought Beersheba. Under Armfield, Beersheba transitioned into a spa attracting Deep South visitors. Analogously, Mississippian plantation owner Asa Watson improved the infrastructure and landscaping for Montvale to entice wealthy southerners. Both Armfield and Watson employed French cooks ("French" implied a cosmopolitan ambiance), built elegant hotels with wide verandahs and grounds for promenades, and provided upper-class pursuits such as hunts, billiards, and soirees.[5]

As a counterpoint to the sophisticated, fashionable Montvale and Beersheba, the more modest Rhea Springs—charging in 1858 about one third of Beersheba's weekly rate—lay in a different topography, the Piney River valley east of the Cumberland Plateau escarpment. Rhea Springs' three-and-one-half mile proximity to the Tennessee River allowed guests to travel leisurely by steamboat from either Chattanooga or Knoxville, just as Deep South planters traveled by steamer on the Tennessee River to Louisville, sixteen miles from Montvale.[6]

Travelers also reached Rhea Springs by carriage from Athens, about twenty-five miles to the southeast of Rhea. From Athens, they paid the same livery stable to provide a carriage to White Cliff Springs, a budding rival to Rhea Springs in the early postbellum period. White Cliff Springs stood at an elevation of over 2,000 feet on Starr Mountain in Monroe County, about sixteen miles to the southeast of Athens.[7] Although White Cliff Springs touted its "dry, pure and very invigorating stratosphere," it also publicized its three springs for the treatment of "diseases of the liver, kidneys & stomach and … as a sovereign remedy in chlorosis & dysmenorrhea … [and] in scrofulous affections of the skin, & chronic diseases of the eye."[8] Rhea Springs water allegedly provided relief from many of the same conditions. The resident physician at each resort most likely convinced perplexed patients as to why his resort's spring water provided superior therapy.

Over sixty miles to the northeast of White Cliff Springs lay Montvale Springs as well as over a dozen other postbellum mineral spring resorts in the Smokies, among them Alleghany Springs, Wildwood Springs, Line Spring, and Doyle Springs. Most of the Smoky Mountain health resorts possessed modest vernacular, wooden architecture that attracted locals from Knox, Blount, and Sevier counties. Some Smoky Mountain resorts via their advertisements appear to have strained to find attributes to set them apart from others. Line Spring on Round-Top Mountain overlooking Wear's Valley in Sevier County offered "as good Mineral Water as can be found in the state."[9] Wildwood Springs, twelve miles from Knoxville, boasted of its "fried chicken [as] a specialty" and its "unexcelled mineral water" (like Line Spring, offering no mineral analysis).[10] Many of these Smoky Mountain resorts opened for business circa 1870s-1910s when railroad guides publicized retreats accessible from their depots and when Knoxville businessmen sent their families to the resorts for the summer, joining them on the weekends.

In the Tennessee Valley, northeast of the confluence of the Holston and French Broad rivers that forms the Tennessee River, lay another cluster of mineral springs resorts in Grainger and Hawkins counties, including Tate Spring, Galbraith's Springs, Hale's Red and White Sulphur Springs, and Mooresburg Springs. Hawkins County's Galbraith's Springs resort was located less than a mile from the Holston River near Short Mountain.[11] Its hotel was cleverly positioned about fifty to seventy-five yards below the spring: As one smitten guest wrote, "Reaching the hotel, [the spring water] passes right under it, chanting a lullaby to the sleepers."[12] Mooresburg Spring, about three miles west from Galbraith's, offered chalybeate water. Although Mooresburg Spring primarily attracted locals, Tennessee Governor Ben W. Hooper rested there to recover his health.[13] Closer to Rogersville stood Hale's Red and White Sulphur Springs, which like Galbraith's Springs, originated in the antebellum period and billed itself as "a quiet home-like place" in a pastoral setting with cool, invigorating temperatures.[14] Tate Spring attracted a wealthy crowd, including those who traveled by private railcar.

Several health resorts dotted the valleys and ridges of Northeast Tennessee. At the Southwest Virginia border, stood Avoca Spring, now part of suburban Bristol. Perhaps as a nod to the famous western Virginia spa, the waters were praised in antebellum times as the "celebrated White Sulphur Springs"; into the early twentieth century, a small hotel served a local populace.[15] From Washington County's Johnson City, one could travel by the East Tennessee, Virginia, and Georgia (ETV&G) Railroad north to Austin's Springs along the Watauga River or take a hack two miles east to Carter County's Easley's Spring where "a plain Boarding House" stood by water "Chalybeate cold and pure, with good proportion, of Magnesia and Sulphur."[16]

To the southwest of Jonesborough in Washington County, locals and occasionally Knoxville residents visited the rustic resorts of Yeager's Springs and Clark Spring (or Clark's Springs).[17] About a mile from the ETV&G at Limestone (about eighteen miles from Jonesborough), a regional newspaper in 1874 announced that J.J. Yeager's sulphur and chalybeate waters cured "Scrofula, Dispepsia [sic], Sore Eyes, Bronchial Diseases [and] Eruptions."[18] Clark Spring, farther to the south in a hollow at the Nolichucky River in the foothills of the Unaka Mountains, provided guests with sulphur water deemed by one visitor as a "never ending source of pleasure to sit and drink not less than a half dozen glasses."[19]

Following the Nolichucky River upstream about sixteen miles from Clark Spring, largely along the old Jonesborough Road (State Route 107), travelers reached Unaka Springs, deep within the Unaka Mountains' Nolichucky River Gorge. Alternatively, guests forded the river from the direction of Erwin or, after the completion of the Clinchfield Railroad, hazarded a walk across the river railroad bridge to reach the hotel. For travelers from Johnson City or from Asheville who wished to travel to the Unaka Mountains to enjoy a spectacular panoramic view or to find relief from hay fever, Roan Mountain's Cloudland Hotel straddling Tennessee and North Carolina promoted both.

The resorts selected for closer examination, Rhea Springs, Montvale Springs, Tate Spring, Austin's Springs, Unaka Springs, and the Cloudland Hotel, represent a variety of topographies, geographies, clientele, and historical periods. All shared an interest, to a greater or lesser degree, in the promotion of their health benefits and leisure activities. Moreover, some served as places of refuge during yellow fever epidemics in other parts of the South.

Despite reports and rumors of the mountains as an impenetrable barrier to outsiders, travelers crisscrossed the Unaka Mountains. Montvale in the rugged Great Smokies attracted visitors before any other Southern Appalachian Tennessee resort east of the Cumberland Plateau. European botanists collected specimens on the Roan Highlands in the 1790s. These examples dramatically demonstrate the cross-connectivity between the Southern Appalachian mountains and other regions such as the Deep South and even western Europe despite the terrain and poor wagon roads prior to and during the antebellum era.

Especially in the postbellum period, railroad construction permitted more efficient access to resorts even if guests still endured jarring hack rides of several miles from the depot to the resort hotel. Railroads also accounted for several farmhouse retreats, such as Yeager's, that sprang up along the tracks; the railroad companies eagerly promoted these in their travel brochure to encourage rail passengers. Some mineral springs resorts located near the river valleys, notably Montvale, Rhea, and Austin's, received visitors from the navigable parts of the Tennessee and Watauga rivers. Unaka Springs, however, although on the banks of the Nolichucky River, stood upstream of Erwin in an area subject to fast currents and white water.

Ads and articles published in such newspapers as the *Savannah Morning News* and private communications brought "outsiders" into Southern Appalachian Tennessee. In addition, hotel proprietorship or resort ownership played a key role in attracting guests from a variety of places. Montvale Springs' Sterling Lanier likely brought in some of his former clientele from Georgia where he had operated Rowland Springs and Macon hotels. Clisbe Austin founded a resort in northern Georgia and operated lodging houses in Hawkins County prior to opening Austin's Springs. Wilder drew visitors to the Cloudland hotel based on his business connections in the iron ore trade, as former mayor of Chattanooga, as Union army hero, and perhaps via his ties with health resorts through his ownership of a Rhea Springs cottage.

Today, the six resorts are no more. TVA dam waters now cover Rhea Springs and the area around Tate Spring; Austin's Springs, now private property, lies at the upper end of the Boone Dam impoundment. The U.S. Forest Service owns the former Cloudland property; the National Park Service administers the Appalachian National Scenic Trail (AT) that runs close to the hotel site. The Unaka Springs hotel, still standing with modifications as of 2022, serves as a private residence close to the Chestoa AT trailhead that lies within the Cherokee National Forest. Tate Spring and Montvale have transitioned into establishments serving young people. Tate operates as a private Christian academy for neglected youth. The Montvale grounds are now home to the Harmony Family Center, which provides therapeutic services and camps to youth, families, and communities.

Austin's Springs

The Watauga River flows eighty miles from the western slopes of North Carolina's Grandfather Mountain to its confluence with the South Fork of the Holston River at TVA's Boone Dam in Northeast Tennessee. The river meanders northwesterly through North Carolina's Avery and Watauga counties into Tennessee's Johnson and Carter counties, forming reservoirs at both TVA's Wilbur Dam (built in 1912 and acquired by TVA in 1945) and Watauga Dam. After leaving Watauga Lake, the river courses southwesterly near Hampton, twists into an ox-bow bend west of Elizabethton, and then flows past the small community of Watauga. It curves again to the northwest to delineate the boundary between Washington and Sullivan counties at Boone Lake near the Austin Springs community.[20]

The river figured in early American history. Daniel Boone roamed the Watauga region, famously carving his boast of "cill[ing] a bar in the year 1760" on a tree that stood in current Washington County near the eponymous Boone's Creek, a tributary of the Watauga. The Watauga Association, considered the first white autonomous government in the British colonies, was formed in modern Carter County in 1772, and served as the site for the Transylvania Purchase, in which the Cherokee Nation ceded control of the Cumberland River Valley and most of Kentucky, about twenty million acres, for trade goods valued at £10,000. In the same area, the Overmountain Men mustered at the Watauga's Sycamore Shoals in 1780 before crossing Yellow Mountain Gap to defeat the British at South Carolina's Battle of King's Mountain.[21]

By 1836, the Washington County seat of Jonesboro, as the town's name was then spelled, could claim about twenty-five professionals, including two physicians, six mechanics, three tanners, and two tavernkeepers. The St. John Milling Company near the Watauga River in the modern community of Watauga had been in operation at that time for almost sixty years. Upper East Tennessee, however, remained largely agrarian, but the coming of rail promised increased commercialization and market access.[22]

In 1848 and 1849, the East Tennessee and Georgia (ET&G) Railroad and the East Tennessee and Virginia (ET&V) Railroad were respectively chartered to connect north Georgia to the major East Tennessee city of Knoxville and to link Knoxville with Bristol at the upper East Tennessee and Southwest Virginia border. By 1855, the ET&G ran from Dalton, Georgia, to Knoxville. Two years later, ET&V rail construction from Knoxville had reached Washington County where an astute Henry Johnson purchased property along the stage road in anticipation of the railroad route. Johnson's construction of a store on this land led to the railroad's erection of a water tank nearby. "Johnson's Tank" served as the hub of commercial development that resulted in the incorporation of Johnson City in 1869. The ET&V crossed the Watauga River at Carter's Depot (now the community of Watauga) and reached Bristol in 1858, resulting in rail reaching across Tennessee, from Georgia to Virginia.[23]

In 1861, a Jewish Jonesboro merchant originally from Bavaria, Jacob Adler, purchased two tracts of farmland totaling almost 850 acres for over $16,000 in northeastern Washington County along the south bank of the Watauga River as a hedge against potential financial downturn during the Civil War. Adler worked enslaved laborers on his farm under the supervision of another German immigrant family while he and his brother-in-law and business partner, Herman Cone, also a Bavarian Jew, remained in Jonesboro.[24] Twelve years later, in spring 1873, Adler sold the land (known as the "Rhea farm") to F.H. and Clisbe Austin, Jr., for $9,000 to be paid in installments over a decade.[25]

F.H. (Frederick H.) and Clisbe, Jr., were two of the more than fifteen children of the controversial, flamboyant Clisbe (Clysby) Austin, Sr. Clisbe, Sr., was born in 1802 in Hawkins County, Tennessee, a county bordering Washington and Sullivan counties on the west.[26] His early primary occupation is unknown (most likely, farming); secondarily, he served as a Methodist deacon after the Methodist Episcopal Church's Holston Conference in 1836 approved his election.[27] By 1848, Clisbe had moved his family to Tunnelsville (now Tunnel Hill), Georgia. There, he built an elegant two-story brick mansion christened "Meadowlawn," opened a store and hotel, became active in the Whig party, and funded the construction of the town's Methodist church.[28]

In 1859, the *Albany Patriot* noted that Clisbe had opened his house as a resort that he called "Limestone Springs."[29] Clisbe advertised his resort for those "desiring to use *pure Limestone Water* [italics original]" and "seeking health, comfort and a *quiet* [italics original] retreat … in a plain, comfortable style."[30] Perhaps the financial success of Catoosa Springs five miles away on the Western & Atlantic Railroad inspired him to compete. He also may have deliberately worded his publicity to contrast his resort's simple and presumably Methodist teetotaling attributes against those of Catoosa, which boasted a variety of fashionable amusements and a bar. In addition, Clisbe may have been attempting to lure those from coastal Georgia traveling from Atlanta to North Georgia to consider a stop first at his resort by billing his location as a mere fifty rods (about 825 feet), all by a convenient boardwalk, from the Tunnel Hill station.[31]

Whatever Clisbe's business intent, within a year he decided to sell the Tunnel Hill property and cryptically gave as his rationale that he was determined to go west.[32] No immediate buyer appeared, but Clisbe continued to advertise the property for sale. In July 1862, he succeeded and headed, not west, but back to Hawkins County where he and some family members established a hotel and eating house at Rogersville Junction (Bull's Gap) by the ET&V railroad.[33]

By 1872, he had sold the Bull's Gap establishment and had moved to Johnson City where he leased a thirty-room hotel and bought the residence of W.H. Taylor, Johnson City's second mayor following its founder, Henry Johnson.[34] In March 1873, his sons purchased "Adler Springs" while Clisbe bought land at Walhalla, South Carolina, for yet another railroad resort, this one to be built by the proposed terminus of the Blue Ridge Railroad.[35]

The Austins initially operated daily hacks to Austin's (Austin) Springs from the Johnson City hotel, the Austin House, itself situated next to "one of the best and largest springs of pure, cold limestone water that ever run from under the mountains."[36] Austin's Springs' chalybeate (iron) spring contained alkaline salts that purportedly treated "neuralgia, rheumatism, nervous dyspepsia and eresypelas (a skin infection)."[37] Indeed, Austin's iron salt and magnesium sulfate (Epsom salt) concentrations ranked near the highest of the Tennessee mineral water analyses listed in Albert Charles Peale's authoritative treatise on mineral waters.[38]

The springs bubbled close to Hyder's Bluff, over one hundred feet high, "overlooking the elegant flowing [Watauga] river and all the valleys and mountains around."[39] Newspapers eagerly reported in spring and summer 1873 that the Austins intended to erect "suitable buildings and to construct a good road from Johnson City."[40]

In the same summer, scattered cholera cases inflicted upper East Tennessee.

At Bull's Gap, Clisbe's son-in-law, the hotelkeeper, died in July while nearby Greenville concurrently breathed a sigh of relief as cases there diminished.[41] In August, F.H. published a short letter taking task with false reports of cholera fatalities at the Bull's Gap house: "We don't mind having the credit of a cholera death once and a while, but don't want to take them all."[42] Likewise, his father announced that the Johnson City Austin hotel and the chalybeate springs showed no sign of cholera and was able to accommodate guests.[43] Going a step further, Clisbe, the resourceful entrepreneur, turned the cholera scare into a business opportunity for a homegrown product.

To prevent a person from contracting cholera, Clisbe patented his "Austin's Liver Regulator," a concoction of apple vinegar and medicinal plant extracts.[44] Whether the Austins ever dispensed the nonalcoholic bitters at Austin's Springs is not known; Clisbe did sell the Liver Regulator in Johnson City and advertised prominent Johnson Citians' testimonials outside the region.[45] Clisbe's medicinal interest and business was sufficiently impactful that he changed his occupation from hotel broker in the 1870 federal census to medical compounder in the next decennial census.[46]

Once the Austins completed the resort hotel, visitors could travel by the ETV&G to Carter's Depot and then take a short ride westerly to the three-storied, white frame hotel with porches wrapped around the first two floors.[47] For the 1874 Fourth of July celebration, the first one since the Civil War to "have elicited much interest in the Southern States," according to a local newspaper, guests from Bristol and Union (modern Bluff City) disembarked at Carter's Depot and then traveled to Austin's largely by hack, only a few by boat because of the Watauga River's shoals and low water level.[48]

A multitude of organized events and activities occurred at the resort in the first dozen years. Tea parties hosted auctions where bachelors bid on supper baskets prepared by eligible young ladies. Civic and church groups organized baseball games, picnics, and day outings.[49] River activities included fishing, boating, and swimming. Publicized also were horseback riding, hunting, and the usual resort activities of ten pins and croquet.[50] Implied in an 1874 advertisement that promised a good time "among plain substantial people," was a simple informality, no designated hours to take promenades on the verandah or down to the springs to sip the waters.[51] Missing from the festivities in this era was alcohol due to the Austins' Methodist teetotalism: Not "cursed with a whiskey saloon," they promised conduct "about the place in a strictly moral manner."[52]

Visitors in the resort's early years included those from the South, one Georgian exuding that "the springs have already attained in notoriety and a reputation equal to many of the older watering places."[53] Jack Plane, prolific travel correspondent for the Georgia press, noted that guests during his stay were mainly Tennesseans, with some from Mississippi and Alabama, along with a few from Savannah and Macon. Plane also observed that the resort lacked many of the amenities of more established resorts but that the Austins were making improvements as their means allowed.[54] Accordingly, Austin's 1878 monthly rate was $20, a third lower than the $30 monthly fee charged by the *grande dame* watering hole of the Smokies, Montvale Springs, which could command a higher price from its clientele.[55]

The 1879 southern yellow fever epidemic brought scores of visitors to Austin's. Mineral spring resorts such as Bon Aqua in Middle Tennessee denied entry to Memphians fleeing from the poorly-understood disease.[56] Austin's Springs welcomed Memphians even as press rumors grew of Memphians' dissatisfaction with bad fare and high lodging rates in East Tennessee.[57] One Memphian countered the criticism: "Reports from Austin Springs, Hale Springs, Tate Springs, Montvale, White Cliff and various other places [are] equally favorable.... Those who have to refugee from Memphis can hardly do better than come to East Tennessee."[58] Rubbing elbows at Austin's with the refugees, literally at poker games, were prominent locals such as Judge John Allison, future author of *Dropped Stitches in Tennessee History,* and Congressman (and future Tennessee Governor and Senator) Bob Taylor.[59]

Although the press reported favorably on Austin's Springs, the Austin brothers lacked income to spend on the resort and explored various options to increase their capital. In 1876, F.H. unsuccessfully sought a resort partner to invest $3,000 to $5,000 (over $84,000 in 2022 dollars) while working as a Remington sewing machine agent.[60] The same year he publicized openings for his short-lived Watauga Institute for Young Ladies ("Chalybeate water [for] pupils of delicate constitution").[61] The ventures failed to secure enough money to pay Adler the $1,000 payment due in 1877; the parties renegotiated the deed.[62]

The Austins persevered in their business ventures, perhaps as much as to keep the resort as to simply generate income. In 1880, Clisbe Jr., produced the first commercial chewing tobacco in East Tennessee at Austin's Springs and later moved his successful operation to Greeneville.[63] By the mid–1880s, F.H. was also managing the Banner House near the Elk Park, North Carolina, depot of the East Tennessee and Western North Carolina (ET&WNC) that ran from Johnson City to magnetite iron ore mines in Cranberry, North Carolina. F.H. also operated a Cranberry timber mill that provided lumber for the Austins' Johnson City furniture factory; he had forfeited an earlier creative vision of building a boat with a steam-saw mill and a dwelling house that he planned to float from Austin's Springs to Knoxville.[64]

Tragedy and subsequent financial hardship, however, fell to the Austins in the next few years. In 1883, Clisbe died at Austin's Springs. H.C. (Henry Clay), the youngest son, who in 1880 managed a venerable antebellum-era built hotel near the Smokies' Montvale Springs, moved to Austin's Springs, presumably to assist in the Austin operations. After F.H.'s death in 1886 from a logging train accident on the ET&WNC, the Austin finances declined precipitously.[65]

The Austins' downturn was evidenced in several commercial and legal actions. The family sold the furniture factory in November 1887 and forfeited a city lot next to the ET&WNC because of failure to pay back taxes.[66] A week later, notice of a Tennessee Supreme Court decree advertised an upcoming auction for the resort because of judgment in favor of Adler against the Austins for loan default.[67] The Washington County Chancery Court instructed creditors to file claims against the Austins' legal entity, Austin & Co., in 1889. In August that year, John H. Caldwell, cashier of Bristol's First National Bank bought the resort for $2,500.[68]

The resort began a renaissance over the next three decades, not only via owner investment, but also by area hotels' publicity and municipal boosterism. Johnson

City's Hotel Carnegie, for example, itself advertised as a summer resort, emphasized its location as "convenient to the 'celebrated' Kings Springs and Austin's Springs."[69] Jonesboro, billing itself as "perhaps the most desirable place ... in East Tennessee at which to spend the heated term," highlighted "one to two hour drives" to "Clark's and Austin's celebrated springs, all on good roads."[70] Six years later, in 1898, Johnson City businessmen advertised their town as a summer resort in part due to its proximity to Austin's, "considered the purest chalybeate water in the country."[71]

Accordingly, Austin's saw a minor revival in the 1890s. In 1893 it arranged to deliver its chalybeate water to Johnson City for sale. In 1896, Johnson City physician Walter J. Miller bought the resort and contracted two years later for a new hotel, the Riverside Inn, more commonly known as the Austin's Springs Hotel, to be built close to the bluff, a few hundred yards west of the current one. Miller, appointed by Governor Bob Taylor to the State Board of Health in 1897 and his personal physician, may have received the ailing governor at the new hotel in 1898 amid press speculation that there he could enjoy absolute rest and obtain the benefit of the chalybeate water.[72]

Although one guest at the turn of the century reported that she was "practically restored to her normal weight" during her resort stay, Austin's Springs' primary emphasis, as was the case for most watering holes of that era, lay in its amusements and recreation.[73] Austin's organized a colt show in 1893 that also included a baseball game between two local teams. Several prominent Johnson City citizens, including H.D. Gump, W.W. Faw, and Dr. J.W. Cox, organized a three-day fair in 1897. The 1903 Fourth of July celebration featured swimming and foot races, a clay pigeon shoot, bowling, table tennis, trolley barge rides for bathers to cross to the Watauga's far side, and an evening ball.[74]

Overnight visitors from the early 1900s appear to have been largely regional, possibly indicating the desire for a modest vacation near home. In 1902 and 1903, for example, guests listed in the hotel register came from almost one hundred locales, about one fifth of them in upper East Tennessee, especially Johnson City. Local guests in that two-year period included the Deadericks, owners of neighboring Unicoi County's Unaka Springs resort, established less than eight years earlier and beginning to vie with Austin's Springs as a venue for health and recreation. The "War of the Roses" gubernatorial rivals, the Taylor brothers, the Democrat Bob from Knoxville and the Republican Alf (Alfred) from Johnson City, recorded their stay in August 1903. Out-of-state guests for this two-year period included a few from Georgia, Mississippi, and Alabama. Outnumbering them, however, were visitors from central and northern Virginia and north into Philadelphia and New York City. Probably most of these northern guests came by the Southern Railway; the Virginia town addresses largely coincide with the railroad's depots.[75] The number of overnight guests appears to have decreased during this period; the ledger records only seventeen parties for 1902's Fourth of July.[76] Despite lower resort numbers, however, opening season galas continued: a Knoxville newspaper lauded the opening of the 1903 resort season for its pomp and splendor, and a large crowd of Johnson City society attended the 1905 grand ball.[77] Locals continued their day trips for picnics. One participant as a young boy in the early 1910s recalled that his mother required two days

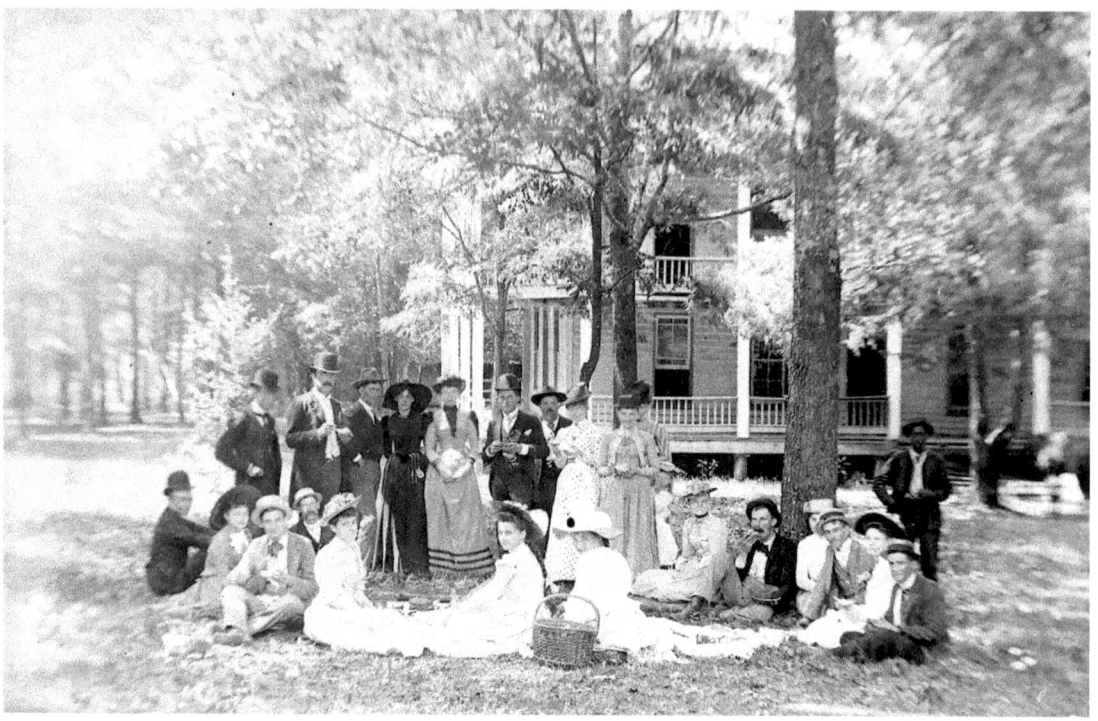

"Austin Springs," Washington County, Tennessee (image courtesy of the John Goodin Papers, Archives of Appalachia, East Tennessee State University, *https://archivesofappalachia.omeka.net/items/show/12268*. ID: 0297_00449).

to prepare his family's elaborate picnic basket; his family then traveled by gravel road in a buggy, fording two creeks, to reach the resort from Johnson City.[78]

The 1920s and early 1930s saw the denouement of the resort even as local roads improved to take travelers to Austin's or elsewhere. In 1920, "Good Road" bond sales funded road construction. A bridge replaced the ferry crossing at Hyder's Bluff, and a new road shortened by eight miles the distance between Johnson City and Bristol in neighboring Sullivan County.[79]

Despite better roads, various lessees and owners failed to recapture Austin's Springs' former prestige, perhaps because potential guests could motor to other resorts. In 1923, Jacob Alder's son recalled a stop at the "delapidated [sic] building of the old Austin Springs Hotel."[80] Castle Heights Military Academy built study halls, athletic courts, and barracks on the property for a boys' summer camp in 1924 but declared bankruptcy in 1925 after only thirty boys instead of the planned one hundred attended the camp.[81] Johnson City made plans to host a tourist camp there in 1927 to replace one four miles away.[82] In the early 1930s, a dirt track racing venture began near the resort, and a night club and dancing pavilion, the Country Kitchen, opened on the site of the old hotel, which had burned down.[83]

Austin's Springs' last chapter was written in the mid–1930s. In summer 1935, a fire destroyed the Country Kitchen.[84] The Works Progress Administration built a school on the racetrack, as recalled by a few former students. In 1937 the Riverside

Park development (formerly the Austin Springs Land Company) divided the former resort and area into lots for sale. Today, the Austin's Springs property that includes the two springs is privately owned.[85]

Cloudland Hotel

Roan Mountain, or "the Roan," straddles the easternmost section of Carter County in Tennessee and the westernmost section of Mitchell County in North Carolina. The Roan does not consist of a single peak: its undulating ridgeline varies from 5,512 feet at Carver's Gap to 6,285 feet at Roan High Knob. The peaks or knobs are generally called "balds" because of a preponderance of sedges and grasses, the cause of which is debated in scientific circles.[86] As a result of the lack of wooded cover, one may hike for hours and admire unobstructed panoramic vistas. Elisha Mitchell, the nineteenth-century University of North Carolina science professor for whom Mount Mitchell is named, wrote that "a person may gallop his horse for a mile or two, with Carolina at his feet on one side, and Tennessee on the other, and a green ocean of mountains raised into tremendous billows immediately about him."[87]

Mitchell was one of many scientists and travelers who trekked to the Roan in the antebellum era, thus dispelling the idea of a mountainous area shunned by the outside world. André Michaux, royal botanist to Louis XVI, named the famous *Rhododendron catawbiense*, whose 600 acres on the Roan constitutes the largest natural rhododendron gardens in the world.[88] In 1796 Methodist bishop Francis Asbury rode fourteen hours from North Carolina's Toe River across the Roan Highlands to the Doe River in Tennessee where he preached the following day.[89] About the same time, botanist John Fraser collected plant specimens on the Roan for Catherine the Great; his name now denotes the *Abies fraseri*, the Fraser fir, whose dark green color may have given the Black Mountains their name. François-André Michaux, son of André, botanized on the Roan and later published *Forest Trees of North America* (1857).[90] In 1841, Harvard University botanist Asa Gray, honored later by the eponymously named *Lilium grayi*, the orange-red Gray's lily, wrote that "it was just sunset when we reached the bald and grassy summit [and enjoyed] for a moment the magnificent view it affords...."[91] Seven years later, travel writer Charles Lanman observed that the same balds' "fine and luxuriant grass" served as pastureland for the "immense numbers" of local farmers' cattle and horses, therefore pointing out the increased populace of the Roan valley.[92]

In addition to agriculture, area residents engaged in extractive industries, particularly iron-ore mining. Iron works built by such regional notables as Elijah Embree and John Sevier proliferated in antebellum times.[93] Elizabethton lobbied as early as 1835 for a proposed Cincinnati and Charleston railroad to pass through Carter County and western North Carolina because of the town's boast that the area then could manufacture enough iron to supply the entire country.[94] An 1858 East Tennessee newspaper quoted the *American Railroad Times* that "North-eastern Tennessee and North-western North Carolina ... [possess] incalculable resources for iron making, and must become at some distant day one of the great centres."[95]

The excellent iron ore grade attracted General John T. Wilder, the builder of the Cloudland Hotel, to the Roan Mountain area in the 1870s. Wilder, born in New York in 1830, moved to Ohio as a young man where he gained experience in mill-wright and foundry work and began geological studies. In 1857, Wilder resettled in Indiana where he opened a foundry and used his knowledge on hydraulics to build plants in several states, including Tennessee and Virginia.[96]

When the Civil War broke out, Wilder converted his foundry to cannon ball production for the Union army. He also served as a Union captain and then as colonel of a light artillery company that became known as Wilder's Lighting Brigade for its decisive battle actions.[97] After the Battle of Chickamauga in 1863, Wilder received promotion to brigadier general for his military leadership.[98]

After studying a Tennessee state geological report during campaign lulls, Wilder decided after the war to move to Chattanooga for its proximity to mineral resources and for its milder climate (his poor health had forced him to resign from the military in 1864). He formed the Roane (after Roane County, Tennessee) Iron Company with two former military associates, which built the first blast furnace operated in the South. Wilder also engaged in other foundry and machine-tooling enterprises, largely in the Chattanooga area.[99]

Around 1870, after engaging in various business and political ventures in Chattanooga, including a brief tenure as mayor, Wilder purchased 7,000 acres at the Roan's higher elevation for $25.15 per acre (four million dollars in 2022).[100] He spent part of the next few years at the base of Roan Mountain in a hamlet that he eventually named Roan Mountain Station in anticipation of the railroad reaching it from Johnson City. According to one local, he laid out and named all the streets, planted all the trees, and, succinctly put, "gave spark to the town."[101] Four years later, he moved to Johnson City, presumably to be closer to his varied business affairs, among them, organization of the Carnegie Land and Improvement Company and serving as vice-president of the Charleston, Cincinnati & Chicago (Three C's) Railroad.[102] In the 1870s, Wilder purchased iron-ore tracts in western North Carolina where he operated a blast furnace at Cranberry and established a mine at what is now Buladean. After the completion of the narrow-gauge East Tennessee and Western North Carolina Railroad in 1882 from Hampton, Tennessee, to Cranberry, Wilder's mines shipped pig iron and ore on the railroad from Cranberry to Johnson City.[103]

Wilder as an entrepreneur recognized another revenue stream: travelers to the mountains. In the early- to mid–1870s, Wilder built a family cottage on top of the Roan, which became the first of his three hotels on the ridge. In August 1877, he turned the cottage into a boarding house, christened as the "Cloudland" that month by a visiting professor's wife.[104] In November 1878, he began to construct nearby the second Cloudland, a modest spruce lodge of fifteen or twenty rooms, with a covered front porch and swinging hammocks.[105] The spruce lodge proved so popular that Wilder began construction within the next six years of the third and best known of his Roan resorts.[106] He erected a steam saw mill near the new hotel site to process nearby spruce timber for the envisioned three-story hotel, at a rate of 10,000 board-feet per day.[107] Built at a cost of over $40,000 (well over $15 million estimated for a construction project in 2022 dollars), the new Cloudland Hotel opened for business in 1885.[108]

Cloudland management operated the spruce lodge in tandem with the new hotel for at least four years. A Johnson City newspaper observed that W.S. Ayers of Richmond, the proprietor with his brother for the 1889 season, "has already received hundreds of letters from parties engaging rooms for the summer, and he expects to have both hotels full during the entire season."[109] A hotel pamphlet in the 1880s noted that "Tennis Courts will be added to both Hotels for the pleasure of guests."[110]

The new Cloudland's white-frame vernacular construction on the top of a bald dominated the horizon. Its front faced into North Carolina; its back and two ells stood in Tennessee. A line painted across the dining room hardwood floor to indicate the states' boundaries served as more than just a point of interest: the line allowed North Carolina authorities to monitor drinking guests on the wet Tennessee side who accidentally wandered onto the dry North Carolina side. First-story verandahs extending almost 400 feet along the front and the two ells of the hotel permitted vast views of the neighboring mountain peaks.[111] An 1884 newspaper article on the hotel construction's progress marveled at the structure's dimensions: each hotel wing was to measure 42 by 414 feet (longer than a modern football field), with 218 bedrooms, "four more than that of [the resort at] Warm Springs, NC."[112]

The final number of guest rooms fluctuates wildly among sources consulted. A floor plan, however, appears to show sixty-six bedrooms on each of the two higher stories and perhaps another thirty on the first floor for a total close to the 166 rooms cited by some sources, including Frank Shell who worked there as a clerk, 1900–1905.[113]

The hotel rooms provided an ambiance of warmth and luxury amid the Roan's lofty height and relative remoteness. Central steam heating supplemented the rooms' fireplaces in the chilly summer evenings and early mornings, and oil lamps provided additional light. Each room contained several pieces of solid cherry furniture, a washstand with an ornate porcelain bowl and pitcher, and a copper bathtub. Telephone service, installed in 1885, soon failed because of unusual static charges at the Cloudland's high elevation; a telegraph line replaced it, allowing businessmen to keep apprised of office affairs.[114]

Access to the Roan summit and later to the Cloudland proved to be a formidable challenge prior to rail service. In 1873 Wilder and his partners built the first road, later called the Calf Pen Road, the Roan Road, or the Glen Ayre Road, from Little Rock Creek in North Carolina. In 1875, Wilder ordered the construction of a hack or buggy road, known as the Ball Road or Bald Road, from Wilder's Forge (modern Buladean) near Big Rock Creek, North Carolina, to the vicinity of Roan High Bluff. Eventually, additional minor routes from North Carolina to Cloudland were built to the Roan.[115] The most notable road, however, sections of it still in use today as both the Burbank Road and as a U.S. Forest Service Trail, is the Hack Line Road on the Tennessee side of the Roan.[116]

The Hack Line Road began at Roan Mountain Station and snaked up the side of the Roan. Given the extreme ruggedness of the area coupled with the primitive equipment available in the 1870s, building the road constituted no insignificant civil engineering project. As he did for his hotel construction projects, Wilder employed locals as his work crew, who used dynamite in conjunction with mattocks, axes, and other hand tools to dig and blast along the mountain to build the Hack Line.[117] A Mitchell County resident recalled that his father, Riley McKinney, "went to work when it was light enough to see and worked till dark. They got fifty cents a day to build the road to the old hotel on the Roan."[118]

Both the Hack Line Road and the Bald Road sharply narrowed in places because of the rocky terrain. The Bald Road is probably the carriage road which two sources stated needed trussed and stilted construction to widen the road so that carriages could pass along bluff edges.[119] Sherman Pippen, who drove guests from Roan Mountain Station to the Cloudland in the early 1900s, recalled that the Hack Line's blind curves forced him to rely on his horse's ears perking up to know when a wagon from the other direction was approaching.[120]

With the completion of the railroad to Roan Mountain Station and to selected points in western North Carolina, guests coming from Tennessee found the journey less time-consuming (and bumpy) but still an adventure on the hack rides. About a year after the spruce lodge opened, visitors could ride the East Tennessee, Virginia, and Georgia Railroad to Johnson City (then known as Johnson's Depot) and then take one of the thrice-weekly hacks for the thirty-two mile ride to the Cloudland.[121] Once the East Tennessee and Western North Carolina, or Stemwinder, narrow-gauge railroad was completed in 1882 to Cranberry, travelers enjoyed a two and one-half hour rail trip through the Doe River Gorge, "the wildest gorge of the Alleghanies," to Roan Mountain Station.[122]

Access to the Cloudland from North Carolina generally required more time and transfers. Guests could ride the Western North Carolina Railroad to Marion where they procured a hack for a forty-five mile ride to the Cloudland via Linville Falls, fifteen miles southeast of the Roan. From Asheville, sixty miles from the Roan, guests paid a driver to take them to Bakersville where they spent the night before embarking on a several-hours journey the next day to the Cloudland.[123] Alternatively, guests could disembark at the Clinchfield railroad station at Toecane, about fifteen miles from Buladean and about ten miles from Bakersville, to ride a hack up the Bald Road.[124]

Visitors stopping at the Roan Mountain depot typically spent the night across the rail tracks at the Roan Mountain Inn, a three-story, white-frame structure built by Wilder, before taking the Roan Mountain Stage Line the next day over the twelve-mile Hack Line Road.[125] The hack charge in 1885 was $4 roundtrip with the first fifty pounds of luggage free (about the cost of two nights' lodging at the Cloudland or about $126 in 2022 dollars).[126] At about the halfway point on the road, the hack driver pulled off to the left at a spring for his passengers to enjoy water "cold enough to frost a glass."[127]

Of course, walking to the hotel was always an option, either for tourists or for local residents. It appears that an ongoing challenge of sorts existed: an 1885 newspaper account noted that three men walked the Hack Line in two hours and fifty-eight minutes, the "best time on record."[128]

Among visitors in 1879 to the Cloudland spruce lodge were Asa Gray and nationally prominent botanists William Canby, John Redfield, and Charles Sprague Sargent. They found the hotel "comfortable and well kept." Redfield noted that the forest that had been encroaching upon the bald at the Cloudland had been checked by the cutting of firewood and fencing materials.[129]

Four years later, a member of Boston's Appalachian Mountain Club journeyed to Johnson City and rode the Stemwinder to Roan Mountain Station where he planned to act upon a rail table footnote that promised "Carriages at Roan Mountain Station for Cloudland Hotel" and to obtain a room at the Cloudland spruce lodge because he had received assurance that the Cloudland was open all year. To his chagrin, he discovered that the one wagon at Roan Mountain Station was broken, that the hotel had not been open for several years, and that the Hack Line Road remained unfinished. He secured a horse, however, and later reported to his club that "from the base of the summit a road is nearly completed.... It was a delightful stroll through the finest forest that I ever saw, through a magnificent flower garden, from base to summit." The Cloudland was a "low picturesque building, rudely constructed, but sufficiently large to make a party of thirty or more comfortable." He encountered a workman repairing lodge shingles and had a "comfortable [night] on a bed of shavings in front of the log fire" inside the lodge.[130]

Charles Dudley Warner, a collaborator of Mark Twain's and a humorist in his own right, also visited the Cloudland spruce lodge. In his travel essay, he wrote that "the hotel (since replaced by a good house) was a rude mountain structure, with a couple of comfortable rooms for office and sitting room, in which big wood fires were blazing; for though the thermometer might record 60°, as it did when we arrived, fire was welcome."[131] Warner encountered visitors from as far south as New Orleans and a few female botanists, the latter uncommon in the 1880s, but all of whom were "delightful company." After a day of rain, Warner and his traveling companion rode about a mile away to Roan High Bluff to see the sunset. He wrote: "In every direction the mountains were clear, and a view was obtained of the vast horizon and the hills and lowlands of several states—a continental prospect, scarcely anywhere else equaled for variety or distance."[132]

Cloudland occupies a unique niche among Southern Appalachian resorts for its large number of botanist visitors. The resort appealed as well to a later clientele based on its health and leisure offerings. Its promotional materials paid homage to the nineteenth-century obsession with mineral springs: one brochure succinctly noted "that several springs of mineral water ... within a few minutes' walk of the Hotel ... have excellent medicinal properties."[133] Furthermore, the Cloudland's high altitude enabled its ads to boast of the absence of heat, humidity, and malaria, and respite from hay fever.

Although one travel brochure for western North Carolina cautioned against recuperating from hay fever at an altitude over 6,000 feet because of the possibilities of a diminished appetite and "frequently disordered" digestive organs, the Cloudland heavily promoted its "6,394 feet above sea level" to hay fever sufferers. Indeed, it grandly branded itself as "The Great Southern Resort for Hay Fever."[134] So many guests afflicted by asthma, hay fever, and other pollen-induced illnesses trekked to the Cloudland in the late nineteenth century that they became known as the "Hay Fever Brigade." A Tennessee State Board of Health report pointed to the Cloudland as an example for prospective hotels and sanitaria to follow to attract guests suffering from summer asthma and similar afflictions. Just as mineral springs visitors made grand tours, so evidently did hay fever patients. For example, a Pennsylvania woman in one testimonial averred that the Cloudland air completely eradicated her hay fever as contrasted to her stays at Caesars Head in South Carolina and in the White Mountains in New Hampshire.[135]

The Hay Fever Brigade that gathered at the Cloudland paid tribute to a national preoccupation with the illness in the latter part of the nineteenth century. Hay fever—also known as summer catarrh, autumnal catarrh, Peach Cold, Rose Cold, June Cold, or July Cold, depending on the time of year—became a fashionable disease in the postbellum period. Hay fever sufferers visited exclusive resorts, for example, in the White Mountains, to seek relief from their symptoms.[136] In the early 1870s, physicians began to publish their hypotheses as to the epidemiology of the disease. A British doctor, Charles H. Blackley speculated that hay fever was "almost wholly confined to the upper classes of society, it is rarely, if ever, met with but among the educated."[137] American doctor George M. Beard three years later echoed Blackley in *Hay-Fever; or, Summer Catarrh* (1876). He commented that hay fever prevailed among those with "nervous diasthesis," a condition most commonly found in the

> organization of the civilized, refined, and educated, rather than of the barbarous and low-born and untrained—of women more than of men. It is developed, fostered, and perpetuated with the progress of civilization, with the advance of culture and refinement, and the corresponding preponderance of labor of the brain over that of the muscles.[138]

Beard's observation that hay fever was "a disease of the fashionable and the thoughtful—the price of wealth and culture," indicative of the opinion of many physicians, encouraged many to believe that they suffered from the ailment.[139] In 1874 hay fever sufferers meeting in the White Mountains organized the U.S. Hay Fever Association, whose goals *The New York Times* dryly hypothesized in 1898 related to handkerchiefs.[140] The newspaper in 1880 belittled the group's existence: "People who have small-pox or scarlet fever, or even gout, have never formed a small-pox club, a scarlet fever society, or a gouty men's association."[141]

The aristocratic hay fever patients' assertion that certain resorts effected a cure led *The New York Times* to ponder rhetorically why a typical catarrh sufferer believed that he would recover in the "cool and picturesque region of the White Mountains" but "would rapidly sneeze his life away" in Coxsackie. The article blamed hotelkeepers for promoting their resorts, particularly those in the White Mountains, as each surrounded by a "peculiar brand of air that is an infallible remedy for the disease." In short, stated the newspaper, "hay fever is simply the creation of hotel-keepers ... kept alive and spread by their exertions."[142]

The resort and its hay fever trade, in a larger sense, followed a national trend in American travel. The hay fever craze resulted from and enhanced a burgeoning tourist industry already offering services to the educated elite, particularly those in the urban and industrial East.[143] Unlike consumption, for which doctors also prescribed "perfectly pure air, away from towns or even villages, on some height for choice," a hay fever diagnosis served as an honorable class distinction.[144] As Beard wrote, "tuberculous diathesis frequently appears in the coarsely organized, the plethoric, and the muscular.... [T]uberculosis also afflicts the day-laborer and the savage." Accordingly, the Cloudland billed itself as a resort where "[c]onsumption is unknown."[145]

At the Cloudland in the late 1800s, a substantial number of guests, even those with their fashionable handkerchiefs, enjoyed nature with at least limited physical exertion. During the day, guests collected plant specimens, fished in one of Cloudland's two ponds, golfed (requiring weighted balls at the high elevation), or hiked. The daughter of the last proprietor recalled that her mother often led hikes; unfazed by the dress protocol of the day, women participants wore skirts hemmed above their ankles and laced on high-topped shoes. Excursions to the "little bluff" at ten cents and the "big bluff" at twenty-five cents occurred at regular intervals. The Cloudland occasionally retained a couple of western North Carolina mountain fiddlers to serenade the hikers at the bluffs.[146]

Famous guests at the second Cloudland hotel included Judge Grafton Greene (a future Tennessee State Supreme Court Chief Justice), Brownlow family members from Knoxville, Harvey Firestone, Henry Ford, and the naturalist John Muir, founder of the Sierra Club. Sherman Pippen remembered transporting dignitaries from Great Britain, Ireland, and France to the Cloudland. The colorful Pippen once grabbed a wild turkey strutting next to his hack and tossed it into the lap of his passenger, an upright bishop, whom he charged with holding the squirming bird until they reached the hotel. Among the more exotic guests were a Madame Yznaga from New Orleans and her daughter Consuelo, named after a Vanderbilt family friend's daughter, and a princess from Spain, who evidently spent too much time on the Tennessee side of the dining hall one night.[147]

Other notables visiting the Cloudland included George Washington Vanderbilt, grandson of the Commodore, and most likely John Jacob Astor. Vanderbilt bought land near Asheville for his eventual Biltmore château in 1888 after he had brought his ailing mother to the area to be seen by Dr. S.W. Battle. By 1890, Vanderbilt was also a shareholder in Asheville's Kenilworth Inn, demonstrating his interest in the local tourist industry.[148] In June 1892, Vanderbilt and several others, including Battle and Charles McNamee (the Biltmore construction supervisor), left Asheville on horseback, registered at the Young's Hotel, a Victorian house located in Bakersville, North Carolina, for the night and then traveled with a guide to Roan Mountain.[149] Several in Vanderbilt's party then went to Johnson City where they boarded Vanderbilt's private train car for New York.[150] John Jacob Astor signed the Young's Hotel register in fall 1883 either for himself or on behalf of his family and may have traveled from Bakersville to the Cloudland.[151]

Notable groups convening at the Cloudland included the Tennessee Press Association. The group met there in 1887 to hear John Allison vividly paint the Roan as "a Niagara of color flashing from the rhododendron and Mountain Magnolia." The press association once again gathered at the hotel in 1896 to "indulge in genial converse and comradeship ... forgetful of the dust and din of the printing office."[152] For newspapermen to travel to the Roan from across the state points to the resort's prominence.

Meals often constituted extravagant affairs in the large dining room. A typical breakfast, according to Nannie Snyder Murrell, wife of the proprietor in the early 1900s, consisted of bacon, liver, steak, fried apples, fried potatoes, biscuits, coffee, eggs, and flannel cakes (pancakes). Dinner, served at noon, offered a choice of two soups, two entrées, at least two meats, six vegetables, and a choice of four desserts. Mountain trout was evidently a specialty, for hundreds of pounds were served each season. Supper was often dinner leftovers accompanied by cereal, meats, flannel cakes, and eggs.[153]

In the evening, guests adjourned to the basement and either amused themselves with bowling or with dances accompanied by a piano, violin, and cornet. During the 1885 season, the niece of the Tennessee governor taught young children in the basement playroom.[154]

To indulge aristocratic guests with banquets and a wide array of activities required the services of many porters, maids, and cooks, who were white for at least the first decade, as one prejudiced Memphis woman noted pleasingly in 1894. The head chef was a Frenchman who directed the White House culinary staff during President Grant's administration. Young ladies from an Asheville academy served the elites in the dining room.[155] In later years, Blacks, who may or may not have been local, worked in the kitchen and in the barbershop.[156]

Mountaineers also found employment at the Cloudland, largely behind the scenes and in subservient or menial roles. Bill Hughes worked as a butcher at the Cloudland in the summer and as a caretaker in the winter.[157] John Gouge in the early 1900s brought his family from the North Carolina side of the Roan to live at the Cloudland while he served as caretaker and as buyer for produce and livestock, earning a meager income of $40 per year (about $6,560 in 2022 dollars) plus free rent for his family.[158] One Roan Mountain town resident recalled her father's experiences as a 14-year-old who fired the stoves for the kitchen staff, who in turn taught him how to bake potato-yeast bread, a recipe which he passed on to his children.[159] Local girls and women walked several miles every day up the mountain to the Cloudland to work as chamber maids and to iron and mend clothes.[160] Other residents took the Bald Road to the Cloudland to sell produce and vegetables. Wilder ate meals at the home of a Cove Creek family near the Hack Line Road and in turn bought honey, vegetables, fruits, and other foods from them.[161]

A New York visitor wrote that "the poverty of these people is startling, and sometimes pathetic. A man walked eight miles to bring 60 cents' worth of corn to the hotel, and another day two girls walked twelve miles to bring 15 cents' worth of beets!"[162] A man whose father had helped construct the Hack Line Road stated that his father and other locals "didn't get but about twenty cents a dozen for corn. Everyone who had anything to sell took it up there. They didn't get much for it, but no one had any money at all and they were so glad to get some."[163]

During the Panic of 1893, Wilder suffered monetary setbacks, including incurring debts of $125,000 from his Johnson City Carnegie businesses, which prompted the robber baron Henry Clay Frick to disavow any relationship between his Carnegie Steel operation and that of Wilder's.[164] Perhaps still financially recovering three years later, Wilder almost lost the Cloudland Hotel for failure to pay delinquent property taxes of $11,615 ($418,000 in 2022 dollars).[165]

Wilder eventually lost interest in the Cloudland Hotel and offered the property to the Murrells for $20,000, which they declined.[166] John and Mary Gouge and their dozen children stayed at the Cloudland as caretakers for several years after the Murrells' lease expired in 1905. Often the winter weather proved so severe that they remained at the Cloudland rather than risk the three-mile round trip down to their cabin on the North Carolina side of the Roan.[167] Lack of sufficient funds and attention from Wilder prompted a visitor in 1913 to note the building's dirty condition. The hotel was eventually abandoned. In 1915 a hiker described in his journal the Cloudland's "glassless windows, leaking roofs, [and] sagging floors."[168]

Wilder died at his summer retreat in Jacksonville, Florida, in 1917.[169] In 1919 Wilder's heirs sold the hotel to a local, who then parceled it off room by room. One family bought the kitchen for thirty dollars in 1919 and reassembled the timber into a house five miles down the mountain. A lawyer in Burbank obtained the barn and livery stable and rebuilt them on his property. Locals took the fine cherry furniture and other furnishings. Several sources stated that many homeowners eventually replaced their front doors with hotel bedroom doors painted with the Cloudland room numbers.[170]

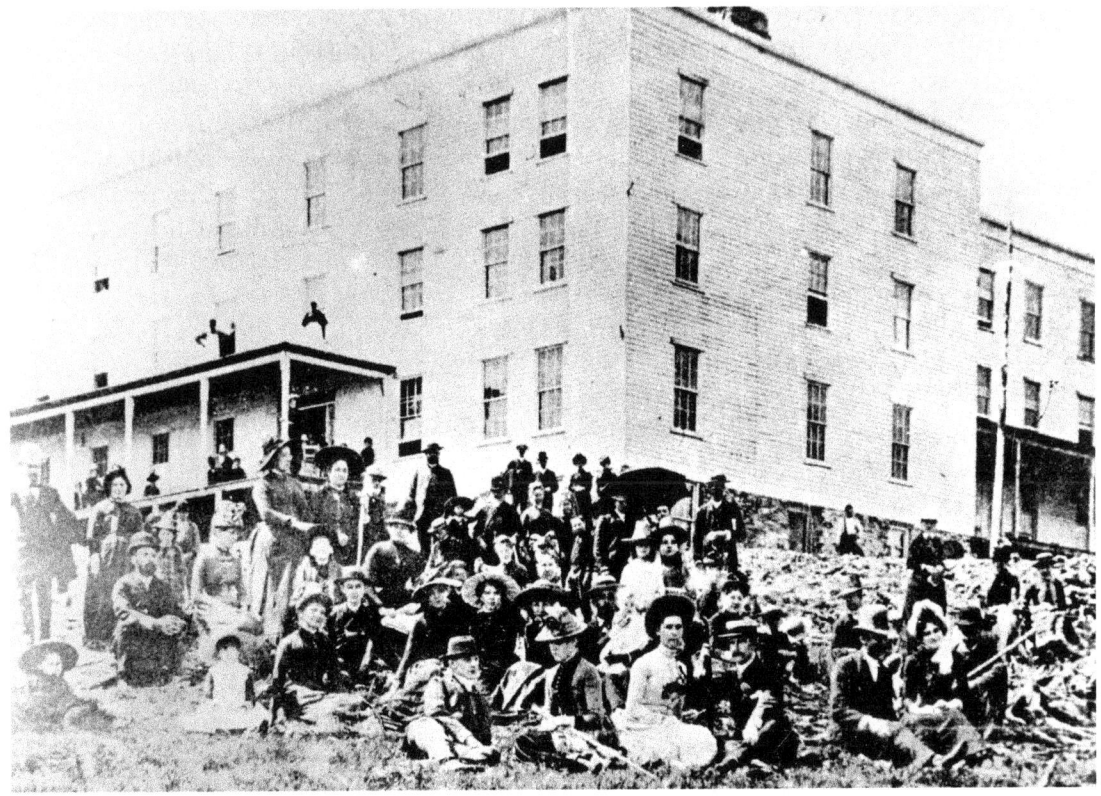

Cloudland Hotel [~1890–1895], Carter County, Tennessee; Mitchell County, North Carolina (image courtesy of the Kim Hendrix Collection, Archives of the City of Elizabethton, Elizabethton-Carter County Public Library, Elizabethton, TN. ID: ACE-CC12-01).

Residents in Carter County, such as those living in the Simerly and Tiger creek communities near present-day State Highway 173, continued to hike or take wagons to the Cloudland site for camping or Sunday picnics. A few enterprising Johnson City businessmen in the early 1930s set up a toll road on the Burbank Road, the name given to a section of the Hack Line Road, and hired a Burbank Road resident to collect a one-dollar fare for each car and driver and twenty-five cents for each passenger; J.C. Penney was one elite who paid the toll. Even during the Depression, occasionally a few hundred cars a day bounced their way up the road.[171]

In 1941, the U.S. Forest Service acquired almost 3,000 acres across the Roan. By spring 1955, the government agency had constructed a paved road from Carver's Gap to the Cloudland site.[172]

The Roan Mountain Inn that Wilder owned in conjunction with the Cloudland was sold in 1905 to S.B. Wood, a doctor for the Forge Mining Company, whose drug store stood as of 2018 next to U.S. Highway 19E; Wood operated the inn for ten years. After a state of neglect, it reopened in 1949 but was torn down in 1952.[173]

Today the Roan Mountain Inn is gone; the Roan Mountain Station depot is now a bank; and U.S. Highway 19E covers much of the narrow-gauge rail past Elizabethton. Tourists wandering on top of the Roan through a grassy expanse may stop to read a U.S. Forest Service sign commemorating the Cloudland. Where guests once feasted at the magnificent dining room banquet table now grows wheat-colored grass broken only by the Appalachian Trail. Where naturalist John Muir wrote to his family over a century ago that "I have been quite miserable but this air has healed me," now stands a copse of red spruce and Fraser fir.[174] And, within this group of trees lies a rubble of fieldstone, the only remnant of the summer home above the clouds.

Montvale Springs

More than twelve million visitors come to the Great Smoky Mountains National Park in a typical year, but most likely only a few knew of the nearby location of one of the most famous Southern Appalachian antebellum health resorts. Montvale Springs, the oldest watering hole in East Tennessee, dating back to 1832, stands in Blount County at an elevation of about 1,400 feet at the foot of the Chilhowee ridgeline on the park's western border, about nine miles south of Maryville and twenty-four miles south of Knoxville. At the summit of Chilhowee Mountain, about three miles by trail from Montvale, is a large rock formation, Look Rock or View Rock, offering a spectacular view of Happy Valley and the Smokies to the east and foothills and rolling country to the west.[175]

As happened at many Southern Appalachian mineral spring resorts, Montvale's springs were rediscovered by whites after having been used by Native Americans. In 1829, Jesse Wallace and Jesse Thompson stumbled upon twin springs while searching for lost cattle; they subsequently bought a land tract that included the springs.

In 1831, Daniel D. Foute, who had moved into the Great Smoky Mountains' Cades Cove area in the 1820s, acquired the springs tract; the next year he opened near the springs a two-story, ten-room log hotel fronted by a porch across its length. Probably because Sam Houston a few decades earlier had supposedly christened the area "Montvale," Foute advertised his newly opened establishment with a hand-written bill for "Montvale or Modern Bethesda Springs." In 1834, he also bought another tract of land a few miles away, which contained the "Black Sulphur Spring," to provide additional mineral water to his guests.[176]

No doubt to encourage resort business and to allow access to his vast land holdings, Foute in the 1830s constructed several pack trails or roads. He built, with hired Cherokee labor, a road from Montvale across the mountain and down Rhea Valley (Happy Valley) to intersect with the Calloway and Parson's Turnpike, which then led to the Unicoi Turnpike to Georgia and North Carolina. He dug out a pack trail that went by way of Look Rock into Cades Cove and built the Foute Trail crossing through Happy Valley that reached Gregory Bald at the North Carolina border.[177]

Business at the hotel, in part due to Foute's trails, increased to the point that Foute obtained the right to open a post office in 1837, evidence that even in that period, the Smokies did not isolate the area from other regions as popular lore has had it. Possibly due to problems stemming from an 1840 lawsuit or perhaps to devote time to other business concerns, Foute stepped down as postmaster in 1847 while continuing to own the resort, billing its attributes as "equally renovating to the dyspeptic and hypochondriac."[178] Three years later, Foute sold 3,840 acres, including the Black Sulphur Springs tract, to a wealthy Mississippi planter, Asa Watson, who believed that the water had cured his chronic diarrhea and dyspepsia.[179]

In 1853, Watson built several dozen guest cottages and replaced Foute's rustic lodge with the most famous of Montvale's four hotels: a seven-gabled, three-story frame inn with a 200-foot-long verandah on each floor front.[180] The hotel contained 125 rooms, which allowed for about 300–400 guests total to stay in the inn and cottages. Watson landscaped the resort's ten or more acres with non-native plantings from his visits to Asia, California, and other locales outside Southern Appalachia.[181]

In late 1856, Sterling Lanier, a career hotelman who previously had managed both the Rowland Springs resort in northwestern Georgia and the Lanier House in Macon, moved to Knoxville to join his brother Sampson, from Tuskegee, Alabama, to run the 250-person capacity Lamar House.[182] The following year, Sterling and his son-in-law, Abram P. Watts, became joint proprietors of Montvale. A few years later, the two, along with Sterling's sons Sidney and William, founded the Montvale Springs Company to purchase Montvale and over 4,000 acres for $25,674, a sum in 2022 worth about $888,000.[183] The Laniers divided some of the land into quarter-acre lots for homes and began to advertise widely the availability of lodging. The Laniers expended about $15,000 to improve Montvale, including hiring two landscape gardeners and a French cook. The two younger Laniers and Watt spent part of the year in Alabama managing Montgomery's Exchange Hotel; the elder Laniers stayed at Montvale. Sterling, calling Montvale "one of the prettiest places I have ever seen," proclaimed that he intended to "[enjoy] the balance of my days here."[184]

Guests at Montvale in the antebellum period, as elsewhere across the country, were typically the elite in society. They came from the Deep South—Georgia, Alabama, Mississippi, and South Carolina—undaunted by rough roads and the lack of rail access before the 1855 completion of the East Tennessee and Georgia Railroad through Knoxville.[185] Guests before that time could hire a stagecoach from Athens, Tennessee, about fifty miles away, or they could "[s]team to Loudon, on the Railroad, and up the [Tennessee] River to Louisville [TN] on Boats, and thence by private conveyance, only 14 miles."[186]

An 1857 guest from Columbus, Georgia, wrote that the Laniers were determined to transform Montvale into "the Saratoga of the South," an antebellum honorific also used by Georgia's Catoosa Springs. Montvale's potential visitors read of it in largely southern newspapers; it found its way, however, into a British publication and a German handbook for those interested in immigrating to the area.[187]

The Deep South planters flocked to Montvale's high altitude to escape the hot humid summer weather and perhaps to find refuge from such epidemics as cholera or the "Tennessee Itch" as described by François-André Michaux.[188] The 1832 cholera epidemic, which caused many elites to head for the mountainous Virginia springs, may have inspired Foute to build Montvale that same year to appeal to a similar clientele.[189]

Interestingly, the antebellum testimonials published in an 1867 Montvale promotional pamphlet came not from the Deep South elites but from East Tennessee residents who hailed from a variety of backgrounds. A well-traveled Charleston, Tennessee, elite wrote in 1853, for example, that he preferred Montvale's therapeutic water to that of Saratoga, the Virginia springs, and "all the celebrated watering-places of the West." Slaveholders took or sent ailing slaves to the springs. A Blount County slaveowner arranged for an enslaved boy ill with scrofula to rest at Montvale for five weeks in 1851. Likewise, a Knoxville slaveowner paid a six-week bill for a "little negro [sic] girl" with the same affliction to stay at the springs the following year.[190]

A Knoxville physician observed that the springs "owed their celebrity … to the wants and sufferings of the country people among whom they are situated." For example, a Blount County blacksmith stayed at Montvale for three months. A house carpenter from Knoxville in 1851 went to Montvale to be cured of chronic diarrhea.[191] Therefore, while the Charleston visitor and the slaveholders belonged to the upper class, Montvale appealed as well to those with modest incomes, who could afford the time and expense of traveling a short distance.

Future Tennessee Governor and Unionist William G. "Parson" Brownlow often lodged at the resort where he cultivated a friendship, perhaps partially based on a common ardent Methodist faith, with Sterling Lanier that ended when Lanier professed Confederate sympathies.[192] Another antebellum politician, South Carolina Senator Robert Y. Hayne allegedly drafted his debate speech at Montvale before he confronted Daniel Webster on states' rights; lore also has it that he and Brownlow practiced their oratory at Look Rock.[193]

Other antebellum notables included fiction writers and scientists, among others. Charles Todd wrote *Woodville* (1832), the first novel published in Tennessee, and

Sidney Lanier, Sterling's grandson, published *Tiger-Lilies* (1867), both loosely based on Montvale.[194] Although a reviewer called *Tiger-Lilies* "one of those novels, the chief wonder of which is, that they ever got published at all," *Tiger-Lilies* does afford a look at Montvale in the antebellum period with its description of a masque ball, shooting matches, and other activities at Montvale and the surrounding area.[195] The Swiss geologist Arnold Guyot resided at Montvale in 1859 while measuring peaks to produce a topographical map of the region's Appalachian mountains.[196] John Mitchel, Irish nationalist and ardent defender of slavery, wrote around 1856 from Montvale to his sister: "Montvale Springs is one of the great watering-places of the South. It is a vast wooden house with accommodations for three or four hundred guests."[197] In another letter, he opined that Montvale's evening dances were attended by such gorgeous dressing that he had never seen in America or anywhere else.[198]

As at Saratoga and the Virginia springs, many guests enjoyed a wide variety of outdoor sports and indoor socializing. Montvale's wide verandahs provided opportunities for healthful promenades, socializing, and to be seen by other elites. As Burns states, "smokers, loungers, and flirters" flocked there.[199] Other public spaces, which allowed the fashionable to be admired, existed on the path leading to an elaborately enclosed spring house and at benches scattered across the vast lawn.[200]

In contrast, the locals interacted in a very different way. Mountaineers sold game, garden vegetables, dairy products, and eggs to the resort.[201] Some may have found work at the resort itself although enslaved persons maintained the croquet grounds, billiard parlor, bar, and ten-pin alley; cleaned the hotel and cottage rooms; and guided guests on hunting, fishing or hiking expeditions.[202]

When the Civil War broke out, the Confederate-supporting Laniers continued to stay at Montvale. Montvale opened for the season of 1861, but a newspaper ad the following year informed potential guests that Montvale "will not be opened for visitors this summer." The older Laniers moved to Alabama while Sterling's grandson Sidney joined the Confederate army.[203]

Montvale served both as an informal infirmary and as a health resort during at least part of the Civil War. In March 1863, Joseph L. King of Knoxville bought Montvale from Sterling Lanier and Abram Watt for $40,000 ($962,000 in 2022 dollars).[204] King reopened the resort, charging an exorbitant $150 per month, a sign of the war's inflationary impact, and advertised that he had refitted it to the best standards that the current state of the country would permit.[205] In the spring of that year, Confederate General Daniel Smith Donelson, nephew and adopted son of Andrew and Rachel Jackson, died there of chronic diarrhea after suffering from poor health for several months.[206]

After the Civil War ended, King continued to operate the health resort for almost another decade. In 1867, King renovated the structure and furnished it with new furniture and revived the antebellum activities of dancing, billiards, and bowling.[207] The following year, King and two associates incorporated the resort under the same title the Laniers had used, the Montvale Springs Company, and undoubtedly hoped to increase their business because of a spur laid by the Knoxville and Charleston Railroad to Montvale Station, three miles from the hotel.[208]

Ownership exchanged hands several times from the mid–1870s to 1889. In 1876

Charles S. King, who succeeded his father as proprietor, lowered the 1875 rates of $40 for three months and $50 for one month to $10 per week for stays of at least three weeks.[209] The rate decrease apparently did not attract sufficient visitors to avoid a loan default; in 1877, R.N. Hood, trustee for a trust deed made out to both Kings and to two others, bought the resort at auction and leased it out for the 1878 season.[210] In December 1879, the property again was sold by court decree to two men from Maryland, who had a claim due to an inheritance; in 1882, J.C. (Jesse) Engel of Maryland bought Montvale and sold it seven years later to D.H. Sims and James Birks, who opened the resort for the winter as well as for the summer, promising to be first class in every particular.[211]

During this period, the 1878 and 1879 yellow fever epidemics that swept across the lower Mississippi River Valley brought West Tennessee refugees to the resort. Memphians settled into a "jolly and lively time" despite the "distressing yellow fever news from day to day [causing] a depressing effect."[212] Although Montvale advised that it had half the danger of the contagion that existed in Knoxville, one guest reported only about 200 boarders, half of the resort's 400-person capacity, causing a momentary downturn in profit for the hotel.[213]

Concurrently, the wealthy and notable continued to dominate Montvale clientele. Brownlow continued his visits to Montvale; there in 1869 for a recuperative stay, he wrote that "this is a beautiful watering place.... I sleep better, have steadier nerves, [and] an improved appetite...."[214] Mary Noailles Murfree drew upon Montvale's mountain culture for *The Prophet of the Smokies*, controversial today for its misleading stereotypical mountaineer images. Physician and naturalist Felix L. Oswald spent the summer of 1885 at Montvale and stayed the next two summers writing *Household Remedies* in a house nearby built especially for him.[215] Wealthy regional residents continued to "make the circuit"; an elderly Knoxville resident in the 1950s recollected her family's annual summer tours in the late 1880s to Montvale, to Virginia, and back to Montvale as a child with the family nurse.[216] Although the 1870s saw Montvale welcoming guests largely from Memphis, Nashville, Savannah, Atlanta, and Montgomery, the year 1901 brought visitors from twelve states, a geographic expansion of its clientele. Later years, however, found more locals frequenting the resort.[217]

Sim and Birks defaulted on their payments; in an 1894 foreclosure, New York City newspaper publisher and famed horse enthusiast Robert Bonner, Jr., of New York City bid the highest for Montvale.[218] In May 1896 the seven-gabled hotel burned down with a reported loss of $50,000 and insurance of only $15,000.[219] In 1901 Andrew Gamble, who had purchased the property through a court sale, built a two-story, five-gabled frame hotel with ell, which could accommodate 200 guests, about half the number of the previous hotel. Gamble sold the property in 1904 to Thomas F. Cooper, who then resold it to Ludwig Pflanze, who built on the property a small lake, christening it "Lake Sidney Lanier."[220]

The popularity of the resort diminished during this time. A 1901 typhoid epidemic contaminated the spring water and severely hampered business for several years.[221] While the season of 1884 saw over 250 boarders early in the summer, the second week of June 1904 found only seventy-two guests, forty of whom were

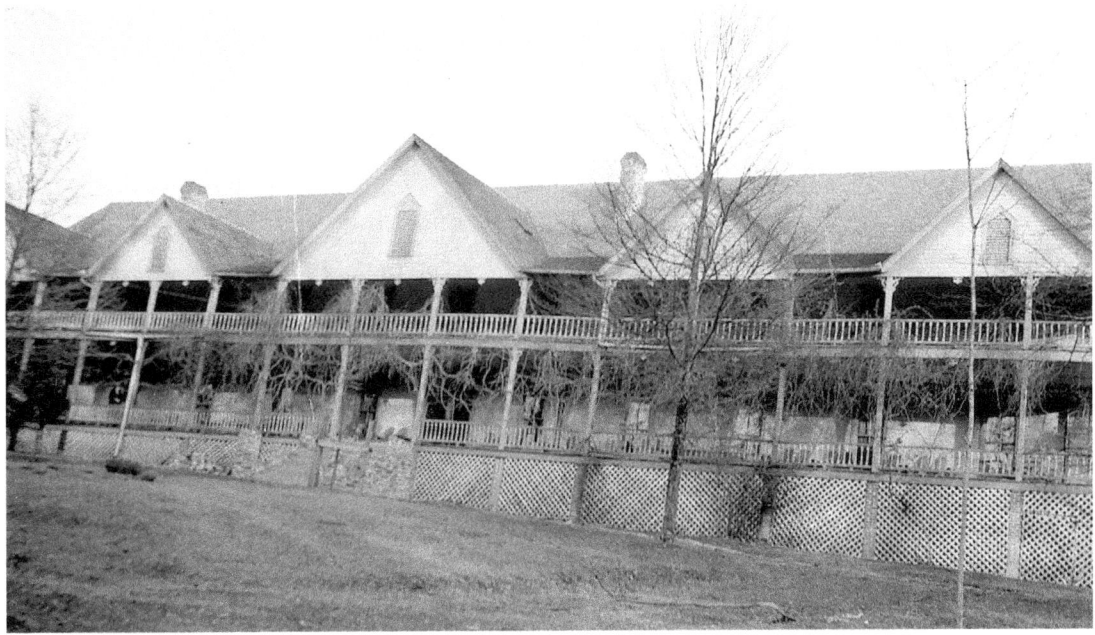

"Montvale Springs Hotel in Montvale, Tennessee [1927]," Blount County, Tennessee (Albert Roth, photographer (image courtesy of the A.G. "Dutch" and Margaret Ann Roth Papers, University of Tennessee, Knoxville Libraries, *https://digital.lib.utk.edu/collections/islandora/object/roth%3A2862/*. ID: roth:2862).

campers.[222] In addition, other Great Smoky watering holes such as Henderson Springs, Mt. Nebo Springs, and Line Spring provided local competition.

Pflanze operated the hotel from 1911 until it burned down in late November 1933 along with his research for a history on Montvale.[223] Undeterred, Pflanze continued to host events, including a Thanksgiving meal (dinner was 75 cents) the same November, using a two-story house and several cabins untouched by the fire.[224]

After Pflanze's death almost a year later, the resort continued for a dozen years as the Montvale Inn. In 1947, the Knoxville YMCA acquired the property and opened a boys' camp in 1949. After the YMCA camp closed in 2005, a conservation easement was placed on the property that restricts use to programs benefiting children, families, and the community. Today, the Harmony Family Center owns the property to provide opportunities for personal growth and fellowship.[225]

Rhea Springs

In Southeast Tennessee lies rural Rhea County, about fifty miles north of Chattanooga and eighty miles southwest of Knoxville. From Interstate 75 between these two metro areas, one can exit west onto State Route 68 in Meigs County and in less than thirty minutes espy the Tennessee River's looming Watts Bar Dam, the major utility for World War II's Manhattan Project at Oak Ridge. Crossing the dam on the state route immediately puts one in Rhea County where the road eventually tees into

U.S. Highway 27. Heading north on U.S. Highway 27 soon brings one to the small community of Spring City, a rail town in the late nineteenth century. Heading south on the highway leads to the county seat of Dayton, site of the 1925 Scopes "Monkey" Trial that pit famed defense team attorney Clarence Darrow against three-time presidential candidate and gifted orator William Jennings Bryan to determine if local teacher John T. Scopes had violated state law for teaching the theory of evolution. Another part of county history has disappeared under the waters of Watts Bar Dam, the resort of Rhea Springs.[226]

The Rhea Springs health resort stood at an elevation of 1,200 feet about two miles east of Spring City. To the west of its former site soars the 2,000-foot tall, eight-to-ten-mile-wide Walden Ridge on the Cumberland Plateau's eastern escarpment.[227] The Piney River drains the ridge into the Spring City and Rhea Springs area. As a writer remarked in 1872 about Rhea Springs: "The location is a beautiful one, lying in a small valley, at the foot of Cumberland mountain [sic], through which runs a considerable stream, with a range of hills on either side."[228]

In common with several Southern Appalachian mineral springs that developed into health resorts, Native Americans used the Rhea Springs waters before whites drove them from their homes (one of the routes for the Trail of Tears crossed through the county at Blythe Ferry on the Tennessee River). Cherokees who occupied lands near Rhea Springs drank the waters from long gum tree troughs that they had fashioned. After the federal government's negotiations with the Cherokees of the 1798 First Treaty of Tellico and the disputed 1835 Treaty of New Echota, white settlers displaced the Cherokees.[229]

Subsequently, Rhea County, named for U.S. Congressman John Rhea of Sullivan County, was established in 1807. Between 1810 and 1830, its population more than tripled from 2,504 to almost 8,200.[230]

The county's location on the mineral-rich Cumberland Plateau's eastern escarpment and in the fertile Tennessee Valley and Ridge helped to catalyze economic growth. Antebellum settlers mined coal and extracted iron ore from Walden Ridge's bituminous seams and dyestone deposits (a type of hematite iron ore). State geologist James M. Safford later praised the county's iron and noted the presence of several bloomeries established in the antebellum period at Smith's Cross Roads (modern Dayton). By 1854, local mining enterprises were extracting coal for local use and for export to Chattanooga and Georgia forges.[231] Cultivated in the valleys were wheat, oats, corn, and cotton, which gave impetus to the village of Cottonport on the Tennessee River from where cotton staple was shipped. The original county seat of Washington, about seven miles northeast of modern Dayton, in the late 1820s contained three cotton gins in addition to ten stores and several blacksmith operations.[232]

Concurrent with the growth of Washington was increased interest in (Rhea) Sulphur Springs, as Rhea Springs was known until 1878. Musters occurred there as early as 1809. In 1833, the federal government established a postal stop, evidence of an increasing population in the Sulphur Springs community; a year later, a school began in a church meeting house.[233]

In 1838 Edward E. Wasson bought from John Noblett over 200 acres that included the springs but exempted the church meeting house property.[234] Wasson, born in Rhea County in 1804, was a slaveholder engaged in both farming and the mercantile business.[235] In 1845 Wasson allowed local Methodists to organize the Sulphur Springs Camp Ground on his property; he deeded the campground's two acres in 1851 to the Methodist church trustees for $100. A few years later, in 1854, he sold to John Rhea II, possibly the bachelor Congressman's nephew, about 210 acres that included the springs, for $3,200, considerably less per acre than what he had charged the church trustees.[236]

John Rhea II pocketed a profit of about 12 percent when he sold the property only a year later for $3,586 to F.P. Stanton and physician W.S. Horr, one of whom, unspecified in an *Athens Post* article detailing the transaction, had been at death's door with weak lungs until drinking the spring waters.[237] Within a year of purchase, in 1856, Horr and Stanton opened a newly built hotel, winning praise in the local newspaper for having "fitted [the springs] up in superior style."[238]

The resort expanded within a year of its opening. The first lodging consisted of a two-story frame structure with nearby cottages. A piping system supplied limestone water from a source close to the Piney River to a fountain fronting the hotel and to guests.[239] In 1856 the resort advertised that lodging was "being improved in a comfortable and substantial manner, for the accommodation of the public" with boarding available.[240] In 1857 a visitor reported that a "large Hotel, 90 by 40 feet one way, and 80 by 32 another," shortly would open along with twenty-five or thirty cottages for accommodation of 150 to 200 boarders.[241]

The financial panic in the autumn of 1857, however, probably contributed to monetary woes for Stanton and Horr. The owners reduced rates for the 1858 season, possibly from lack of guests. During the same timeframe, they expended over $30,000 (over $1 million in 2022 dollars) to improve the hotel and grounds.[242]

With the loss of cash on hand, Horr and Stanton found themselves as defendants in a complicated title dispute with Wasson, Rhea, and others who accused them of defaulting on property payments and apparent loans. In November 1858 the local chancery court advertised the property for auction, including the hotel's "Marble Top Tables, Mahogony [sic] Sofas … one very fine Piano Forte … in fact everything necessary to the furnishing and carrying on of a first class hotel."[243] Winner of the property in July 1860 with a bid of roughly $6,000 was Edward Wasson's son, physician J.C. (Jeremiah Chapman) Wasson.[244]

The hotel thrived despite any effect from the litigation. Its local popularity in 1860 allowed it to charge $5 weekly, more than the $3 weekly rate of Chilhowee Springs, about twelve miles southeast of Athens. Compared with Georgia's fashionable Catoosa Springs resort, however, Sulphur Springs faltered: Catoosa's popularity with southern elite allowed it to command a princely $10 weekly rate.[245]

Visitors in the antebellum era mainly hailed from such Southeast Tennessee towns as Charleston and Cleveland. Notables included Chattanooga's James A. Whiteside, who in 1858 built his own resort, the Lookout Mountain Hotel, and U.S. Congressman Samuel A. Smith of Cleveland. Slaveholders, probably also from Southeast Tennessee, brought their enslaved persons to the springs to rest to increase their worth before an auction or a sale.[246]

The promise of restorative health attracted antebellum Southeast Tennesseans to Rhea more than less frequently publicized social events such as party suppers.[247] One ad promoted the water as a "powerful diuretic cathartic and alterative" for skin infections, "torpidity of the liver," and "habitual costiveness [constipation]."[248] A guest suffering from both bleeding lungs and a torpid liver (an ambiguous phrase for concerns such as general malaise, flatulence, or dyspepsia) regained his health through use of the water and praised its curative power for a host of other ailments, including deleterious side effects of mercury (commonly used at the time in the drug calomel). For those ailing from dyspepsia and weak stomachs who drank the water for one to two weeks, the guest advised that they could then "eat a hearty meal of bacon and beans" with no inconvenience.[249]

The perceived therapeutic effects were noted over a period of at least seventy years. In the antebellum period, the water was found to contain Epsom salts (magnesium sulfate); the Smithsonian Institution in 1858 also recorded iodine and magnesia (magnesium oxide), the latter traditionally used as a mild laxative or antacid. An 1880 American Medical Association committee noted the water's calcium sulfate's laxative effect. Fitch in 1927 described the large amount of carbon dioxide bubbling through the water, which may have relieved dyspepsia.[250]

Even though Rhea Countians had supported the Constitutional Union Party that largely opposed secession, they by and large aligned themselves with the Confederacy. Of the eight military units formed in Rhea County, seven joined the Confederacy, of which three mustered at Sulphur Springs. J.C. Wasson joined one of the three in 1861, quickly earning the position of regimental sutler. The county's one Union regiment mustered at the porch of a general store near the resort, evidence of the war's divisiveness even in such a small community as Sulphur Springs. Early in the war, the Sulphur Springs community women provided 200 blankets for Confederate soldiers, and a group of teenage girls formed the "Rhea County Spartans," a female Confederate company that delivered food and other essentials to the soldiers.[251] According to one old-timer, locals dug up the lead pipe bringing water to the Sulphur Springs hotel and refashioned it into presumably Confederate bullets.[252]

The war left Rhea Countians embittered. A Confederate veteran remarked in his memoirs about the county's desolation: "The yankees [sic] had stripped the country of everything to live upon.... Some of these widows had lost husbands and sons."[253] A Confederate lieutenant prisoner of war wrote home from a Delaware prison: "What has become of the Negroes? I suppose you are aware of the fact that they are as free now as the whites. Do the people realize the fact that the Confederacy has 'played out'?"[254] As for J.C. Wasson, he returned to Sulphur Springs where he apparently transitioned back into civilian life without due hardship: he operated a mercantile store at the site of the old Methodist campground, sold real estate, and reopened the resort.[255]

Resort attendees during the next several years included those who built cottages near the property, a sign of the watering hole's enduring appeal. One such postbellum visitor was Union General John T. Wilder, who won fame with his Lightning Brigade at Chickamauga and who co-founded in 1868 the Roane Iron Works in neighboring Roane County. Wilder, who suffered from several bouts of dysentery during the war, found so much therapeutic benefit at Sulphur Springs that he built a summer cottage near the resort (about a decade later, he built Roan Mountain's Cloudland Hotel straddling the western North Carolina and upper East Tennessee border).[256] Another cottage owner was U.S. Congressman John Randolph Neal, an Athens lawyer and former Confederate officer, whose son John Jr., served as chief defense counsel during the Scopes trial.[257]

Wasson's medical training and credo of service to others came into play in the late 1870s when he welcomed summer fever refugees during a time when other hotels turned away desperate travelers. During the 1878 yellow fever epidemic that raged through Memphis and other areas of the South, Wasson hospitably received at the resort 140 Chattanoogans, some of whom were infected before their arrival. Wasson and a fellow physician successfully treated them; upon their leaving Rhea Springs several months later, they signed the hotel register attesting that the mineral water assisted their convalescence.[258] Consequently, the following year, Wasson "receiv[ed] letters from persons all over the South as to summer board ... [who] intend this year to flee in advance of danger."[259]

Depending on the era and the traveler's point of origin, guests arrived by buggy, boat, rail, or automobile. Horr and Stanton advised that southerners could proceed to Athens to ride in a carriage about twenty miles to a landing to then hire a ferry to cross the Tennessee River and then engage a hack to reach the resort.[260] Travelers on the Cumberland Plateau could veer off the Walton Road, running between Knoxville and Nashville via Kingston, to descend through rocky gaps along Walden Ridge to reach Sulphur Springs. Steamboats provided a comfortable and scenic way to travel. In the 1870s, Rhea Springs publicized that it could be reached by steamboats from Chattanooga, Loudon, and Knoxville from its location about three and one-half miles away from the river. Boats such as the *J.T. Wilder* and the *City of Knoxville* sounded a steam whistle to notify the livery stables that a stop was imminent.[261] In 1879, the Cincinnati Southern Railway came through the area, thanks in part to a donation of $1,000 from the Rhea Springs community for the construction of a depot about two miles away that formed the nexus of Spring City.[262] By the early twentieth century, the Queen and Crescent Route published special rates that included a stopover for the resort.[263] Within ten years, so-called "automobile parties" drove the fifty miles from Chattanooga for a weekend at Rhea Springs.[264] A 1920 newspaper account observed that since "the roads are in much better traveling condition than they were last month, the inn has a number of tourists stopping almost daily."[265]

The resort's mineral waters continued to attract guests into the twentieth century, but more so its recreational opportunities. In the 1910s, ads enumerated the usual mineral spring resort activities of music, dancing, golf, tennis, croquet, fishing, boating, and board walks while secondarily acknowledging the resort's origin as the "home of the Old Reliable Rhea Springs Water ... tried for a century."[266]

Even as weekend dances, some held on flatboats on the Tennessee River, seemed to be a major drawing card for guests, Rhea Springs found another source of profit for its water.[267] In 1885, Rhea Springs was one of eight Tennessee resorts (four of them situated in Southern Appalachia) selling mineral water.[268] In the 1910s through at least the early 1930s, the resort occasionally publicized its water in ads separate from ones that focused on the resort activities.[269]

Resort ownership changed hands several times after a local chancery court sale occurred in 1880.[270] Proprietors and owners included a hotelman with experience at North Carolina's Warm Springs, a developer investigated for mail fraud, and the last owner, Chapman Wasson, son of J.C.[271]

Ironically, both fire and water caused Rhea Springs' demise. In January 1916, the resort, by then a three-story building with 300 rooms and twenty adjoining cottages, burned at a loss estimated at $50,000.[272] Another hotel with cottages was built; again, fire completely destroyed the structures in late fall 1921.[273] The last hotel, constructed from logs harvested from an adjoining forest, contained modern conveniences such as private baths piped with cold and hot water.[274] In 1941, as construction of Watts Bar Dam neared its end, Rhea Springs residents left their community. In January of the following year, the reservoir submerged the area, but not remembrances. A committee headed by Thompson Owen Wasson, a descendant of the resort owners, built a community memorial, incorporating the resort's spring house columns, at the entrance to the Spring City Park.[275]

Tate Spring

Tate Spring stood near the crossroads of two Native American trails, the Great Warriors' Path and one of its arteries, the Catawba Trail, close to today's intersection of U.S. Highway 11W and U.S. Highway 25E in Grainger County.[276] From Tate Spring, one can drive forty miles north to reach Cumberland Gap on U.S. Highway 25E, largely following the Great Warriors' Path, which Daniel Boone also traveled before he blazed the legendary Wilderness Road to the Gap from Long Island (modern Kingsport) in 1775.[277] Driving fifty miles south from Tate on U.S. Highway 11W, one will enter Knoxville. Both highways closely parallel major nineteenth-century thoroughfares that followed the Native American paths, linking Southern Appalachia with outside markets. Kentucky drovers herded their livestock and fowl through Cumberland Gap on the Kentucky Road (Wilderness Road) to reach both southern and eastern markets; eastern traders also followed in part the Great Stage Road (mainly U.S. Highway 11W) to take goods to Knoxville markets or beyond to destinations such as Nashville.[278]

Grainger County lies in the Great Valley of East Tennessee, the state's Valley and Ridge physiographic province, which runs in a northeasterly to southwesterly direction.[279] Between the Clinch River to the north and the Holston River to the south lies a series of ridges and contrasting valleys such as Bean's Station Valley and Poor Valley, the former described by an 1874 state agricultural bulletin as one of the most beautiful spots in the world and the latter described by the same source as "sterile, sandy, with desolation presiding over its whole length."[280] Throughout Poor Valley Ridge are gaps on the ridge's southeastern slope containing largely sulphur springs, from which Tate Spring and other watering holes developed in the nineteenth century.[281] Lea Springs, enjoyed by guests into at least the 1930s, is twenty-three miles southwest of Tate Spring on U.S. Highway 11W.[282] In the other direction on the highway, about one mile northeast of Tate Spring, stood the resort of Mineral Hill Springs, which lived up to its name by providing Epsom, chalybeate, and red, black, and white sulfur waters.[283] In neighboring Hawkins County, about eleven miles east of Tate, was Galbraith's Springs near the Holston River and Hale's Red and White Sulphur Springs six miles northeast of Rogersville.[284]

Information is sketchy about Tate Spring before the early 1870s. Native Americans first used the waters, considered particularly efficacious for the treatment of eye diseases.[285] In 1853 Samuel B. Tate, a prosperous farmer and slaveowner, acquired 300 acres through his father-in-law, Stephen W. Senter; sometime before 1857, the earliest date for which information about the health resort can be found, Tate built the original hotel. During the Civil War, Tate received a few southern invalids.[286]

In spring and summer 1873, a cholera epidemic swept through much of the country, including East Tennessee. Fear of the disease prompted the city recorder of Morristown, Tennessee, a town near Tate, to advertise in July that the town and Tate Spring were cholera-free.[287] After Tate's daughter Harriet died that same month from what the Mineral Hill physician diagnosed as a congestive chill but which many Tate guests assumed was cholera, almost all guests quickly evacuated. The Tates moved to Morristown in the wake of the hotel's plummeting business.[288]

In 1876 Thomas Tomlinson, son of a wealthy South Carolina merchant and planter, and a merchant and farm owner in Mooresburg, Hawkins County, along with twenty-two others, paid $25,000 to Tate for the hotel. In 1879 the joint stock company advertised a need to sell the property due to apparent disagreement among the twenty-three partners. Tomlinson bought the resort for $30,000 from his partners in 1882.[289]

Upon Tomlinson's death in 1909, his four surviving children, Dr. Oscar R. Tomlinson, Clement Tomlinson, Mrs. Annie M. Ragsdale, and Mrs. John R. Jarnagin, co-managed the hotel at first, followed by a series of owners for the next three decades. In 1926 one newspaper reported that its editor was invited to attend the May 1 opening of the resort under new management, which had bought it for more than one million dollars.[290] Oscar and Clement Tomlinson may have been involved with the new management, or they may have bought the resort back: when Oscar died in 1930; two obituaries listed him as joint owner with Clement. At some point Fidelity Bankers Trust gained control of the property. In 1938 a small group of capitalists led by S.G. Gluck of Indianapolis then managed the resort for a few years.[291]

In 1941 the resort closed. The following year, TVA bought much of the property for the creation of Cherokee Lake. In 1945 Kingswood School, a Christian-based institution for needy and neglected children, was incorporated in Tennessee. Its founder, the Reverend A.E. Wachtel, moved the school from Springfield, Virginia, to Tate Spring upon his purchase of the property. In 1958 much of the main hotel was condemned; the upper three floors were torn down and students relocated eventually to newly constructed cottages on the property. The remaining structure burned down in 1963. Today, Kingswood Home for Children operates on the Tate Spring property; the springhouse, in the form of a two-story white-frame, red-roof gazebo, stands to the right of U.S. Highway 11W going towards Knoxville.[292]

Travelers to the Tate Spring region could venture there year round from the time of Tomlinson's ownership, perhaps partially because of better transportation. Before the completion of the East Tennessee and Virginia Railroad in 1858, guests reached the health resort via the two main roads that intersected near it. Once the rail extended to Morristown, visitors took a hack or stage to Tate, about nine miles away.[293] By the turn of the century, guests could reach Tate Spring Station from Corryton, northeast of Knoxville, on the Knoxville and Bristol ("Peavine") Railroad from Morristown.[294] Visitors arriving on the Cumberland Gap and Louisville Railroad from the North or Midwest changed trains at Corryton to go to the Tate Spring Station.[295] The very rich went by rail in private railroad cars. By 1919 the Morristown-Tate Spring train had ceased service. By the mid-1920s, the new Lee Highway (U.S. Highway 11W) traversed the hotel property and intersected with the Dixie Highway (U.S. Highway 25E); visitors now could travel by automobile from many parts of the country without a need for train service. One of the wealthiest families who visited, the Studebakers from Indiana, drove the biggest model their company manufactured. Those who came by train in the early 1930s, called "high society" by one interviewee, were picked up at the depot by a touring car driver.[296]

Tate's prices provide clues to the socioeconomic status of the guests. In 1880 the hotel monthly summer (high season) rate of $35 was almost 60 percent higher than the $20 charged by Lea Springs and almost on par with Montvale Springs' constant monthly rate of $35.[297] By 1926, however, Tate had eclipsed Montvale in exclusivity: Montvale in 1911 was charging $7 weekly, less than half of Tate's cheapest rate in the early twentieth century.[298] Montvale, in other words, was in the mid-1910s much more affordable to the middle class than Tate.

Tate's rising exclusivity is shown in the increasing services and leisure activities it offered guests. In 1879, Tomlinson improved the bowling alley and bath house and contracted for a brass band.[299] Just three years later, Tate was offering horses for riding and driving, hiking, fishing, climbing, cavern exploration, archery, and other outdoor activities; a string and bass band for outdoor and ballroom music; nightly concerts; masquerades and evening balls; and the usual bowling, croquet, and billiard games.[300] About ten years later, morning dances and dramatic entertainments constituted part of the leisure activities.[301] "Clock golf" (a game in which golfers putt from the circumference of a circle to a hole in the middle) was added a few years later.[302]

Perhaps the activity that distinguished Tate from other Southern Appalachian resorts was golf. By the 1910s, the resort boasted a nine-hole golf course, with the first and last holes near the spring gazebo or pavilion, an inadvertent symbolic juxtaposition of the leisure pursuit adjacent to the health pursuit.[303] In 1926 a Donald Ross–designed eighteen-hole golf course opened for members of a Tate management-sponsored club.[304] In the early 1930s, caddies made twenty-five cents to fifty cents daily, carrying the bags of the likes of Sam Snead and Ben Hogan. Helping to maintain the course at some point were sheep, which kept the grass trimmed.[305]

As at other resorts, Tate provided public spaces for its clientele to promenade, to see and to be seen. Not only did verandahs adorn the perimeters of both floors of the two-story structure built by Tate, but they also wrapped around the sides of the four-story Victorian gingerbread rambling structure Tomlinson erected before the 1898 summer season. From the verandahs, the fanciful turrets, and balconies of Tomlinson's 200-person main hotel, guests absorbed panoramic views of the hills behind the hotel as well as the train depot over a mile away in front of the hotel. Before the start of the 1906 season, Tate added a 200-foot-long dining room and over twenty "elegant rooms, en suite, with private bath," indicating the increasing popularity of the resort. Guests occasionally bought lots to erect Queen Anne–styled mansions with turrets and wraparound porches. Bachelors and those planning on a rowdy time stayed in one of the row cottages, all with verandahs, named after such southern states as Alabama, Mississippi, and Louisiana.[306]

Although recreation made up a significant part of a typical guest's day, health activities attracted a steady stream of clientele up to the 1930s when Tate Spring began to decline.[307] Tate promoted its waters for a variety of illnesses, primarily gastrointestinal in origin. Clientele in the 1870s, for example, sought its waters for dyspepsia, chronic diarrhea, and, in the case of the president of a Mississippi railroad, for a "torpid liver, indigestion, and diseased kidneys, accompanied by general nervous prostration."[308] Thirty years later, Tate had extended its range of afflictions curable by the water to include "nervous diseases, insomnia, [and] female diseases."[309]

Tate enhanced its health offerings with a medical technique that by the 1880s was gaining acceptance in established medical circles, electricity-based therapy. In 1883, it publicized Electro Therapeutic Baths, a method of applying electricity to purportedly cure disease.[310] Tate's treatment appears to have been in vogue with similar electrotherapies in use in the late 1800s across the country. The First Brooklyn Light and Water Cure Institute in New York, for example, advertised blue and white electric light baths and electric vibration massage.[311] Similarly, the Atlanta Health Institute, founded by a former Rowland Springs physician, publicized its "Hygienic, Movement, and Electrical Water-Cure."[312] Contrary to the popular stereotype of the insularity of Southern Appalachia, Tate Spring exemplified health trends occurring elsewhere in the country.

Tate's focus on health manifested itself in another way that continued for decades—its sale of bottled water. By billing itself as the "Carlsbad of America," Tate sought to compare its waters with those of the famous German spa.[313] For at least thirty years, Tate sold its water at a consistent $5 per barrel.[314] In 1875, the resort received a weekly order for at least one barrel; by 1881, Tomlinson claimed that he was shipping 2,000 barrels yearly to Boston, Chicago, and other destinations removed from Southern Appalachia.[315] By 1926 distributors for Tate water operated out of much of the country; Tate also continued to ship directly from a small operation located at the gazebo.[316]

Tate saw several waves of guests over the years. In the early antebellum period, locals most likely frequented the waters. As Tate Spring's reputation spread, it attracted Deep South planters seeking refuge from summer heat and fevers in the shade of Tate's 800 trees at the resort's 1,400-foot elevation.[317] Although the 1870s perhaps saw more guests from Tennessee than from other states, by the mid–1880s, the states most represented at Tate were Georgia, Alabama, Mississippi, Louisiana, and South Carolina.[318] Notable visitors in this period included former Confederate

Vice-President Alexander Stephens, Mrs. W.G. Brownlow of Knoxville, General J.B. Hood of New Orleans, J.M. Studebaker of South Bend, Indiana, and former Georgia Governor Joseph E. Brown.[319] Adolph and Effie Ochs of Chattanooga stayed there in the late 1880s when Adolph owned the *Chattanooga Daily Times*; in 1896, he became owner and publisher of *The New York Times*.[320]

By 1886, Tate experienced as much business from New York and Pennsylvania residents as from Louisiana and South Carolina residents, for example.[321] Tate's proximity to two major rail lines with access to the South, Midwest, and North helps to explain the geographical diversity of guests during this period. In addition, "word of mouth" probably was important; for example, the increase in guests from Indiana may have originated with the praise for the health resort lavished by J.M. Studebaker, who made an annual pilgrimage there (the Studebaker family made an unsuccessful pitch to buy the resort in the late 1920s or early 1930s).[322]

A different guest geographic pattern emerged in the 1920s. Visitors in June 1923 were chiefly regional, including J. Fred Johnson, a founding father of modern

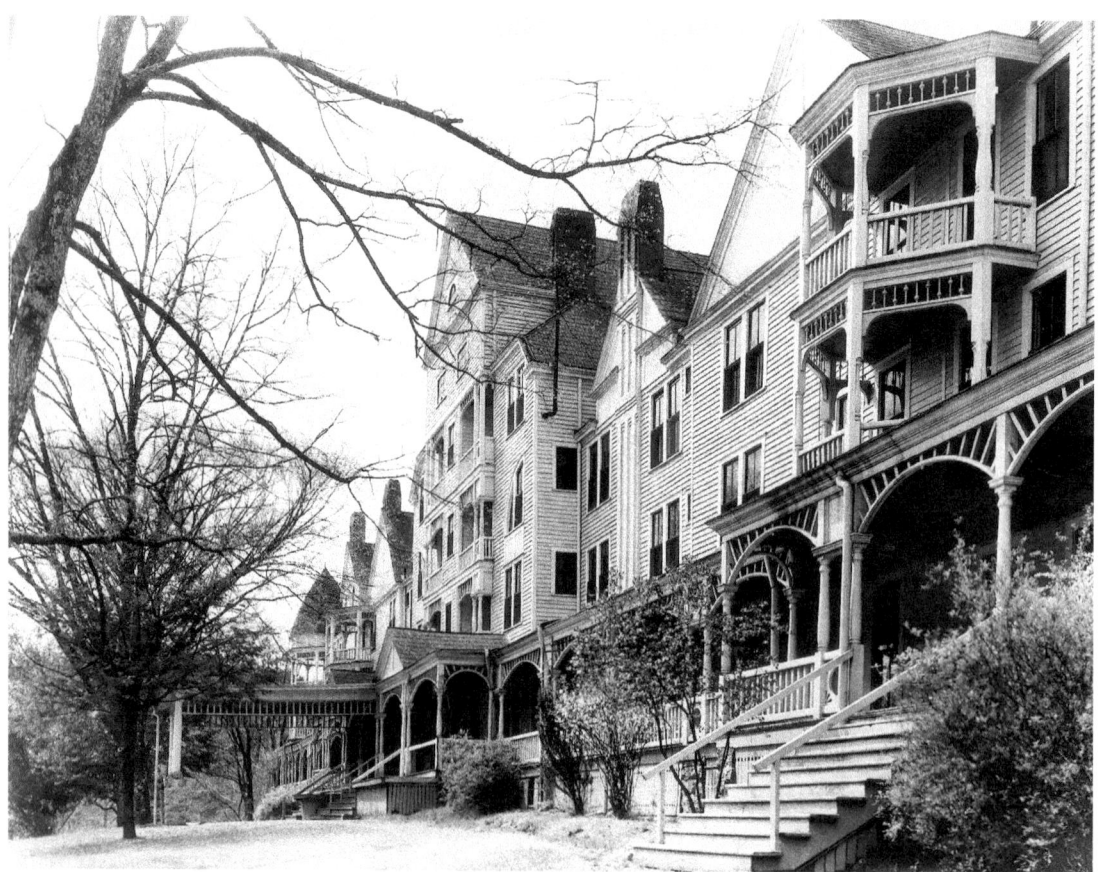

"Tate Springs buildings," Grainger County, Tennessee (Thompson Brothers, photographer. Thompson Photograph Collection, McClung Historical Collection, Knox County Public Library, Knoxville, TN, https://cmdc.knoxlib.org/digital/collection/p265301coll7/id/129/rec/1. ID: N-0071 A5).

Kingsport, Tennessee, noted for successfully lobbying George Eastman to establish a Kodak chemical plant in Kingsport three years earlier. Some visitors hailed from Alabama, Toledo, and Atlanta and a few from locales farther removed, New York, California, and Ontario.[323]

The Great Depression saw lower numbers at Tate, which reduced its operations to only summer months.[324] In June 1923, for example, about 736 parties had registered at the Tate; in June 1934, the number had fallen to about 493 parties. Tate guests now limited their stays to a few days, rather than weeks, thus decreasing the resort's revenue further.[325]

As happened at other health resorts, Tate found that its elite clientele were seeking other climes: the Great Depression did not hamper the vacation habits of the truly rich.[326] In addition, the wealthy sought more exclusive retreats once the middle class began to travel to the same resorts; Saratoga elites "escaped" eventually to the private compounds of Newport.[327] The growing availability of the automobile, coupled with better roads, especially at Tate's location at the intersection of two major highways, led many people to travel elsewhere. In addition, as one interviewee noted, by 1938, the "old folks" who owned it had passed away, and the younger generation had other interests.[328]

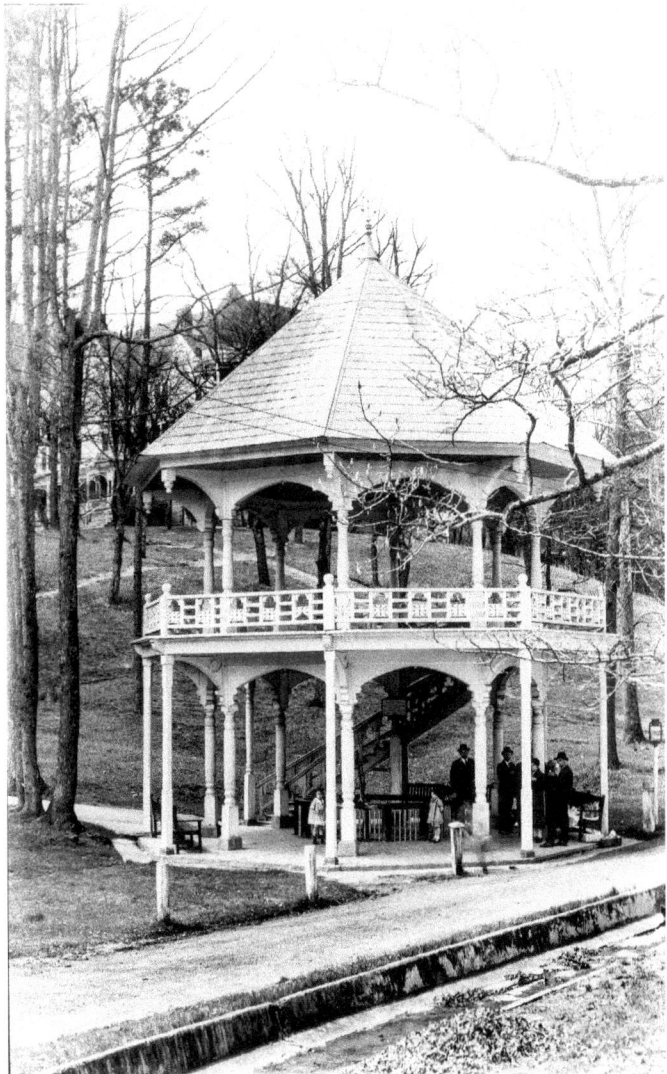

"Tate Springs gazebo," Grainger County, Tennessee (Thompson Brothers, photographer. Thompson Photograph Collection, McClung Historical Collection, Knox County Public Library, Knoxville, TN, *https://cmdc.knoxlib.org/digital/collection/p265301coll7/id/128/rec/1.* ID: N-0071 A4).

Several observations can be offered about Tate Spring's role as a health resort in Southern Appalachia. First, the very wealthy found exclusivity in upper East Tennessee, a region often perceived in the popular media to be populated with isolated mountain folk. Tate's prominent location at the crossroads of major routes enhanced its ability to attract elite from beyond the South. Second, Tate not only offered the usual mineral water springs' curative or palliative therapy but extended a range of health services such as electrotherapy even after it had begun to offer a smorgasbord of leisure activities. Third, similar to other health resorts, only the elite first frequented Tate Spring, followed by a regional less affluent clientele, via improved railroad networks and paved roads. Ironically, the same roads that allowed entrance for the elite took them elsewhere as regional visitors began to displace them at Tate Spring.

Unaka Springs

Unaka Springs in upper East Tennessee's Unicoi County developed in the late 1800s, long after many fashionable antebellum health resorts had faded away. The Unaka Springs Hotel, today a private residence, stands in the Nolichucky River Gorge, about four miles south of the town of Erwin near Interstate 26 before the road begins roughly a 2,100-foot ascent to Sams Gap at the Tennessee–North Carolina border. The CSX railroad crosses the river at the site of the hotel, making the resort's location easy to spot from the other side of the Nolichucky. The mineral springs around the resort are slightly more than one-half mile behind the hotel on a steep hill.

In the mid–1880s, Arthur V. Deaderick and his wife, Mary Adeline Walker Deaderick, built a small hotel next to the Nolichucky River, greatly improved in 1886 from the 1885 season.[329] Arthur was the son of James W. Deaderick of Jonesboro (as the town's name was then spelled), the chief justice of the Tennessee State Supreme Court from 1876 to 1886, and Adeline McDowell, granddaughter of Tennessee Governor Isaac Shelby. Arthur and Mary's son Henry, or "Mac," who ran the hotel after his parents, was a photographer for the Carolina, Clinchfield, & Ohio Railway, now part of CSX.[330]

Business prospered, for in June 1886 a post office opened at Unaka Springs. The resort's popularity did not, however, result from easy access to the hotel. Most early guests reached the hotel by fording the Nolichucky. The intrepid who arrived on the same side of the river as the hotel carefully negotiated a path dug into the hill behind the hotel.[331]

The completion of the Charleston, Cincinnati & Chicago Railroad (the "Three C's") and its trestle bridge at Unaka Springs in August 1890 greatly facilitated transportation to the resort.[332] Rather than engage a hack at Johnson City, the nearest train depot seventeen miles away, visitors traveled the Three C's from Johnson City to Erwin within two hours, and then arrived at the resort twenty-five minutes later.[333]

In July 1895, the Unicoi County Commissioners, one of whom was General John T. Wilder, founder of Roan Mountain's Cloudland Hotel and investor in the Three C's, partitioned lots in the Unaka Springs community at the request of the owners of the Unaka Springs tract.[334] Tract owners at this time included Arthur Deaderick, Henry Deaderick, and the heirs of Robert Love, a well-known elite of the late

1700s.³³⁵ The commissioners designated two lots to Arthur Deaderick—the southern boundary of one stood eighty-three feet north of the mineral springs—and two to Henry Deaderick, one of which adjoined one of his father's lots.³³⁶

The importance of the mineral springs is evident in the detail that the commissioners devoted to the topic in the deed. The commissioners sectioned off an esplanade along the Nolichucky near the railroad bridge, established streets and alleys according to an annexed plat, and set apart one lot that included the mineral springs. The commissioners declared that the lot with the mineral springs, the planned esplanade, and the planned streets and alleys were to "remain unpartitioned and to remain the property of all the owners," who were to be "equally liable for the taxes and improvement of the park or lot." The springs were to be "free and equal to all the owners" and to be accessible via piped water to a first basin connected to a second basin to receive overflow. More than likely a dispute had taken place about the ownership and right to the springs for the commissioners to put such stress on these concerns in the deed.³³⁷

In 1901 the Deadericks razed the hotel and planned to build a new hotel on its site, but a massive May flood, one that attracted national attention, swept away the building materials. After the flood clean-up, the Deadericks built a three-story, white-frame hotel with a first-floor verandah fronting the river and first- and second-story side verandahs. Adding to the structure's rustic appearance were rhododendron-branch latticework porch rails and a landscaping of benches and paths, one leading uphill to the springs.³³⁸

In 1907 the rail from Johnson City to Spruce Pine, North Carolina, was improved. Known as the South and Western Railway, under the leadership of George L. Carter who had bought the Ohio River and Charleston line, the new management eliminated the railroad's sharp curves in the mountains. At Unaka Springs, a steel girder bridge replaced the old timber truss bridge. To accommodate the railroad renovations, the Deadericks moved the hotel sixty feet back from its river location. The repositioning of the hotel blocked its previous first-floor view of the Nolichucky; a railroad bank now stood about ten feet above the ground along the river. The hotel was set on moorings high enough to avoid contact with a small creek that ran under the hotel. The Deadericks built a boardwalk with latticework railings from the railroad bank to the hotel verandah about forty feet away. A pond with two gushing fountains, one on each side of the boardwalk, completed the scene guests saw upon arrival.³³⁹

Visitors entering the second hotel saw a relatively elaborate interior. Near a large lobby was a 130-person dining room with a victrola and piano. Behind the lobby staircase was a marble- and quartz-decorated hallway leading to parlors. Chandeliers with oil lamps lit the first-floor hallway and main rooms, which included a railroad ticket and telegraph office. Most of the forty upstairs guestrooms were decorated with wallpaper and with high bead-board ceilings. One bathroom served each floor, with water provided through a gravity-flow pipe from a freestone spring uphill from the hotel.³⁴⁰

The springs purportedly provided the usual health benefits. Hotel stationery stated that the waters would benefit indigestion. Several sources disagree about the mineral content of the springs, whether iron, sulfur, or a combination, but the water most likely, by personal observation of its reddish hue, contains largely iron.[341]

A spring drinking ritual constituted part of the daily resort activities. Every afternoon, female guests filled their guestroom pitchers at the mineral springs for their evening servings. Occasionally, a Deaderick grandchild lay in wait in the thickets surrounding the springs, screeching like a wildcat, to frighten the ladies away.[342]

Guests participated in a variety of amusements, many also popular at other contemporary health resorts. Indoor activities included board games, talent shows, dancing, and Sunday sermons although parents' late Saturday night hours often meant that their children attended services alone. Outdoors, guests might hike, swim in a sheltered area downstream from the hotel, ride horses, and play croquet or miniature golf. In the summer humidity, visitors especially enjoyed blasts of cool air from a nearby shallow opening in the ground known as the "Cold Storage" or "Ice Cave," where the hotel chilled lemonade. Occasionally resort visitors rode the train to Erwin to sight-see.[343]

The hotel received most of its visitors in summer because the winter shadows of the mountains kept ice and snow from melting around the resort. Although the hotel remained open year-round for up to two years in the late 1920s, by the late 1940s, the resort officially opened only for weekends.[344]

Visitors to Unaka Springs prior to the Great Depression ranged from area residents to travelers from the eastern coast. Several interviewees stated that guests came from various regions of the country, apparently because of heavy railroad advertising. The Southern Railway and the Seaboard Air Line Railway, for example, listed the health resort in their summer promotions. The Cotton Belt Route extolled to Texas newspaper readers Unaka Springs' cool temperature.[345] The hotel during this time often teemed with visitors; overflow crowds camped on the lawn.[346]

Before the Depression, locals frequented the resort for day trips. They came to the hotel for Sunday dinner by train from Johnson City and Erwin; this tradition continued to the 1950s. Area residents also swam, picnicked, hiked, and camped there.[347] In the 1920s, elites from Johnson City, Kingsport, and Erwin sometimes arrived on the "Jitney," a special passenger train.[348] Erwin elites constructed summer cottages near the hotel on lots that they bought from the Deadericks. Some working-class locals also lived near the hotel; one interviewee's father, for example, labored on a nearby section of the railroad.[349]

The elites, who typically were lawyers, doctors, and railroad corporate managers, did not socialize much with what one interviewee called Erwin's "lower class," those who worked in the pottery, timber, or railroad industries. As a youngster, the interviewee believed that the local elites did not want to associate with the "common people." He did, however, as did several other interviewees or their parents as youth, play either with some of the cottage owners' children or with the Deaderick grandchildren. Another interviewee recalled that hotel management in the late 1920s through early 1930s did not allow locals on the weekends to mingle freely with guests; conversely, guests, who during that period came mainly from Florida, chose not to mix very much with the locals.[350]

One interviewee recalled, however, that her mother, an orphan whose grandmother cared for her and several other siblings, received paternalistic attention from the elites. A guest from either Maryland or New York wanted to adopt a younger sibling; the grandmother refused, but the interviewee's mother reflected that her younger sibling would have enjoyed a better life through the adoption. One cottage owner, aware of the family's precarious financial situation, paid the interviewee's mother fifty cents daily to wash his family's dishes and bought shoes and socks for her.[351]

Walking and driving augmented the train rides to reach the resort. Local young people lacking money or unwilling to splurge on a train ticket from Erwin walked across the Nolichucky railroad bridge to attend Unaka Springs' weekend dances or to indulge in the swimming hole. A narrow walkway along the bridge's underside provided an escape route if a train approached. With the advent of the car, some locals and guests parked their vehicles next to the river and then navigated the bridge to reach the resort. After the Civilian Conservation Corps (CCC) chiseled a narrow road bed out of the steep hill behind the hotel, guests could access the hotel via that route.[352]

Interviewees were adamant that the CCC road ironically greatly diminished the hotel's business, not the Great Depression alone; they stated that the road providing ease of access to the resort was also responsible for its decline. After the road was

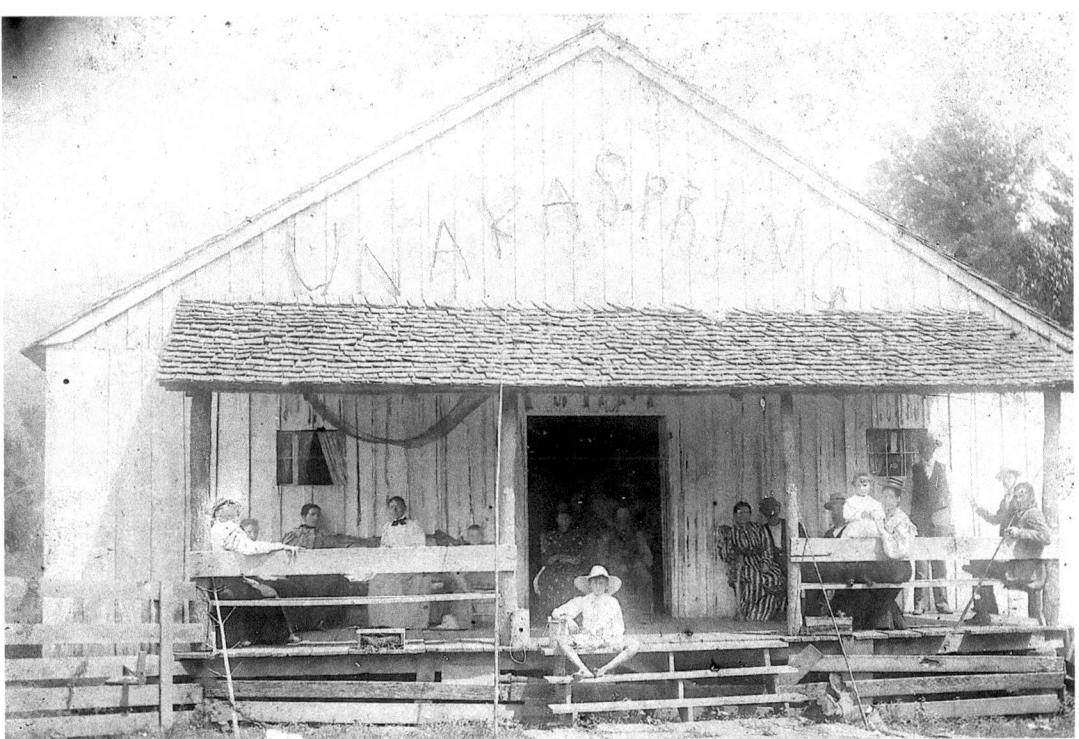

"Unaka Springs 1st hotel," Unicoi County, Tennessee. Compare this structure with the expanded hotel in later years (Henry R. and Mary Deaderick Duncan Collection, McClung Historical Collection, Knox County Public Library, Knoxville, TN, *https://cmdc.knoxlib.org/digital/collection/p265301coll9/id/576/rec/3*. ID: Duncan_003).

constructed, those who enjoyed to tipple found the property a place of rambunctious weekend entertainment, which likely resulted in a loss of the resort's aura of exclusivity. One interviewee reared in the Unaka Springs community could recall only Deaderick family members and a retired New York judge visiting the resort in the early 1930s.[353] And, as happened at other resorts, vacationers began to travel elsewhere.

The resort lingered on during and for a few more decades after the Depression. Henry "Mac" Deaderick ran the hotel when his father became elderly. Arthur, unfortunately, borrowed $1,403.35 against the hotel and defaulted on the loan; C.B. Rumbley of Johnson City, who owned the debt on the hotel, bought the resort at auction for only $200 in 1936. He conveyed the property to J.E. Rumbley, who then conveyed deed to Dr. Aura Barrowman. Stella Hopson bought the hotel and its furnishings in 1946 for $7,000 from Barrowman.[354] She operated the hotel year-round for four years as a dance hall and bar and then sold the property for $2,000 in 1950. Gradually, the

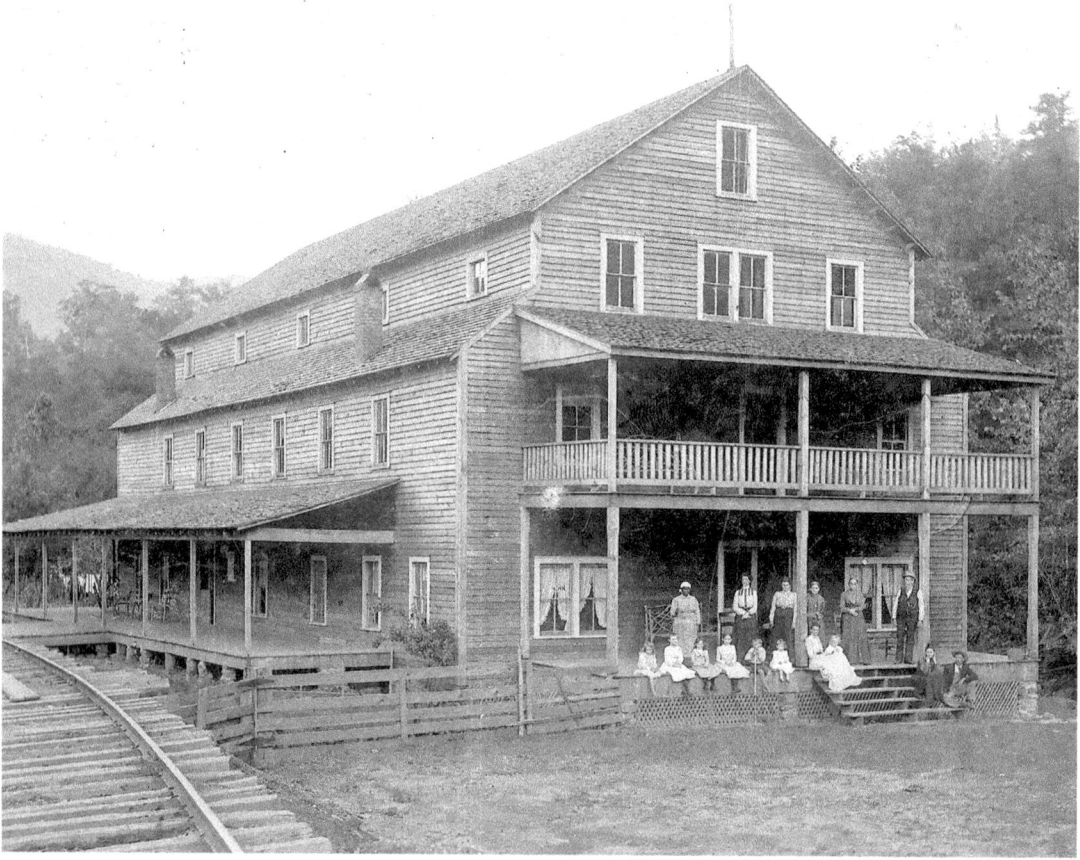

"Unaka Springs Hotel," [~1890–1906], Unicoi County, Tennessee. The railroad when this photograph was taken ran immediately in front of the hotel. On the side porch, a Black woman stands behind several seated white children, suggesting the wealth of the family that possibly engaged her as a domestic (image courtesy of the Burr Harrison Photographs, Archives of Appalachia, East Tennessee State University, *https://archivesofappalachia.omeka.net/items/show/404*. ID: 0064_334).

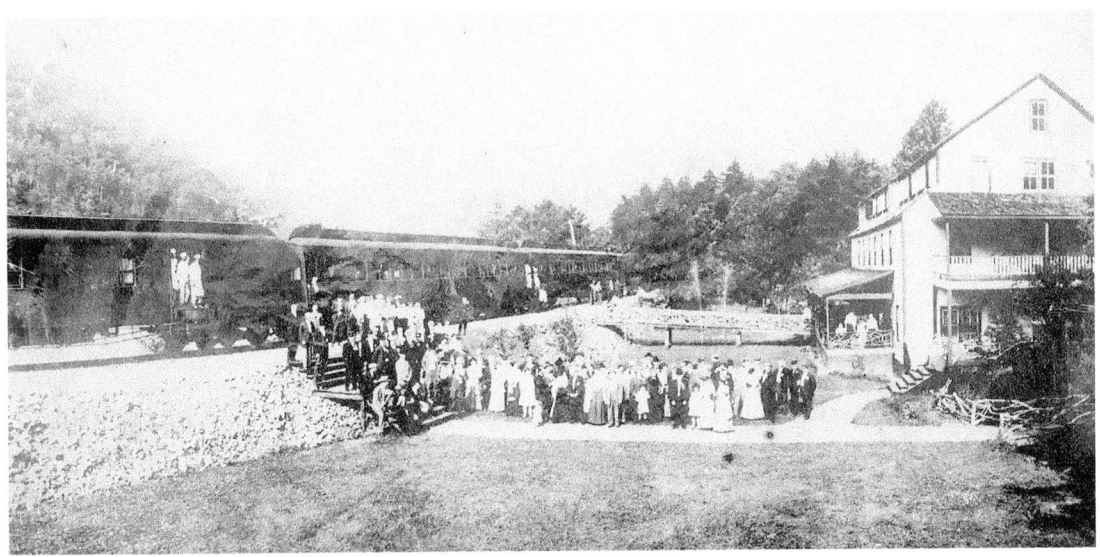

"Postcard—Unaka Springs Hotel," 1910, Unicoi County, Tennessee. Note that the hotel by this time had been moved back from the railroad (image courtesy of the John Goodin Papers, Archives of Appalachia, East Tennessee State University, *https://archivesofappalachia.omeka.net/items/show/14343*. ID: 0482_B02_F02_001a).

original cottage owners moved out; they sold some homes to residents relocating from Lost Cove, North Carolina, when that community dissolved after its train service ended in 1955.[355]

The hotel saw several more owners after Hopson. Sometime in the 1950s, the owner of the hotel removed its third story and its middle section so that he could rent out two separate houses. In the mid- to late–1970s, a rafting company rented the facility for overnight stays and as a convenient place for rafters to change clothes. From 1982 through at least 2007, a family in New Jersey with relatives in the area owned the former hotel.[356]

In late September 2024, Hurricane Helene unleashed torrential rains that resulted in devastating and deadly flooding in the Nolichucky River Gorge and its environs. Sadly, at least eleven people drowned in the Erwin area. The Unaka Springs hotel remained standing. In September 2025, CSX announced the completion of its rebuilding of sixty miles of severely damaged rail, including that by the hotel.

Virginia

Introduction

"No state in the Union perhaps has as many health resorts as Virginia."[1] This 1886 pronouncement from a federal commerce report's commentary on mineral springs summarizes the state's complex landscape of watering holes. The Virginia springs run from the southwestern panhandle of the state to its border with western Maryland and Pennsylvania, where the Mason-Dixon line demarcates Campbell's northern border of Southern Appalachia. This chapter will focus on the Virginia springs and will also include watering holes in West Virginia, part of antebellum Virginia, and home to Southern Appalachia's premier spa, Greenbrier County's White Sulphur Springs.[2] Fitch in 1927 listed for both states over 160 named mineral springs, of which almost half enjoyed at one time a reputation as a health resort. Stan Cohen's 1994 *Historic Springs of the Virginias* describes 75 resorts.[3] Most places identified in both works were in Southern Appalachia's Allegheny or Blue Ridge mountains or in the Valley of Virginia. Fitch and Cohen did not cover many minor Southern Appalachian resorts, such as Bland County's Sharon Springs and Tazewell County's Iron Lithia Springs, which add a local dimension to the sprawling network of Virginia watering holes available to travelers.[4]

The White Sulphur Springs in the antebellum western Virginia interior region served as the nexus for the popular Virginia springs circuit. The circuit consisted of a series of descriptively named resorts such as Warm Springs, Hot Springs, the Red Sulphur, the Red Sweet, the Salt Sulphur, and the Blue Sulphur, prescribed by physicians in a certain order of visitation depending on their patients' ailments.[5] William Burke, a physician who owned the Red Sulphur, unabashedly praised his resort's water: "We can prove beyond a doubt that this water exerts an influence over the circulation that no other agent has been known to exert."[6] Burke's rival in the 1840s, John J. Moorman, the White Sulphur's resident physician, recommended the White's water for such varied afflictions as dyspepsia, "chronic inflammation and congestion" of the brain, and hepatic ailments: "Volumes might be filled with details of gratifying results [of those] who visited these waters as sort of 'last resort' for liver disease."[7] Other physicians extolled the medicinal properties of individual resorts in publications devoted to a single spa such as the Gray Sulphur, the Salt Sulphur, and the Healing Springs. The Medical Society of Virginia met annually at one of the Virginia springs to debate the therapeutic values of the various watering holes;

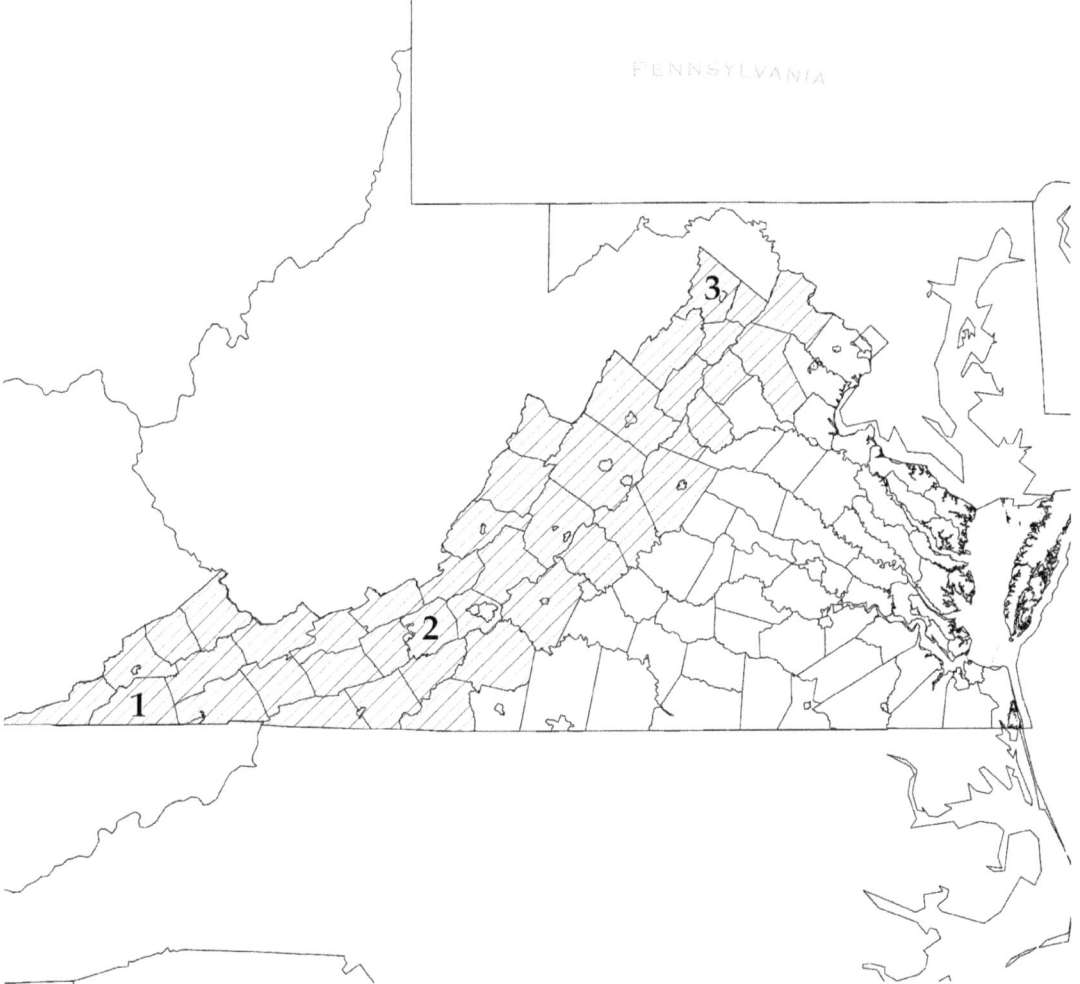

Virginia counties with featured health resorts: (1) Scott County, Holston Springs; (2) Montgomery County, Yellow Sulphur Springs, Alleghany Springs and Montgomery White Sulphur Springs; (3) Frederick County, Jordan's White Sulphur Springs and Rock Enon (Sources: Esri, NOAA, USGS, The Living Atlas. Cartographer: Sayona Turner, East Tennessee State University).

not until 1875 did a scant bit of disbelief in the springs' claims appear in medical journals.[8]

In addition to the ill, the Virginia springs also attracted those in search of matrimony, socialization and relaxation, and those wishing to curry favor with national politicians.[9] The White Sulphur's master of ceremonies in the early 1830s, Colonel William Pope, initiated the match-making "Billing, Wooing and Cooing Society" to ensure proper introductions and fitting behaviors at balls.[10] A Virginia Military Institute cadet in 1843, hale in health and likely in search of fashionable dance partners, wrote to his father that his classmates and he intended "to visit all the different Springs, the Warm, the White Sulphur, etc."[11] Some popular belles announced their stay at a particular resort to which male admirers then flocked; some spas promised

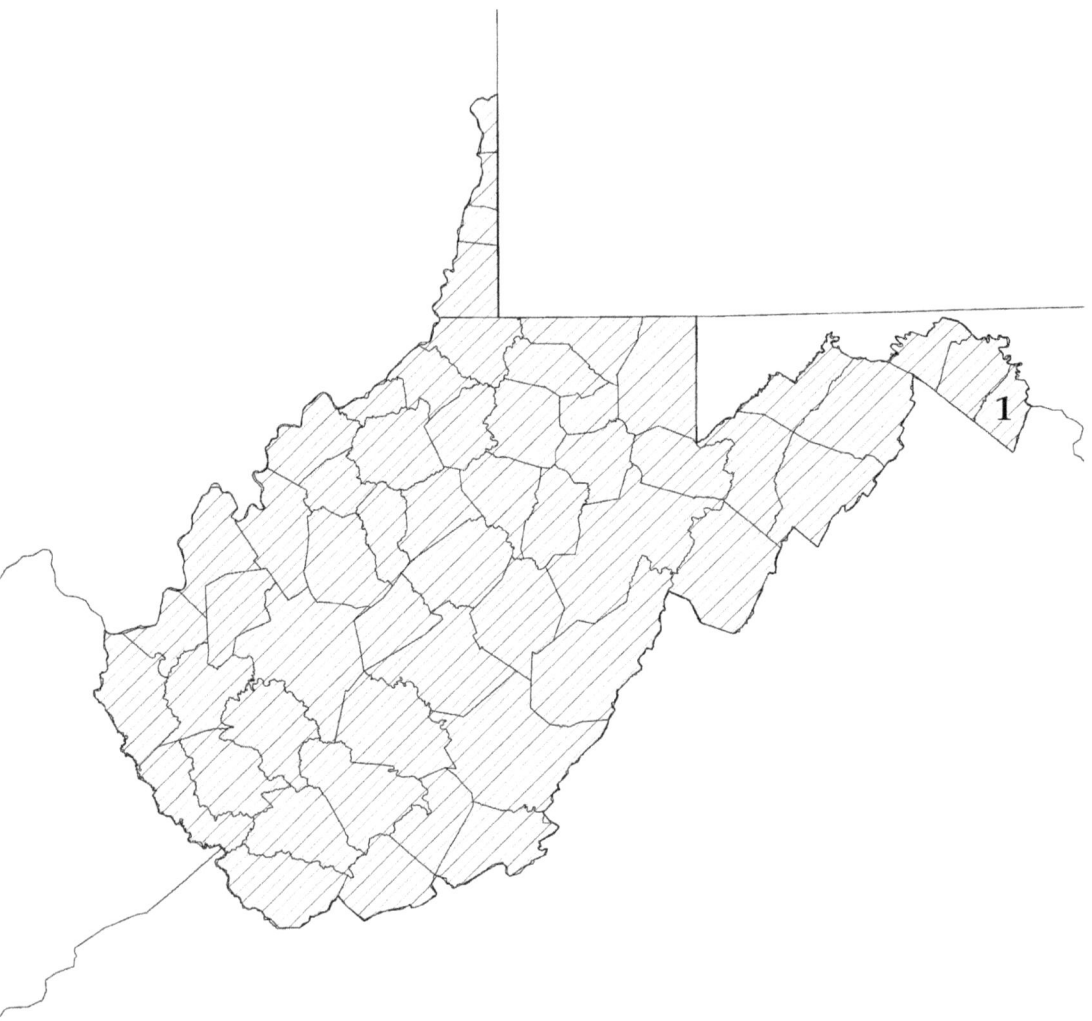

West Virginia county with featured health resort: (1) Jefferson County, Shannondale Springs (Sources: Esri, NOAA, USGS, The Living Atlas. Cartographer: Sayona Turner, East Tennessee State University).

good matches and ample matrimonial chances for guests.[12] Henry Clay, who always culminated his semiannual or annual Virginia springs tour with a visit at the White Sulphur, acted as that resort's unofficial host for its assorted visitors, including the young unattached, the southern planters, the northern elite, office-seekers, and national politicians. His presence served as such a drawing card that he received free room and board.[13]

The state's preeminent Southern Appalachian spas, including several located closer to Washington, D.C., than to the White Sulphur and its environs, welcomed other national political figures who came for health, socialization, and political discourse. Notables included Clay's fellow members of the "Great Triumvirate," Senators John C. Calhoun and Daniel Webster; U.S. presidents and cabinet members; and higher level members of the judiciary. Calhoun visited the Salt Sulphur and the White Sulphur, ostensibly for health concerns, but also to gain a political pulse from southern agrarian elite around issues such as the country's intensifying sectionalism.[14] Webster, to applause at northern Virginia's Capon Springs, thundered that "to preserve the Union we must observe, in good faith, the Constitution in all its parts."[15] The White Sulphur received U.S. Presidents James Monroe, Martin van Buren, John Tyler, Millard Fillmore, Franklin Pierce, and James Buchanan, a few of whom also toured such other Virginia spas as Jefferson County's Shannondale Springs.[16] Supreme Court Chief Justice Roger Taney and his wife professed after their six-week visit to the Red Sulphur Springs that they were in "much better health than we had known for years before."[17] Taney also retired with the Virginia governor to the Rockbridge Baths, thirty-five miles southeast of Warm Springs; recreated at Shannondale Springs; and frequented the Fauquier White Sulphur Springs, about seventy miles from Washington, D.C., where he mingled with ex–President Pierce and Kentucky Senator John Crittenden in 1857, three years before the senator drafted his famous compromise in a failed attempt to keep the Union peaceably intact.[18]

Traveling to and among any of the Virginia springs was arduous and time-consuming before improvement and expansion of the state's turnpike, canal, and railroad systems in the 1830s. Lowcountry planters might travel by a network of stage lines along roads following such Native American trails as the Great Indian Warpath through the Great Valley of Virginia.[19] Elites from New Orleans and other southern ports disembarked from steamboats at Guyandotte, Virginia (Huntington, West Virginia), for stages heading southeast to the springs.[20] Washingtonians and elites farther north, across the Potomac River in Maryland, traveled by stage to sojourn at Fauquier White Sulphur, Berkeley Springs (Bath) or at Shannondale Springs before perhaps continuing on to the White Sulphur. On the one hand, Berkeley Springs in 1838 reassured potential guests that coaches traveled on "county roads [that] are in a very good state of repair."[21] On the other hand, a stage carrying Tennessee politician and former Secretary of the Treasury George W. Campbell from the White Sulphur to the Blue Sulphur flipped on its side on the road's downhill, injuring several as the horses bolted.[22] Travel by horse-drawn coaches averaged about four miles an hour if no mishaps. Proprietor Erasmus Stribling of Augusta Springs advertised that hacks could reach his watering hole in three hours from Staunton, a mere thirteen miles to the northwest.[23] Prolix noted that his party left Bath County's Hot Springs on a fine afternoon to reach the county's Warm Springs four miles away after an hour's drive where the group lodged for the night.[24]

Ease of travel greatly improved after the mid–1830s.[25] By 1835, the Chesapeake & Ohio Canal, the Baltimore & Ohio Railroad, and the Winchester and Potomac Railroad had all reached Harpers Ferry, allowing for more visitors to northern Virginia spas and connections to those more southern.[26] To reach Shannondale Springs, in what might be considered a frustration today but which was an improvement in 1838, Washington or Baltimore residents could leave by railroad in the morning, arrive at Harpers Ferry for dinner, continue on railroad to Charlestown where stagecoaches transported them the five miles to a landing at the Shenandoah River, where they then crossed by ferry to reach the hotel before sunset.[27] Construction of the Virginia and Tennessee Railroad through the Great Valley of Virginia aided the development of minor resorts such as Washington Springs two miles from the Glade Springs depot and Coyner's Springs one mile from Roanoke's station.[28] In addition, the railroad expansion and improved road construction near Christiansburg allowed Montgomery County's resorts of Yellow Sulphur Springs and Montgomery White Sulphur Springs to be more accessible to travelers on the traditional Virginia springs circuit. Farther north in the Shenandoah Valley, the Virginia and Central Railroad in 1853 ran stages from Staunton to stop for the night at Warm Springs or other nearby resorts before reaching the White Sulphur the next evening.[29] By 1858, the Virginia and Central could boast that any passenger could "take from Staunton almost any road [to] come soon to a mineral spring."[30]

Traffic to the Virginia springs increased remarkably because of the improved transportation infrastructure. Bath County in 1800 received about 6,000 visitors to its spring resorts; fifty years later, for one week alone, Capon, White Sulphur, and Jordan's White Sulphur Springs were housing a collective 1,200 guests.[31] To keep the numerous mineral spring resorts operating smoothly for elite guests required much skilled and unskilled labor, much of it from Black enslaved persons.[32]

Slave labor at the Virginia springs came chiefly from venues such as the Richmond slave exchanges, through the hiring of slaves in the off-season from local farmers, or from the resort owners themselves.[33] Two agents, for example, in one 1860 Richmond newspaper advertised for thirty to forty cabin and dining room servants for the Old Sweet; in addition, a Black enslaved person named Fields wrote in his memoirs that he had to leave Richmond for the four-month season of the Virginia springs.[34] Branch Jordan of Jordan's White Sulphur Springs and William Crow of the Shannondale Springs stock company were slave traders, and several co-proprietors of those resorts owned enslaved people.

Some Virginia antebellum resorts hired free Black workers.[35] Fauquier White Sulphur employed both free and enslaved Black workers.[36] In 1860, White Sulphur Springs employed sixty-three free Black males in its main hotel dining room; the resort in March of that year had advertised for 200 "servants."[37] The payment of wages to the Black waiters must have jarred the southern sensibilities of planter guests entrenched in an economic system established on slave labor even as the continued use of Black workers in a service role reinforced white domination. In addition, the intermingling of free Black employees and slaves in unsupervised contact as they journeyed to and from White Sulphur posed a dangerous situation of potential collusion to the agrarian elite.[38]

The rationale for the employment of free Black workers at the White Sulphur remains an open question, but three conjectures may partially provide an answer. First, slaveowners may have become increasingly reluctant to hire out their enslaved persons to the resort once they recognized that their slaves' disgruntlement upon their return to arduous plantation work was due to the White Sulphur's less-taxing duties, the slaves' ability to earn money such as tips from resort guests, and the resort's somewhat freer ambiance in which slaves might socialize with other Black persons away from plantation overseers.[39] Second, perhaps the crush of visitors at the springs necessitated more workers than could be had with the supply of slave labor. Third, Fain notes that White Sulphur Springs in 1850 moved towards to a slave-leasing model from a slave-owning model to curb expenses.[40] Extrapolating from Fain, I can speculate that the cost of hiring free Black workers for an hourly wage may have been cheaper than contracting enslaved persons for an entire season from a profit-motivated slaveowner experienced in price negotiation, particularly if the free Black waiters had limited options for other income.[41] An analysis based on research into free worker wages, hired-slave contracts, and other economic factors is required to explore further these conjectures.[42]

During the Civil War, Virginia experienced more major battles than any other state. Consequently, probably all of its mineral spring resorts closed to guests at some point during the war. Some became army headquarters such as Shenandoah County's Orkney Springs for the Confederates and the Salt Sulphur for both sides, depending on the victor of the latest skirmish.[43] More of the major resorts, however, saw service as military hospitals. In the northern Shenandoah Valley, Jordan's White Sulphur Springs functioned as a hospital for both sides as nearby strategic Winchester changed hands over seventy times during the war.[44] Over 200 miles to the southwest, the Confederacy established a hospital at the New River Valley's Montgomery White Sulphur and another one 150 miles farther southwest at Scott County's Holston Springs. Resorts prominent on the fashionable Virginia springs circuit tour such as the Blue Sulphur, Red Sulphur, Hot Springs, Warm Springs, and Healing Springs also were converted to hospitals, the latter three only briefly in fall 1861 due to Confederate repositioning from Bath County to Staunton.[45] As for the White Sulphur, it temporarily served as a Confederate hospital in fall 1861 and escaped destruction during the 1863 Battle of White Sulphur Springs fought nearby.[46]

A Kentucky Confederate officer observed the condition of several of the resorts as his troops marched north from Holston Springs in November 1864. By then, the Warm Springs' large buildings were vacant, "quite a melancholy appearance"; Hot Springs was "all deserted"; and the Healing "[m]ore elegant" than the Warm and the Hot. The Old Sweet's large hotel "far exceed[ed] anything have yet seen"; a few of the officer's superiors paused there to enjoy a bath. By the time his troops reached the Salt Sulphur in early December, he commented that its hotel was "not so elegant as many we have passed, but substantial & commodious. We are heartily tired of Springs. Satiated with them."[47]

In the postbellum era, many of the resorts reopened. Some, such as the Greenbrier White Sulphur and the Homestead (Hot Springs), continued to enjoy sophisticated reputations. Destroyed during the war, however, were a few prominent resorts such as the Blue Sulphur, never rebuilt, and the Fauquier White Sulphur, revived in 1877 by an influx of capital from a stock company.[48]

Other Virginia spring resorts that reopened after the war either gained or ebbed in popularity. Coming into its own after the war was Rock Enon in northern Virginia, an inconsequential antebellum watering hole known as Capper's Springs, that vied after the 1860s with fellow Frederick County resort Jordan's White Sulphur Springs to receive prominent Washingtonians and Baltimoreans. Receding into the background was nearby Jefferson County's Shannondale Springs, popular with elites such as James Monroe in the 1820s, but which never regained a considerable clientele even after its hotel was rebuilt in 1888 from a fire thirty years earlier. To the southwest, the New River Valley's Montgomery County resorts of Yellow Sulphur and Montgomery White Sulphur continued their antebellum tradition of receiving Deep South visitors but, along with their fellow Montgomery County postbellum resort, Alleghany Springs, now drew more visitors from the local area. Holston Springs became the summer home of the state attorney general, Rufus Ayers, but also welcomed a few guests.

These seven resorts, Rock Enon, Shannondale Springs, Jordan's White Sulphur Springs, Montgomery White Sulphur Springs, Alleghany Springs, Yellow Sulphur Springs, and Holston Springs, are the subjects of this chapter. I selected them from the myriad of Virginia spas based on four factors. First, their unfamiliarity to most readers compared to the White Sulphur Springs and its companion resorts on the traditional Virginia springs circuit seemed likely to pique curiosity. Second, as a corollary, little has been published on them relative to the vast literature on some of the Virginia springs (but not so little that a substantive story could not be told). Third, their geographic variances—the state's southwestern panhandle, the New River Valley, and the northern region—ensured coverage of the length of western antebellum Virginia. Fourth, the research initiated by Virginia Tech's Brian Katen on Black ownership and fellowship at mineral springs, what he terms "places of congregation" as opposed to "places of segregation," prompted inclusion of one of the mineral springs he researched for its Black heritage, Yellow Sulphur Springs.[49]

The history of these resorts provides some nuance to counter the traditional image of the Virginia springs as a monolithic julep-sipping society. Holston Springs, obscure today, attracted coverage in the Lowcountry press in the 1810s but declined in popularity after railroad expansion through the Great Valley of Virginia provided travelers with accessibility to other resorts. The New River Valley's Yellow Sulphur Springs, Montgomery White, and Alleghany Springs served as postbellum forums for former Confederate generals Jubal Early and P.G.T. Beauregard to shape their perceptions of the "Lost Cause," but they also welcomed guests as varied as New Orleans Jewish families and Roanoke-area businessmen and physicians. In the 1920s, Yellow Sulphur shifted from secessionist reminisces to Black empowerment when African American businessmen bought the property to provide Black guests a safe and sociable retreat. Shannondale Springs, Jordan White Sulphur Springs, and Rock Enon largely drew from the Atlantic cities, Washington, D.C., Baltimore, and Alexandria, appealing to high-level functionaries and to the occasional Cabinet or Congressional member.

The details of the resorts in this chapter provide a brief glimpse into their social histories. Exploration of additional resorts in the state and research into the social fabric of Black and white relations centered around mineral springs not yet researched are (reluctantly) beyond the scope of this work. Both topics would, however, enhance the multifaceted understanding of Virginia's health resorts.

Holston Springs

In the southwestern corner of Virginia lies hilly Scott County, about seventy miles east of Cumberland Gap and homeplace of the internationally known Carter

Family of country music fame.⁵⁰ Named for General Winfield Scott upon its establishment in 1814, Scott County is surrounded by Lee County to the west, Washington County to the east, Russell County to the northeast, Wise County to the northwest, and the Tennessee counties of Sullivan, Hawkins, and Hancock to its south. The Clinch River and the North Fork of the Holston River flow in a general northeasterly to southwesterly direction near such Clinch Mountain high points as Possum Knobs (2,010 feet tall) and Copper Creek Knobs (2,090 feet tall).⁵¹ A tributary of the Clinch in Scott County is Stock Creek, which passes through the impressive ten-story high Natural Tunnel, described by William Jennings Bryan as the "Eighth Wonder of the World."⁵² The North Fork of the Holston, south of the Clinch, curves in a series of horseshoe bends on its way to merge with the South Fork of the Holston near Kingsport, Tennessee's Historic Boat Yard District and the Long Island of the Holston, a sacred Cherokee gathering place.

Scott County was home to three resorts recognized for their waters. The Mountain Springs Hotel resort, a two-story framed building with an ell extension, stood on Yuma Road (Virginia State Route 614) near Kermit and enjoyed largely a local community reputation in the late 1800s through the mid-twentieth century for its nearby cluster of chalybeate, alum and magnesia springs.⁵³ Thirty miles to the northeast where Hunters Valley East Road (Virginia State Route 653) crosses Staunton Creek is Hagan Springs. Also known as (Blue) Sulphur Springs, Hagan Springs bubbles near the ruins of Hagan Hall, the mid-nineteenth-century two-story brick home of prosperous land owner and attorney Patrick Hagan, who christened the area "Dungannon" after his Irish hometown.⁵⁴ The sulphur springs along with nearby chalybeate springs served as a "local resort," according to the nineteenth-century mineral water authority Albert C. Peale.⁵⁵ The most well-known mineral springs resort, and the topic of this chapter, is Holston Springs, about four miles east of Mountain Springs on modern Yuma Road near modern Weber City, which received about 170 guests during its opening season of 1809 and advertised in the Savannah and Charleston press 400 miles away.⁵⁶

One might wonder why a seemingly isolated resort on the frontier in its early years attracted Lowcountry patrons. Although Scott County today is largely considered a rural area off the beaten path, in the early nineteenth century, a network of roads crisscrossed its region based in part on Native American trails such as the Great Indian Warrior Path. Abingdon, about 45 miles to the northeast of Holston Springs, saw its first tavern in 1778, thanks in part to its location on the Wilderness Road, a branch of the Great Wagon Road that extended from Philadelphia to South Carolina and Georgia. The Wilderness Road, also later known in various locations as the Reedy Creek Road, Kentucky Road, or Bloomingdale Pike, ran to the Long Island from where Daniel Boone and his team of ax men blazed a section in 1775 through Scott County's Moccasin Gap, near modern Gate City, westward to Cumberland Gap and into Kentucky.⁵⁷

Thirty-four years later, in April 1809, Andrew McHenry opened a rude lodge (a "house of entertainment") supplemented by a row of cabins on property fronting the North Fork of the Holston River about "five miles from the Boat-Yard ... two miles from Moquesin [sic] Gap [and] about one mile from the Kentucky Road."⁵⁸ Andrew's coproprietor was David McHenry, who may have been his younger brother, who died in 1816 as acting sheriff of neighboring Lee County. The McHenrys advertised three springs that purportedly cured or benefited 159 of the 168 guests for the season of 1809 for such ailments as "Dead Palsy," "Sore Legs," "Hysterick Cholick," "Consumption," "Piles" (hemorrhoids), and "Hypochondria." The springs also allegedly healed horses ailing from "the Scratches," "Yellow Water," and "Throat Kernels."[59]

Andrew McHenry, a native of Washington County, Virginia, was active in area politics and business, serving as a commissioner, for example, to select the location of Scott County's county seat and serving as an attorney for the commonwealth.[60] His business and legal acumen may have prompted him to improve transportation to Holston Springs to increase resort revenue. McHenry and his three partners of "Andrew McHenry's spring" joined with other potential stock subscribers, chiefly in Abingdon and Wythe County's Saltville, to persuade the Virginia General Assembly in 1821 to pass an act to incorporate "The North Fork of Holstein [sic] River Company" at a capital investment of $15,000 to improve the navigation of the North Fork "from the Tennessee line … to Tate's mill in [Washington County]" and to charge tolls to recover expenses.[61] Whether the corporation succeeded is unclear, but in any event, sufficient funding from the river company or from McHenry and his partners resulted in the construction of "McHenry's Bridge," which prompted the 1823 rerouting of the Kentucky Road from an old ford crossing upstream on the North Fork.[62]

McHenry may have died in the mid–1830s; he is not listed in the 1840 U.S. Census but appears in the 60–70-year-old age category in the 1830 census.[63] According to a family narrative, he died at Holston Springs.[64] If he did die in the mid–1830s, that timeframe would serve as a plausible explanation as to why the McHenry family sold Holston Springs in 1837 to John Montgomery Preston of Abingdon.[65]

Preston was a wealthy member of prominent families associated with both the Walnut Grove Plantation in Washington County and Smithfield Plantation in present-day Montgomery County, Virginia.[66] He was a founding father of Abingdon, serving as its first mayor, and also a large early donor to Emory and Henry College, a Methodist-affiliated institution north of Abingdon.[67] As a businessman, he sold goods in Abingdon and, perhaps in a nod to his Holston Springs business, built a two-story Greek and Federal Revival brick house as a stagecoach inn at Seven Mile Ford in 1842 off the Wilderness Road (near the Virginia State Route 645 and U.S. Highway 11 intersection in Smyth County, Virginia).[68]

Preston improved the Holston Springs property, possibly using Native American laborers to supplement other workers to burn the bricks for the eventual three-story hotel fronted by verandahs across the first two stories and by two great side chimneys that David Hunter Strother sketched in the mid–1850s.[69] No source consulted describes resort activities, whether recreational or therapeutic, that occurred at Holston Springs through Preston's eight-year ownership. The multiple springs, however, must have been the major attraction as a detailed chemical analysis of the springs that appeared in an 1843 ad was widely republished in subsequent years.[70]

Although Preston lived in Abingdon during this period because of his business and civic affairs, he maintained a personal interest in property in southwest Virginia and upper East Tennessee.[71] In 1845, as part of a larger transaction, he traded Holston Springs to John Strother Gaines of Sullivan County, a North Carolina native who had served in the Tennessee Militia during the War of 1812. Gaines was descended from a wealthy, distinguished clan, which included Edmund Pendleton, chairman of the Second Continental Congress, who had received a land grant in 1756 in the environs of Reedy Creek in present-day Kingsport. Upon Pendleton's death in 1805, Gaines' father and uncle came into possession of 2,400 acres of the grant.[72]

Gaines had developed a self-sufficient plantation, known colloquially as the Exchange Place because of its use as a location to exchange state currencies or to exchange fatigued horses for fresh horses during journeys.[73] According to family tradition, Gaines's sons had spent their father's money lavishly, necessitating Gaines's 1845 transaction with Preston.[74] The transaction included the sale of 1,182 acres of the Gaines plantation on its western side to Preston; part of the contract included Gaines receiving Holston Springs.[75] Interestingly, $900 of the payment from Preston to Gaines for 108 acres of the total, covered in an addendum to the original contract, could be paid by cash and / or the sale of a "yellow boy" valued at $454.50; by Holston Springs farming implements, livestock, and wagon; and by merchandise from Preston's Abingdon store.[76] No further information can be located on the status or fate of the enslaved boy.

Gaines owned Holston Springs for about a dozen years but after four years returned to Sullivan County to live on the eastern tract of 1,200 acres that he had not sold to Preston.[77] A relative, Samuel M. Gaines, apparently tended to daily operations during part of this period.[78] Gaines, however, continued to place ads that publicized the "extraordinary cures" of the "delightful medicated warm bath" of the "Warm Spring"; the "White Sulphur, very pure and pleasant to the taste"; the "chalybeate of excellent quality"; and a "cold Limestone Spring."[79]

Antebellum guests attested to the waters' powers described in the advertisements. One visitor, on his way to the White Sulphur Springs, stopped at Gaines' Sullivan County property in 1847 where Gaines shrewdly persuaded him to try first Holston Springs; the traveler subsequently spent the remaining part of the summer there and gained a healthy thirty-five pounds after his "diseased liver" was cured.[80] A travel guide writer in 1855 also favorably compared Holston Springs water to that of the *belle dame* of the Virginia springs: The "medicinal qualities of the water are excellent, containing all the ingredients of the White Sulphur."[81] A visitor from Wetumpka, Alabama, exalted "the clear dashing river," the "fresh, bracing" air, and the "mineral draught" that he recommended for all "in quest of health" or "pleasant summer retreat."[82]

The Wetumpka visitor, however, writing in 1856, also noted the "isolated situation of this place" and "its inaccessibility" and hoped that the "hindrances" would be overcome.[83] By 1856, wagon roads and railroads had opened in several other regions of the South but lagged in development around Holston Springs and its environs. As one historian has noted, the lack of adequate roads isolated southwestern Virginia from the rest of the state (Abingdon was an exception), and a turnpike proposed by the state in the 1840s through southwestern Virginia was never implemented.[84]

The first passenger train did not reach Estillville (Gate City) until 1887; the first rail through the Natural Tunnel was not laid until 1890.[85]

Accordingly, Gaines family tradition has it that Gaines' move back to Sullivan County resulted from poor business at Holston Springs.[86] Lack of good roads constituted one factor. The other rationale, however, for the unfavorable profit margin lies in the clientele, who can be segmented into three categories: Familial and friend; those traveling for business, sight-seeing, or desiring a local meal; and regional and Deep South elite.

According to an interviewee, Gaines' kin did not typically pay for their board and lodging.[87] The Holston Springs hotel register, however, shows some family charges but includes apparent discounts such as an eight dollar charge for Gaines' wife's four week stay in May 1856 instead of the customary twenty dollar billing rate.[88] The register does not indicate if Gaines actually paid or wrote off his kin's bills but does record his personal charges, such as $4.50 for three hot baths.[89] In addition, the hotel hosted for days at a time Preston's relations, including the Greenways, Cummings, and Campbells from the Abingdon area and their children and "servants" (likely slaves). Gaines may have also granted discounts to them: The hotel charged $47.00 to a Russell County, Virginia, family and servant in 1854 for a two-week stay but only $22.50 to Mrs. E. Cummings of Abingdon in 1853 who was accompanied by three servants (possibly enslaved persons) for the same length of time.[90]

Most guests spent one or two nights or came only for "dinner" or "supper" because they resided within a day's travel of the hotel.[91] These clientele largely hailed from the border counties of Sullivan or Hawkins in Tennessee through Washington County, Virginia, northeasterly to Russell County. Less frequent regional visitors, who also spent a night or a few days at the hotel, came from Knoxville and Blountville in Tennessee and Virginia's Lee County, Tazewell, Wytheville, and Lynchburg. Several of those who spent only a night (about $1.00–$1.25) or took a single meal (~50–75 cents) were judges, lawyers, physicians, and presumed merchants apparently traveling in the area on a routine basis from the Abingdon area and to a much lesser extent from Knoxville.[92] Possibly, a few sight-seeing travelers may have stopped for one night or a meal on their way to or back from a visit to Stock Creek and Natural Tunnel.[93] In fact, sample counts across the five-year period show that the resort averaged only about two guests daily, including those who came for only a meal as part of a group of fifteen to twenty, indicating a narrow profit margin.[94]

The local and Deep South elite who stayed at Holston Springs did not include, with a few exceptions, the political or business leaders who congregated at some antebellum Southern Appalachian resorts to discuss tariffs, abolition, or other economic issues during the summer season. Notable local elites included Thomas Fain of Sullivan County's Arcadia Plantation, Patrick Hagan, and "Gov. Floid" (Governor John B. Floyd and a Preston relative by marriage), who stayed independently for only one to two nights or who paid for a single meal, hardly the time needed to engage in protracted discourse with fellow guests.[95] The Deep South elite who did travel to Holston Springs constituted a relatively small number of visitors compared to local or regional guests. In 1853, none of the six families who stayed for two weeks or longer hailed from the Deep South; all were local with the exception of an Asheville family with two servants (possibly enslaved persons).[96] In 1854, three families, one from the Deep South (Mississippi), stayed at least two weeks; in 1856, the number of groups paying for two or more weeks had risen to fifteen, of which three hailed from Mississippi, one from New Market, North Carolina, and the others largely from Abingdon.[97] Therefore, although a Richmond newspaper in 1889 described Holston Springs as a "popular resort in the fifties" where "belles of old Virginia and our dear Southland [met] in the halcyon days of their sunlit girlhood," the hotel ledger indicates that at least after 1852, the resort appears to have functioned more as a wayside hotel than as a recreative or restorative retreat in the tradition of other antebellum health resorts.[98]

Because of the financial difficulties of Holston Springs, Gaines in 1858 sold the property to a partnership consisting of the Reverend William D. Jones, former president of both Kentucky's Centre College and Rogersville, Tennessee's, Female College and a professor, Thomas B. Bailey, of Columbus, Mississippi. Both Jones and Bailey had boarded at Holston Springs several times so knew the property well.[99] Billing themselves as "both Southerners by birth and education," they organized a short-lived female academy.[100] The institute failed, and the resort was sold at auction in 1860 to local minister and slaveowner Jonathan Draper, who continued to operate it through the Civil War as a Confederate hospital and as headquarters for Brigadier General Humphrey Marshall.[101]

Draper's reputation may have differed between the perspectives of the officers and those of his enslaved persons. Several Confederates complained that the contract that they had negotiated with Draper for room and board saw "too much of the profits falling on Mr. Draper's side…. [One officer stated that] Draper would trade his golden harp-strings off."[102] William Davis, one of Draper's former enslaved persons (all being in the same immediate family), remarked that Draper and his wife were "mighty good to us" with "no whuppin' on our place."[103] The former slave recalled that as a boy before the war, Draper allowed him to keep coins given to him by guests for his assistance in helping them disembark from stagecoaches and permitted him to bathe in or drink the spring water. After the war, Draper paid the ex-slave family $120 annually to tend to the hotel's orchards and fields until the father of the family died in 1868. Draper's wife's warning to the ex-slave family, however, about "carpet baggers and liars [causing you to] be worse off den you ever has been, if you has anythin' to do with dem" may have prompted the family to remain at Holston Springs rather than because of any good will felt towards the Drapers.[104]

In 1870, Draper declared bankruptcy, and the property was then offered for rent.[105] One traveler bemoaned that the "property was very much out of repair" and hoped that "an enterprising proprietor" [might improve it to take advantage of the] "virtues of its various waters, its bold, rugged mountain scenery … and unsurpassed facilities afforded here for the sportsman."[106]

A series of owners followed Draper. Around 1884, Holston Springs received its last owner, Rufus Ayers, a lawyer and business executive, who was elected attorney general of Virginia in 1885.[107] The twenty-four-room hotel received paying guests into at least the early 1890s and even hosted weddings. Ayers then maintained

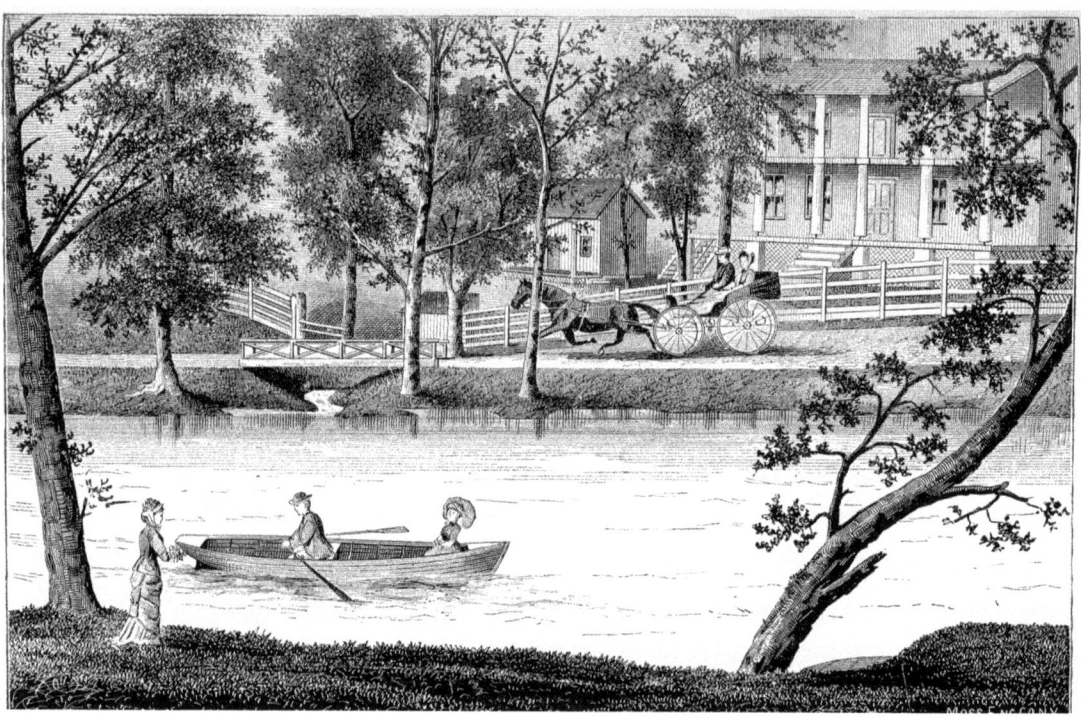

Holston Springs, Scott County, Virginia. Charles Rufus Boyd, *Resources of South-West Virginia: Showing the Mineral Deposits of Iron, Coal, Zinc, Copper and Lead*, 3rd ed. (New York: John Wiley & Sons, 1881), 208 (Library of Congress; image courtesy of the Archives of Appalachia, East Tennessee State University).

Holston Springs as a summer home once his stately stone mansion in Big Stone Gap in southwestern Virginia was finished in 1895.[108] Ayers' use of Holston Springs, however, ended abruptly in 1913. In December of that year, a fire that began in the resort's heating system destroyed the building and household furnishings.[109]

The Holston Springs mansion was never rebuilt. For the next several years, camping, picnics, and other outings, including the curiously named "bacon bat," were intermittently held at the property.[110] In 1941, the land was auctioned off into smaller farms and lots.[111] Today, a private home sits on the site of the former resort at the intersection of Warm Springs Road and Yuma Road.

Montgomery County: Yellow Sulphur Springs, Alleghany Springs, Montgomery White Sulphur Springs

As one drives north on Interstate 81 from Bristol at the Tennessee / Virginia state line, the elevation gradually increases from around 1,670 feet to about 2,130 feet in Christiansburg 115 miles away. Christiansburg, in the highlands of the Blue Ridge Mountains, part of the greater Appalachian Ridge and Valley physiographic region, is the county seat of Montgomery County. Along with Floyd, Giles, and Pulaski counties, Montgomery County lies within Virginia's New River Valley.[112]

This region today is associated with FloydFest, Blacksburg's Virginia Tech Hokies, and Giles County's Mountain Lake, location for much of the 1987 film "Dirty Dancing." In the nineteenth century, the Virginia New River Valley contained several mineral spring resorts secondary to the aristocratic White Sulphur and other elite resorts in the mountains around present-day Greenbrier County, West Virginia, and the aptly named Bath County, Virginia. Peale's 1886 treatise on American mineral spring resorts, for example, included Giles County's Eggleston Springs (New River White Sulphur Springs) and Pulaski County's Pulaski Alum Springs.[113]

Montgomery County was home to at least four health resorts: Crockett Springs, Alleghany Springs, Montgomery White Sulphur Springs, and Yellow Sulphur Springs. Crockett Springs, a modest hotel with a bottling operation near the South Fork Roanoke River, received guests from about 1889 until the 1930s when the Great Depression decimated business. Today the Alta Mons church camp stands on the property, which fronts Virginia State Route 637.[114] About three miles northwest on the same road stood the more fashionable Alleghany Springs. Another posh property, Montgomery White Sulphur Springs, was located about four miles northwest from Alleghany, off today's State Route 641. Yellow Sulphur Springs, farther to the west, lies on State Route 643, about five miles north of Christiansburg and three and one-half miles south of Blacksburg, and fifteen miles northwest of Alleghany Springs.[115]

This chapter focuses on the latter three resorts, all of which began in antebellum times. Two of the mineral spring hotels, Montgomery White Sulphur and Alleghany Springs, shared a proprietor for several years, which partially explains the lack of rivalry among the three Montgomery County resorts. The third, Yellow Sulphur Springs, the oldest of the county resorts, received fewer visitors than the Montgomery White and Alleghany but continued to operate under different business models into the twenty-first century, including three years as a safe vacation stop for Black travelers during the Jim Crow era in the 1920s. All three resorts welcomed guests from the Deep South in antebellum times and prospered with the construction of the Virginia and Tennessee Railroad through the county in the 1850s. In the postbellum period, contingents of former Confederate officers visited the watering spas where they relived their battle tactics and reminisced about the "Lost Cause" with fellow visitors, many of whom hailed from Louisiana, Mississippi, and other former slave states.

The Yellow Sulphur Springs health resort originated as a two-story frame hotel, built around 1810 by Charles Taylor, who had rented the property to build housing for invalids seeking the waters. Known originally as Taylor Springs or Yellow Springs, the hotel and its outbuildings stood at the intersection of three ravines near the head waters of Wilson Creek, a tributary of the North Fork Roanoke River.[116] At an elevation of about 1,900 feet, at what the nineteenth-century traveler Edward A. Pollard described as the "great altitude of the spring" ... [rendering] the air ... "elastic, pure and invigorating," the Yellow Sulphur perched about 500 feet above both the Alleghany Springs and Montgomery White Sulphur resorts.[117]

Visitors initially came from North Carolina and eastern Virginia.[118] John Guerrant of Richmond, for example, recovered in 1806 from bowel difficulties, apparently staying in a crude shelter that predated Taylor's hotel.[119] A writer expounded in a Richmond newspaper in 1810 on the sulphur's taste ("somewhat astringent ... not unlike the first impression of ink upon the tongue ... often drunk by healthy, laborious persons in preference to the common Limestone water") and its curative effects on leg ulcers, cutaneous disorders, eye inflammations, and "obstructions of the Viscera."[120]

Taylor bought the property in 1812 and for reasons unclear decided to sell or lease it within two years. From 1814 through 1826, he intermittently publicized the sale of its 600 acres, pleading in 1826 that he had "been long rendered incapable of attending to business from indisposition."[121] By 1833, he found a stable lessee in Creed Taylor (relationship not known between the two Taylors) who operated the resort for at least three seasons, publicizing in 1835 the springs' curative powers "to remove the causes of impaired digestion [and] to give tone and strength to the human constitution."[122]

In 1842 an owner emerged with sufficient income to extensively improve the property over the next decade. Armistead (Armstead) W. Forrest acquired the property's 728 acres for $2,000.[123] He remodeled the hotel to include a two-story portico across its length and constructed cottage rows, each consisting of a series of one-story, six-unit structures, along the lower slopes of the ravines. Behind the rows, named for cities such as Petersburg and Memphis, stood one-story, double-servant frame cottages for enslaved persons accompanying owners occupying the main rows.[124]

In 1853, Forrest sold the hotel and 274 acres to a syndicate that rechristened the property as "Yellow Sulphur Springs," perhaps as a nod to the Greenbrier White Sulphur and its nearby resorts about ninety miles to the northwest of Christiansburg.[125] The Yellow Sulphur Springs Company continued to renovate the property; Edward Beyer's 1857 lithograph in his *Album of Virginia* depicts a central fountain fronting the hotel and its cottage rows and several large shade trees dotting the fenced manicured lawns and riding paths.[126]

The arrival of the Virginia and Tennessee Railroad to Montgomery County in the mid–1850s marked a boom era for the county's health resort development as the new railroad linked to other regional rail systems. Originating in Lynchburg with a transfer line to Petersburg and Richmond, the Virginia and Tennessee Railroad reached Wytheville in 1855 and Bristol in fall 1856 where it joined with the East Tennessee and Virginia Railroad, which led southerly to Knoxville and beyond.[127] In response to the completion of the railroad in its vicinity, the Yellow Sulphur Springs Company built a three-mile turnpike, with twice-daily hack service, to the Christiansburg depot.[128] Nearly concurrent with the construction of the railroad through the county was the establishment of Alleghany Springs in the early 1850s, about three miles south of the Shawsville railroad stop built in 1854, followed by the 1855 incorporation of Montgomery White Sulphur Springs, which lobbied the railroad for a depot two miles away at Big Tunnel.[129] The Montgomery White Sulphur could then boast that "[p]assengers leaving Richmond or Petersburg after breakfast reach the Springs by 5 o'clock, P.M., same day, all the way by Rail Road."[130] Likewise, Alleghany Springs advertised "Four-Horse Omnibuses" to meet guests arriving the same day from Baltimore, Washington, Richmond, and Petersburg, with "the same conveyance on the arrival of each train" from the south.[131] To boost its passenger traffic, the Virginia and Tennessee Railroad publicized train travel from Petersburg through Lynchburg to Salem, Virginia. After an overnight stay in Salem, passengers traveled "only sixty one miles of Staging" to reach the White Sulphur Springs or to visit "other delightful watering places immediately on the line," such as the Yellow Sulphur Springs and the Alleghany Springs.[132]

Antebellum details on Alleghany Springs' origin are few. The exact year of the Alleghany Springs resort's opening is unclear although a letter writer in 1852 penned that he would delay his travels home due to his longer use of the water, and the proprietorship of Holt, Colhoun & Co. erected "all new" improvements "of the most comfortable character" in 1853, implying that a hotel existed before 1852 or 1853.[133] Also unknown is the early appearance of the resort. By 1859, however, the 400-acre property consisted of a working farm, a bath house, and accommodations for 500 visitors in cabins and the hotel.[134] An 1870 illustration drawn from the nearby peak of Fisher's View gives a bird's-eye perspective of about a dozen buildings, including two multi-storied structures, upslope from the South Fork Roanoke River.[135]

Better known is the purported therapeutic value of the Alleghany's water. Prior to the resort development, locals frequented the springs. John J. Moorman, resident physician at the elite White Sulphur Springs, in 1855 wrote that the mineral spring waters had "long been esteemed valuable by persons in their immediate neighborhood."[136] Antebellum visitors supposedly found relief for "*Nervous or Cutaneous Diseases* [italics original], Dyspepsia, or any disease originating from a disordered state of the stomach or liver."[137] A New Orleans newspaper in 1860 suggested to its readers "who may contemplate a trip to the mountains of Old Virginia" to consider the Alleghany: "There are instances of men who have been rescued almost from the grave and restored to perfect health in a few weeks by a visit to Alleghany Springs."[138] An enterprise to ship the water began in the antebellum period, which "extended to every State in the Union."[139]

Ownership of the Alleghany from at least 1854 through its demise in the early twentieth century remained in part or in entirety with C.A. (Charles Alexander) Colhoun (Calhoun). Colhoun in 1850 was a merchant in Nelson County, northeast of Lynchburg, with real estate valued at $5,000 who by the 1860 federal census had parlayed his occupation of "Proprietor watering place" to $60,000 in real estate with $10,000 in personal estate. By 1870, Colhoun was worth $100,000 (over $2.3 million in 2022 dollars) in real estate and a not insignificant personal estate at $12,000.[140] Part of Colhoun's monetary worth in 1870, however, lay in his partial ownership at that time of the third Montgomery County resort, the Montgomery White Sulphur.

The Montgomery White Sulphur originated as part of an 1835 tract purchase by James Kent, Montgomery County's largest antebellum slaveowner.[141] Like Alleghany Springs and Yellow Sulphur Springs, "people of the neighborhood" had used the springs since the early 1800s.[142] Prompted most likely by the building of the Virginia and Tennessee Railroad, Kent and several others incorporated the Montgomery White Sulphur Company in 1855 to hold "lands not exceeding three thousand acres," "to erect buildings for the accommodation of visitors and others, to provide for their entertainment ... to improve and cultivate its lands ... and to conduct and erect saw and other mills."[143]

The Montgomery White Sulphur Company first built in spring 1855 a two-story frame reception house at the springs, about sixty by forty feet, with a porch wrapped around the four sides. Within two years, the resort had greatly expanded, according to Beyer's 1857 lithograph.[144] The resort as drawn by Beyer consisted of a "V"-shaped formation, two-story cottages forming the flanks of the V. At the intersection of the two rows of cottages stood the "elegant reception house ... most agreeable to the tired traveler, after a long journey on the rail."[145] Travelers literally rode in railcars straight to the reception house: Once they disembarked at the Big Tunnel depot, they transferred to engineless railcars on the resort's private railroad for a two-mile ride, "along an easy descending grade ... without trouble or fatigue," to the building entrance.[146] A three-story structure topped by a cupola, possibly the main hotel, stood centered in one of the flanks. A central pond and fountain stood within the complex connected with shady paths to the cottage rows and to a circular drive through which carriages entered the compound.[147]

The water, like an exquisite wine, was favorably compared to that of the Greenbrier White Sulphur and other sulphur springs. An 1855 Montgomery White ad offered that its water was "more pleasant to the taste, and equally effective" than the Greenbrier's.[148] Pollard considered it "of like effects and qualities with the famous Greenbrier White Sulphur."[149] Moorman, intimately familiar with the Greenbrier's waters in his role as that resort's medical consultant, wrote that the Montgomery White's "bland and pleasant" taste was "less cathartic" than many sulphurs so "may be used with more freedom and with greater safety than such waters, by delicate and excitable persons."[150]

The sulphur springs and two chalybeate springs, the latter described by Pollard as of a "strongly tonic character," were advertised to benefit a variety of ailments.[151] Newspaper ads confidently assured that almost all afflictions were treatable: "Diseases of the Liver and Kidneys, all Diseases of the Stomach, especially of a Chronic character; and in all Cutaneous Diseases, tetter [ringworm or eczema], Scald Head [scalp disease], Erysipelas, Salt Rhem, &c, &c."[152] A visitor in 1858 wrote that "[m]any persons, the present season, declare themselves highly benefitted by [the sulphur water]. There is also a very excellent chalybeate spring close by which is much used and esteemed."[153] A guest a year later opined that the "waters are decidedly good for disease of the liver, bowels and dyspepsia. I was greatly benefitted from my short stay."[154]

The focal point of Montgomery White Sulphur, however, lay not in the water but in its fashionable society. The same guest who commented about the curative nature of the water for liver and bowel diseases also wrote that the "place is patronized almost entirely by the wealthy merchants and planters of the South ... dresses costing from $500 to $2,000 are very common sight.... I saw one pyramid julep prepared, ordered by a lady, that cost $2 50 [sic], for which cash was paid right down."[155] A Richmond commentator noted that the Alleghany Springs were "celebrated for their medicinal qualities," that the Yellow Sulphur Springs was frequented by those who visited a nearby alum springs, but that the Montgomery White "promise[d] to eclipse even its namesake of Greenbrier."[156] Another observer agreed: "The Montgomery White Sulphur Springs ... have grown to a degree of vastness and importance out-rivalling the far famed Greenbrier.... [N]ot in the mere matter of improving health alone that they should command a preference."[157] Although both Alleghany Springs and the Yellow Sulphur advertised in the southern press and Yellow Sulphur received future C.S.A. Brigadier General P.G.T. Beauregard, Fire-Eater planter Edmund Ruffin and Whig Congressman T.S. Flournoy, the Montgomery White Sulphur attracted more of the aristocratic southern elite for conviviality and less for health objectives than did the other two resorts.[158]

The advent of the Civil War did not immediately close the three resorts. Yellow Sulphur Springs remained open for the early years of the war but closed by 1864 with some furnishings auctioned off.[159] Alleghany Springs continued to sell water in at least the early war days and, via extensive advertising in the southern press, welcomed Virginia springs circuit guests such as New Orleans cotton broker Henry S. Gilmour who traveled there and to the White Sulphur for the summer of 1861.[160] To reassure Richmond-area residents, the Alleghany in spring 1862 promised the "best security for families."[161] The soothing words apparently had the desired effect, for the resort in early July 1862, about the time of Richmond's Seven Days' Battles from June 25–July 1, announced that the "great number of applications for board had induced the Proprietors to open this place" to "be kept in as a good style as the circumstances of the country will admit."[162] Likewise, the Montgomery White Sulphur promised in the southern press in 1861 and early summer 1862 that it remained a "delightful summer resort, but in these exciting times, a safe retreat for ladies and children."[163]

Circumstances changed, however, for the Alleghany and the Montgomery White Sulphur in late summer 1862. In September, a wounded Confederate officer sojourning at Alleghany Springs wrote that it would close in a few days despite a small "pleasant society" that included a Confederate general's wife, a couple from Mobile, and a Virginia judge.[164] The Confederate government converted the Montgomery White that summer into an army hospital, administered by the Sisters of Mercy Catholic order, where most of the six hundred patients that October were "without clothing, shoes, under-shirt."[165] A smallpox epidemic swept through the unvaccinated at the army hospital, contributing to the 265 or more troop burials on the grounds.[166] One-third interests of both resort properties were put on the market in late 1863 and early 1864 (no information available if actually sold); the Confederate hospital remained in service until the end of the war, with several dozen Union military patients there.[167]

After the war, the resorts had reopened by the time of Pollard's visits in 1869. Pollard noted that the Yellow Sulphur accommodated about one hundred guests in "new and comfortable" buildings but lamented that it could receive more visitors if additional rooms were available.[168] In 1871, as if in response to Pollard's appeal, new owners John and James Wade, who had bought the resort in November 1870 for $25,000 from a seller unknown, built an additional forty-room, two and one half story mansard-roof hotel, which unfortunately burned down the following year.[169] Colhoun by 1867 had reopened the Alleghany, having made "thorough repairs," and by 1868 had partnered with John T. Cowan to own the Montgomery White

Sulphur.[170] Under "the energetic efforts" of Cowan and Colhoun, Pollard wrote that the Montgomery White's transformation from hospital to mineral springs spa was "absolutely astounding."[171]

In the postbellum period, all three resorts prospered, continuing their pre-war tradition of catering to regional clientele and visitors from the Deep South. Both Yellow Sulphur Springs and the Montgomery White hosted early regional board meetings of the newly developed Virginia Agricultural and Mechanical College (Virginia Tech) in nearby Blacksburg.[172] The Alleghany Springs in 1866 reopened both its water shipping business and its hotel, prompting a jubilant New Orleans visitor in summer 1868 to exclaim that the "end of the war found me a confirmed dyspeptic.... [After drinking the water,] I can now pitch a three-pound quilt sixty feet, and jump over a sixteen-hand horse."[173]

The resorts' ambiance now largely centered around the "Lost Cause." Many former Confederate officers and politicians gathered at the watering holes with wealthy planters and southern businessmen, particularly at Alleghany Springs and Montgomery White Sulphur, which each offered accommodations for over 1,000 guests.[174] At Alleghany Springs in 1872, the unreconstructed Major General Samuel G. French from Mississippi debated Lieutenant General John Bell Hood over the latter's halt at Cassville, Georgia, in May 1864, part of the larger Atlanta Campaign.[175] The resort also received Lieutenant General James Longstreet, "avoided like a leper" as a consequence of his controversial delayed offensive at Gettysburg and his support of U.S. Grant in the 1868 presidential election.[176] Jefferson Davis attended a meeting of the Southern Historical Society, devoted to preserving a sympathetic and heroic Confederate perspective of the Civil War, which Lieutenant General Jubal Early reorganized at the Montgomery White.[177] The society, which met at both the Montgomery White and Yellow Sulphur in subsequent years, commanded a slate of offices held by former Confederates such as Major General M.C. Butler and General J.B. Hood.[178] Yellow Sulphur Springs and the Montgomery White hosted fancy tournament balls respectively in 1868 and 1869, a throwback to a popular antebellum resort activity, sponsored in part by such well known Confederate generals as Robert E. Lee at the Montgomery White and P.G.T. Beauregard and William Mahone at both.[179]

Ownership remained stable at the Alleghany Springs under Colhoun in the 1880s but changed hands at the other two resorts. In 1881, a lawsuit precipitated a county court to sell Montgomery White Sulphur Springs; George W. Fagg, associated with the previous resort management, bought the property's 1,439 acres with other businessmen for $19,000, a bargain as the original cost was estimated at $160,000.[180] In 1886 ex–Confederate Captain Ridgway (Ridgeway) Holt assumed ownership of Yellow Sulphur Springs and constructed a sixty-room shingle-style hotel with bowling alley, ballroom, and a pool room. In the next three years, in anticipation of future growth, the resort management built additional cottages for 300 more guests, dredged a lake and fishpond, and installed "[e]legant bath houses, with all the conveniences for hot and cold mineral baths."[181]

During the 1880s and 1890s, guests continued to arrive at the Montgomery County resorts largely from the Deep South and the nearby Virginia region. A browsing of Alleghany advertisements and newspaper society sections from this era indicates that the resort remained popular with southern travelers from Memphis, Atlanta, Vicksburg, and New Orleans and visitors from eastern Virginia. To a lesser extent, patrons arrived from Knoxville and the Tallahassee area.[182] Hotel ledgers from both the Montgomery White and Yellow Sulphur resorts also confirm the Deep South and regional residences of guests.

The Montgomery White and Yellow Sulphur ledgers provide more nuance than can be discerned from newspaper society sections alone. As noted below, I examined ledger entries from selected years.[183] First, guests at one resort periodically traveled to others in the region. For instance, a Pulaski, Virginia, resident stayed at Yellow Sulphur Springs on August 31, 1887, then traveled to the Montgomery White two days later. Conversely, a Portsmouth, Virginia, resident stayed at the Montgomery White on September 2, 1887, and then three days later signed in at the Yellow Sulphur. Colhoun's sons occasionally traveled from Alleghany Springs to the other two resorts in the late 1880s and again in the 1893–1894 period. The merchant J.J. Fagg, whose father owned the Montgomery White, registered at the Yellow Sulphur in addition to boarding at the Montgomery White. Guests from the Greenbrier White Sulphur visited the Yellow Sulphur in August 1887; guests from the Alleghany traveled to the Montgomery White in 1888.

Second, Deep South elite continued to summer or spend a few weeks at the

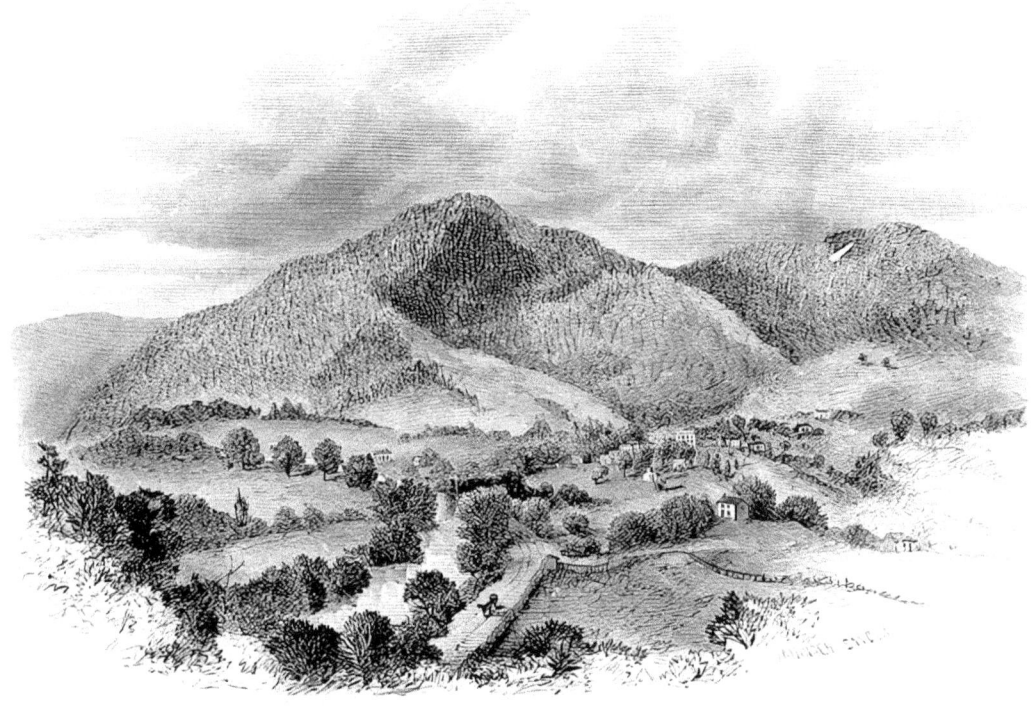

"Fisher's View—Alleghany Springs." Pollard states that the view was named after an artist who had studied in Europe and sketched the scene, declaring that he had seen nothing in Europe to equal its "wild and unkept variety." Edward A. Pollard and Joseph Meredith Toner Collection, *The Virginia Tourist: Sketches of the Springs and Mountains of Virginia...* (Philadelphia: J.R. Lippincott & Co., 1870), 89; Library of Congress, *https://lccn.loc.gov/rc01002850*).

resorts. Varina Davis, daughter of Jefferson, traveled from Beauvoir, Mississippi, in summer 1888 to visit both the Yellow Sulphur and the Montgomery White. Jubal Early built a cottage at Yellow Sulphur Springs; the resort maintained a permanent room for Beauregard during his summer visits from New Orleans (the ledger records several entries for each).[184] Other southern notables at Yellow Sulphur Springs, several of whom made repeat visits, included the family of Benson Blake, chair of the Vicksburg Cotton Exchange; the New Orleans Hanna merchant family; and the family of Richard Pritchard, New Orleans businessman and director of a regional railroad. In addition, frequent visitors in 1894 and 1895 were two prominent Jewish families, the R.W. Levy family of New York and New Orleans, engaged in the cotton exchange business, and the family of Rabbi I.L. Leucht, of one of New Orleans' "more important" congregations, the Judah Touro Synagogue.[185] Montgomery White Sulphur received Napoleon Hill, the so-called "merchant prince of Memphis"; New Orleans Mayor William J. Behan; and Macon, Georgia's R.S. Lanier, father of the poet Sidney Lanier and son of Sterling Lanier, the antebellum proprietor of East Tennessee's famed Montvale Springs.

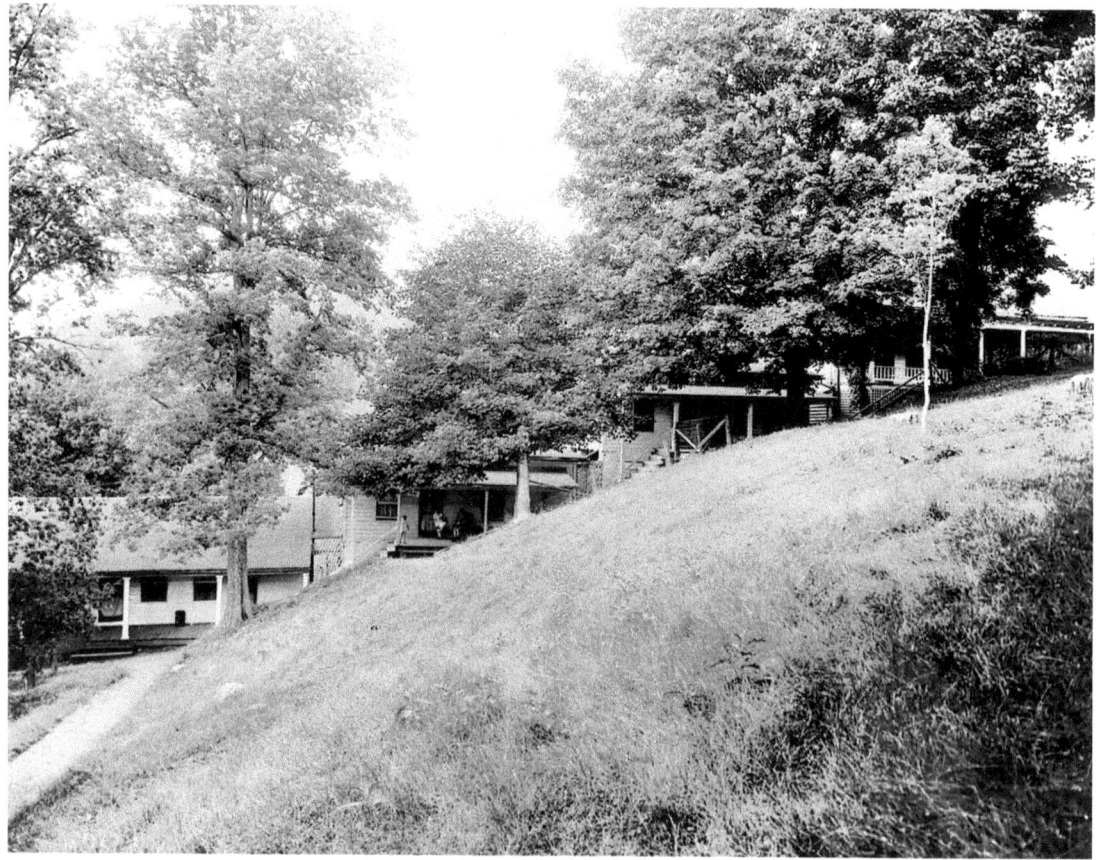

"Cottages of Alleghany Springs," Montgomery County, Virginia (image from the Collection of the Historical Society of Western Virginia, Roanoke, *https://hswv.pastperfectonline.com/photo/6AFD9AD5-34DC-4246-8179-648484006189*. ID: 1967.24.1).

Third, during the periods analyzed, both the Yellow Sulphur and Montgomery White resorts attracted more visitors from the nearby regions of Virginia and North Carolina than from other parts of the South. Data from the last week of August 1887 show that the Montgomery White received forty-three guests from Virginia, twenty-one from other parts of the South, and six from other geographies such as Washington, D.C. Likewise, Yellow Sulphur Springs, a much smaller resort, for the same period registered twenty-three regional visitors, two from other southern geographies, and four from outside the South. The Fourth of July for 1888 entries show 170 regional guests and three guests from other parts of the South for the Montgomery White Sulphur; the Yellow Sulphur the same day received only eight regional guests and one from outside the South. Regional visitors to both resorts included professors, ministers, tobacco capitalists, judges, and a textile mill magnate.

Fourth, a glance at the Yellow Sulphur Springs ledger for its last recorded ten days, July 1–10, 1895, illustrates the greater capacity for travel by the late 1890s. The register shows, exclusive of the registration of three Lynchburg musicians hired to provide entertainment, twenty-six regional guests; fifteen visitors from other parts of the South, including Knoxville, Texas, New Orleans, and Natchez; and twelve from other locales, including Hong Kong, San Francisco, London, Paris, and Canada. Probably some of the visitors were related or friends (e.g., the Parisian roomed with the San Franciscan), but the diversity of home locations shows the increased mobility of the late nineteenth century.

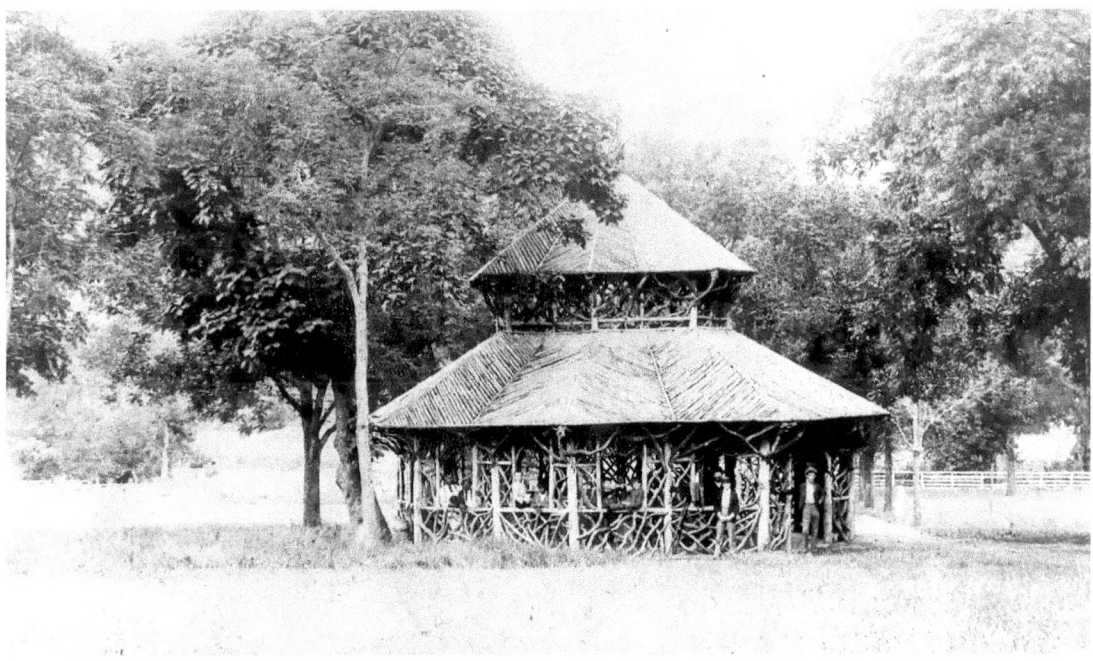

"The Spring House Gazebo at Alleghany Springs [1890s]," Montgomery County, Virginia (image from the Collection of the Historical Society of Western Virginia, Roanoke, *https://hswv.pastperfectonline.com/photo/029041E0-0C65-4C16-AAA7-252917511770/*. ID: 1967.24.2).

The three resorts declined during the next three decades. A fire in 1900 destroyed the hotel and mountain row of cottages at Alleghany Springs.[186] In 1903, James C. Crockett, who had bought the Montgomery White Sulphur just the year before, auctioned off hotel furniture and dismantled the remaining structures in 1904 after a flood and a fire devasted the resort.[187] Yellow Sulphur Springs floundered as well due to the rerouting of the main route between Christiansburg and Blacksburg in the 1910s.[188]

Yellow Sulphur, however, saw a brief renaissance in spring 1926 when a group of ten Black Roanoke businessmen purchased the resort.[189] The members of the Yellow Sulphur Springs, Inc., represented a variety of occupations essential to the funding and operation of the resort at a time when self-reliance in the Black community was imperative. Members included the Magic City Building and Loan Association's president William H. Burwell and treasurer/secretary Henry C. Johnson, realty owner Albert F. Brooks, railroad porter C.W. Thompson, and the Hotel Roanoke's chief bellman Alvin L. Coleman.[190] The businessmen were closely connected to Roanoke's Henry Street, a major economic hub and social community for regional Blacks across several decades and recognized today by an annual street festival.[191]

The Yellow Sulphur Springs syndicate may have envisioned the resort as a restful

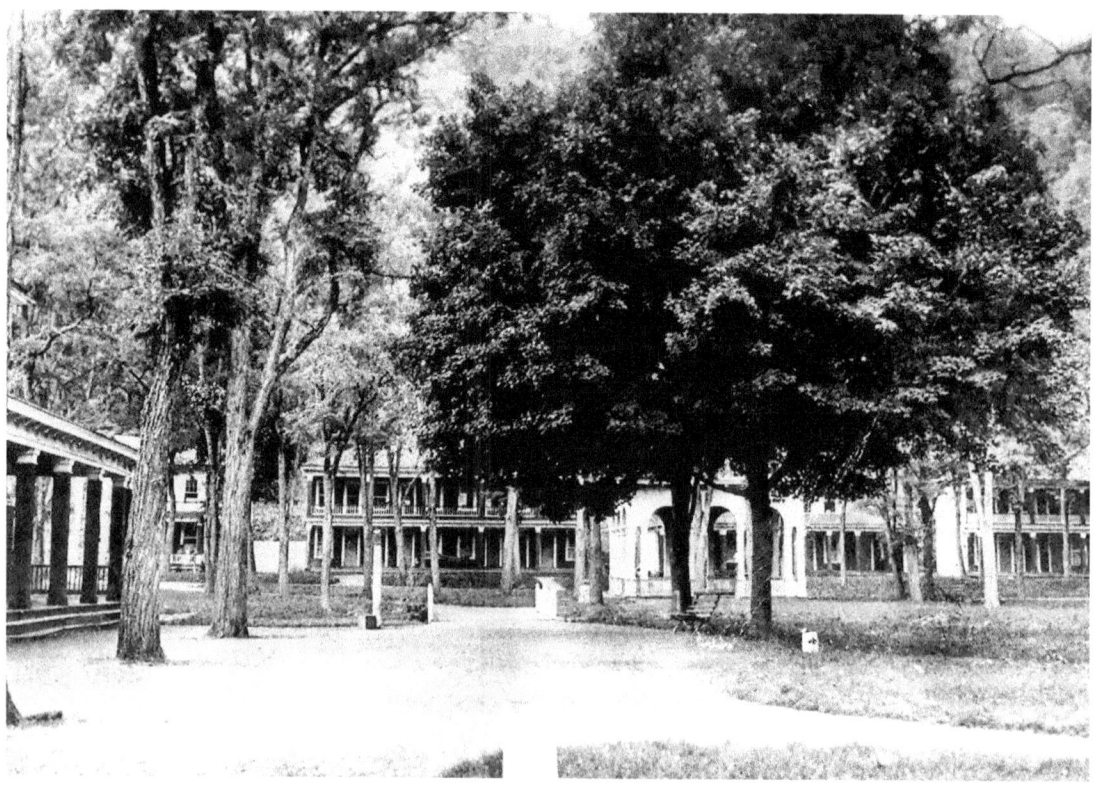

"White Sulphur Springs [1900]," Montgomery County, Virginia (image courtesy of the Harry Downing Temple, Jr. Papers (Ms1988-039), Special Collections and University Archives, University Libraries, Virginia Polytechnic Institute and State University, *https://digitalsc.lib.vt.edu/Ms1988_039_/t016*. ID: t016).

respite from a white-dominated society and as a safe overnight stop for Blacks traveling elsewhere. The Black publication *Norfolk Journal and Guide* billed it as a place "where the air is pure and invigorating with an environment where race prejudice is not likely to arise."[192] Black travelers passing through Virginia stayed at Yellow Sulphur Springs in an era of racial hostility and segregation. As an example, a young Black male from Kingsport, Tennessee, about 140 miles away, spent one night there on his automobile trip to another destination.[193] Speculatively, because Roanoke was part of the "Chitlin' Circuit," a series of safe places for Black entertainers and musicians to perform and "bed down" during segregation, perhaps the Yellow Sulphur Springs syndicate saw its resort, about thirty-five miles away from Roanoke, as a stop as well.[194]

Aubrey Mills, however, a Black male born at the resort in 1927, recalled in 2010 that more racial intermingling may have occurred than is assumed. Black and white musicians apparently played together for presumably mixed audiences. He remembered hearing of interracial weddings at the resort although the U.S. Supreme Court would not strike down anti-miscegenation marriage state laws until 1967 in the famous *Loving v. Virginia* case.[195]

Unfortunately, the Black-operated resort was short-lived. In 1929, for

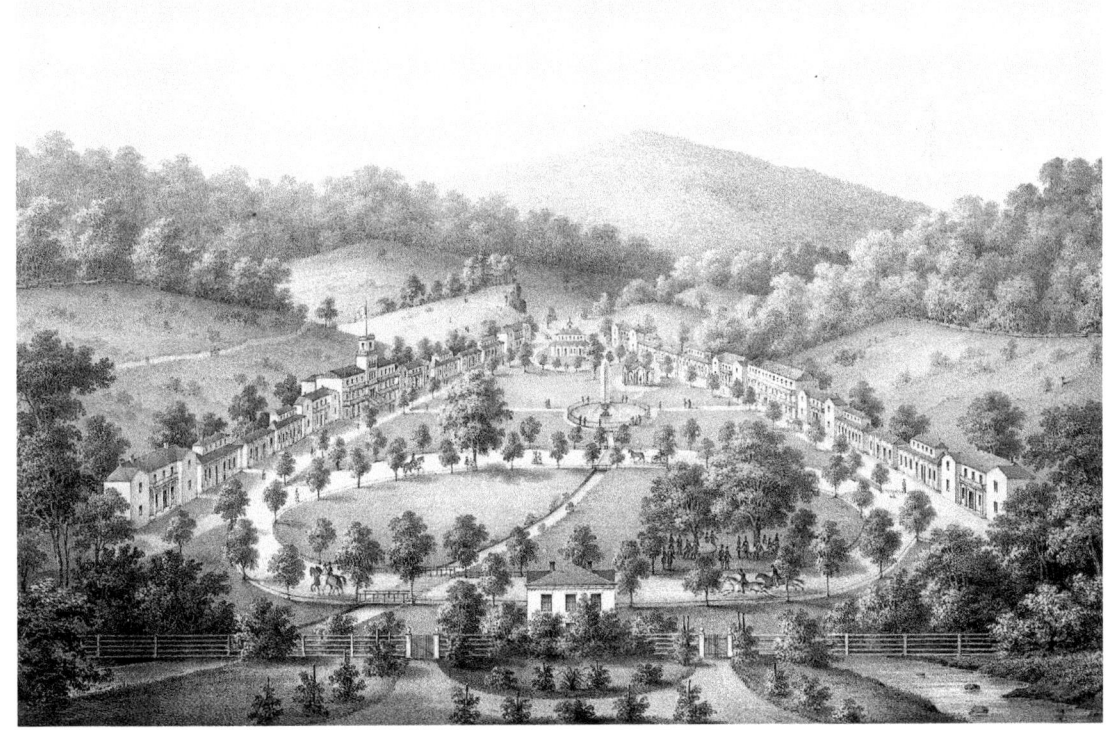

"White Sulphur Spring, Montgomery County, VA from 'Album of Virginia' [1858]." Edward Beyer, artist. W. Loeillot, lithographer (image courtesy of American Art Collection, Virginia Museum of Fine Arts, Richmond, Virginiana Fund, *https://vmfa.museum/picttion/6027262-8090171/*. ID: 71.13.2).

reasons unclear, Montgomery County auctioned off the Yellow Sulphur Springs resort.[196]

After the 1929 sale, Yellow Sulphur Springs experienced several changes in ownership. In 1932, the Yellow Sulphur Springs Recreative Sanatorium received a charter for the site as a health and pleasure retreat, but the sanatorium never opened.[197] The same year, the Virginia Transient Bureau reconfigured the resort to house homeless men, who restored the buildings and grounds during the Great Depression.[198] Charles A. Crumpacker bought the springs after the 1930s; after his death in 1942, his daughter owned the property until she passed away in 1994.[199] In 1997, Bernard Ross and his wife Victoria Taylor bought the property, renovated much of it, and established a healing arts center on the premises. As of October 2021, they were seeking a new steward for its fifty-four acres.[200]

The three major mineral spring resorts of Montgomery County catered to white southern elites who summered there and also provided travelers with a spa circuit before they continued on to the more fashionable Virginia (and postbellum West Virginia) spring resorts to the northwest. Southern visitors to the Montgomery County mineral spring resorts often continued to "take the waters" by traveling by turnpike to the New River White Sulphur and then to either the Red Sulphur or to Salt Sulphur via Mountain Lake and then beyond to the Greenbrier White Sulphur

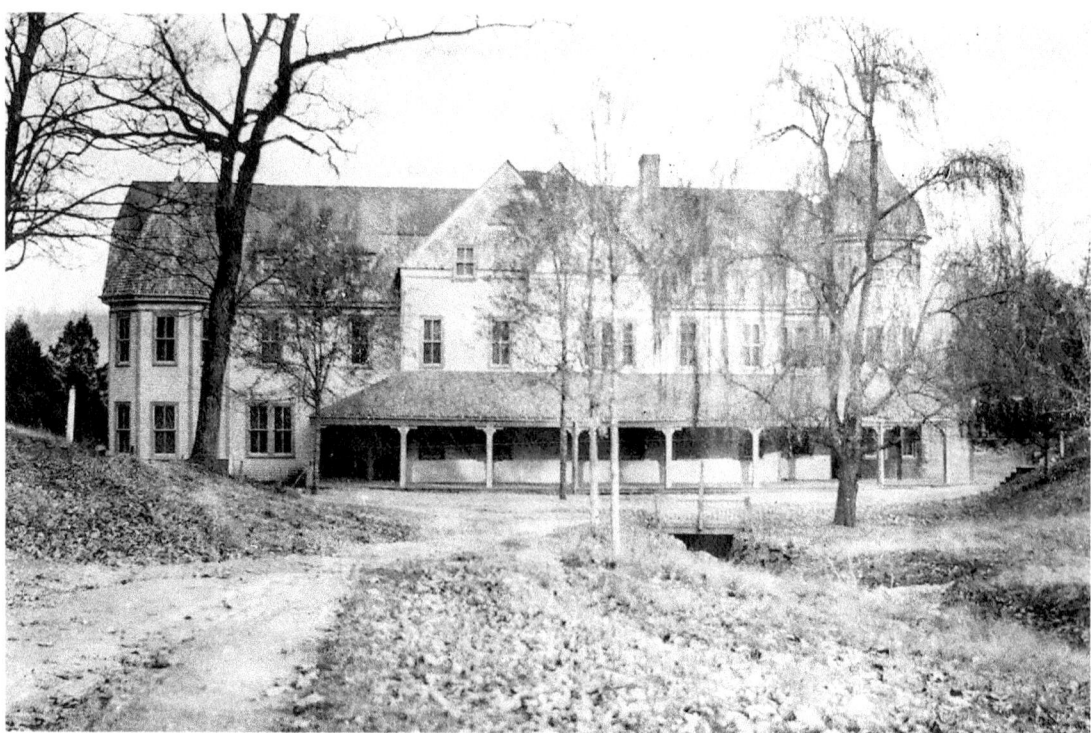

"Old Hotel at Yellow Sulphur Springs," Montgomery County, Virginia (image courtesy of the Historical Photograph Collection, Special Collections and University Archives, University Libraries, Virginia Polytechnic Institute and State University, *https://digitalsc.lib.vt.edu/items/show/17686*. ID: YSS003-old-hotel).

and the Sweet Springs.[201] Conversely, guests from the Greenbrier White Sulphur might register at the Montgomery County resorts. Beauregard and Pritchard, frequent guests at the Yellow Sulphur, endorsed a proprietor whom they knew from visits to Bath County's exclusive Warm Springs and Healing Springs.[202]

The Montgomery County mineral springs resorts also provided a comforting and familiar ambiance for southern noblesse after the Civil War. At the Montgomery White Sulphur and Yellow Sulphur Springs, Early and other Confederate sympathizers welcomed the "Daughter of the Confederacy," Varina "Winnie" Davis, and defended their military decisions to other aging Confederates at Southern Historical Society gatherings.[203] At the Alleghany Springs, Beauregard and fellow generals Hardee and Gordon debated the merits of the opposing sides in the 1870 Franco-Prussian War in front of an eager crowd.[204]

Perhaps the most intriguing of the three resorts is Yellow Sulphur Springs due to the evolution of Black roles at the spa, from slave to resort owner. In 1850, Armistead Forrest held an enslaved adult female and three enslaved children and in 1860, three enslaved adult women, one enslaved 20-year-old adult male, and nine enslaved children thirteen and under.[205] The ages and genders suggest that the nuclear families were separated, an additional hardship under bondage. The last known antebellum owners, the Yellow Sulphur Springs Company's three partners, Thomas H. Foulkes, Charles B. Gardner, and James P. Edmundson, collectively owned 45 slaves in 1860.[206] Although more research is needed to confirm, it can be speculated that some of the enslaved persons worked at the resort, the younger ones perhaps fanning the guests as they ate and the older ones perhaps maintaining the property. In the postbellum period, Jubal Early, frequent visitor to the resort, penned that "domestic slavery

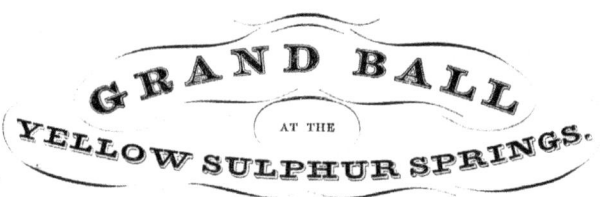
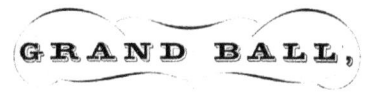
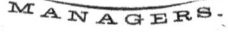

Grand Ball at the Yellow Sulphur Springs invitation (1871) (image courtesy of Virginia Ball Invitations, Special Collections and University Archives, University Libraries, Virginia Polytechnic Institute and State University, *https://aspace.lib.vt.edu/repositories/2/resources/2522/collection_organization#tree::archival_object_58553.* **ID: Ms2009-103).**

… had not only resulted in a great improvement in the moral and physical condition of the negro [sic] race, but had furnished a class of laborers as happy and content as any in the world, if not more so."[207] Eighty years after Armistead Forrest had purchased the property, with more than a tinge of irony and perhaps with an edge of triumph, Yellow Sulphur Springs had transitioned from a slaveowner proprietorship and as a postbellum retreat for Lost Cause apologists to a Black-owned vacation haven for descendants of enslaved persons.

Shannondale, Jordan White Sulphur Springs, Rock Enon

The northern Shenandoah Valley extends from Rockingham County, Virginia, to the Potomac River, about 140 miles away. It lies in the Valley and Ridge physiographic province of Southern Appalachia in what some commentators term as "the Great Valley of Virginia."[208] To the valley's east rise the ridges of the undulating Blue Ridge Mountains; the Allegheny Mountains border the valley on its west. Sprinkling the northern Shenandoah Valley and its surrounding mountains beginning in the eighteenth century were numerous health resorts, a few almost as prestigious as the Greenbrier White Sulphur Springs, about 200 miles to the south of Winchester. Winchester was a major market and transportation hub beginning in the early 1800s and witnessed many Civil War skirmishes and battles, thanks to its strategic location at the head of the northern Shenandoah Valley, thirty miles and eighty miles respectively from Harpers Ferry and Gettysburg to the northeast and eighty miles southeast of Washington, D.C.

The health resorts in the northern Shenandoah Valley and in the adjacent mountains included the prestigious Berkeley Springs (Bath), perhaps the earliest American spring resort, forty miles north of Winchester in West Virginia's Eastern Panhandle.[209] About twenty-two miles west of Winchester in West Virginia's Hardy County was the famed Capon Springs on the slope of the Great North Mountain, boasting at one time the South's largest resort hotel, erected in 1850.[210] Antebellum railroad ads and newspaper articles provided travelers in search of health or leisure detailed schedules of how to reach these two resorts as well as a dozen others in the vicinity such as Hardy White Sulphur Springs, Rockbridge Alum Springs, and Rawley Springs.[211]

Probably less well known in this region are three other resorts: West Virginia's Shannondale Springs of Jefferson County and Virginia's Jordan's White Sulphur Springs and Rock Enon of Frederick County. These resorts began in the late 1700s for those in search of better health to try their waters. Likely using the labor of enslaved persons, as was common at southern resorts, Shannondale and Jordan's provided antebellum elites, including national politicians, with the comfort and leisure they expected of the established, fashionable Virginia spring resorts.[212] Rock Enon, known as Capper's Springs in the antebellum period, catered to less prestigious guests. In the postbellum era, the three resorts served as recreative retreats for Washington, D.C.'s, middle- and upper-level civilian and military workforce and for the regional elite from such cities as Baltimore, Alexandria, and Fredericksburg. This chapter will explore their connected histories as well as their unique stories.

Jordan's White Sulphur Springs, about five miles north of Winchester, originally was a Catawba gathering place for rituals and drinking the waters.[213] Denied by the Catawbas to allow one of his guests to use the springs as had been customary, a local tavernkeeper appealed to a court in 1747, which resulted in the Native Americans abandoning use of the water.[214] Probably after 1790, local resident Rezin Duvall (Duval) purchased the spring tract, built a few cabins, and hired a Dr. Williams to serve as resident physician.[215] The watering hole then became largely known as Duval's or Duvall's (White) Sulphur Spring and less frequently as Williams' Sulphur Spring after Dr. Williams' brother Allan purchased the mineral spring from Duvall in the late 1820s or by 1831 at the latest.[216]

Allen and Leroy P. Williams, coproprietors, greatly improved the spring property.[217] They constructed additional rooms to accommodate a total of one hundred boarders and a large bath house that provided plunge or shower sulphur baths in either cold or warm water.[218] Although it is not known in the 1830s if they owned slaves (the 1850 census records show that they were wealthy farmers and slaveowners), they likely used either their own enslaved persons or hired slaves for outdoor labor on the "good slate land" and in the garden nearby.[219] In addition, they advertised that they had "procured attentive servants" in 1831 and two years later, assured potential guests that the "best servants ... have been provided," most probably referencing Black domestic slaves.[220]

In 1836 the Williamses sold the resort, by now known as Frederick White Sulphur Springs, to Branch Jordan, patriarch of a large clan that operated the mineral spring resort for the next 70 years.[221] Branch, a wealthy Frederick County farmer and slave trader, bought the spring tract based on his beneficial use of the water.[222] Branch employed Granville Jordan to serve as proprietor to manage his growing resort, which by 1837 included a 150-foot long, three-story brick colonnaded hotel with fifty guest rooms on the upper levels and a large dining room and ballroom on the first floor.[223] Brothers R.M. (Robert), G.N. (German) Jordan, and E.C. (Edwin) succeeded Granville as co-proprietors and unsuccessfully sought in 1859 to sell the resort, rebranded as "Jordan's White Sulphur Springs," under the moniker "R.M. Jordan & Bro.," probably because R.M., a physician, had relocated his medical office to Baltimore.[224]

By the time of the unsuccessful 1859 sale, visitors strolling on the ivy-covered brick house's "fine promenade" could admire the lawn "dotted with lambs," plantation fields with grazing cattle, and "the neat building of the slaves belonging to the establishment."[225] The enslaved persons most likely tilled the fields, served as domestic servants, and may have helped to construct several wood-frame cottages, a second hotel, and a springhouse encircled by massive Doric columns in place by 1855.[226] Oblivious to the fate of the enslaved persons, one antebellum writer observed that the property resembled "an excursion ... with Sir Walter Scott, in some fairy spot of his beloved Highlands."[227]

Contemporaneous with Jordan's as a mineral springs resort in the antebellum period was Shannondale Springs. Located in a horseshoe bend of the Shenandoah River, Shannondale Springs stood in the Blue Ridge foothills, about thirty miles northeast of Winchester. In 1814, Ferdinando Fairfax, a descendant of Thomas, Lord Fairfax, began to auction off his debt-laden properties, including a tract containing a sulphur spring, due to a failed iron ore extractive enterprise on his land and possibly other unsuccessful business ventures.[228] In 1820, after two property transactions, Shannondale opened with guest accommodations found in about a dozen wood-frame cottages and other crude buildings.[229] Ownership changed hands several times until the Shannondale Springs Corporation, whose shareholders included several slaveowners such as Samuel W. Lackland and slave trader William Crow, bought the property to "accommodate invalids and others who may resort."[230] The corporation unsuccessfully attempted to sell the resort in an 1847 downturn, hiring out slaves underutilized as hotel domestic servants, and failed to rent out the property in 1855, forcing the resort's temporary closure.[231] The hotel burned down in 1858 due to a chimney fire and was not rebuilt until after the Civil War.[232]

Shannondale, like Jordan's White Sulphur Springs in the antebellum era, consisted of a hotel, cottages, and outbuildings on manicured lawns. The two-story brick and frame hotel, with a porch fronting its 133-foot-long first floor, provided a view of the Shenandoah River and its tree-covered banks for promenading guests.[233] The hotel, together with several white-painted single-story cottages and other lodging houses behind it on a gentle slope, accommodated a modest 150 visitors.[234] Howe in the antebellum period called Shannondale's locale on the river with the Blue Ridge as a backdrop "beautiful and majestic"; two decades later, Moorman concurred that the site was "unsurpassed for its varied beauty."[235]

As also was the case with Jordan's, Shannondale relied on enslaved labor to maintain the property and to provide services to guests.[236] Visitors captured their observations of the Black enslaved persons at work, employing pejoratives common to the time. Dinner in general, according to one guest, was a "grand military movement of black [sic] waiters, and the elegant ladies and gentlemen are merely by-figures upon which the African army exercise their [sic] skill."[237] The bath attendant, a "negro [sic] man," curiously never known to sleep, was an "inoffensive obliging creature."[238] An observer in 1848 wrote that an "old colored woman seated near the Spring" dipped up water for tips.[239]

The latter two observations connect to the original attraction of Jordan's, Shannondale Springs, and Capper's Springs (as Rock Enon was first known): the therapeutic use of the water. A plantation owner's wife as testament to Shannondale's drawing power wrote in 1820 that "I would have liked to drink them for a whole week, but all the houses were full."[240] Jordan's sulphur water and Capper's primary spring, flowing out beneath a cliff over eighty feet high, were both alleged to treat liver "derangement," dyspepsia, and other afflictions.[241] Both Jordan's and Capper's waters were noted by prominent physicians: Jordan's by John Bell and Capper's by H.H. McGuire.[242]

Visitors to Jordan's, Shannondale, and Capper's Springs made the rounds of other springs in the region in search of health or social activities. Resort proprietors, newspapers, and railroads happily obliged to promote the springs circuit to increase profits. Proprietor Leroy Williams of Capper's advertised that Capon and Berkeley were each "one day's ride" from his resort.[243] A newspaper journalist in 1845 asked that the reader not be "satisfied with a visit merely to Shannondale: There are Jourdon's [sic] White Sulphur Springs ... within three hours' ride, by Stages and Cars, of the former."[244] A *Richmond Dispatch* article reprinted in other Virginia newspapers lauded the state's transportation system of railroad and turnpike for reaching Shannondale, Jordan's, and about two dozen other Virginia mineral spring resorts.[245] Discriminating visitors could then more efficiently tour the regional resorts and compare the waters: Shannondale's to that of Pennsylvania's Bedford Springs, Jordan's to the Greenbrier White Sulphur's, and Capper's to its neighbor, Capon Springs.[246]

Attracted to Shannondale Springs and Jordan's, probably less due to the springs than to their relatively close location to Washington, D.C., were national political elites (and presumably those who wished to burnish their images by socializing with the national politicians). President James Monroe and his family stayed at Shannondale in 1821; Monroe also considered Shannondale as a summer White House for his cabinet.[247] Shannondale additionally received Democrat President Martin Van Buren in 1843 and Whig President Millard Fillmore and Secretary of War Charles Magill Conrad in 1851.[248] Whig President John Tyler, Supreme Court Chief Justice Roger Taney, and Reverdy Johnson, Maryland Senator and Attorney General under Zachary Taylor, visited Jordan's for several years.[249] Other well-known antebellum guests at Shannondale included John C. Calhoun and William H. Crawford and Jacksonian Maine politician Edward Kavanagh and Massachusetts Whig Congressman William B. Calhoun at Jordan's.[250] Although neither resort appears to have advertised in the Lowcountry newspapers, both attracted guests outside the Virginia region who desired to socialize with the political elite or to tour the fashionable Virginia spring circuit; a brief 1843 newspaper article references Shannondale guests arriving from Louisiana, Mississippi, Georgia, and Florida.[251]

Antebellum guests at Jordan's and Shannondale Springs participated in activities similar to those of other regional springs resorts.[252] Jordan's sponsored a jockey club as did Fauquier White Sulphur Springs ten miles to the south.[253] Inspired by the popular novels of Sir Walter Scott, ring tournaments, replete with knights competing for the honor of crowning the "Queen of Love and Beauty," followed by a "Fancy Ball," were held at Fauquier, Capon, Berkeley, Jordan's, and at Shannondale, where at the latter Black servants dressed in livery and sounded the tournament bugle.[254] Band music, waltzes involving intimate "wreathing of arms and clasping of waists," outdoor excursions, and gentlemanly conversations over cordials (Jordan's advertised in 1831 "the best wine and liquors") composed other social activities.[255] Perhaps a Shannondale guest in 1841 best summed up visitors at these resorts as "all descriptions of persons, from the grave seeker of health ... to the gay, gossiping, sprightly belles and beaus, who go husband or wife-hunting."[256]

Less well documented, and by extrapolation less frequented by notables than either Jordan's or Shannondale in the antebellum era, was Rock Enon, located in a gorge of the western slope of the Great North Mountain, sixteen miles west of

Winchester and nine miles northeast of Capon Springs.[257] John Capper (1734–1808), a Frederick County resident, is credited with being the first white person to use the springs.[258] In 1828 the owner, Hardy County's Daniel Babb, in an advertisement to sell "Caper's Springs" (Capper's Springs) noted that the springs' "continuity to Winchester and the valley of Virginia would entitle them to rank (when improved) among the first watering places in this section of the country."[259] In 1856, after the springs tract had exchanged several hands, William F. Marker, a carpenter, bought the property for about $3,000 and built a two-story hotel with a 100-foot-long double porch across its full length for its inaugural season of 1857.[260] A regional newspaper in 1859 reported that Capper's and Jordan's were attracting "a fair company" although not as many visitors as Capon or Berkeley.[261] Capper's continued to prosper; for the following year, Marker had amassed real estate valued over $10,400 and personal estate at almost $1,300.[262]

During the Civil War, both the Shannondale's cottages spared from the 1858 hotel fire and the Capper's Springs hotel most likely closed.[263] Jordan's White Sulphur, however, served as a military hospital at various times for the Union and Confederate forces, but most notably for the Confederates after their casualties at Antietam, Gettysburg, and several losses at Winchester.[264] E.C. Jordan, Branch's nephew, operated the resort during and following the war; he invited Confederate troops to breakfast after Union Brigadier General Robert Milroy's defeat at the Second Battle of Winchester in mid–June 1863.[265] Several weeks later, during Lee's retreat into Virginia following Gettysburg, over 1,000 wounded soldiers arrived at Jordan's to be ministered to by the relatively large hospital staff of four ward masters and 26 nurses.[266]

Reestablishing Jordan's as a profitable resort proved challenging from 1865 to 1867. In June 1865, (Brevet) Major General Alfred Torbett, victor of the Third Battle of Winchester in fall 1864 under Major General Phillip Sheridan, moved his headquarters from Winchester to Jordan's where his soldiers planned picnics with the young Winchester ladies not averse to Union troops.[267] At the same time, E.C. planned to receive a limited number of acquaintances by July 1 as he had auctioned off furniture from both hotels, which along with the springs, had fallen into minor disrepair.[268] In 1866, E.C. at the request of R.M. (the legal resort owner) unsuccessfully tried to sell the resort, advertising that the still somewhat dilapidated property could be "ready for visitors within 30 days."[269] The following year, E.C. bought the resort from R.M. and began extensive renovations.[270]

Under E.C.'s and other family members' management, the resort regained its footing. The "accommodating, energetic and gentlemanly" E.C. and his "accomplished wife," enthused one newspaper, spared nothing to "provide for the comfort and pleasure of visitors," and as an unintended nod to antebellum ads, kept "the best servants and waiters that can be obtained."[271] The newspaper's characterization of E.C.'s nature appears accurate, for within two years, he built new cottages, a "new and commodious" bowling alley, a billiards saloon, and installed lights to illuminate the relandscaped grounds and walks.[272] Although the large brick hotel built by Branch Jordan burned down in winter 1876, E.C. kept the resort open for the season at reduced rates, likely due more to lingering effects from the Panic of 1873 than from the fire.²⁷³ Following E.C.'s death in 1889 from an unusual accident, blood poisoning from a pet squirrel's bite, his son, E.C. Jr., expanded the resort, building a new brick three-story, sixty-room hotel in 1894 with capacity for 250.²⁷⁴ In 1902, E.C. Jr., sold the property to his brother-in-law, Colonel Harry H. Baker, a member of Virginia Governor A.J. Montague's staff, after which the property left the family in 1911, falling into a period of gradual decline.²⁷⁵

Shannondale after the Civil War hosted church services on its grounds but lacked a hotel until after 1888 when Colonel J. Garland Hurst paid roughly $6,200 for the 189 acres, a pittance according to a local newspaper.²⁷⁶ Hurst and his partner, Eugene Baker, constructed new bathrooms and pavilions and provided fifty guest rooms through the new three-story hotel and cottages.²⁷⁷ In 1902, after Hurst and Baker defaulted on their loan for the property, H.C. Getzendanner bought Shannondale at a public auction.²⁷⁸ A November 1909 fire left the hotel in disuse although the cottages were used for the next thirty years until they became unsound.²⁷⁹

Capper's Springs languished after the Civil War until a Washington, D.C.–based company purchased the property for $11,100 at a trustee sale in 1869.²⁸⁰ The company branded itself as the Rock Enon Springs Company after its incorporation two years later and consequently also changed the name of the resort. In addition to the Biblical connotation, the resort advertised "no bar" for the next several decades.²⁸¹ In 1875, A.S. (Adam) Pratt, one of the original stockholders, bought the resort at almost the same price that the stock company had paid.²⁸²

Pratt oversaw the resort in its prime years. In response to its growing popularity, he added a three-story ell of thirty rooms and an enlarged parlor to the hotel, expanded the promenade to run the entire building length of 800 feet, and improved bathing facilities.²⁸³ A jet fountain, outdoor dancing pavilion, croquet lawn, and cottages with names such as Pavilion and Maple graced the grounds.²⁸⁴ The hotel now accommodated 300 guests compared to Jordan's 250; Shannondale did well to see forty to fifty guests at this time.²⁸⁵ Although Rock Enon was considered a "favorite of Washingtonians" in 1896, the resort was sold, for reasons unclear, by a decree of court in 1899.²⁸⁶

The three resorts in this period, from the late 1860s through the early 1900s, attracted mainly Washingtonians and other regional visitors in search of relief from summer heat and in search of an escape from business and political concerns. Rock Enon's stock owners sought those who wished to "secure a healthful, quiet and attractive retreat, free from the trammels of fashion and from temptations to vice and dissipation" and published ads calling for "those seeking health, pleasure or a quiet retreat from the cares of business and the scorching heat of Summer."²⁸⁷ Jordan's White Sulphur, according to an attendee at the Association of Maryland Editors that met there in 1869, was "not a resort of the sporting fraternity or the votaries of fashion, but a quiet, healthful place, all the more inviting for the absence of such visitors."²⁸⁸ Shannondale Springs also appealed to those wishing for a tranquil atmosphere in a mountain setting: hosting family camping and Sunday School picnics on its grounds, providing bass fishing and boating in the peaceful Shenandoah River, and offering general "rusticating."²⁸⁹

The Washingtonians fleeing to the resorts in a "regular stampede" during federal governmental summer recesses included an array of military officers, judges, civil service bureaucrats, businessmen, appointed officials, and other professionals or their families and occasionally children's nurses.[290] A few of the innumerable examples of the regional visitors follow. Rock Enon in August 1878 welcomed the chaplain for the U.S. House of Representatives and a military colonel and his family from the District.[291] A Washington, D.C., newspaper article in 1887 listed a general, colonel, and captain among other guests at Jordan's and an admiral and several physician families with others at Rock Enon.[292] In summer 1890, regional newspapers reported that Rock Enon's list of visitors included professors, physicians, civil service employees, and military officers from the District and that Shannondale Springs welcomed in early September two Washington judges.[293]

Well-known personages accounted for a few of the postbellum visitors at the three resorts. Former Confederate General Joseph E. Johnston, making a tour of mineral spring resorts, left Bedford Springs to stay at Jordan's in 1883.[294] Shannondale welcomed West Virginia Congressman Thomas B. Davis.[295] Rock Enon received John Philip Sousa recovering from an illness and acclaimed Hudson River Valley artist Eliza Pratt Greatorex, sister to proprietor A.S. Pratt.[296] U.S. Attorney General Augustus Hill Garland in 1885 purportedly declared that Rock Enon's water "was beneficial to me beyond anything I ever used … wonderful in its action on the liver and kidneys."[297]

Garland's comment demonstrates the staying power of the waters of the three resorts. Although the three mineral spring resorts provided the typical resort amusements such as swimming, croquet, and bowling, and Rock Enon and Shannondale

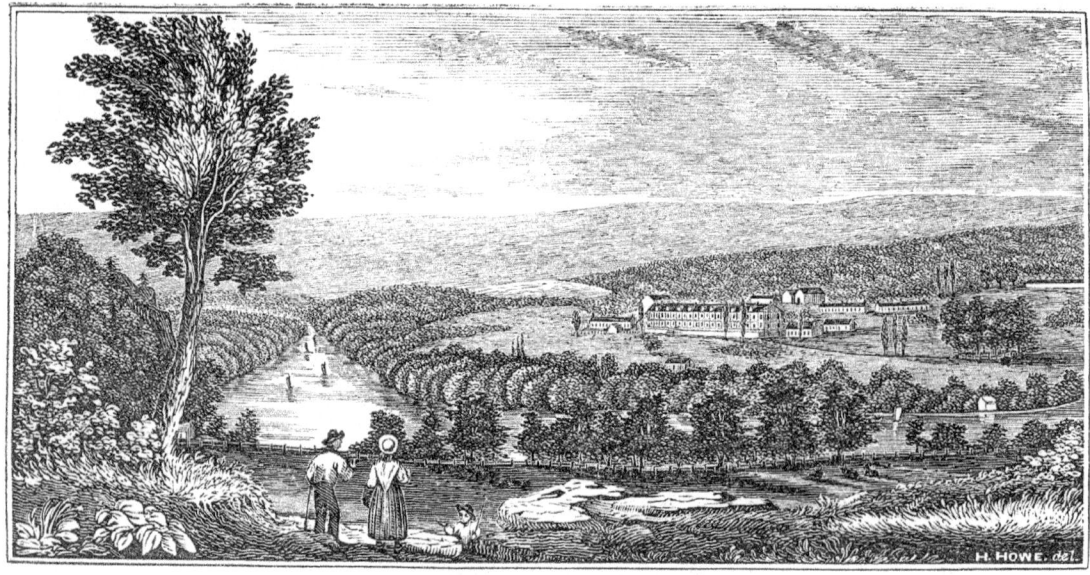

"The Shannondale Springs," Jefferson County, West Virginia. Henry Howe, *Historical Collections of Virginia* (Charleston, SC: Babcock & Co., 1847), unnumbered page following page 34 (image from the American Antiquarian Society, Worcester, MA).

hosted tournaments, the resorts continually highlighted their mineral waters' attributes, also endorsed by medical professionals.[298] Jordan's in 1874 touted a newly discovered chalybeate spring as a "success" just as its white sulphur water had "proved of much value to invalids."[299] In 1891, Shannondale Springs publicized in large boldface its "3 Fine Mineral Springs" ("Saline Chalybeate and Red and Blue Sulphur").[300] As if to substantiate the two health resorts' claims, an American Medical Association committee included both waters in its report of recognized American mineral waters.[301] Rock Enon advertised in 1889 its "strengthening, healing waters" and its mineral baths 16 years later.[302] In the interim, physician James K. Crook recommended Rock Enon's water in his authoritative 1899 mineral spring treatise for "rheumatism, diseases of the skin, and certain of the intestinal worms."[303]

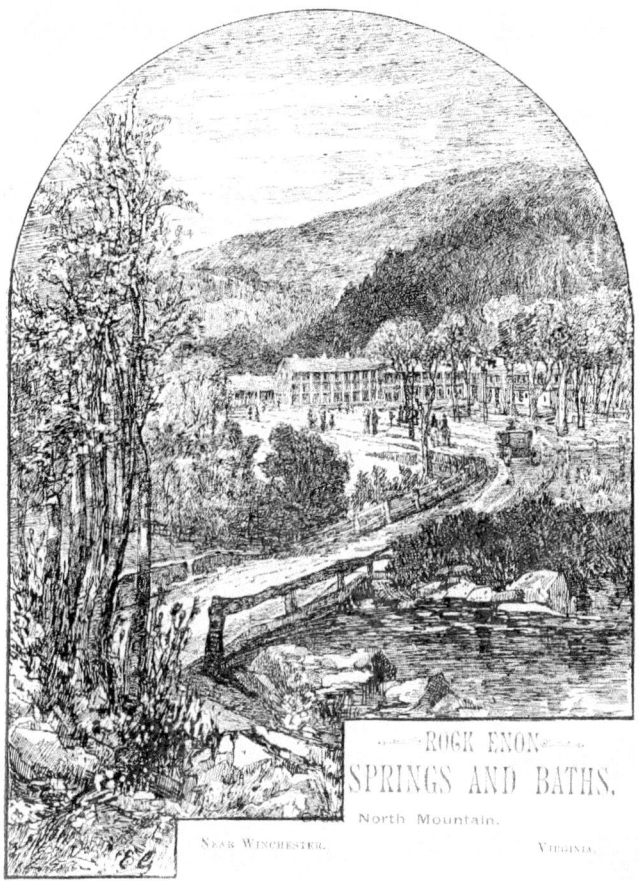

Rock Enon, Frederick County, Virginia. *The Rock Enon Springs and Baths* (Washington, D.C.: 1883), drawing located between pages 2 and 3 (Library of Congress, *https://www.loc.gov/item/tmp92001735/*).

Guests less prominent than Garland found their well-being enhanced by taking the waters. A Maryland insurance company executive officer, after making the rounds of Berkeley and Jordan's in 1890, reported his health much improved.[304] Visiting Shannondale the same year was a Virginia lady who came as "almost a helpless invalid" but returned home after three weeks, able to dispense with a servant and do her own housework.[305] The demand for the resorts' mineral water was so great that Jordan's and Shannondale sold their water at druggists or by shipments during the late 1800s, Shannondale continuing to sell, perhaps sporadically, as late as 1931.[306]

After the demise of the resorts in the early 1900s, the properties found new uses. Jordan's served briefly as an academy instructing students from Iron Curtain countries in precepts of anti–Communism followed by turns as a Catholic seminary / monastery and as a drug rehabilitation center.[307] Today, the property is known as Historic Jordan Springs, an event center and the headquarters for several private companies.³⁰⁸ The last owner of Rock Enon sold the property to the Shenandoah Area Council of the Boy Scouts of America. The council salvaged materials from what remained of the old hotel and now oversees the grounds as part of Camp Rock Enon.³⁰⁹ Shannondale Springs now lies within a West Virginia Wildlife Management Area of the same name, continuing the tradition of fishing and other outdoor activities associated with the former watering hole.³¹⁰

Chapter Notes

General Introduction

1. Fanslow, "Resorts of Southern Appalachia."
2. Campbell, *Southern Highlander and His Homeland*, 10–12. For an online map of Campbell's Southern Appalachia in comparison with other definitions of Southern Appalachia, see University of South Carolina, College of Arts and Sciences, "Where is Appalachia?" https://artsandsciences.sc.edu/appalachianenglish/node/783.
3. Sears, *Sacred Places*, 10, 222n11.
4. Nineteenth-century authorities either omitted Maryland or provided short entries for only five resorts for the entire state. See Crook, *Mineral Waters of the United States*, 269, 270–71.
5. Stoll, 22. Isolation continues to be discussed in ARC-related reports. A 2016 report, for example, authored by The University of Tennessee, Knoxville (UTK) for the ARC states that "the long-term concern for Appalachia must be one of becoming more isolated and disconnected from domestic and global markets and opportunities—essentially becoming an economic island unto itself." See UTK, "Access vs. Isolation: Preserving Appalachia's Rail Connectivity in the Twenty-First Century, Part One (Jan. 2016), 4, https://www.arc.gov/wp-content/uploads/2017/03/RailAccessinAppalachiaPartOneFinal.pdf.
6. "Dumb Hillbillies? Media Portrayal in the Age of Trump" (PhD diss., Georgia State University, 2023), 6, https://doi.org/10.57709/34765631. Following are two other recent publications demonstrating the persistence of the myth of isolationism. Stokes and Atkins-Sayre explore Southern Appalachian cuisine, noting the lingering stereotype of insularity in a seemingly backwards and isolated region. Wykoff enumerates eight myths of Appalachia, including isolationism, and posits a ninth myth, disinterest in healthcare. See Ashli Q. Stokes and Wendy Atkins-Sayre, "Lost But Not Found," Dublin Gastronomy Symposium, Session 11 (2024): 1–2, https://doi.org/10.21427/9nw9-9h77; Randall Wykoff, "The Ninth Myth of Appalachia," *Journal of Appalachian Health* 5 no. 2 (2023):1–4, https://doi.org/10.13023/jah.0502.01.
7. Batteau, *Invention of Appalachia*, 40; Hsiung, *Two Worlds in the Tennessee Mountains*, 162–63; Shapiro, *Appalachia on Our Mind*, 69–70. Murfree's color stemmed in part from her family's sojourns at Tennessee's Beersheba Springs and her travels to Montvale Springs. See Durwood Dunn, "Mary Noailles Murfree: A Reappraisal," *Appalachian Journal* 6, no. 3 (1979): 196–204, JSTOR; Allison Ensor, "Mary Noailles Murfree ("Charles Egbert Craddock")," *Tennessee Encyclopedia* (Nashville: Tennessee Historical Society; Knoxville: University of Tennessee Press, updated 1 Mar. 2018), http://tennesseeencyclopedia.net/entries/mary-noailles-murfree/.
8. *American Journal of Sociology*, 4 (July 1898), 1, https://www.journals.uchicago.edu/doi/pdf/10.1086/2107671.
9. Batteau, 40.
10. Shapiro, 63.
11. "Our Contemporary Ancestors in the Southern Mountains," *Atlantic Monthly* 83 (Mar. 1899): 311, 319.
12. *Ibid.*, 311; Batteau, 74.
13. Fickey and Samers, "Developing Appalachia," in *Studying Appalachian Studies*, 125.
14. Stoll, *Ramp Hollow*, 6–7.
15. Appalachian Studies scholars have explored economic development in the region since the field began in the 1970s. Dunaway's analysis has been widely used since its 1996 publication that stemmed from her 1994 dissertation. See, for example, Elizabeth Avery Moore, "The Vanishing Frontier: Economic and Social Change in Western North Carolina, 1945–1970" (PhD diss, West Virginia University, 2022), 28–29, https://researchrepository.wvu.edu/etd/11295.
16. *First American Frontier*, 305.
17. *Ibid.*, 307.
18. Williams, *Appalachia*, 133. Williams notes that Ulrich B. Phillips considered the White Sulphur Springs as the summer capital of the Old South because of the number of pro-secessionists and slave-holding planters who congregated there.
19. Hilliard, *Hog Meat and Hoe Cake*, 192–94. Page references are to the 2014 ed.
20. *Two Worlds in the Tennessee Mountains*, 10.
21. Dunaway, *Slavery in the American Mountain South*, 2–3, 70, 150–51.
22. Purcell, "'A Damned Piece of Rascality,'" 5, 10, 13.

23. Savitt, *Medicine and Slavery*, 152.
24. Works Projects Administration for the State of Tennessee, *Tennessee*, 363; *Montvale Springs*, 14, 20–21, "Montvale Springs, Blount County, An Analysis of the Springs 1867."
25. "Northeast Tennessee" began to replace "upper East Tennessee" in the media in the late 1970s to drive a regional identity to promote tourism and industry. "Upper East Tennessee" had been in use since the 1840s. See John Morgan and Leonard W. Brinkman, "The Renaming of a Tennessee Region," *Geographical Bulletin* 37, no. 1 (1995): 49.
26. "Catoosa Springs," *Georgia Citizen* (Macon), 2 Aug 1851; Genovese, *Sweetness of Life*, 203.
27. "Correspondence of the Enterprise," *Southern Enterprise* (Greenville, SC), 26 June 1856.
28. "Cherokee Georgia and Its Resources," *Rome Tri-Weekly Courier* (GA), 10 Feb. 1866.
29. Wilson, *Baptized in Blood*, x.
30. *Journal and Tribune* (Knoxville), 3 Aug. 1898; *Evening Bulletin* (Maysville, KY), 15 July 1898. Sources consulted do not connect the two waiter strikes.
31. Hsiung, 18.
32. Fletcher, *Ashe County*, 94–95.

Alabama

Introduction

1. King, *Great South*, 339.
2. Mike Neilson, "Physiographic Sections of Alabama" in *Encyclopedia of Alabama*, updated July 12, 2023, https://encyclopediaofalabama.org/article/physiographic-sections-of-alabama/, Numerous classifications characterize the terrain of Alabama. I chose to rely on Nelson and intersperse among its classifications place names found in other geological and geographical descriptions. See, for example, the USGS topo quadrangles found at data.us.fs.usda.gov; Eugene Allen Smith, prepared in co-operation with the U.S. Geological Survey, *Underground Water Resources of Alabama* (Montgomery: Brown Printing Co., 1907), 4–10.
3. De Land and Smith, *Northern Alabama*, 13–17.
4. Riley, *Alabama As It Is*, 44–50, 84, 99, 102. Riley divides the state into four "grand divisions": Timber, Cotton (Black), Mineral, and Cereal Belts. Southern Appalachian counties fall into the Cereal and Mineral Belts.
5. Tuomey, *First Biennial Report*, 63.
6. Smith, *Underground Water Resources*, 67.
7. Nuermberger, *Clays of Alabama*, 84, 111–12, 129, 185; Clay-Clopton, *Belle of the Fifties*, 153.
8. Gaines, *Reminiscences*, 112–13. Gaines was a member of the prominent Gaines and Pendleton families of Virginia, of which one branch owned the historic Exchange Place in Kingsport, TN, and Holston Springs in Scott County, VA.
9. "Alonzo E. Skaggs," *Our Mountain Home* (Talladega, AL), 16 July 1879.

10. Horsman, *Josiah Nott*, 229, 259–60, 266. Nott permitted the Battle House to use his name as endorsement that the area had been immune to the 1853 yellow fever epidemic.
11. Bassett, "On the Climate and Diseases," 317n [editor's note]; Bassett, "Report on the Topography," 263. See "Report" for "all that is essential" quote.
12. Webb, "The Livingston Artesian Well Water," 322–23, 326, 328.
13. Partin, "Alabama's Yellow Fever Epidemic," 35–36. I examined all *Transactions* available from the Library of Congress on microfilm; the gaps of several years, notably 1850–1868, necessitate that my conclusions are not definitive but rather suggest *Association* meeting themes.
14. Bassett, "Report on the Topography," 262.
15. Michel, "Haemorrhagic Malarial Fever," 35–40.
16. Mabry, "Miasmatic Fevers," 124; Donald, Reese, and Furness, "Report on Medical Topography," 95; McDaniel, "Report on Topography," 104.
17. Johnston, "The Antipyretic Treatment of Fevers," 235–36; Mattheson, "Treatment of Relapses of Malarial Fevers," 128; Brockway, "Hemorrhagic Malarial Fever," 372; Dixon, "Epidemic of Jaundice in Talladega," 443; Fahs, "Report on Medicinal Properties of the Sulphites," 121.
18. Michel, 35–53 (quote, p. 53).
19. Kumpe and Abernathy, "Report on Climatology and Diseases," 71–82.
20. Oakes and Sumner, *Angels of Mercy*, 24; *Home Journal* (Winchester, TN), 23 Feb. 1867.
21. Inzer, *Diary*, 143, 151–52.
22. Resources of Alabama (from the *Montgomery Advertiser*) [letter by Gov. Patton, 5 July 1867, Montgomery, AL]," *Union Springs Herald* (AL), 24 July 1867.
23. "Alabama," *Times-Picayune* (New Orleans), 21 July 1865.

Blount Springs

24. Brewster, *Alabama*, 138.
25. Powell, "Description and History of Blount County," 99, 101.
26. *Ibid.*, 131.
27. Burden, *Blount Springs*, 3–5. Burden's book provides rich detail on the resort's history.
28. Nuermberger, 70.
29. Burden, 12; Brewster, *Alabama*, 138; Sulzby, *Historic Alabama Hotels*, 59–60.
30. Mitchell, *Accompaniment to Mitchell's Reference and Distance*, 281.
31. *Appletons'* (1857), 289; Disturnell, *Springs, Water-Falls*, 150. Later *Appletons'* editions used similar phraseology.
32. Sulzby, 60; Hanes, *State of Alabama*, 114.
33. "Blount Springs, [ALA.]," *Southern Argus* (Columbus, MS), 27 July 1841.
34. *Ibid.*
35. "Blount Springs [ad]," *Southern Argus* (Columbus, MS), 2 Aug. 1842.

36. Letter from B. Smith in Blount Springs, AL, to R.G. Hazard, Peace Dale, RI, 15 Aug. 1844.
37. Gayle, *Journal of Sarah Haynsworth Gayle*, 110, 252; Wiggins, "Sarah Ann Haynsworth Gayle."
38. "A Poet Plunderer: Mary Gordon Duffee's Theft from the Confederate Government," *Indianapolis Journal*, 1 July 1889.
39. *Ibid.*; Sulzby, 61.
40. Burden, 53; Jonathan M. Atkins, "John Bell," in *Tennessee Encyclopedia* (Nashville: Tennessee Historical Society; Knoxville: University of Tennessee Press, last updated Mar. 1, 2018), http://tennesseeencyclopedia.net/entries/john-bell.
41. "Hon. John Bell," *Memphis Daily Appeal*, 9 July 1862.
42. "A Poet Plunderer."
43. Sulzby, 61–62; *Birmingham Iron Age*, 10 July 1878.
44. Sulzby, 64; *Cullman Southern Immigrant* (AL), 15 Aug. 1878; "Local News in Alabama," 49.
45. *Birmingham Iron Age*, 10 July 1878.
46. Gatewood, *Aristocrats of Color*, 87.
47. Palmer, "Alabama Notes," 246–247, 249–250.
48. Powell, "Description and History of Blount County," 131–32.
49. "Excursion South," *Fort Wayne Gazette* (IN), 25 June 1873.
50. *Commonwealth* (Greenwood, MS), 18 Aug. 1899.
51. "Gov. Johnston Foils the Lynchers," *Semi-Weekly Times-Democrat* (New Orleans), 28 July 1899.
52. *Minneapolis Tribune*, 17 July 1877.
53. *Brazil Register* (IN), 23 Oct. 1882.
54. Sulzby, 62.
55. "Latest from Savannah: What An Atlanta Man Saw and Heard There About Yellow Fever," *Atlanta Constitution*, 6 Sept. 1876.
56. Sulzby, 62.
57. "Its Backbone Broken: The Fever, It is Hoped, Will Soon Be Exterminated in New Orleans," *Sunday Tribune* (Minneapolis), 7 Nov. 1897.
58. Sulzby, 68; "Blount Springs Peaceful Setting for Residential Growth," *Athens News Courier* (AL), 5 Mar. 2006.
59. "Swept by Fire: Two Hotels and Several Stores at Summer Resort are Destroyed," *Columbia Herald* (TN), 11 June 1915; "Hotels and Cottages Burn at Blount Springs," *Cullman Times Democrat* (AL), 10 June 1915.
60. Burden, 193; *Cullman Times Democrat* (AL), 3 July 1924; "Cullman People at Blount Springs," *Ibid.*, 25 July 1925; "Mel Drennen," Bhamwiki, https://www.bhamwiki.com/w/Mel_Drennen; "Walter Melville Drennen," "Alabama Deaths, 1908-1974," www.familysearch.org; Arthur J. Ellis, "Mineral Waters," in Smith, *Statistics*, 89.
61. Fitch, *Mineral Waters of the United States and American Spas*, 204–05.
62. "Blount Springs Peaceful Setting for Residential Growth"; "Blount Springs," https://www.blountsprings.com/history; Burden, 198.

DeKalb County:
Mentone, Alabama
White Sulphur Springs

63. Riley, 30. The handbooks of the mineral spring authorities of the nineteenth and early twentieth century—Bell (1855), Moorman (1873), Walton (1874), Peale (1886), Crook (1899), Fitch (1927)—list no resort for Jackson County. Michael Tuomey, the state geologist, also lacks information on any health resort in Jackson County. See M. Tuomey, *First Biennial Report of the Geology of Alabama* (Tuskaloosa: M.D.J. Slade, Printer, 1850).
64. Sprague, "Alabama," 85–86; Berney, *Hand-Book of Alabama*, 372–74; "Fort Payne: The Boston Excursion on Hand and a Royal Reception," *Montgomery Advertiser*, 26 Jan. 1890; "Fort Payne, Ala.: Its Manufacturing Industries," *Iron Age* (June 5, 1890): 943; "The Booming South," *Lenoir Topic* (NC), 18 Sept. 1889; "Notice of Sale," *Fort Payne Journal* (AL), 10 Jan. 1894.
65. For a history of the railroad names in Wills Valley, see "Alabama & Chattanooga Railroad," https://www.bhamwiki.com.
66. "Lookout Mountain, Mentone Mineral Springs Hotel [ad]," *Sunny South* (Atlanta), 4 July 1891.
67. Sulzby, 176; Strayhorn, "Mentone."
68. Sulzby, 176.
69. *Dublin University Calendar*, 442, 690; "'Mrs. John E. Purdon,' *Cullman Democrat*, 9 May 1907, v.6 no. 3," in Sterling, *Newspaper Clippings*, 89.
70. Purdon, "Correspondence," 1049–52.
71. "Mystery of the Sphygmograph," 407. The sphygmograph was placed on the wrist to record on paper any changes in the pulse frequency when the wearer was communicating with spirits.
72. *Chattooga News* (GA), 23 Oct. 1895; "Cloudland," *Summerville News* (GA), 4 Aug. 1897. Planning begun in 1895 called for an additional 100 rooms that by 1897 had been scaled back to 30 rooms.
73. U.S. Dept. of the Interior, NPS, National Register of Historic Places, "Mentone Springs Hotel."
74. "Mentone Mineral Springs Hotel [ad]," *Montgomery Advertiser*, 30 April 1893; *Summerville News* (GA), 30 Mar. 1905.
75. "Mentone Popular Resort in Summer," *Birmingham News*, 9 July 1923; "In Alabama's Land of the Sky," *Ibid.*, 20 Sept. 1925.
76. See, for example, *Ft. Payne Journal*, 7 Mar. 1894; *Ibid.*, 16 May 1894; *Cullman* [AL] *Times Democrat*, 7 Aug. 1919; "Mentone Springs Visitors," *Anniston Star*, 6 July 1919; *Chattanooga News*, 1 Sept. 1919.
77. King, *Where to Stop*, 165; *Montgomery Advertiser*, 30 Apr. 1893.
78. Sulzby, 177; Strayhorn, "Mentone."
79. "Baptists Purchase Site at Mentone for Encampments," *Anniston Star*, 17 Mar. 1921; "Baptists Have Secured Menton [sic] for Assemblies," *Anniston Star*, 9 July 1921; Strayhorn, "Mentone."

80. National Register of Historic Places, "Mentone Springs Hotel."
81. *Ibid.*
82. "A Tribute to the Grand Old Lady." The entire newsletter is devoted to the hotel.
83. *North Georgia Citizen* (Dalton), 31 May 1877; Sulzby, 5; *Official Guide of the Railways*, "Queen and Crescent Route," 689.
84. *Montgomery Daily Advertiser*, 10 May 1876.
85. Sulzby, 5.
86. *Ibid.*; *Daily Times* (Chattanooga), 2 Aug. 1873.
87. Sulzby, 5.
88. *Montgomery Daily Advertiser*, 10 May 1876; "Hanna Mineral Springs [ad]," *Atlanta Constitution*, 7 June 1878; *Vicksburg Herald*, "Alabama White Sulphur Springs. Formerly Hanna Springs," *Tuscaloosa Weekly Times*, 26 May 1880.
89. "A Popular Summer Resort," *Chattanooga Daily Times*, 21 Feb. 1880; "Alabama White Sulphur Springs. Formerly Hanna Springs."
90. "Alabama White Sulphur Springs. Formerly Hanna Springs."
91. "Hanna Mineral Springs [ad]," *Atlanta Constitution*, 7 June 1878.
92. "Ala. White Sulphur Springs Hotel [ad]," *Anniston Star*, 12 July 1922.
93. "About Hanna Springs," *Montgomery Advertiser*, 31 Aug. 1877.
94. "Summer Resorts: Hotel Lamine," *Tuscaloosa News*, 7 July 1906.
95. *Montgomery Advertiser*, 1 Aug. 1877; *Chattanooga News*, 9 July 1919; *Times* (Richmond, VA), 28 July 1901.
96. "Alabama White Sulphur Springs [ad]," *Clarion-Ledger* (Jackson, MS), 30 June 1880.
97. Hall, *Cincinnati Southern Railway*, 188.
98. Sulzby, 6. Several newspaper society sections and ads refer to the resort as (Alabama) White Sulphur Springs after 1901. See, for example, *Chattanooga News*, 29 July 1919; "Ala. White Sulphur Springs Hotel [ad]," *Anniston Star*, 19 July 1922.
99. Fitch, 202–03.
100. Sulzby, 6. Newspaper society and community news show that girls attended the YWCA camp, Camp Elizabeth Lupton, past 1948. For additional information on Lupton's business and philanthropic ventures, see Ned L. Irwin, "John Thomas Lupton," in *Tennessee Encyclopedia* (Nashville: Tennessee Historical Society; Knoxville: University of Tennessee Press, last updated Mar. 1, 2018), http://tennesseeencyclopedia.net/entries/john-thomas-lupton/.
101. Sulzby, 7; "Auction Sale [ad]," *Fort Payne Journal*, 5 Mar. 1956. No source consulted provides information on the auction outcome.
102. Landmarks of DeKalb County, "DeKalb Communities: Sulphur Springs."

Monte Sano

103. Taylor, "Early History of Madison County," 149, 167–68.
104. Brewster, *Alabama*, 346–47; U.S. Census Bureau, *Population…1860: Alabama*, 5; USDA, "Census…, 1860."
105. De Land and Smith, 243.
106. "Robert Fearn (1795)," HCC; Thomas Fearn," *Ibid.*; "George Fearn," *Ibid.*; Hill, "History of the Development," 65. One writer notes that Thomas and George established Viduta and that Thomas may have christened the mountain as "Monte Sano" (Mountain of Health) after taking a sick child to the mountain for several days where the child recovered. See Lynn Murray, "Dr. Thomas Fearn: Pioneer Builder of Huntsville," *Huntsville Historical Review* 1 (Jan. 1971): 6, 8, HCC.
107. Nuermberger, 84, 167; Clay-Copton, 157.
108. "Robert Fearn (1795)"; "Dr. Thomas Fearn"; "George Fearn."
109. "No. 176, An Act To Regulate Tolls on the Monte Sano Turnpike Company," in *Acts of the Seventh Biennial Session*, 196.
110. Fleming, *Civil War and Reconstruction*, 62; Clay-Copton, 183.
111. Roberts, "Romance and Realism of Monte Sano," 4–5; Nuermberger, 84.
112. Roberts, 5.
113. Sulzby, 181; "Huntsville—Receives the First and Second North Alabama New Bales of Cotton, which bring Good Prices—Crops Looking Well —- the Agricultural Fair, Etc.," *Memphis Daily Appeal*, 2 Sept. 1879; Johnson, "Epidemic Cholera at Huntsville, 1873," 21–22.
114. Sulzby, 181–82; Roberts, 5–6; Hill, 68.
115. "Huntsville, Alabama: As Viewed by a Terre Haute Lady," *Terre Haute Saturday Evening Mail*, 5 Mar. 1887.
116. P.K.M., "Editorial Correspondence: Monte Sano Hotel," *Pascagoula Democrat-Star* (MS), 23 Sept. 1887. The number of rooms varies as so often is the case among accounts of old resorts. Sulzby and Hill give the number as 233; Roberts, as 200. See Sulzby, 182; Roberts, 6; Hill, 68.
117. Sulzby, 184.
118. *Atlanta Constitution*, 6 July 1890.
119. "Editorial Correspondence," *Pascagoula Democrat-Star* (MS), 23 Sept. 1887; "At Monte Sano: The Season is in Full Blast, and Everything Seems Delightful," *Atlanta Constitution*, 27 July 1890.
120. Sulzby, 183; Hill, 70.
121. Sulzby, 182–83; Roberts, 6; "At Monte Sano: The Season is in Full Blast"; "Editorial Correspondence," *Pascagoula Democrat-Star* (MS), 23 Sept. 1887.
122. "A Big Deal: A Six Million Dollar Real Estate Transfer in Which Cedar Rapids Parties are interested—The Details of the Transaction," *Cedar Rapids Evening Gazette* (IA), 21 Jan. 1892. The headline gives the property sale at $6M; the lead paragraph values the "largest deal ever consummated in the south" at $5M.
123. Hill, 70–71.
124. Sulzby, 185; Roberts, 7.
125. *Hattiesburg News* (MS), 1 April 1909.

126. Sulzby, 184–85; Roberts, 9; Luttrell, "Society Wins Award," 28; Thomas V. Ress, "Monte Sano State Park," in *Encyclopedia of Alabama*, updated July 25, 2023, http://www.encyclopediaofalabama.org/article/h-2903.

Talladega County: Chandler Springs, Talladega Springs, and Shocco Springs

127. Mike Neilson, "Physiographic Sections of Alabama," updated July 12, 2023, https://encyclopediaofalabama.org/article/physiographic-sections-of-alabama/; Donna J. Siebenthaler, "Talladega County," updated May 30, 2023, https://encyclopediaofalabama.org/article/talladega-county/; Mike Neilson, "Tennessee Valley and Ridge Physiographic Section, *Ibid.*, updated July 12, 2023, https://encyclopediaofalabama.org/article/tennessee-valley-and-ridge-physiographic-section/.

128. George Garner, "Gold Production in Alabama," *Ibid.*, updated July 26, 2023, https://encyclopediaofalabama.org/article/gold-production-in-alabama/; Adams, "A Century of Gold Mining in Alabama," 272; Young, "The Southern Gold Rush," 389. The year and place of discovery of gold in Alabama is unclear. Garner states that gold was discovered in 1836 in Chilton County. Adams comments that gold was discovered most likely in Alabama in 1830, a year after its discovery in Georgia, hence the occasion for his paper on the centennial.

129. Brewster, *Alabama*, 534; Riley, 73.

130. McKinney, "Vernon Courier, Lamar County"; McKinney, "Gold."

131. Dean, "Alabama Gold," 28.

132. T. Logan, "Talladega. Alabama's Beautiful 'Bride of the Mountains' and Her Resources," *Atlanta Constitution*, 8 May 1887.

133. Armes, *Story of Coal and Iron*, 82–83.

134. U.S. Population Census 1850, FamilySearch, www.familysearch.org/; "James Chandler and Catharine Perry, 17 May 1832," in *Georgia, County Marriages, 1785-1950*, FamilySearch, https://www.familysearch.org/ark:/61903/1:1:-KXJB-PHC; Hahn, "Creeks in Alabama"; Sulzby, 93–94; Eureka, "Chandler's Springs," *Our Mountain Home* (Talladega), 3 Mar. 1886; Crook, *Mineral Waters of the United States*, 87. Both Crook and the 1886 *Our Mountain Home* article state that Chandler settled at the springs and / or opened the resort in 1838. Sulzby states that Chandler settled at the springs in 1832 and that a post office, Mountain Spring, opened in 1838.

135. Sulzby, 94; Crook, *Mineral Waters of the United States*, 87.

136. *Independent Monitor* (Tuscaloosa), 12 Jan. 1842.

137. Rambler, "The Minerals of Talladega County," *Alabama State Sentinel* (Selma), 15 Oct. 1853.

138. "Chandler's Springs." Perhaps the "impure state of blood" refers to iron-deficiency anemia.

139. L.P.C.M., "Chandler Springs Correspondence," *Tuskegee Republican*, 7 Oct. 1858.

140. Sulzby, 229–30.

141. *Ibid.*, 231.

142. *Ibid.*

143. *Ibid.*

144. "Talladega Sulphur Springs [ad]," *Weekly Advertiser* (Montgomery), 2 June 1852.

145. Bell, *Mineral and Thermal Springs*, 295–96.

146. Isaac M. Thomas, "Talladega Springs, Talladega Co., [testimonial for Dr. Spencer's Vegetable Pills]," *Mississippi Free Trader* (Natchez), 27 July 1844.

147. Sellers, "1852 and 1859 Alabama Tax Assessment Records, 7. The planter survived the trip but died in the next two years.

148. Stockdale, "The Early Days," 407–09.

149. "Public Attention," *State Guard* (Wetumpka, AL), 5 Sept. 1848.

150. Curry, "Reminiscences of Talladega," 368; "More Withdrawals from the Order in Alabama," *Wilmington Journal* (NC), 3 Aug. 1855. The Know-Nothing Party in Alabama was a complicated mix of ideologies. By fall 1855, the state Democratic Party's platform rhetoric, denouncing the national Know-Nothings as promoting free-soilism, abolitionism, and state aid, had begun to catalyze a precipitous drop in Alabama American Party membership. For more discussion, see Jeff Frederick, "Unintended Consequences: The Rise and Fall of the Know-Nothing Party in Alabama." *Alabama Review* 55 (Jan. 2002): 3–33.

151. Vandiver, "Pioneer Talladega," 163.

152. *Ibid.*, 164.

153. *Democratic Watchtower* (Talladega), 17 June 1863.

154. Vandiver, 166.

155. Barclay, "Reminiscences of Rousseau's Raid," 7.

156. "Shocco Springs Conference Center: Who We Are," www.shocco.org/who-we-are/.

157. McMillan, "The Name of Shocco Springs," 12.

158. Busey and Busey, *Confederate Casualties*, 109; "Shocco Springs [ad]," *Montgomery Advertiser*, 12 July 1878.

159. "Shocco Springs Conference Center: Who We Are." The website in 2017 stated that the resort was a "well-known health spa by 1874."

160. T.M.R., "Shocco Springs," *Montgomery Advertiser*, 10 July 1878.

161. *Ibid.*

162. "Shocco Springs!," *Our Mountain Home* (Talladega), 5 Aug. 1885; "Shocco Springs," *Ibid.*, 5 June 1895.

163. T.M.R., "Shocco Springs," *Montgomery Advertiser*, 10 July 1878.

164. *Our Mountain Home* (Talladega), 22 Jan. 1879.

165. *Ibid.*, 31 Mar. 1909.

166. Shocco Springs Co. Is Organized," *Ibid.*, 20 Sept. 1916.

167. "Coca Cola Bottled in Talladega," 4.

168. Fitch, 213.

169. *Our Mountain Home* (Talladega), 28 Aug. 1895.

170. *Our Mountain Home* (Talladega), 12 July 1882; "Distinguished Arrival," *Ibid.*, 3 July 1872; *Ibid.*, 21 June 1882; "Good Speeches and a Big Jollyfication!," *Ibid.*, 26 July 1882.

171. *Ibid.*, 16 July 1879.

172. *Ibid.*, 16 Apr. 1884; "Chandler Springs," *Montgomery Advertiser* 18 June 1881; "Chandler Springs: Now Open to Summer Boarders," *Our Mountain Home* (Talladega), 31 Aug. 1892.

173. "Talladega Springs!," *Our Mountain Home* (Talladega), 18 June 1879; "Talladega Springs," *Anniston Evening Star*, 3 June 1901; Sulzby, 233.

174. "Observations on Talladega County," *Our Mountain Home* (Talladega), 27 Aug. 1884; N.W. Ayer & Son, *American Newspaper Annual*, 425.

175. "Chandler Springs," *Our Mountain Home* (Talladega), 31 Aug. 1892; "Talladega Springs!," *Ibid.*, 18 June 1879; *Our Mountain Home* (Talladega), 22 Jan. 1879.

176. "Shocco Springs," *Ibid.*, 5 June 1895.

177. McCord, *Baptists of Bibb County*, 85–86; F.J. Katz, *Mineral Resources*, 115; Powell, "Landreth Inducted," 12.

178. Anderson, "Cora Porter," 3; "Shocco Springs Conference Center: Who We Are."

179. *Anniston Evening Star*, 29 June 1907.

180. "The Opening of the Talladega Springs Hotel," *Montgomery Advertiser*, 15 May 1907.

181. *Ibid.*; *Anniston Evening Star*, 8 July 1907.

182. *Anniston Evening Star*, 29 June 1907; "[Furniture ad]," *Union Banner* (Clanton, AL), 22 Dec. 1921; Sulzby, 236; "Pursell Farms: History of Talladega Springs," https://pursellfarms.com/talladega-springs/. The Pursell Farms resort lies within 5 miles of Talladega Springs. Its website shows some early photos of the mineral spring resort and its environs.

183. Sulzby, 96; Pasquill, *Civilian Conservation Corps*, 52; "Restores Ond [sic] Home," *Anniston Star*, 5 Aug. 1958.

Valhermoso Springs

184. "Summary Report: Brindley Mountain," in U.S. Dept. of the Interior, USGS, U.S. Board on Geographic Names, https://edits.nationalmap.gov/apps/gaz-domestic/public/search/names/162832; "Valhermoso Springs [spring]," *Ibid.*, https://edits.nationalmap.gov/apps/gaz-domestic/public/search/names/153826.

185. Riley, 26, 40.

186. *Ibid.*, 38.

187. Harris, *Dead Towns*, 108. In 1823, Lancelot did deed 100 acres "and the houses and buildings thereon" to William, but more research is needed to determine if this parcel constituted any part of the resort lands. See *Valley Leaves* 12 (Dec. 1977): 48, Alabama Dept. of Archives & History, https://digital.archives.alabama.gov/digital/collection/hgpub/id/23916/rec/43.

188. Perkins, "Morgan Deed Book," 43.

189. "Valhermoso Springs," *Alabama Enquirer* (Hartselle, AL), 19 Sept. 1895.

190. *Ibid.*

191. Harris, 108.

192. "Valhermoso Springs."

193. *Ibid.*; "White Sulphur Springs, Morgan County, Alabama [ad]," *Democrat* (Huntsville, AL), 7 Sept. 1839.

194. "White Sulphur Springs, Morgan County, Alabama [ad]."

195. *Ibid.*

196. "Rates of Charge at the Morgan White Sulphur Springs [ad]," *Democrat* (Huntsville, AL), 7 Sept. 1839; "Morgan White Sulphur Springs [ad]," *Columbus Democrat* (MS), 6 June 1840.

197. "Valhermoso Springs."

198. Sulzby, 92.

199. "Immigration to North Alabama," *Tennessean* (Nashville), 20 Jan. 1870.

200. Sulzby, 90; Foscue, *Place Names in Alabama*, 141; "Valhermoso Springs."

201. *Historic Alabama Hotels*, 92; "The Reign of Terror," *Liberator* (Boston), 16 Nov. 1860.

202. "The Reign of Terror."

203. A Grand Railroad Victory: Eighty-Three Miles of Iron Rail Reclaimed—The American Flag Waving over Ten Towns in Alabama," *Philadelphia Inquirer*, 15 Apr. 1862.

204. "Huntsville," *Ibid.*, 15 Apr. 1862.

205. Sulzby, 92.

206. "From Huntsville," *Weekly Advertiser* (Montgomery), 30 Sept. 1863. The Civil War, as in many parts of Southern Appalachia, tore neighbors and families apart. Morgan County voted against secession before the war. To learn more about the complex situation in Morgan County, see Dave Tabler, "New Exhibit: The Civil War in Morgan County, AL," Sept. 23, 2014, Appalachian History: Stories, Quotes, and Anecdotes, http://www.appalachianhistory.net/2014/09/new-exhibit-civil-war-morgan-county-al.html.

207. "Valhermoso Springs (formerly Manning's) Morgan County, Alabama," *Daily State Sentinel* (Montgomery), 23 May 1867; "Valhermoso Springs, In the Mountains of Morgan County, in Alabama," *Memphis Daily Appeal*, 1 July 1869.

208. "Valhermoso Springs, Morgan Co., Alabama," *Memphis Daily Appeal*, 12 Aug. 1873.

209. "Valhermoso Springs, In the Mountains of Morgan County, in Alabama."

210. "Help Wanted," *Valley Leaves* 35 (Mar. 2001): 52, Alabama Dept. of Archives & History, https://digital.archives.alabama.gov/digital/collection/hgpub/id/31029/rec/144.

211. "Valhermoso Springs, In the Mountains of Morgan County, in Alabama."; "Montvale Springs, 1869," *Ibid.*, 1 July 1869.

212. "White Sulphur Springs, Morgan County, Alabama [ad]," *Democrat* (Huntsville, AL), 7 Sept.

1839; "Valhermoso Springs, In the Mountains of Morgan County, in Alabama"; "Valhermoso Summer Resort," *New Decatur Advertiser* (AL), 24 June 1904; Williamson, "Seven Ways." The CPI calculator was used.

213. "Valhermoso Springs."

214. Sulzby, 92; "Wanted—A Partner or Lessee for Valhermoso Spring," *Alabama Enquirer*, 19 Feb. 1891; "For Sale—the Valhermoso Springs Property Consisting of 281 acres," *Albany-Decatur Daily* (AL), 26 Nov. 1917; "Hotel-Oldest Health Resort in South, for Sale or Lease," *Indiana Weekly Messenger* (PA), 15 Mar. 1928.

215. Sulzby, 92.

216. Alabama Historical Association—Historical Markers—Morgan County, "Valhermoso Springs: Vale of Beauty," https://www.alabamahistory.net/copy-of-montgomery.

Georgia

Introduction

1. E. Lynn Usery, "Geographic Regions of Georgia: Overview," in *New Georgia Encyclopedia*, updated July 19, 2018, https://www.georgiaencyclopedia.org/articles/geography-environment/geographic-regions-of-georgia-overview/.

2. Timothy Chowns, "Appalachian Plateau Geologic Province," *Ibid.*, updated July 9, 2018, https://www.georgiaencyclopedia.org/articles/science-medicine/appalachian-plateau-geologic-province/.

3. Chowns, "Valley and Ridge Geologic Province," *Ibid.*, updated Aug. 10, 2018, https://www.georgiaencyclopedia.org/articles/science-medicine/valley-and-ridge-geologic-province/.

4. Frank B. Golley, "Piedmont Geographic Region," *Ibid.*, updated July 26, 2017, https://www.georgiaencyclopedia.org/articles/geography-environment/piedmont-geographic-region/.

5. Charles Seabrook, "Blue Ridge Mountains," *Ibid.*, updated July 15, 2020, https://www.georgiaencyclopedia.org/articles/geography-environment/blue-ridge-mountains/.

6. Sidney Lanier, "The Song of the Chattahoochee," www.poets.org.

7. Posey, "Report upon the Topography and Epidemic Diseases of the State of Georgia," 133.

8. "McCallie, *Preliminary Report of the Mineral Springs of Georgia*, 130, 148, 150, 214.

9. "Mineral Resources of Georgia," *De Bow's Review*, 61.

10. McCallie, 123, 127.

11. Posey, "Report on the Topography," 184.

12. Pepper et al., "Report by Committee on Sanitaria and on Mineral Springs," 538.

13. *Ibid.*, 549, 556, 559.

14. "Proposals," *Tri-Weekly Nashville Union*, 26 Aug. 1837; C., "Editorial Correspondence: Spring Place, Murray Co., July 5, 1848," *Federal Union* (Milledgeville), 11 July 1848.

15. "Gordon Springs, Located in Northern Georgia, Near Tunnel Hill, on State Railroad [ad]," *Augusta Evening Dispatch*, 11 Aug. 1858.

16. "Grand Fancy Ball at Catoosa [ad]," *Columbus Enquirer* (GA), 12 Aug. 1851.

17. "Medical Intelligence: Notes of the Mineral Springs in the State of Georgia," 443. In 1849, Meriwether County's Warm Springs, associated with FDR in the twentieth century, was not as developed as the other Georgia mineral spring resorts mentioned.

18. "Gordon Springs, Near Tunnel Hill Station, Georgia, For Sale [ad]," *Southern Confederacy* (Atlanta), 30 Apr. 1862.

19. Georgia Historical Commission, "Cherokee Springs Confederate Hospital," Waymarking.com, http://www.waymarking.com/gallery/image.aspx?f=1&guid=0116c6c8-dda9-4495-9a45-77d8910c9d82; Freemon, "The Medical Support System for the Confederate Army of Tennessee," 45; "Cherokee Springs [ad]," *Daily Chronicle and Sentinel* (Augusta), 20 May 1853.

20. Crook, *Mineral Waters of the United States*, 208, 211, 213.

21. *Ibid.*, 218.

22. Sawyer, *Northeast Georgia*, 48.

23. Western and Atlantic Railroad, "W & A," 2.

24. Albert S. Hardy, "In North Georgia: A Visit to that Delightful Resort, Porter Springs, 'Queen of the Mountains,'" *Barnesville Gazette*, 12 Sept. 1895.

25. "Dissolution of Mt. Airy Hotel Company," *Weekly Constitution* (Atlanta), 2 Jan. 1877. E.W. Holland signed the notice, who may have been the same Holland who owned New Holland Springs.

26. "Mount Airy Hotel," *Athens Banner* (GA), 28 June 1881; "The Gem of the Mountains. Mt. Airy Hotel, Mt. Airy, GA. [ad]," *Gainesville Eagle* (GA), 7 Sept. 1882.

27. Mary E. Bryan, "The Southern Switzerland," *Sunny South* (Atlanta), 14 Jan. 1882.

28. Burke, *Reminiscences of Georgia*, 22–28. Not until 1949 was the school year mandated at 9 months across Georgia. See Denise S. Mewborn, "Public Education," in *New Georgia Encyclopedia*, updated July 21, 2020, https://www.georgiaencyclopedia.org/articles/education/public-education-prek-12/.

29. O.M., "Porter Springs. The Impressions of a Thomasville Young Lady, Who is Visiting That Resort," *Daily Times-Enterprise* (Thomasville), 11 Sept. 1897.

30. Fletcher M. Johnson, "A Defense of the Mountaineers," *Georgia Cracker* (Gainesville), 22 Mar. 1902. For more information on educational uplift in northern Georgia, see William A. Link, *The Paradox of Southern Progressivism, 1880–1930* (Chapel Hill: University of North Carolina Press, 1992), 79–80.

31. "Stay At Home," *Southern Sentinel* (Columbus, GA), 13 June 1850.

32. "Chalybeate Springs," *Daily Chronicle & Sentinel* (Augusta), 18 Apr. 1860.

33. Jack Plane, "Life at the Springs and Where

Shall We Go?" *Macon Telegraph and Messenger*, 20 June 1879.

34. *The Saratoga of the Confederate States: Catoosa Springs, Catoosa County, Georgia, Harman & Nichols, Proprietors* (n.p.: [1861]), 2, www.archive.org.

Catoosa Springs

35. Elizabeth B. Cooksey, "Catoosa County," in *New Georgia Encyclopedia*, updated June 16, 2022, https://www.georgiaencyclopedia.org/articles/counties-cities-neighborhoods/catoosa-county/.; Mary E. Johnson, "Cherokee County," *Ibid.*, updated June 16, 2022, https://www.georgiaencyclopedia.org/articles/counties-cities-neighborhoods/cherokee-county/. The Cherokee who escaped removal joined the North Carolina (Qualla Boundary) Cherokee, who in 1870 came to be known as the Eastern Band of the Cherokee Indians. See John R. Finger, *The Eastern Band of Cherokees 1819-1900* (Knoxville: University of Tennessee Press, 1984), especially Chapters 1–2 and p. 113 for reference to the first mention of the Eastern Band of Cherokee Indians.

36. Goff, [no title] *Georgia Mineral Newsletter*, reprinted in *Placenames of Georgia*, 147.

37. William J. Frazier, "Geologic Regions of Georgia: Overview," in *New Georgia Encyclopedia*, updated Mar. 7, 2022, https://www.georgiaencyclopedia.org/articles/science-medicine/geologic-regions-georgia-overview/; Timothy Chowns, "Valley and Ridge Geologic Province," *Ibid.*, updated Aug. 10, 2018, https://www.georgiaencyclopedia.org/articles/science-medicine/valley-and-ridge-geologic-province/; "1946 Ringgold 7.5 Minute Topo Map," https://www.pickatrail.com/topo-map/r/7.5x7.5/ringgold-ga.html.

38. McCallie, *Preliminary Report on the Mineral Resources of Georgia* (1910), 118.

39. *Ibid.*, 123; Derry and Wright, *Advantages of Georgia*, 37.

40. *Preliminary Report on the Mineral Resources of Georgia* (1910), 169; Joseph E. Willet, "Salt Springs in Georgia, and How to Find Them," *Southern Confederacy* (Atlanta), 13 May 1862; "Alum Spring," *Georgia Journal and Messenger* (Macon), 7 Oct. 1857.

41. Crook, *Mineral Waters of the United States*, 208; McCallie, *Preliminary Report of the Mineral Springs of Georgia* (1913), 49–51, 54–55.

42. McCallie, *Preliminary Report of the Mineral Springs of Georgia* (1913), 49.

43. "Irish Potatoes [*sic*] from Slips," 63–64.

44. "Medical Intelligence: Notice of the Mineral Springs in the State of Georgia," 443.

45. *Daily Chronicle & Sentinel* (Augusta), 27 Aug. 1849; *Ibid.*, 27 Sept. 1849.

46. O'Bryant, *Brief History of Catoosa County*, 50–51.

47. "Cherokee Springs [ad]," *Daily Constitutionalist and Republic* (Augusta), 1 July 1853; "Cherokee Springs for Sale [ad]," *Ibid.*, 3 July 1857.

48. DINKS, "Letter from Cherokee," *Georgia Citizen* (Macon), 26 July 1850; Williamson, "Seven Ways." The CPI calculator was used for dollar conversions in this chapter.

49. Kennesaw, "(Correspondence) Marietta, Sept. 11th, 1850," *Albany Patriot* (GA), 20 Sept. 1850.

50. F., "Editors [*sic*] Correspondence, Warm Springs, Meriwether Co., August 8, 1850," *Columbus Times* (GA), 13 Aug. 1850.

51. "Letter from Cherokee."

52. "View of Cotoosa Springs," in White, *Historical Collections of Georgia*, 668.

53. "Letter from Cherokee"; Kennesaw, "(Correspondence) Marietta."

54. Visitor, "Catoosa Springs, Aug. 24, 1857," *Daily Morning News* (Savannah), 29 Aug. 1857.

55. "Letter from Cherokee"; "Cotoosa Springs [ad]," *Daily Chronicle & Sentinel* (Augusta), 23 May 1851; "Catoosa Springs, Georgia [ad]," *Weekly Chronicle & Sentinel* (Augusta), 2 June 1852.

56. "Catoosa Springs, Georgia [ad]," *Weekly Chronicle & Sentinel* (Augusta), 2 June 1852.

57. "Catoosa County, Ga. [ad]," *Georgia Citizen* (Macon), 25 June 1858.

58. Crook, *Mineral Waters of the United States*, 208.

59. *Ibid.*, 208; Kennesaw, "(Correspondence) Marietta."

60. Visitor, "Catoosa Springs, Aug. 24, 1857."

61. *Ibid.*; John H. Seals, "Editorial Correspondence, Catoosa Springs, Aug. 13th, 1855," *Temperance Banner* (Penfield, GA), 18 Aug. 1855.

62. Henry Campbell, "A Hoosier's Civil War Diary," *Jasper Dubois County Daily Herald* (Jasper, IN), 3 Oct. 1961.

63. Ferguson, *On to Atlanta*, 28; Royse, *History of the Story of the 115th Regiment Illinois Volunteer Infantry*, 200.

64. "Catoosa Springs," *Southern Federal Union* (Milledgeville), 9 July 1861; Kennesaw, "(Correspondence) Marietta."

65. "Catoosa Springs, Aug. 1, 1855," *Atlanta Weekly Intelligencer and Cherokee Advocate* (Atlanta and Marietta), 3 Aug. 1855; Seals, "Editorial Correspondence, Catoosa Springs, Aug. 13th, 1855."

66. "Grand Fancy Ball at Catoosa [ad]," *Columbus Enquirer* (GA), 12 Aug. 1851; "Grand Tournament and Fancy Ball at Catoosa Springs [ad]," *Savannah Daily Republican*, 29 Aug. 1856.

67. "A Grand Fancy Ball [ad]," *Daily Chronicle & Sentinel* (Augusta), Aug 19, 1855; "Grand Doings at Catoosa Springs," *Ibid.*, 22 Aug. 1856; "Catoosa Springs—Grand Fancy Dress Ball," *Telegraph and Messenger* (Macon), 8 Aug. 1872.

68. "Cotoosa Springs [ad]," *Daily Chronicle & Sentinel* (Augusta), 23 May 1851; *Saratoga of the Confederate States*, 2.

69. "Letter from Cherokee."

70. *Saratoga of the Confederate States*, 1.

71. "Catoosa Springs," *Savannah Daily Republican*, 27 May 1861.
72. "Catoosa Springs," *Ibid.*, 20 Aug. 1861.
73. "Catoosa Springs, GA. [ad]," *Southern Confederacy* (Atlanta), 7 June 1862; *Daily Morning News* (Savannah), 27 Sept. 1862; "The Late Captain Wm. H. Battey," *Weekly Constitutionalist* (Augusta), 10 Dec. 1862.
74. Schroeder-Lein, *Confederate Hospitals*, 63, 98.
75. "Auction Sale of Hotel Furniture [ad]," *Southern Confederacy* (Atlanta) 21 Jan. 1863; B., "Communicated, Bachelor Hall, Room 24, Catoosa, Georgia, August 14, 1871," *Weekly Sumter Republican* (Americus), 19 Aug. 1871.
76. "The Situation in Front," *Southern Banner* (Athens, GA), 16 Sept. 1863; Schroeder-Lein, 124-25, 177, 197.
77. "Letter from 'Rambler,'" *New Albany Daily Ledger* (Albany, IN), 21 May 1864.
78. E.M. Cravatt, "Camp near Catoosa Springs, Ga.," *Sandusky Daily Commercial Register* (Ohio), 16 May 1864.
79. B.F.C., "Letter from the Mountains, Ringgold, Ga., April 5, 1872," *Telegraph and Messenger* (Macon), 7 Apr. 1872.
80. F., "Letter from Georgia, Ringgold, Ga., May 14," *Janesville Gazette* (WI), 12 June 1867.
81. *Atlanta Daily Sun*, 14 Oct. 1871.
82. Alpha, "Letter from Cotoosa Springs," *Savannah Morning News*, 15 Aug. 1872; S.A.A., "Catoosa Springs, July 16th," *Southern Banner* (Athens, GA), 19 July 1872; B.L.C., "From Catoosa Springs," *Telegraph and Messenger* (Macon), 30 July 1872; Williamson, "Seven Ways."
83. *Albany News* (GA), 14 June 1872; "Montvale Springs [ad]," *Savannah Morning News*, 6 July 1872; "Reduction of Rates at Catoosa Springs," *Albany News*, 2 Aug. 1872.
84. "Letter from Cotoosa Springs."
85. "Old Virginia Welcome! [ad]," *Albany News*, 10 May 1872; "Sweet Chalybeate Springs [ad]," *Savannah Morning News*, 6 July 1872; "White Sulphur Springs [ad]," *Ibid.*; "Sigma," "Delayed Letter from Catoosa Springs," *Albany News*, 24 Sept. 1874.
86. Henry Sch., "A Trip to Catoosa Springs," *North Georgia Citizen* (Dalton), 22 July 1875; J.B.G., "Catoosa Springs," *Weekly Constitution* (Atlanta), 1 Sept. 1874.
87. *Columbus Daily Enquirer-Sun* (GA), 18 Nov. 1877.
88. Catoosa Springs, Georgia [ad]," *Savannah Morning News*, 22 May 1878; Jack Plane, "Letter from Our Traveling Correspondent, Catoosa Springs, July 29, 1878," *Ibid.*, 1 Aug. 1878; *Savannah Morning News*, 11 July 1879.
89. *Savannah Morning News*, 11 July 1879; *Sunny South* (Atlanta), 23 Aug. 1879.
90. *Macon Telegraph and Messenger*, 8 Aug. 1879; *North Georgia Citizen* (Dalton), 14 Aug. 1879.
91. Hon. Randall Franklin, "There is Nothing Like Being a Legislator," *Sandersville Herald* (GA), 4 Aug. 1881.
92. "Sale of Catoosa Springs," *North Georgia Citizen* (Dalton), 25 Aug. 1881; *Ibid.*, 8 Dec. 1881.
93. *Ibid.*, 11 June 1885; *Ibid.*, 26 May 1887; *Ibid.*, 30 June 1887; *Ibid.*, 14 June 1888.
94. *Morning News* (Savannah), 1 Oct. 1892; *Cedartown Standard* (GA), 2 May 1901.
95. "Gen. Baldwin Buys Catoosa Springs," *Walker County Messenger* (LaFayette, GA), 7 May 1903.
96. *Ibid.*; Cashin, Charles Alexander, and William T. Anderson, *Under Fire*, 286.
97. "Dance at Catoosa Springs," *North Georgia Citizen* (Dalton), 3 Aug. 1911; "Practice March Through Georgia by Max G. Dice," *Washington Court House Herald* (Ohio), 8 Dec. 1917; Snyder, *Tennessee Army National Guard*, 14.
98. Fitch, 327.
99. Patterson, "Theodore Anderson Baldwin"; "BG Samuel Dickerson Rockenbach," *Military Hall of Honor,* https://militaryhallofhonor.com/honoree-record.php?id=3014; *San Antonio Light* (TX), 30 Oct. 1933.
100. O'Bryant, 53.
101. Snyder, 1.

Gainesville: Gower's Spring, New Holland Springs, Oconee White Sulphur Springs

102. Frank B. Golley, "Piedmont Geographic Region," in *New Georgia Encyclopedia*, updated July 26, 2017, https://www.georgiaencyclopedia.org/articles/geography-environment/piedmont-geographic-region/ ; Mack S. Duncan, "Fall Line," *Ibid.*, updated July 23, 2018, https://www.georgiaencyclopedia.org/articles/geography-environment/fall-line/; "Gainesville Topographic Map," https://en-us.topographic-map.com/map-cdfmt/Gainesville/.
103. Thomas Hanley, "Piedmont Geologic Province," in *New Georgia Encyclopedia*, updated Aug. 10, 2018, https://www.georgiaencyclopedia.org/articles/science-medicine/piedmont-geologic-province/.
104. White, *Historical Collections of Georgia*, 490.
105. "Negroes [ad]," *Georgia Telegraph* (Macon), 21 May 1835.
106. "Georgia Gold Region," *Southern Banner* (Athens), 28 Dec. 1838; McCallie, *Preliminary Report on the Mineral Resources of Georgia* (1910), 107, 110, 123, 148; *Gainesville: The Great Health Resort of the South*, 6.
107. Smith, *Story of Georgia*, 331.
108. "The Subscriber [ad]," *Savannah Georgian*, 6 July 1829.
109. "Planters' Hotel [ad]," *Georgia Constitutionalist* (Augusta), 29 June 1832.
110. Examples of other springs, many noted in the press for therapeutic claims, follow. A "Limestone Spring" 3 mi. south of Gainesville attracted M.R. Mitchell, who built a hotel there in 1832

("Limestone Spring," *Georgia Journal* (Milledgeville), 31 May 1832; Dorsey, *History of Hall County,* 34). Deal Spring was located 2 mi. from Gainesville (Crook, *Mineral Waters of the United States,* 213). A "large cluster of mineral springs" was located within 200 yds. of the Air Line depot (Barton & Judson, *Guide-Book and Biographical Sketches of Northeastern Georgia and the Carolinas Adjacent to the Atlanta and Charlotte Air-Line Railway* (Atlanta: James P. Harrison, 1878), 19. A spring with a rock wall stood near the "old Academy … at the head of Washington street [sic]." (Dorsey, 61). The "Gainesville Springs" stood within 200 yds. of the Mansion House, located on the south side of Gainesville on the Lawrenceville Rd. ("Mansion House [ad]," *Tri-Weekly Chronicle & Sentinel* (Augusta), 1 June 1841; Dorsey, 111).

111. Sybil W. McRay, comp., "Hall County Place Names," in Dorsey, 373.

112. "Greenville Coach Factory. Dissolution of Co-Partnership," *Southern Enterprise* (Greenville, SC), 21 Feb. 1856; Dorsey, 397; Huff, *Greenville,* 119; Williamson, "Seven Ways." The CPI calculator was used.

113. "Gainesville Hotel [ad]," *Southern Recorder* (Milledgeville), 16 May 1837; Brockington and Associates, *Gainesville,* 70; *Southern Watchman* (Athens, GA), 23 July 1857.

114. Dorsey, 112–13; "Gower & Lester. Carriage Makers! [ad]," *Southern Banner* [Athens], 23 June 1859; U.S. Population Census 1860, FamilySearch, www.familysearch.org/, all subsequent Census records in this chapter accessed at FamilySearch.

115. "Gainesville Hotel [ad]," *Daily Morning News* (Savannah), 26 July 1861; "Died," *Southern Watchman* (Athens), 14 Jan. 1863.

116. "Iron," *Southern Watchman* (Athens), 14 Oct. 1863.

117. Annie Maria, "A Trip to Gainesville, and Its Incidents Amusing and Practical," *Weekly Constitution* (Atlanta), 23 Sept. 1873. Because Town Spring water was characterized as chalybeate and was located about 1.5 mile from the village of Gainesville in the 1830s, it is plausible that it is the same as Gower's Spring and that overgrowth hid the spring in subsequent decades, thus allowing for its 1873 "discovery." The website "Explore Gainesville" corroborates the hypothesis. See "Explore Gainesville: Historic Green Street," https://www.exploregainesville.org/historic-green-street/.

118. "'Abroad Again'—Letter from Jack Plane," *Georgia Weekly Telegraph and Georgia Journal & Messenger* (Macon), 31 July 1877.

119. "Gower Springs (Near Gainesville, GA.) [ad]," *Columbus Enquirer-Sun* (GA), 30 May 1889. The ad includes a sketch of the hotel.

120. "'Abroad Again'—Letter from Jack Plane."

121. *Gainesville: The Great Health Resort of the South,* 23.

122. "Kit Warren. His Remarks Concerning Gower," *Sunny South* (Atlanta), 15 Aug. 1885.

123. *Mineral Waters of the United States,* 212–13.

124. *Gainesville: The Great Health Resort of the South,* 31.

125. "Gower Springs [ad]," *Morning News* (Savannah), 22 June 1890.

126. J.H.C., "Glances at Gainesville. A North Georgia Town of Great Expectations," *Columbus Daily Enquirer-Sun,* 31 Aug. 1884.

127. Brockington and Associates, 44; U.S. Population Census 1880.

128. Brockington and Associates, 44.

129. *Ibid.*, 44, 72.

130. *Savannah Morning News,* 27 Aug. 1885; U.S. Population Census 1880.

131. "Kit Warren: His Remarks Concerning Georgians, Tennesseans, Floridians, Labor, Land, Law and Loveliness," *Sunny South* (Atlanta), 29 Aug. 1885.

132. *Savannah Morning News,* May 19, 1886; "Gower Springs Hotel Burned," *Morning News* (Savannah), 29 Oct. 1893.

133. *Gainesville: The Great Health Resort of the South,* 29.

134. "The Piedmont Hotel [ad]," *Macon Telegraph and Messenger,* 26 June 1877.

135. "Gower Springs (Near Gainesville, GA.) [ad]," *Columbus Enquirer-Sun,* 30 May 1889.

136. "Gower Springs [ad]," *Morning News* (Savannah), 22 June 1888.

137. "Summer Homes at Gower Springs, Gainesville, Ga.," *Morning News* (Savannah), 29 July 1888.

138. "Gower Springs Hotel Burned," *Morning Sun* (Savannah), 29 Oct. 1893; "For Sale [ad]," *Ibid.*, 25 Feb. 1894.

139. "Foreclosure of Mortgage," *Georgia Cracker* (Gainesville), 8 Sept. 1900; "Why Not Build a New Hotel," *Gainesville News* (GA), 11 Mar. 1903; "Gower Springs," *Georgia Cracker* (Gainesville), 7 Sept. 1901.

140. *Cleveland Progress* (GA), 29 May 1896; "Evans' Livery and Car Line," *Georgia Cracker* (Gainesville), 4 Sept. 1897.

141. "Firemen's Picnic," *Gainesville News,* 13 May 1903; "Union Sunday School at Gower Spring," *Ibid.*, 17 July 1912; "Mr. J.W. Large is Dead," *Ibid.*, 16 Apr. 1913.

142. "Announcement: Green Street Circle is now Open!," *Gainesville News,* 13 Oct. 1909. The article includes a plat of the subdivision.

143. Gower Springs Water," *Ibid.*, 27 Apr. 1910; Deanna M. Gillespie, "'A First-Rate Summer Resort': Gainesville's Mineral Springs and the New South," *Georgia Historical Quarterly* 107(Summer 2023):182; *Dahlonega Nugget,* 16 May 1924.

144. Brockington and Associates, 60; Dorsey, 373. Brockington pinpoints the location as property of the First Baptist Church; Dorsey identifies the Triangle Shopping Center as the site.

145. W.P. Rivers, "Gainesville Long Ago: Interesting Reminiscences by One of the Earliest Settlers," *Gainesville Eagle,* 8 Mar. 1894; White, 490; Dorsey, 61.

146. "Georgia Hotel [ad]," *Southern Recorder*

(Milledgeville), 10 Nov. 1835; "Planters' Hotel [ad]," *Southern Banner* (Athens), 19 June 1832.

147. "From the *Southern Whig*: Gainesville, July 24," *Augusta Chronicle* (GA), 16 Aug. 1834.

148. "Gainesville Long Ago"; U.S. Population Census 1830; *Federal Union* (Milledgeville), 2 May 1833; "A Teacher Wanted," *Southern Banner* (Athens), 28 Dec. 1833.

149. "Gainesville Long Ago"; Bill Arp, "Bill Arp Speaks," *Weekly Constitution* (Atlanta), 21 June 1887; U.S. Population Census 1850. The Census lists Rivers' occupation as "merchant" with property valued at $4,000.

150. "Gainesville Long Ago"; Dorsey, 61.

151. Dr. H.J. Massey, "Men Who Made Atlanta," *Atlanta Constitution*, 6 Jan. 1906.

152. Pioneers' Society of Atlanta, *Pioneer Citizens' History of Atlanta*, 328; "Men Who Made Atlanta."

153. *Pioneer Citizens' History of Atlanta*, 328; Tammy H. Galloway, "Alfred Austell (1814–1881)," in *New Georgia Encyclopedia*, updated Aug. 16, 2013, https://www.georgiaencyclopedia.org/articles/business-economy/alfred-austell-1814-1881/.

154. "New Holland Springs! [ad]," *Macon Telegraph and Messenger*, 7 Apr. 1874.

155. "New Holland Spring, Ga. [ad]," *Atlanta Daily Herald*, 16 Aug. 1874; "Catoosa Springs, Georgia [ad]," *Daily Constitutionalist* (Augusta), 22 July 1874; "Blount Springs!," *Memphis Daily Appeal*, 7 June 1874; "Montvale Springs, Blount County, East Tenn. [ad]," *Daily Press and Herald* (Knoxville), 15 July 1874; "Easley's Spring [ad]," *Herald and Tribune* (Jonesborough, TN), 13 Aug. 1874.

156. Sidney Herbert, "Letter from New Holland Springs," *Troy Messenger* (AL), 22 July 1875; Chatham, "Letter from Atlanta," *Savannah Morning News*, 26 June 1882; "Savannahians at the Springs," *Ibid.*, 11 Aug. 1881; "New Holland Spring [ad]," *Macon Telegraph and Messenger*, 18 May 1875; *Weekly Sumter Republican* (Americus), 13 Aug. 1875; *Weekly News and Advertiser* (Albany, GA), 1 Aug. 1885.

157. "Savannahians Booked for the Springs," *Savannah Morning News*, 14 June 1876; *Home Journal* (Perry, GA), 7 Aug. 1879.

158. Chatham, "New Holland Springs. Ball in Honor of the Georgia Agricultural Society," *Savannah Morning News*, 15 Aug. 1876.

159. Chatham, "New Holland Springs."

160. "Dinner at New Holland," *Banner-Watchman* (Athens), 4 Aug. 1885.

161. *Savannah Daily Republican*, 7 May 1845; New Holland Springs Now Open [ad]," *Sandersville Herald* (GA), 2 July 1891.

162. Timothy Harley, "Southward, Ho! From Athens to Tallulah and the Scenes Along the Way," *Savannah Morning News*, 3 Dec. 1885; John S. Billings, *The National Medical Dictionary*, vol. 2, *K to Z*. (Philadelphia: Lea Brothers, 1890), 213, 378, 384.

163. "New Holland Springs! Headquarters for Health [ad]," *Savannah Morning News*, 26 May 1879.

164. *Ibid.*; "Southward, Ho!."

165. Chatham, "New Holland Springs."

166. "Southward, Ho!."

167. "New Holland Springs. A Cool and Inviting Summer Resort," *Thomasville Times*, 14 Aug. 1886.

168. Peale, *Lists and Analyses of the Mineral Springs of the United States*, 81. Crook estimated New Holland's flow at 200 gal./min., which corresponds to 12,000 gal./hr., most likely an error. See *Mineral Waters of the United States*, 213. Another observer of the water velocity reported it at 100 gal./min., but still less than Crook's report. See *Savannah Morning News*, 1 July 1885.

169. "New Holland Springs. A Cool and Inviting Summer Resort."

170. Crawford, "Breezes Blow. A Banner Man in the Switzerland of Georgia," *Athens Weekly Banner* (GA), 20 Aug. 1889.

171. *Savannah Morning News*, 10 Aug. 1875; "A Flourishing Resort. A Few Points About New Holland Springs," *Ibid.*, 20 Aug. 1884.

172. "New Holland Spring [ad]."

173. "Affairs in Georgia," *Savannah Morning News*, 26 May 1875.

174. "New Holland Springs: A Cool and Inviting Summer Resort"; "Northeastern R.R. of Ga.," *Jackson Herald* (Jefferson, GA), 3 Sept. 1886; "Richmond & Danville R.R. Piedmont Air-Line Route," *Hartwell Sun* (GA), 22 Oct. 1886.

175. Brockington and Associates, 7.

176. "New Holland Springs! Headquarters for Health," *Savannah Morning News*, 26 May 1879.

177. *Ibid.*; "New Holland Springs: The 'Queen of the Mountains,'" *Savannah Morning News*, 1 July 1885; "Southward, Ho!."

178. "Atlanta Gossip," *Savannah Morning News*, 21 June 1882; "Gate City Gossip," *Ibid.*, 13 July 1882.

179. Georgia Historical Society, "Struggles of the Late 19th Century: Yellow Fever," https://georgiahistory.com/education-outreach/online-exhibits/online-exhibits/three-centuries-of-georgia-history/nineteenth-century/struggles-of-the-late-19th-century/.

180. "Yellow Fever. The Disease in Georgia," *Columbus Daily Enquirer* (GA), 23 Sept. 1876.

181. "Letter from Atlanta," *Savannah Morning News*, 4 Sept. 1876.

182. W.A. Greene, "Dr. Thomas and the State Board of Health," *Macon Telegraph and Messenger*, 13 Sept. 1876.

183. *Macon Telegraph and Messenger*, 22 Sept. 1876.

184. *Barnesville Gazette* (GA), 17 Dec. 1885.

185. *Savannah Morning News*, 10 Feb. 1887; "Another Watering Place In Trouble," *Weekly Banner-Watchman* (Athens, GA), 22 Feb. 1887.

186. *Columbus Enquirer-Sun*, 25 Aug. 1888; Garrett, *Atlanta and Environs*, 120.

187. "Big Sale of Land," *Daily Times-Enterprise* (Thomasville, GA), 25 Sept. 1890.

188. Mr. R. Wink Taylor, Proprietor of the

Arlington, Gainesville, Ga. [ad]," *Morning News* (Savannah), 18 June 1891.

189. "Items of General Interest From the Capital of Hall," *Macon Telegraph*, 1 Sept. 1898.

190. *Morning News* (Savannah), 29 Dec. 1899.

191. "A $1,000,000. Mill," *Georgia Cracker* (Gainesville), 17 Mar. 1900. Tragedy struck the site in 1903 when a tornado killed 33 workers and children at the mill and its cottages. See "Estimate of Property Loss," *Fayetteville News* (GA), 5 June 1903.

192. "New Holland Spring Cared For," *Georgia Cracker* (Gainesville), 22 June 1901; "American Springs," 267; Alyson Shields, "New Holland: 'If You Met the Standard, You Worked Hard,'" https://accesswdun.com/article/2019/12/862511/crossroads-new-holland.

193. McRay, 391.

194. "Mansion House [ad]," *Daily Chronicle & Sentinel* (Augusta), May 18, 1841.

195. *Acts of the General Assembly of the State of Georgia*, 44–45; Elizabeth Cooksey, "Banks County," in *New Georgia Encyclopedia*, updated June 8, 2022, https://www.georgiaencyclopedia.org/articles/counties-cities-neighborhoods/banks-county/.

196. U.S. Population Census 1840.

197. Dorsey, 76, 185.

198. "Unrivalled Medicine," *Southern Recorder* (Milledgeville), 12 Jan. 1847.

199. "To Summer Visitors [ad]," *Southern Banner* (Athens), 23 May 1844.

200. "White Sulphur Spring. Hall County, Ga. [ad]," *Daily Chronicle & Sentinel* (Augusta), 21 May 1846.

201. White, 308.

202. Medicus, "Letter from a Watering Place," *Southern Literary Gazette* (Charleston), 8 June 1850.

203. "White Sulpher [sic] Springs [ad]," *Weekly Republic* (Augusta), 4 June 1851; U.S. Population Census 1850; "Ewsiel Pace," Find a Grave, https://www.findagrave.com/memorial/118296425/ewsiel-pace.

204. J.A.G., "Editorial Correspondence. White Sulphur Springs, Hall Co., June 28, 1855," *Southern Banner*, 5 July 1855.

205. *Ibid.*; "Letter from a Watering Place."

206. "'Abroad Again'—A Letter from Jack Plane."

207. "Hall County White Sulphur Springs," *Atlanta Constitution*, 9 June 1907.

208. "White Sulphur Closes Tomorrow," *Gainesville News*, 24 Sept. 1919.

209. "Letter from a Watering Place."

210. J.A.G., "Editorial Correspondence. White Sulphur Springs."

211. McRay, 388; Dorsey, 160, 423; U.S. Population Census 1860.

212. "Gainesville Hotel [ad]," *Savannah Daily Morning News*, 3 June 1861.

213. M.S., "Mineral Spring," *Southern Watchman* (Athens), 14 July 1869.

214. "Oh, for a Lodge in Some Vast Wilderness," *Southern Watchman* (Athens), 28 June 1871.

215. "Gilt-Edge Property at Executor's Sale," *Savannah Morning News*, 4 Dec. 1874.

216. *Savannah Morning News*, 26 Apr. 1877; *Athens Weekly Georgian*, 8 May 1877.

217. *Savannah Morning News*, 4 Mar. 1878; *Ibid.*, 1 Aug. 1878; *Ibid.*, 21 Aug. 1878; "Death of Colonel James D. Mathews," *Ibid.*, 28 Aug. 1878.

218. T. Larry Gantt, "Mr. Jacob Phinizy Amplifies Gantt's Story of the Late Ferdinand Phinizy," *Athens Banner*, 26 Nov. 1922; "Ferdinand Phinizy," *Athens Daily Banner*, 16 June 1901.

219. G.G.S., "Gainesville Letter," *Union and Recorder* (Milledgeville), 9 Mar. 1880.

220. "Muscogee," "White Sulphur Springs. Hall County, Ga.—Location—Scenery—Personals—Guests," *Columbus Daily Enquirer-Sun*, 21 July 1880. Muscogee comments that Phinizy bought the resort because the water cured a family member, but Phinizy's son recalled to the Athens newspaper in 1922 that his father acquired the property due to a debt.

221. Muscogee, "White Sulphur Springs."

222. Mildred Loring, "The Oconee White," *Athens Banner*, 10 Aug. 1880.

223. *Ibid.*; *Savannah Morning News*, 18 Aug. 1880.

224. "Sale of White Sulphur Springs," *Athens Daily Banner*, 6 Apr. 1900; "Sale of the White Sulphur Springs Property," *Georgia Cracker* (Gainesville), 10 Mar. 1900.

225. "Big Sale of Land," *Daily Times-Enterprise* (Thomasville, GA), 25 Sept. 1890; Emory Eye Center, "Our History," www.eyecenter.emory.edu/our_history.htm.

226. "Sale of the White Sulphur Springs Property," *Georgia Cracker* (Gainesville), 10 Mar. 1900.

227. "Sale of White Sulphur Springs"; "For Sale—Real Estate [ad]," *Morning News* (Savannah), 12 Apr. 1900.

228. Sawyer, 77.

229. "Hall County White Sulphur Springs," *Atlanta Constitution*, 9 June 1907.

230. Sawyer, 78; "Famed Resort Burns Near Gainesville," *Forsyth County News* (Cumming, GA), 26 Jan. 1933; "White Sulphur Community was Home to Resort for Wealthy," *Gainesville Times*, https://www.gainesvilletimes.com/life/white-sulphur-community-was-home-to-resort-for-wealthy/.

Porter's Springs

231. Miss F.G.L., "Beautiful Mountain Scenery—Dahlonega, Ga.—Graphic Description," *Sunny South* (Atlanta), 18 May 1878.

232. "Appalachian Trail Community: Dahlonega, GA," Appalachian Trail Conservancy, https://www.appalachiantrail.org/home/conservation/a-t-community-program/at-community-partners/dahlonega-ga; Robert Sutherland, "Filming Locations for A Walk

in the Woods with Robert Redford," https://appalachiantrail.com/20151001/filming-locations-for-a-walk-in-the-woods-with-robert-redford/; "Georgia Appalachian Trail Club: Trail Guide," https://georgia-atclub.org/hike-the-a-t/trail-guide.

233. Charles Seabrook, "Blue Ridge Mountains," in *New Georgia Encyclopedia*, updated July 15, 2020, https://www.georgiaencyclopedia.org/articles/geography-environment/blue-ridge-mountains/; Timothy E. LaTour, "Blue Ridge Geologic Province," *Ibid.*, updated July 23, 2018, https://www.georgiaencyclopedia.org/articles/science-medicine/blue-ridge-geologic-province.

234. Green, "Georgia's Forgotten Industry, Part I," 96–97.

235. *Ibid.*, 99. For names of others credited with first discovering gold during this period, see S.W. McCallie, *Preliminary Report on the Mineral Resources of Georgia* (1910), 97–8; Dorsey, *History of Hall County*, 23; Sawyer, *Northeast Georgia*, 34.

236. *Ibid.*, 100; Lumpkin County, GA, "Southern Living, Southern Charm—History," http://www.lumpkincounty.gov/305/History. For information on other original names for Dahlonega, see also E. Melton Coulter, *Auraria: The Story of a Gold-Mining Town* (Athens: University of Georgia Press, 2009), 99; Green, "Georgia's Forgotten Industry, Part I," 109.

237. Green, "Georgia's Forgotten Industry, Part II," 210–11.

238. Williams, "Georgia's Forgotten Miners," 80.

239. Green, "Georgia's Forgotten Industry, Part II," 223.

240. Wanderer, "From the Up-Country," *Southern Watchman* (Athens), 4 Aug. 1869.

241. Cain, *History of Lumpkin County*, 191; "Historical Markers—Trahlyta's Grave," http://dahlonega.org/tours-a-scenic-drives-2/historical-markers; Pine, "Uncovering Trahlyta, 18–25.

242. Walton, *Mineral Springs of the United States*, 336; Cain, 190. Walton lists the "Bethesda Hotel" as the lodging available at Bethesda Springs, a little used name for Porter Springs. No research uncovered any other usage of this name although Cain states that it was infrequently used in the resort's early years.

243. Wanderer, "From the Up-Country."

244. Ibid.

245. "New Fountain of Health," *Weekly Georgia Telegraph* (Macon), 25 June 1869.

246. W.H. McA., "North East Georgia," *Weekly Sun* (Atlanta), 10 June 1873.

247. M.P.C., "The Lumpkin Springs," *Southern Watchman* (Athens), 4 Aug. 1869; Cain, 199.

248. W.H. McA., "North East Georgia."

249. "Proceedings of the Georgia Legislature," 20 Aug. 1872.

250. Johnny Vardeman, "'Ghost Town' Health Resort in Lumpkin County Drew Crowds," *Gainesville Times*, https://www.gainesvilletimes.com/columnists/johnny-vardemans-column/ghost-town-health-resort-in-lumpkin-county-drew-crowds/; *Savannah Morning News*, 24 Oct. 1874; "Col. H. P. Farrow Dead," *Gainesville News*, 13 Feb. 1907; *Gainesville News*, 29 Mar. 1905; Cain, 200, 202.

251. *Gainesville: The Great Health Resort of the South*, 33–34; Cain, 203; Albert S. Hardy, "In North Georgia. A Visit to That Delightful Resort: Porter Springs, 'Queen of the Mountains,'" *Barnesville Gazette*, 12 Sept. 1895.

252. "Porter Springs, Lumpkin County, Georgia [ad]," *Savannah Morning News*, 16 May 1876.

253. "Porter Springs, Near Dahlonega, Ga. [ad]," *Ibid.*, 19 May 1875; Porter Springs [ad]," *Ibid.*, 9 May 1879; "In North Georgia"; "Porter Springs [ad]," *Ibid.*, 9 May 1879; "Porter Springs, Georgia [ad]," *Ibid.*, 25 May 1877.

254. "In North Georgia."

255. Ibid.

256. "Porter Springs [ad]," *Morning News* (Savannah), 28 June 1889.

257. Hardy, "In North Georgia"; *Gainesville News*, 29 Mar. 1905; *Dahlonega Nugget*, 3 Mar. 1905.

258. M.T.D., "Porter Springs," *Advertiser and Appeal* (Brunswick), 23 June 1883.

259. E.R. Callaway and Mrs. S.P.C., "Letter from Porter Springs," *La Grange Reporter*, 13 Aug. 1897.

260. *Gainesville: The Great Health Resort of the South*, 33.

261. "New Holland Springs (Near Gainesville, Georgia) [ad]," *Washington Gazette* (GA), 18 Aug. 1875; "Porter Springs, Near Dahlonega, GA. [ad]," *Savannah Morning News*, 19 May 1875.

262. "Away to the Mountains! Grand Opening of the Piedmont Hotel, Gainesville, Georgia [ad]," *Macon Telegraph and Messenger*, 8 June 1876; "Porter Springs, Lumpkin County, Georgia [ad]," *Savannah Morning News*, 16 May 1876; "Porter Springs and Piedmont Hotel," *Macon Telegraph and Messenger*, 1 June 1878.

263. M.T.D., "A Voice from the Mountains," *Brunswick Advertiser*, 30 Oct. 1880.

264. "Porter's Springs [ad]," *Southern Watchman* (Athens), 16 July 1873.

265. O.M., "Porter Springs. The Impressions of a Thomasville Young Lady."

266. "Editorial Correspondence: Letter III., Porter Springs, Ga., August 21, 1883," *Advertiser and Appeal* (Brunswick), 8 Sept. 1883.

267. L., "A Trip to the Mountains," *Forest News* (Jefferson, GA), 28 Aug. 1875.

268. "Further from Dahlonega. What 'Specs' Has to Say," *Atlanta Daily Herald*, 12 July 1873; *Telegraph and Messenger* (Macon), 24 Aug. 1873; "The General and His Young Bride," *Brunswick Times*, 9 Sept. 1892.

269. "Porter Springs, Near Dahlonega, GA. [ad]," *Savannah Morning News*, 19 May 1875.

270. Cain, *History of Lumpkin County*, 190, 192–93.

271. Ads publicizing onsite physicians were located periodically from 1879 through 1898. See,

for example, "Porter Springs [ad]," *Macon Telegraph and Messenger*, 11 June 1879; "Queen of the Mountains. Porter Springs[ad]," *Georgia Cracker*, 18 June 1898.

272. "Porter Springs," *Advertiser and Appeal* (Brunswick), 17 May 1884. No further information on the sanitarium has been located.

273. Ed. Republican, "Porter Springs," *Weekly Sumter Republican* (Americus), 16 May 1884.

274. A.S. Hardy, "Nature's Own Retreat: Such is Porter Springs—"Queen of the Mountains," *Barnesville Gazette*, 13 Sept. 1894.

275. E.R. Callaway and Mrs. S.P.C., "Letter from Porter Springs," *La Grange Reporter* (GA), 13 Aug. 1897.

276. O.M., "Porter Springs. The Impressions of a Thomasville Young Lady."

277. "In North Georgia.

278. Wanderer, "From the Up-Country"; "A Strange Land and a Peculiar People," 429–38.

279. "In North Georgia."

280. R., "The Up Country. Summer Resorts of Georgia—A Pleasant Land and a Spicy Letter," *Savannah Morning News*, 25 July 1877. The English in colonial America and in England by the 1760s were using the term "cracker" for back country Scots-Irish settlers in the South. One definition evolved to mean a poor rural South Georgian or North Floridian. For more on the etymology, see John A. Burrison, "Crackers," in *New Georgia Encyclopedia*, updated Aug. 6, 2013, https://www.georgiaencyclopedia.org/articles/arts-culture/crackers/.

281. O.M., "Porter Springs. The Impressions of a Thomasville Young Lady."

282. The Georgia Cracker, "Porter Springs: The Queen of the Mountains," *La Grange Reporter*, 13 Oct. 1899.

283. *Ibid*. Farrow may have chosen the nickname, "Queen of the Mountains," in response to Tallulah Falls Hotel's branding as "King of the Mountains" or to Gainesville's title as "Queen City of the Mountains. For examples of Tallulah and Gainesville's branding, see, for example, "The King of the Mountains, 3182 Feet Above the Sea [ad]," *Macon Telegraph and Messenger*, 19 June 1879 and Cousin Annie, "Letter from Cousin Annie: Gainesville—Its Present and Future Prospects—Entertainment for the Fever Sufferers," *Savannah Morning News*, 25 Sept. 1878.

284. Amerson, "Joseph Whitner," 225.

285. *Dahlonega Nugget*, 14 July 1922; *Ibid*., 24 Apr. 1925.

286. Amerson, "Porter Springs," 124; Amerson, "Joseph Whitner," 230.

287. "Auction [ad]," *Dawson County Advertiser*, 18 Nov. 1960; "'Ghost Town' Health Resort."

Rowland Springs

288. Cunyus, *History of Bartow County*, 177; Croft, "Geology and Ground-Water," FF2-FF3.

289. Cunyus, 177; "Bartow County, Georgia: Geography and Climate," https://www.bartowcountyga.gov/departments/government/geography_and_climate/index.php.

290. "Bartow County, Georgia: Geography and Climate"; William J. Frazier, "Geologic Regions of Georgia: Overview," in *New Georgia Encyclopedia*, updated Mar. 7, 2022, https://www.georgiaencyclopedia.org/articles/science-medicine/geologic-regions-georgia-overview; Croft, FF3.

291. Cunyus, 21, 33–35; "Biographies of the Secretaries of State: Lewis Cass (1782–1866)," https://history.state.gov/departmenthistory/people/cass-lewis; Chantel Parker, "Bartow County," in *New Georgia Encyclopedia*, updated June 8, 2022, https://www.georgiaencyclopedia.org/articles/counties-cities-neighborhoods/bartow-county/.

292. Cunyus, 3, 12–13; Hébert, "Civil War and Reconstruction Era, 24.

293. Cunyus, 14, 17, 101, 180.

294. *Ibid*., 89; Livingston, *Circular*, 267.

295. R., "Correspondence of the Daily Morning News: Rowland Springs, Ga., Aug. 29, 1855," *Daily Morning News* (Savannah), 1 Sept. 1855.

296. *Ibid*.

297. Cunyus, 273, 329–337. Cunyus published an abbreviated form of the 1840 Cass County Census in her book. Of about 1,200 households in the county, probably one third owned enslaved persons. Most of the 400 households owned only a few.

298. Cunyus, 273; Wilma Dunaway, "Slavery and Emancipation in the Mountain South: Sources, Evidence, Methods," Table 1.9, "Twenty-Five of Southern Appalachia's Richest Planters," https://scholar.lib.vt.edu/faculty_archives/mountain_slavery/1tab.pdf.

299. White, *Historical Collections of Georgia*, 299; Livingston, 267. White gives the year as 1843; Livingston, as 1840.

300. Rambler, "Miscellany. For the Times. A Ramble in North-Western Georgia," *Columbus Times* (GA), 29 Dec. 1846.

301. G., "Rowland Springs, Cass County, Sept. 10th, 1846," *Savannah Daily Republican*, 18 Sept. 1846.

302. "Rowland Springs, Cass County [ad]," *Daily Georgian* (Savannah), 7 May 1847; "Rowland's Springs, Cass County, Ga. [ad]," *Daily Constitutionalist* (Augusta), 21 July 1847.

303. "Summer Resorts," *Savannah Georgian*, 7 June 1848; "Rowland Springs," *Georgia Journal and Messenger* (Macon), 17 May 1848.

304. Rowland Springs, Cass County [ad]"; Macon, "To the Editors of the *Journal & Mercury*," *Georgia Journal and Messenger* (Macon), 26 May 1847; A Visitor, "The Rowland Springs," *Savannah Daily Republican*, 31 July 1847.

305. "Summer Resorts," *Savannah Georgian*, 7 June 1848.

306. "The Rowland Springs," *Georgia Journal and Messenger* (Macon), 14 Aug. 1850.

307. G., "Rowland Springs, Cass County, Sept. 10, 1846."

308. "Rowland Springs, Cass Co., August 16th,

1850," *Southern Recorder* (Milledgeville), 27 Aug. 1850.
309. "Rowland's Springs, Cass county [sic], August 14th, 1848," *Ibid.*, 22 Aug. 1848.
310. Clark, *Memoirs of Judge Richard H. Clark*, 205.
311. "St. Lanier & Son. [ad]," *Georgia Journal and Messenger* (Macon), 2 Aug. 1848.
312. "Rowland's Springs," *Daily Constitutionalist* (Augusta), 15 June 1848.
313. S.T.C., "Editorial Correspondence of the *Macon Journal & Messenger*: Rowland Springs, August 24th," *Daily Chronicle & Sentinel* (Augusta), 3 Sept. 1849.
314. "Rowland Spring Fancy Ball," *Milledgeville Federal Union*, 21 Aug. 1849.
315. "Correspondence of the Recorder. Rowland Springs, Cass Co. August 16th. 1850," *Southern Recorder* (Milledgeville), 27 Aug. 1850.
316. T., "Rowland's Springs, Cass county [sic], August 14th, 1848," *Southern Recorder* (Milledgeville), 22 Aug. 1848.
317. "Correspondence of the Recorder. Rowland Springs, Cass Co. August 16th. 1850," *Ibid.*, 27 Aug. 1850.
318. "Classical Boarding School [ad]," *Ibid.*, 3 Nov. 1846; Cunyus, 139.
319. B., "Cassville, Aug. 10, 1850," *Albany Patriot* (GA), 16 Aug. 1850. See also "Rowland's Springs," *Columbus Times* (GA), 25 July 1848.
320. "(From the Charleston Mercury, 10th inst.) Rowland's Springs," *Daily Georgian* (Savannah), 12 June 1847.
321. "Enon Ala. August 8th. 1851," *Columbus Times* (GA), 19 Aug. 1851.
322. Cunyus, 178.
323. C., "Rowland's Springs, Aug. 17, 1847," *Georgia Journal and Messenger* (Macon), 25 Aug. 1847.
324. "Rowland Springs, Cass Co., Aug. 24, 1850," *Southern Recorder* (Milledgeville), 3 Sept. 1850.
325. C., "Dalton, Aug. 17, 1847," *Federal Union* (Milledgeville), 24 Aug. 1847.
326. *Ibid.*; *Daily Chronicle & Sentinel* (Augusta), 23 July 1850.
327. "Rowland Springs, Sept. 2, 1851," *Columbus Times* (GA), 9 Sept. 1851.
328. T., "Rowland's Springs, Cass county [sic], August 14th, 1848," *Southern Recorder* (Milledgeville), 22 Aug. 1848.
329. Parks, *Joseph E. Brown of Georgia*, 84, 106–07.
330. "Gov. Brown and his Secretary," *Georgia Citizen* (Macon), 9 Sept. 1859; "[From the Federal Union.] Gov. Brown, Col. Waters and the Cassville Meeting," *Atlanta Weekly Intelligencer*, 2 June 1859.
331. Wright and Wheeler, "New Men in the Old South," 380.
332. *Ibid.*, 385; Cunyus, 89.
333. "Rowland Springs for Sale [ad]," *Memphis Daily Appeal*, 8 Sept. 1863; "Rowland Springs for Sale [ad]," *Atlanta Daily Intelligencer*, 11 Sept. 1863; Hébert, 131–32.
334. "Obituary," *Daily Morning News* (Savannah), 3 Oct. 1863.
335. *Atlanta Constitution*, 3 June 1870; *Daily Columbus Enquirer* (GA), 20 May 1873. Research did not uncover additional information about ownership in the early 1870s.
336. Paul, "The State Road," *Weekly Constitution* (Atlanta), 27 July 1875.
337. "Rowland Springs: Rowland Springs Hygienic Institute," *Atlanta Daily Constitution*, 15 Jan. 1878.
338. "Atlanta Health Institute (Electrical Movement and Water Cure [ad])," *Atlanta Constitution*, 19 Feb. 1879.
339. Hébert, 307.
340. "Sheltering Arms Orphans Safe at Summer Home; Matron Thanks Friends," *Atlanta Georgian and News* 26 July 1907; "Sheltering Arms Tots Happy in Fresh Air," *Ibid.*, 6 Aug 1907.
341. McCallie, *Preliminary Report of the Mineral Springs of Georgia* (1913), 138; Jolly, "Old Rowland Springs Resort," 3.
342. Jolly, 4.
343. "Rowland Springs Land Near Cartersville Is Acquired by Floridian," *Atlanta Constitution* 20 Dec. 1925.
344. Jolly, 3.
345. Etowah Valley Historical Society, "Rowland Springs," Historical Marker Database, https://www.hmdb.org/m.asp?m=70986.

Kentucky

Introduction

1. Kentucky Geologic Survey and the University of Kentucky, "The Eastern Kentucky Coal Field," https://www.uky.edu/KGS/geoky/regioneastern.htm.
2. Rennick, *Kentucky Place Names*, 60.
3. Kentucky Geologic Survey and the University of Kentucky, "Physiographic Map of Kentucky," https://www.uky.edu/KGS/geoky/physiographic.htm.
4. Coleman, "Old Kentucky Watering Places," 13, 20.
5. *Mineral Waters of the United States and Their Therapeutic Uses*, 251.
6. *Appletons'* (1857), 323.
7. Coleman, *Springs of Kentucky*, 48; "Old Kentucky Watering Places," 17.
8. *Springs of Kentucky*, 67–68.
9. *Ibid.*, 81.
10. *Ibid.*, 13.
11. Estill Development Alliance, "Green Clay"; U.S. Population Census 1860; U.S. Population Census 1850; U.S. Census 1850 (Slave Schedule), all Census records accessed at FamilySearch, www.familysearch.org.

Lewis County: Esculapia and Glen Springs

12. Kentucky Atlas & Gazatteer, "Lewis County," https://www.kyatlas.com/21135.html; Kentucky Geologic Survey and the University of Kentucky, "Lewis County: Topography," http://www.uky.edu/KGS/water/library/gwatlas/Lewis/Topography.htm.
13. Talley, "Salt Lick Creek and Its Salt Works," 85, 90–91; Talley and Franke, *Lewis County*, 7–8.
14. Kentucky Geological Survey, *Report of the Progress*, 101; "Time's Changes," *News-Herald* (Hillsboro, Ohio), 13 June 1895; "Opening of Glen Sulphur Hotel," *Maysville Evening Bulletin* (KY), 2 Sept. 1889.
15. Ragan, *History of Lewis County*, 17, 324; "Mrs. Lavina Virginia Davis," *Daily Public Ledger* (Maysville, KY), 5 Oct. 1912.
16. Ragan, 24, 271, 291.
17. *Ibid.*, 265; U.S. Population Census 1850, FamilySearch, www.familysearch.org. Subsequent Census records were accessed at FamilySearch.
18. Baldwin and J. Thomas, *New and Complete Gazetteer*, 636; Marla Toncray, "Lewis County—A Land of Virgin Forests and Pure, Sparkling Streams," *Ledger Independent* (Maysville, KY), 21 Sept. 2012, https://maysville-online.com/features/117917/lewis-county-a-land-of-virgin-forests-and-pure-sparkling-streams.
19. U.S. Population Census 1850; U.S. Census, *Kentucky Agricultural Schedule* 1850; Williamson, "Seven Ways." The CPI calculator was used for all dollar conversions in this chapter.
20. U.S. Population Census 1850; Ragan, 41, 79.
21. Beale, *Marcus T.C. Gould, Stenographer*, 38, 45–46.
22. "Lewis County, Kentucky [ad]," *Louisville Journal*, 7 June 1842; Coleman, *Springs of Kentucky*, 53.
23. *Springs of Kentucky*, 53; Ragan, 154; University of Maryland, *Esculapia: or the White Sulphur and Chalybeate Springs*, 20; Esculapia," *Morning Courier* (Louisville), 26 May 1847; "Esculapia," *Ibid.*, 1 June 1848. Coleman gives the date of incorporation as 1846; Ragan, Jan. 1849.
24. Ragan, 154.
25. U.S. Census 1850 (Slave Schedule). Lewis County in the early 1850s had a population of 7,202, of whom 322 were enslaved persons. See Baldwin and Thomas, *A New and Complete Gazetteer*, 598.
26. Collins, *Collins' Historical Sketches of Kentucky*, 465.
27. Baldwin and Thomas, *A New and Complete Gazetteer*, 598.
28. Collins, np before 465; *Esculapia: or the White Sulphur and Chalybeate Springs*, 6–7.
29. "Lewis County, Kentucky [ad]," *Louisville Journal*, 7 June 1842; *Esculapia: or the White Sulphur and Chalybeate Springs*, 10, np before 16.
30. *Esculapia: or the White Sulphur and Chalybeate Springs*, 7, 18–19.
31. *Ibid.*, 20–21.
32. *Ibid.*, np following 11; *Springs of Kentucky*, 53.
33. *Ibid.*, np before 16; Katie Crawford-Lackey, "General James Taylor Home," accessed Apr. 27, 2022, https://explorekyhistory.ky.gov/items/show/525.
34. "A 'Bar' Fight," *Evening Bulletin* (Maysville, KY), 25 Jan. 1890.
35. *Esculapia: or the White Sulphur and Chalybeate Springs*, 9, 11.
36. *Ibid.*, 21; Ragan, 154, 369.
37. "Esculapia [ad]," *Morning Courier* (Louisville), 26 July 1847.
38. John Klee, "Maysville," in *The Encyclopedia of Northern Kentucky*, eds., Paul A. Tenkotte and James C. Claypool (Lexington: University Press of Kentucky, 2009), 595.
39. Ohio History Connection, "Cholera Epidemics," in Ohio History Central, https://ohiohistorycentral.org/w/Cholera_Epidemics.
40. *Louisville Daily Courier*, 24 July 1850; "Cholera at Esculapia," *Southern Press* (Washington, D.C.), 29 July 1850.
41. Beale, 47; "Mr. Dixon's Health," *Louisville Daily Courier*, 2 Aug. 1851; Ragan, 17.
42. Ron D. Bryant, "Lewis County," in *Kentucky Encyclopedia*, ed. John E. Kleber, 549.
43. Toncray, "Lewis County"; *Daily Tribune* (Winfield, KS), 28 Nov. 1886.
44. U.S. Population Census 1870; Williamson, "Seven Ways."
45. "Esculapia Springs [ad]," *Greenville Journal* (Ohio), 28 Aug. 1879; *Courier-Journal* (Louisville), 8 July 1882.
46. "The Best and the Cheapest: Esculapia Springs [ad]," *Daily American* (Nashville), 25 June 1881.
47. *Evening Bulletin* (Maysville, KY), 14 May 1886; U.S. Population Census 1880.
48. *Daily Tribune* (Winfield, KS), 28 Nov. 1886.
49. *Evening Bulletin* (Maysville, KY), 24 July 1886.
50. *American Israelite* (Cincinnati), 13 July 1888; *Evening Bulletin* (Maysville, KY), 26 Aug. 1885.
51. *Evening Bulletin* (Maysville, KY), 24 July 1886; *Ibid.*, 21 July 1891.
52. *Ibid.*, 12 Mar. 1892.
53. "Esculapia," *Ibid.*, 27 Sept. 1892; *Ibid.*, 28 Sept. 1892; *Ibid.*, 5 Dec. 1892.
54. "Litigating Landlords," *Cincinnati Tribune*, 21 Jan. 1893; *Ibid.*, 25 Jan. 1893; *Cincinnati Commercial Gazette*, 25 Jan. 1893.
55. *Evening Bulletin* (Maysville, KY), 28 Mar. 1893; Jack Wessling, "Washington, George, Jr.," in *Encyclopedia of Northern Kentucky*; [no author] "Nelson, Robert W., " in *Encyclopedia of Northern Kentucky*, 647.
56. "Tragedy," *Lexington Leader*, 16 Aug. 1905; "Beach Gives Up; Trial Goes On At Once," *Cincinnati Post*, 20 Jan. 1906; "Dr. Charles Beach Acquitted of Murder," *Courier-Journal* (Louisville), 7 Oct. 1906.

57. Talley and Franke, 9; "Time's Changes," *News-Herald* (Hillsboro, Ohio), 13 June 1895; Barrett, "Lewis County," 118.

58. "Glenn Springs," *Evening Bulletin* (Maysville, KY), 15 July 1890; X., "Glen Springs," *Ibid.*, 19 Aug. 1890; "Glen Springs Hotel, Lewis County, KY. [ad]," *Herald and Presbyter* (Cincinnati), 3 July 1895.

59. "Opening of Glen Sulphur Hotel," *Maysville Evening Bulletin* (KY), 2 Sept. 1889; "Summer Resort for Sale to Settle Estate [ad]," *Cincinnati Enquirer*, 4 May 1913; U.S. Population Census 1880; "From Glen Springs," *Daily Public Ledger* (Maysville, KY), 10 Aug. 1897. I.N. Walker himself died in 1900.

60. "Glenn Springs," *Evening Bulletin* (Maysville, KY), 15 July 1890.

61. X., "Glen Springs," *Ibid.*, 19 Aug. 1890; "Glen Springs, Lewis County," *Daily Public Ledger* (Maysville, KY), 30 June 1894; "Glen Springs Hotel, Lewis County, KY. [ad]," *Herald and Presbyter* (Cincinnati), 3 July 1895.

62. Walter Pluckard, "Mineral Memories: Lewis County's Spas Sign of Yesteryear," *Portsmouth Times* (Ohio), 9 Sept. 1961; "Summer Resort for Sale to Settle Estate [ad]," *Cincinnati Enquirer*, 4 May 1913.

63. X., "Glen Springs"; "Glen Springs Hotel, Lewis County, KY. [ad]," *Herald and Presbyter* (Cincinnati), 3 July 1895.

64. X., "Glen Springs."

65. "A Good Joke," *Evening Bulletin* (Maysville, KY), 4 Sept. 1896.

66. "Time's Changes," *News-Herald* (Hillsboro, Ohio), 13 June 1895; *Evening Bulletin* (Maysville, KY) ,26 Aug. 1898; *Ibid.*, 14 July 1886; *Ibid.*, 18 June 1892.

67. Ruggles was founded in 1873 and is today affiliated with the United Methodist Church as a retreat center and camp. See "Ruggles Camp & Retreat Center," https://www.rugglescamp.org/.

68. "At Ruggles Camp-Meeting," *Daily Public Ledger* (Maysville, KY), 6 Aug. 1892; *Ibid.*, 30 July 1897.

69. "The Best and the Cheapest: Esculapia Springs [ad]," *Daily American* (Nashville), 25 June 1881; "Clen [sic] Springs," *Evening Bulletin* (Maysville, KY), 10 July 1894.

70. "Glen Springs Hotel, Lewis County, KY. [ad]," *Herald and Presbyter* (Cincinnati), 3 July 1895.

71. *News-Herald* (Hillsboro, Ohio), 2 Aug. 1894; *Evening Bulletin* (Maysville, KY), 27 June 1895.

72. "Go to Glen Springs," *Daily Public Ledger* (Maysville, KY), 28 June 1892; *Evening Bulletin* (Maysville, KY), 5 July 1893; *Daily Public Ledger* (Maysville, KY), 17 June 1892.

73. "Esculapia Springs Is Sold By Dr. C.E. [sic] Beach," *Portsmouth Daily Times* (Ohio), 4 Feb. 1910; "Esculapia Springs Burn," *Lexington Leader*, 9 Aug. 1912.

74. "May Build Baptist Academy," *Public Ledger* (Maysville, KY), 2 Sept. 1916; "Glenn Springs College," *Public Ledger* (Maysville, KY), 26 Jan. 1917; "Recent Fires and Their Lessons," *Safety Engineering* 35 (Apr. 1918): 253.

75. Kentucky Historical Society and Kentucky Dept. of Highways, "Esculapia Springs," Historical Marker Database, https://www.hmdb.org/m.asp?m=146849.

Estill Springs

76. University of Kentucky, Kentucky Geological Survey, "Estill County: Topography," http://www.uky.edu/KGS/water/library/gwatlas/Estill/Topography.htm; "Estill Springs," *Louisville Daily Courier*, 27 Aug. 1853.

77. "Estill County KY Peaks List," www.listsofjohn.com.

78. USDA, *Soil Survey of Estill and Lee Counties*, 3–4.

79. "Estill Springs," in *Kentucky Encyclopedia*, ed. John B. Kiener, 299; Ron D. Bryant, "Estill County," *Ibid.*, 298.

80. Ellwanger, "Estill Springs," 45; USDA, 2; Kentucky Historical Society and Kentucky Dept. of Highways, "Estill Springs," Historical Marker Database, https://www.hmdb.org/m.asp?m=136947, hereafter cited as HMD; Thomas Dwaine Riddell, "Estill Springs Hotel—That Grand Old Hotel of the 1800s," *Lexington Herald*, 26 Dec. 1968. Riddell supplied the McAfee quote. Ellwanger was a KY newspaper woman who served as hostess at Estill Springs in 1910. See "Mrs. Ellwanger at Estill," *Cloverport Breckenridge News* (Cloverport, KY), 13 July 1910.

81. Sources that provide a year of establishment give the year anywhere from 1800 to 1814.

82. Estill Development Alliance, "Green Clay"; Harrison, "The Anti-Slavery Career of Cassius M. Clay," 296, 298.

83. "Green Clay"; Hugh, "Letter from Estill Springs," *Louisville Daily Courier*, 21 Aug. 1854.

84. "Estill Springs," HMD; "Estill Springs," *Kentucky Encyclopedia*, 299; Dunn, "Gen. Green Clay in Fayette County Records," 147; "Old Kentucky Watering Places," 7n35. Coleman supplied the quotation on the hotel description from an 1814 Lexington newspaper.

85. Ellwanger, 45; "Green Clay"; Riddell, "Estill Springs Hotel"; "Estill Springs [ad]," *Louisville Morning Courier*, 5 June 1850; U.S. Population Census 1850, FamilySearch, www.familysearch.org; subsequent census citations in this chapter are from FamilySearch.

86. "Estill Springs," *Kentucky Encyclopedia*, 299; U.S. Population Census 1850.

87. Riddell, "Estill Springs Hotel"; "Estill Springs [ad]," *Louisville Morning Courier*, 5 June 1850; Ellwanger, 43.

88. U.S. Population Census 1850; Williamson, "Seven Ways." The CPI calculator was used.

89. Hugh, "Letter from Estill Springs."

90. Collins, *Collins' Historical Sketches of Kentucky*, 167.

91. *Ibid.*; Amicitia, "From Estill County," *Interior Journal* (Stanford, KY), 8 Aug. 1873; The Filson Historical Society Manuscript Database, "Shelby-Bruen Family. Papers, 1761–1916: Content," https://filsonhistorical.org/vcc/card/?id=fec3c81ba017e2af77deb6d017328751.
92. "Shelby-Bruen Family Papers, Content."
93. Mrs. Joe Ohr. Jr., "Estill Springs is a Spot of Beauty, *Lexington Herald-Leader*, 15 Jan. 1956.
94. Matson, *Water Resources of the Blue Grass Region*, 206; Collins, 167.
95. "Shelby-Bruen Family Papers, Content"; "Estill Springs [ad]," *Louisville Daily Courier*, 26 May 1853; *Louisville Daily Courier*, 9 Aug. 1852; "Louisville Beauties Abroad," *Louisville Daily Courier*, 25 Aug. 1855.
96. Ellwanger, 45; "Shelby-Bruen Family Papers, Content"; Hugh, "Letter from Estill Springs."
97. Hugh, "Letter from Estill Springs"; "Correspondence from Estill Springs," *Bourbon News* (Paris, KY), 3 Aug. 1897.
98. Hugh, "Letter from Estill Springs"; "Estill Springs [ad]," *Louisville Daily Courier*, 26 May 1853.
99. Ellwanger, 45; *Louisville Morning Courier*, 14 Aug. 1851; "Health of Mr. Clay," *Daily Chronicle & Sentinel* (Augusta, GA), 14 Aug. 1848.
100. *Louisville Daily Journal*, 30 Aug. 1852.
101. "Estill Springs [ad]," *Louisville Daily Courier*, 27 Aug. 1853; Hugh, "Letter from Estill Springs"; Ellwanger, 45.
102. "Railroads. Through Tickets to Cincinnati [ad]," *Louisville Daily Courier*, 10 Aug. 1855; "Estill Springs," *Ibid.*, 18 July 1855; Hugh, "Letter from Estill Springs."
103. "Estill Springs [ad]," *Louisville Morning Courier*, 5 June 1850; "Estill Springs [ad]," *Louisville Daily Journal*, 25 May 1858; "Estill Springs," *Louisville Daily Courier*, 18 July 1855.
104. Riddell, "Estill Springs Hotel"; "Estill Springs [ad]," *Louisville Daily Journal*, 25 May 1858; *Ibid.*, 14 Oct. 1859.
105. Ellwanger, 50; Estill Development Alliance, "Sidney Barnes," accessed Mar. 12, 2022, https://www.estill.org/sidney-barnes.html; "Troops at Estill Springs," *Louisville Daily Journal*, 23 Nov. 1861; Dyer, *A Compendium of the War of the Rebellion*, 1202.
106. Estill Development Alliance, "Sidney Barnes."
107. *Ibid.*
108. *Big Sandy News* (Louisa, KY), 5 Jan. 1888; *Semi-Weekly Interior Journal* (Stanford, KY), 24 Jan. 1888; Riddell, "Estill Springs Hotel."
109. *Climax* (Richmond, KY), 19 Feb. 1890; "Estill Springs Board Reduced," *Ibid.*, 4 July 1888; *Bourbon News* (Paris, KY), 14 June 1898. The much higher price that Coleman-Bush paid compared to the 1888 transactions may indicate the purchase of additional acreage, which they planned to develop.
110. "Estill Springs," *Climax* (Richmond, KY), 13 July 1887; "Estill Springs," *Ibid.*, 29 June 1887; *Ibid.*, 15 July 1896; *Frankfort Roundabout*, 29 June 1895.
111. *Climax* (Richmond, KY), 26 Sept. 1894.
112. "Y.M.C.A. Excursion [ad]," *Climax* (Richmond, KY), 10 June 1896; *Semi-Weekly Interior Journal* (Stanford, KY), 26 July 1895.
113. Amicitia, "From Estill County."
114. "Estill Springs [ad]," *Climax* (Richmond, KY), 3 June 1896; "How to Tell Her," *Bourbon News* (Paris, KY), 15 June 1900.
115. "Estill Springs [ad]," *Climax* (Richmond, KY), 3 June 1896.
116. "How to Tell Her."
117. *Bourbon News* (Millersburg, KY), 20 July 1883; "Estill Springs," *Louisville Daily Courier*, 27 Aug. 1853. The antebellum visitor reportedly was gaining a robust two pounds weekly.
118. *Evening Bulletin* (Maysville, KY), 23 June 1888; *Bourbon News* (Paris, KY), 26 July 1898.
119. *Semi-Weekly Interior Journal* (Stanford, KY), 7 July 1899; "How to Tell Her"; "Mr. Bryan Invited to Estill," *Bourbon News* (Paris, KY), 21 Dec. 1897. No source consulted mentions that Bryan visited the springs.
120. "Estill Springs Sold to Labe Riddell for $10,936.11," *Mount Sterling Advocate* (KY), 22 Feb. 1911; Riddell, "Estill Springs Hotel"; Ellwanger, 46.
121. Riddell, "Estill Springs Hotel"; Estill Development Alliance, "Lena R. White Wallace," https://www.estill.org/lena-r-white-wallace.html.

Pulaski County: Rockcastle Springs and Sublimity Springs

122. Kentucky Dept. of Fish and Wildlife Resources, "Rockcastle River," https://fw.ky.gov/Education/Pages/Rockcastle-River.aspx.
123. "Pleasure Jaunt to Rockcastle Springs Reveals Nature's Work, *Mountain-Echo*, 1 Sept. 1882," from *Louisville Commercial*," *London Sentinel Echo*, 12 Aug. 1954; Clark, *A History of Laurel County*, 264; Bill Mardis, "Bee Rock Campground Will Re-Open in 2021," *Commonwealth Journal* (Somerset, KY), 3 Apr. 2020, https://www.somerset-kentucky.com/news/bee-rock-campground-will-re-open-in-2021/article_d036d53c-7562-11ea-a88b-131601457cb3.html.
124. U.S. Forest Service, "Overview / Background: Ghost Resorts Along the Rockcastle."
125. Coleman, *Springs of Kentucky*, 60; "Overview / Background: Ghost Resorts Along the Rockcastle." Other sources consulted give the opening year based on postbellum resort letterhead or ads branded with the phrase "XXth season of Rockcastle Springs." For example, 1888 ads state that the resort is in its 48th season, thereby implying that the opening year is 1841. However, the letterhead and ads do not state that the resort was opened *continuously* since its establishment; its closing during the Civil War supports an earlier opening year than 1841.
126. "Rockcastle Springs [ad]," *Kentucky*

Tribune (Danville), 5 Aug. 1853; *Ibid.*, 2 June 1854.

127. "The Premium Springs of Kentucky [ad]," *Danville Weekly Kentucky Tribune*, 7 Sept. 1860; *Ibid.*, 8 Feb. 1861. Sources consulted provided no background information on Lear or McLean.

128. "In the Middle of the Great Cumberland Vacation Empire," *London Sentinel Echo* (KY), 12 Aug. 1954.

129. For background on Graham's ownership of Graham's Springs, see "Old Kentucky Watering Places," 7. For biographies of Graham, see "The Delightful Dr. Graham," *Kentucky Advocate Sunday Magazine* (Danville), 28 Sept. 1969; "Dr. C.C. Graham Dead," *Courier-Journal* (Louisville), 4 Feb. 1885. The *Kentucky Advocate* newspaper supplement article, however, erroneously considers Rockcastle Springs and Sublimity Springs to be the same health resort. Graham was not the inventor of Graham's flour as many sources state. Sylvester Graham, a New England minister and antebellum health reformer, innovated the coarsely ground whole wheat flour.

130. Stephenson, "Old Graham Springs, 34; Williamson, "Seven Ways." The CPI calculator was used.

131. Clark, *History*, 265.

132. "In the Middle of the Great Cumberland Vacation Empire."

133. Jan Sparkman, "Traces of Laurel: Early Resort Period," 23 Apr. 2014, *Sentinel-Echo* (London, KY), https://www.sentinel-echo.com/opinion/traces-of-laurel-early-resort-period/article_0c6aeab6-5aa1-5c57-a0b3-0c06546ca442.html; "Pleasure Jaunt to Rockcastle Springs Reveals Nature's Work"; Clark, "Sublimity Springs," 859; "From Wetmore's Battery," *Cleveland Morning Leader* (Ohio), 25 Feb. 1862.

134. "Traces of Laurel."

135. Brother William, "Sublimity Springs, Pulaski County, Kentucky, Feb. 3d, 1862," *Holmes County Republican* (Millersburg, Ohio), 20 Feb. 1862; "From Wetmore's Battery," *Cleveland Morning Leader* (Ohio), 25 Feb. 1862.

136. Clark, "Sublimity Springs," 859; U.S. Population Census 1860, FamilySearch, www.familysearch.org/; all Census records in this chapter accessed at FamilySearch. The 1860 census gives Campbell's occupation as "hotel keeper" in Pulaski County and lists Montrose as "Mountain Graham" in Campbell's household, perhaps a nickname or given as an irreverent remark to the census taker.

137. "An Act to Incorporate the Town of Sublimity, in Pulaski County," in *Acts of the General Assembly of the Commonwealth of Kentucky*, 175.

138. U.S. Population Census 1870.

139. "In the Middle of the Great Cumberland Vacation Empire."

140. *Semi-Weekly Interior Journal* (Stanford, KY), 24 July 1885.

141. "In the Middle of the Great Cumberland Vacation Empire"; "Death Comes to Col. Montrose Graham In His Mountain Home," *Sunday Leader* (Lexington), 26 Dec. 1897; W.O. McIntyre, "Memories of Dr. Christopher Columbus Graham," *Courier-Journal* (Louisville), 27 Dec. 1931.

142. "Death Comes to Col. Montrose Graham In His Mountain Home."

143. *Springs of Kentucky*, 24, 46.

144. "From Wetmore's Battery."

145. Clark, *History*, 264.

146. "Traces of Laurel."

147. "Traces of Laurel"; W.P.W., "Rock Castle Springs," *Semi-Weekly Interior Journal* (Stanford, KY), 24 July 1888.

148. Clark, *History*, 264.

149. "Sublimity Springs, Pulaski County, Kentucky, Feb. 3d, 1862."

150. "Fighting Them Over," *National Tribune* (Washington, D.C.), 26 Oct. 1899.

151. T.B. Linn, "London, Laurel Co., Ky., Feb. 7th, 1862," *Holmes County Republican* (Millersburg, Ohio), 20 Feb. 1862; "Sublimity Springs, Pulaski County, Kentucky, Feb. 3d, 1862."

152. "From Wetmore's Battery."

153. L.L.W., "The 16th Regiment," *Summit County Beacon* (Akron), 27 Feb. 1862.

154. "Sublimity Springs, Pulaski County, Kentucky, Feb. 3d, 1862."

155. "From Wetmore's Battery." Clark describes the unsatisfactory status of Kentucky education in the nineteenth century, commenting that a state system of schools was not established until 1849 and not funded fully until the twentieth century. See Clark, *History*, 145.

156. Allen, *History of Kentucky*, 322. Allen writes that Graham's establishment of a Sunday school at Sublimity attracted young boys from several miles away, some of whom Graham thought to be "among the brightest little fellows" he had met, appreciating any books given to them.

157. "Oil! Oil! Oil! [ad]," *Frankfort Commonwealth*, 14 Feb. 1865; "In the Middle of the Great Cumberland Vacation Empire."

158. "In the Middle of the Great Cumberland Vacation Empire"; "Sublimity Springs [ad]," *Courier-Journal* (Louisville), 5 June 1874.

159. "Sublimity Springs [ad]."

160. *Semi-Weekly Interior Journal* (Stanford, KY), 11 Oct. 1872; "Old Rockcastle Springs [ad]," *Kentucky Advocate* (Danville), 21 Apr. 1871.

161. "Old Rockcastle Springs [ad]," *Kentucky Advocate* (Danville), 21 Apr. 1871; "Old Rockcastle Springs [ad]," *Courier-Journal* (Louisville), 6 June 1881. The 1881 ad lists W.J. Lyons and the address for the Rockcastle Springs Co. Other ads for "Old Rockcastle Springs" provide similar information about management that discount the Sublimity Springs pseudonym tradition. In addition, some "Old Rockcastle Springs" ads were published after part of the Sublimity hotel had washed away.

162. "Old Rockcastle Springs [ad]," *Kentucky Advocate* (Danville), 21 Apr. 1871.

163. *Semi-Weekly Interior Journal* (Stanford, KY), 24 July 1874; "Rockcastle Springs for Sale," *Kentucky Advocate* (Danville), 29 May 1874.

164. "In the Middle of the Great Cumberland Vacation Empire"; W.P.W., "Rock Castle Springs." Some sources incorrectly list F.J. Campbell's name as "Flavius Josephus Campbell." Information to uncover F.J.'s full name and his tentative relationship to Josephus Campbell was established via research in newspapers, FindAGrave.com, and at FamilySearch. F.J,'s father's name was "John A. Campbell"; Josephus had a brother by the same name. See "Francis Josephus Campbell," FindAGrave.com, https://www.findagrave.com/memorial/61305955/francis-josephus-campbell; U.S. Population Census 1850; "Josephus Campbell Family Tree," FamilySearch, https://www.familysearch.org/tree/pedigree/landscape/K8ZL-D91; "Clair H. Campbell Dies," *Lexington Leader*, 12 June 1931.

165. "In the Middle of the Great Cumberland Vacation Empire"; "Kentucky's Model Health Resort [ad]," *Semi-Weekly Interior Journal* (Stanford, KY), 5 May 1885; "Sublimity, Rockcastle Springs Early Resorts," *Corbin Times Tribune* (KY), 7 Aug. 1993.

166. "Kentucky's Model Health Resort [ad]"; "In the Middle of the Great Cumberland Vacation Empire."

167. *Kentucky Tribune* (Danville), 2 June 1854; B., "From Rockcastle Springs," *Stanford Interior Journal* (KY), 9 Aug. 1872; "In the Middle of the Great Cumberland Vacation Empire."

168. *Semi-Weekly Interior Journal* (Stanford, KY), 18 May 1886; "Old Kentucky Watering Places," 22.

169. E.C.W., "Rock Castle Springs," *Semi-Weekly Interior Journal* (Stanford, KY), 16 July 1886.

170. Crook, *Mineral Waters of the United States*, 258; "Rock Castle Springs: Kentucky's Favorite Resort [ad]," *Climax* (Richmond, KY), 20 June 1894.

171. "Rock Castle Springs: Kentucky's Favorite Resort [ad]"; "Description and Analysis of Rock Castle Springs [ad]," *Semi-Weekly Interior Journal* (Stanford, KY), 5 May 1885.

172. *Semi-Weekly Interior Journal* (Stanford, KY), 1 Aug. 1882; "Pleasure Jaunt to Rockcastle Springs Reveals Nature's Work."

173. W.P.W., "Rock Castle Springs."

174. *Semi-Weekly Interior Journal* (Stanford, KY), 7 July 1885; E.C. Walton, B.M., "Rock Castle Springs," *Ibid.*, 21 July 1885.

175. W.P.W., "Rock Castle Springs"; L.P. McC., "Rock Castle Springs," *Central Record* (Lancaster, KY), 10 Aug. 1899; E.C.W., "Rock Castle Springs." For examples of visitors from Indiana, see *New Albany Ledger Standard* [IN], 23 July 1881; *Ibid.*, 16 July 1883; *Leavenworth Crawford County Democrat* (IN), 12 July 1877.

176. *Frankfort Tri Weekly Kentucky Yeoman*, 1 Aug. 1871; *Memphis Daily Appeal*, 18 Aug. 1873; *Semi-Weekly Interior Journal* (Stanford, KY), 24 April 1885; *Ibid.*, 18 Aug. 1896.

177. J.F.W., "Rock Castle Springs," *Semi-Weekly Interior Journal* (Stanford, KY), 17 July 1885.

178. *Ibid.*; W.P.W., "Rock Castle Springs."

179. "Rock Castle Springs," *Daily Leader* (Lexington), 13 June 1897.

180. "Mr. Morgan Sells Out," *Lexington Herald*, 21 July 1899; *Interior Journal* (Stanford, KY), 24 July 1908.

181. "In the Middle of the Great Cumberland Vacation Empire," *Sentinel-Echo* (London, KY), 12 Aug. 1954; *Semi-Weekly Interior Journal* (Stanford, Ky.), 6 Nov. 1900; *Danville News* (KY), 1 Feb. 1901.

182. *Cincinnati Commercial Tribune*, 14 Sept. 1913; "In the Middle of the Great Cumberland Vacation Empire"; *Courier-Journal* (Louisville), 30 July 1928.

183. "L.F. Hubble Dead," *Lexington Leader*, 10 Nov. 1922.

184. "Traces of Laurel"; "Famous Property Sold," *Courier-Journal* (Louisville), 28 Oct. 1912; "Pleasure Jaunt to Rockcastle Springs Reveals Nature's Works." Searching issues of the *Interior Journal* from 1878–1882 for local river flooding found several articles, but none spoke directly of Sublimity Springs. Therefore, the exact year cannot be pinpointed. For examples of articles found, see *Interior Journal* (Stanford, KY), 17 Jan. 1879; *Ibid.*, 20 Feb. 1880.

185. *Mount Vernon Signal* (KY), 8 Nov. 1912; "Famous Property," *Courier-Journal* (Louisville); "Famous Property Sold," *Lancaster Central Record* (KY), 1 Nov 1912. Both the Mount Vernon and Louisville newspapers used the phrase "Old Sublimity Springs," perhaps analogous to the use of "Old Rockcastle Springs" for Rockcastle Springs. The Lancaster newspaper stated that Sublimity Springs was sold "through" Hubble, implying that he was an agent, not directly the property owner.

186. "Overview / Background: Ghost Resorts Along the Rockcastle."

187. U.S. Forest Service, "Bee Rock Campground," https://www.fs.usda.gov/recarea/dbnf/recarea/?recid=39604; National Forest Foundation, "Daniel Boone National Forest: A Weeks Act Forest Profile," https://www.nationalforests.org/blog/daniel-boone-national-forest-profile.

188. Joe Creason, "The Glories of Kentucky Autumn," *Louisville Courier-Journal*, 4 Nov. 1956.

North Carolina

Introduction

1. Frances Tiernan, under the penname of Christian Reid, wrote *The Land of the Sky, Or Adventures in Mountain By-Ways* as a serialization in *Appleton's Journal* in 1875. For the importance of this work in promoting western North Carolina as a tourist destination, see Starnes, *Creating the Land of the Sky*, 37–42, and Martin, *Tourism in the Mountain South*, 50–51.

2. Blackmun, *Western North Carolina*, 202–03.

3. For the history of Hot Springs, see, for

example, Della Hazel Moore, *Hot Springs of North Carolina*, 2d ed. (Johnson City, TN: Overmountain Press, 2002); Milton Ready, *Mystical Madison: The History of a Mountain Region* (Lynn, NC: EverReady Publications, 2011), 128–38; C. Brenden Martin, "Hot Springs, North Carolina," in Ruby Abramson and Jean Haskell (eds.), *Encyclopedia of Appalachia* (Knoxville: The University of Tennessee Press, 2006), 650.

For a history of Sulphur Springs, see Virginia Gunn Fick and Richard D. Starnes, with additional research provided by David Stick, "Resorts, Part 2: Resorts of Western North Carolina," in *Encyclopedia of North Carolina*, ed. William S. Powell (Chapel Hill: University of North Carolina Press, 2006), NCPedia, https://www.ncpedia.org/resorts-part-2-resorts-western.

4. Brewster, *Summer Migrations*, 87. Warm Springs began in 1781 largely as a drover stand, a waystation for herders driving livestock and fowl from East Tennessee and Kentucky to markets in South Carolina and Georgia, but the hostelry also attracted invalids even before 1800. See William Lee Grissom, *History of Methodism in North Carolina: From 1772 to the Present Time, vol. 1: Introduction of Methodism in North Carolina to the year 1805* (Nashville: Publishing House of the Methodist Episcopal Church, South, 1905), 300; Brewster, *Summer Migrations*, 299–300.

5. "Sulphur Springs [ad]," *Highland Messenger* (Asheville), 28 Aug. 1840.

6. Starnes, *Creating the Land of the Sky*, 15.

7. Trencherman, "Piedmont Springs," *Raleigh News*, 1 Aug. 1879; "Piedmont Sulphur and Chalybeate Springs, Burke County, N.C. [ad]," *Western Democrat* (Charlotte), 15 July 1856.

8. Ruscin, *History of Transportation*, 91. For a full railroad timeline, see pp. 88–99.

9. *Ibid.*, 84–85.

10. Martin, *Tourism*, 29.

11. "Our Story: Estate History," https://www.biltmore.com/our-story/estate-history/.

12. Bishir, Southern, and Martin, *Guide to the Historic Architecture*, 356.

13. H.V.W., "Balsam Mountain, N.C.," *Birmingham News*, 16 Aug. 1905. The hotel, rebuilt in 1908 as a two-and-one-half story resort with Tuscan-columned double porches on each level, became known in 2019 as the Grand Old Lady Hotel. See Bishir, 357; WLOS staff, "At Grand Old Lady Hotel, Ghosts are Like Family," WLOS, https://wlos.com/news/local/at-grand-old-lady-hotel-ghostly-guests-are-like-family.

14. Jobe, *Mountaineer in Motion*, 134. No source consulted indicates that Jobe's vision succeeded; the Taylor spring remained undeveloped.

15. "Skyland Springs [ad]," *Daily Citizen* (Asheville), 28 Feb. 1890; Lindsey, *Lindsey's Guide Book*, 58.

16. Visitor, "Thompson's Spring," *Lenoir Topic*, 22 June 1887; "Mt. Airy White Sulphur Springs [ad]," *Western Sentinel* (Winston, NC), 23 July 1885.

17. "Mt. Airy White Sulphur Springs [ad]," *Wilmington Journal* (NC), 7 May 1875.

18. Mt. Airy White Sulphur Springs by 1914 enjoyed better transportation access, allowing for more pleasure-seekers. A society column for one week alone in 1914 described guests enjoyed bowling, card parties, boating, and dancing. See "White Sulphur Springs," *Greensboro Daily News*, 19 July 1914.

19. Starnes, *Creating the Land of the Sky*, 30; Van Noppen, *Western North Carolina*, 37, 39.

20. Starnes, *Creating the Land of the Sky*, 30.

21. *Ibid.*

22. H.V.W., "Balsam Mountain, N.C.," *Birmingham News*, 16 Aug. 1905; Edwin A. Curley, "The Pure Mountain Air," *Wichita Daily Eagle* (KS), 21 Feb. 1891; "In the Mountain Country," *Charlotte News*, 11 June 1906.

23. "The White Sulphur to Open," *Carolina Mountaineer and Waynesville Courier*, 13 Mar. 1919; "Waynesville, N.C.: Haywood White Sulphur Springs Hotel [ad]," *News and Observer* (Raleigh), 15 June 1919.

24. Phifer, "Slavery in Microcosm," 141–42; Federal Writers' Project: Slave Narrative Project, vol. 11, North Carolina, Part 1, Adams-Hunter, 1936, Manuscript/Mixed Material, "Interview with W.L. Bost," 139–41, https://www.loc.gov/item/mesn111/; "Negroes for Sale [ad]," *Raleigh Register and North-Carolina Gazette*, 7 July 1835. The ad gives the sale venue as an estate near Morganton in Burke County. Bost recounts a slave auction and slave coffle marches through Newton, about 30 miles east of Morganton.

25. U.S. Population Census 1860, U.S. Census 1860 (Slave Schedule), FamilySearch, www.familysearch.org/.

26. "The State Press Convention," *Western Sentinel* (Winston, NC), 12 July 1883; *Journal and Tribune* (Knoxville), 3 Aug. 1898.

27. "Will McNabb Was Killed," *Waynesville Courier* (NC), 23 July 1900.

28. Martin, 39.

29. *News and Observer* (Raleigh), 4 Apr. 1902; *Charlotte Home and Democrat*, 25 Dec. 1885; "Meet in Interest of Shatley Springs," *Ibid.*, 15 Jan. 1927; "Under Trustee's Right," *Charlotte Observer*, 23 Aug. 1927.

Ashe County: Healing Springs and Shatley Springs

30. David Perlmutt, "River Brings Clinton, Gore to a Corner of N.C.," *Charlotte Observer*, 30 July 1998. To read about the 14-year struggle by residents in Ashe, Alleghany, and Grayson counties to save the New River from a hydroelectric dam project that would have flooded 42K acres, see Thomas J. Schoenbaum, with a foreword by former senator Sam J. Ervin, Jr., *The New River Controversy* (Winston-Salem: John F. Blair, 1979). McFarland published a new edition of the book in 2007.

31. For a map of the New River and nearby

towns in North Carolina and for possible explanations on how the New River acquired its name, see Leland R. Cooper and Mary Lee Cooper, comps., *The People of the New River: Oral Histories from the Ashe, Alleghany and Watauga Counties of North Carolina*, Contributions to Southern Appalachian Studies, vol. 3 (Jefferson, NC: McFarland, 2001), 6–7.

32. Ed Anderson, "Famous Spas in North Carolina: Western North Carolina Mineral Springs Still Attract Thousands During Summer," *Charlotte Observer*, 23 July 1939.

33. "Another Pool of Siloam," *Anderson Intelligencer* (Anderson Court House, SC), 27 Oct. 1887; Warmuth, *Washington County*, 63; "Famous Spas,"; Guerrant, *Headquarters Diary*, 128.

34. "Famous Spas"; Williamson, "Seven Ways." The CPI calculator was used.

35. "Healing Springs," *Abingdon Weekly Virginian*, 22 Oct. 1885.

36. *Ibid.*; "Bethesda Healing Springs [ad]," *Lenoir Topic* (NC), 18 Nov. 1885; Bethany May, "Eureka Springs (Carroll County)," in *CALS Encyclopedia of Arkansas*, updated Jan. 29, 2024, https://encyclopediaofarkansas.net/entries/eureka-springs-843/.

37. *Abingdon Weekly Virginian*, 22 July 1886; *Lenoir Topic* (NC), 23 June 1886; *Danbury Reporter and Post* (NC), 14 Apr. 1887. North Carolina was also home to Healing Springs in Davidson County and All Healing Springs near King's Mountain in Gaston County. Virginia's Healing Springs in Bath County was one of the exclusive Virginia Springs. Therefore, pinpointing information salient to Ashe County's Healing Springs in regional newspapers presented challenges. The location of Bethesda Healing Water is not known; Thompson's water's popularity may have shut down the Bethesda Healing Water enterprise as no further information on it can be located.

38. "Famous Spas"; Grayson County, VA, Heritage Foundation, "A Wonderful Spring!"; U.S. Dept. of the Interior, NPS, National Register of Historic Places, "Thompson's Bromine and Arsenic Springs, 7. Description."

39. Visitor, "Thompson's Spring," *Lenoir Topic* (NC), 22 June 1887.

40. *Ibid.*

41. *Ibid.*

42. *Lenoir Topic* (NC), 22 June 1887; "A Wonderful Spring!"; Price, *Holston Methodism*, 179. The *Lenoir Topic* article detailing Thompson's sale ran separately from the "Visitor's" narrative in the same newspaper issue. Thompson's sale was convoluted: He sold a fourth interest in the property for $10 to a local physician, stipulating that the physician should sell the spring and bear all advertising expenses. The doctor sold for $4,000 and made a profit of $990.

43. Visitor, "Thompson's Spring."

44. "Famous Spas."

45. D.D.D., "A Trip Through Ashe," *Watauga Democrat* (NC), 5 Sept. 1889.

46. "A Trip Through Ashe"; Visitor, "Thompson's Spring."

47. Visitor, "Thompson's Spring"; Norfolk and Western, *Virginia Summer Resorts*, 37.

48. *Danbury Reporter and Post* (NC), 17 Feb. 1887; *Ibid.*, 14 Apr. 1887.

49. "A Trip Through Ashe"; "Famous Spas."

50. "That Water," *Columbus Enquirer-Sun* (GA), 3 Apr. 1887; "$4.65 [ad]," *Richmond Dispatch*, 10 June 1887.

51. "Why Take Patent Medicines For [ad]," *Atlanta Constitution*, 17 Apr. 1887.

52. *Danbury Reporter and Post* (NC), 14 Apr. 1887.

53. "Another Pool of Siloam: Thompson's Bromine-Arsenic Spring in Ashe County, N.C., Creating a Sensation, J.W. Hay in *New York World*," *Daily Times* (Richmond), 1 Dec. 1889.

54. "Eager for Its Healing Waters: North Carolina Mountaineers Wrought Up Over a Mineral Spring, From the *New York Sun*," *Morning News* (Savannah), 2 Feb. 1888.

55. "Eager for Its Healing Waters"; "Another Pool of Siloam."

56. "Thompson's Bromine and Arsenic Water," *Morning News* (Savannah), 31 Mar. 1889.

57. "At Our Mineral Water Depot [ad]," *Charlotte Chronicle*, 4 Apr. 1888.

58. Norfolk and Western, 38.

59. Critic, "That Wonderful Spring," *Sunny South* (Atlanta), 11 Aug. 1888.

60. Fletcher, *Ashe County*, 191, 297; "A Trip Through Ashe"; "Natures [sic] Greeting to the Afflicted [ad]," *Daily Times* (Richmond), 10 Oct. 1889.

61. Bud Phillips, "Abram Reynolds was a Builder and Developer in Bristol," *Bristol Herald Courier* (TN), 15 Jan. 2015, https://heraldcourier.com/news/abram-reynolds-was-a-builder-and-developer-in-bristol/article_5c7c4b48-9680-11e4-9993-3b4b8f8d0cc7.html; "Andrew L. Snapp [obituary]," *Bristol News Bulletin* (TN), 22 Mar. 1943.

62. "Fountain of Health! [ad]," *Norfolk Landmark* (VA), 23 May 1890; "Glad Tidings to the Afflicted," *Roanoke Daily Times* (VA), 16 Nov. 1889.

63. "Glad Tidings to the Afflicted."

64. "Water from the Bromine and Arsenic Springs to be Piped to Bristol," *Chattanooga Daily Times*, 24 July 1891.

65. *Washington Weekly Progress* (NC), 1 May 1888; "Thompson's is the Only Genuine [ad]," *Thomasville Times* (GA), 28 Dec. 1888.

66. "Thompson's is the Only Genuine."

67. "A Card," *Richmond Dispatch*, 17 Oct. 1889.

68. J.H. Mills, "A Healing Fountain," *State Chronicle* (Raleigh), 11 Oct. 1889.

69. *Comet* (Johnson City, TN), 14 Aug. 1890.

70. Fletcher, 94–95.

71. "Famous Spas."

72. *Ibid.*; Mills, "A Healing Fountain."

73. "Famous Spas"; Robert E. Lee Plummer Family Tree, FamilySearch, www.familysearch.org/.

74. "Thompson Bromine and Arsenic Springs, Continuation Sheet—Item Number 8—Page 2, National Register of Historic Places Inventory—Application Form; "Fire Destroys Healing Springs Resort Hotel," *Asheville Citizen-Times*, 26 Aug. 1962. The National Register application form lists several owners after George Palmer who are excluded by Anderson in "Famous Spas."

75. "The Cabins at Healing Springs," https://www.cabinsathealingsprings.com/.

76. "Our History," Shatley Springs Restaurant: Smiling Faces in Scenic Places, https://shatleysprings.com/our-history/; "Martin Shatley's Testimonial," *Ibid.*, https://shatleysprings.com/testimonial/.

77. "Our History."

78. "Ashe County Minerals," *Charlotte Sunday Observer*, 12 Aug. 1923; "Shatley Springs is Fast Becoming Large Resort," *Watauga Democrat* (NC), 1 July 1926; "Our History."

79. "Ashe County Minerals," *Charlotte Observer*, 12 Aug. 1923.

80. *News and Observer* (Raleigh), 29 Aug. 1925.

81. "Shatley Springs," *North Wilkesboro Hustler* (NC), 13 Jan. 1926.

82. Fletcher, 297–98; "Shatley Springs—Next to Purest Water in America," *North Wilkesboro Hustler* (NC), 9 June 1926; "Heritage," Froehling & Robertson, https://www.fandr.com/company/#heritage. Froehling & Robertson is still in practice today.

83. "Radium: A Medical Treatment in the Early Twentieth Century," Historical Medical Library of the College of Physicians of Philadelphia, https://histmed.collegeofphysicians.org/for-students/radium/; M.A. Buchholz and M. Cervera, Oak Ridge Institute for Science and Education, *Radium Historical Items Catalog, Final Report, 2008, Prepared for the U.S. Nuclear Regulatory Commission*, 31, 33, https://www.nrc.gov/docs/ML1008/ML100840118.pdf.

84. *Radium Historical Items Catalog*, 31.

85. "Shatley Springs—Next to Purest Water in America."

86. *Ibid.*

87. "Radium Springs Water: This Famous Water Can Now Be Purchased At All Good Drugstores [ad]," *Asheville Citizen*, 6 July 1927.

88. "Radium Springs Water: This Famous Water Can Now Be Purchased."

89. "Meet in Interest of Shatley Springs," *News and Observer* (Raleigh), 15 Jan. 1927; "Radium Springs Incorporated: Group Forms Firm to Develop Health Resort in Ashe County; Stock Held Here," *Charlotte Observer*, 22 Jan. 1927; "$2,000,000 Concern To Develop Shatley Springs," *Watauga Democrat* (NC), 20 Jan. 1927; Fletcher, 297.

90. "Radium Springs Incorporated"; "$2,000,000 Concern."

91. "Shatley Springs Sold Under Trustee's Right," *Charlotte Observer*, 23 Aug. 1927. More research is needed to determine why the venture faltered.

92. "Shatley Springs Distributing Co., Inc.," *Ibid.*, 22 Nov. 1930; "Improvements Under Way at Shatley Springs," *Watauga Democrat* (NC), 8 May 1930.

93. "Famous Spas"; "Our History"; "Resort in Ashe County to Open Saturday, May 13," *Asheville Citizen*, 29 Apr. 1939; "Mr. Collings [sic] Is At Shatley Springs," *Journal-Patriot* (North Wilkesboro, NC), 6 June 1949.

94. "Our History."

95. "Lee Allan Elliott, "Water Is the Main Attraction," *Charlotte Observer*, 27 Aug. 1967.

96. Adams, *Far Appalachia*, 35.

97. *Elkin Tribune* (NC), 21 Aug. 1930; *Ibid.*, 12 July 1934; *Journal-Patriot* (North Wilkesboro, NC), 16 July 1934; "Sands Community Club," *Watauga Democrat* (Boone, NC), 27 Aug. 1936; *Journal-Patriot* (North Wilkesboro, NC), 13 July 1942; "Shatley Springs is Open to the Public," *Ibid.*, 19 June 1944; *Ibid.*, 6 July 1933.

98. "Duke Alumni Banquet To Be Held at Shatley," *Watauga Democrat* (Boone, NC), 22 Aug. 1940; "Alumni To Meet in Sparta Aug. 22," *Ibid.*, 14 Aug. 1941; "Alumni of State to Hear Case 29th, *Journal-Patriot* (North Wilkesboro, NC), 25 Aug. 1949; "Hundreds to See White Top Event," *Kingsport Times* (TN), 14 Aug. 1940; "Congressman Doughton Will Address Editors," *Charlotte Observer*, 21 Aug. 1941; *Statesville Daily Record* (NC), 27 Aug. 1941; *Johnson City Press* (TN), 4 Jan. 1998.

99. "Good Food, Good Water At Old Resort," *Asheville Citizen-Times*, 1 Sept. 1989; "Water's 'Powers' Draw Multitudes to Shatley Springs," *Charlotte Observer*, 16 May 1981.

100. Larry Timbs, "Maybe It's in the Water (and the Good Food)," *Charlotte Observer*, 7 Sept. 1997.

Burke County: Piedmont Springs, Glen Alpine Springs, and Connelly Springs

101. Gerald R. Ford Library & Museum, "Sam Ervin (1896–1985)," The Watergate Files, https://www.fordlibrarymuseum.gov/museum/exhibits/watergate_files/content.php?section=2&page=b; Charles Perry," Sermon on the Hill: A Sam Erwin Sampler," *Rolling Stone*, 13 Sept. 1973, https://www.rollingstone.com/politics/politics-news/sermon-on-the-hill-a-sam-ervin-sampler-70955/.

102. Ervin, *Humor of a Country Lawyer*, 13.

103. "What is Grandfather Mountain?" Grandfather Mountain, https://grandfather.com/about-grandfather-mountain/what-is-grandfather-mountain/; Marcus B. Simpson, Jr., "Linville Gorge," in NCPedia, https://www.ncpedia.org/linville-gorge; National Park Service, "Linville Falls Hiking Trails," Blue Ridge Parkway NC/VA, https://www.nps.gov/blri/planyourvisit/linville-falls-trails.htm.

104. U.S. Forest Service, "Linville Gorge Wilderness," 2014, Linville Gorge Maps and More,

http://lgmaps.org/maps/usfs/NC_LinvilleGorge_Map_2014.pdf.
105. Worldwide Elevation Finder, https://elevation.maplogs.com/.
106. Pratt and Berry, *Mining Industry*, passim 12–20, 38, 105.
107. Willard, *Morganton and Burke County*, 7; Phifer, *Burke County*, 2–3.
108. Willard, 7; Phifer, *Burke County*, 20.
109. Phifer, *Burke County*, 77–78.
110. Walton, *Sketches of the Pioneers*, 36–37.
111. *Ibid.*, 37; Phifer, "Champagne," 492.
112. Phifer, *Burke County*, 79.
113. "Champagne," 500; Phifer, *Burke County*, 79; Willard, 56.
114. Beaumont, "The Mineral Region of North Carolina," *Fayetteville Weekly Observer* (NC), 7 Dec. 1847. Brown Mountain is best known for its "Brown Mountain Lights," orbs of light that dance across the ridges at night and whose sightings appear to have increased with electrification in the region.
115. Beaumont, "To the Editor of the Southerner," *Raleigh Register*, 8 Dec. 1847; Miller, "Piedmont Springs Hotel." Miller cites Grant #6220 as the source for Estes opening the hotel in June 1848.
116. "Piedmont Sulphur and Chalybeate Springs, in Burke County, N.C. [ad]," *Charlotte Democrat*, 20 July 1855. Estes' resort was largely contemporary with the resort of Piedmont Springs in Stokes County, NC. I discounted innumerable newspaper articles where I was not able to determine if the "Piedmont Springs" mentioned was indeed the health resort in Burke County.
117. Hornet's Nest, "Where Shall We Go?" *Semi-Weekly Standard* (Raleigh), 28 June 1851.
118. U.S. Census 1850 (Slave Schedule), "U.S. Census 1860 (Slave Schedule) 1860," both at FamilySearch, www.familysearch.org; subsequent Census records in this chapter accessed at FamilySearch.
119. Phifer, "Certain Aspects of Medical Practice," 40; "Piedmont Sulphur and Chalybeate Springs [ad]," *Western Democrat* (Charlotte), 4 Aug. 1854; "Dr. Michael's Pils [sic]," *Lincoln Courier* (Lincolnton, NC), 7 July 1848. Happoldt owned 12 slaves in 1850; see U.S. Census 1850 (Slave Schedule).
120. "Piedmont Sulphur and Chalybeate Springs [ad]," *Western Democrat* (Charlotte), 29 July 1856.
121. "Piedmont Sulphur Chalybait [sic] Springs of Burke County, N.C. [ad]," *Hornets' Nest* (Charlotte, NC), 30 Aug. 1851.
122. H., "North Carolina Correspondence: Visit to Table Rock," *Charleston Courier*, 17 Aug. 1855.
123. "Piedmont Sulphur Chalybait [sic] Springs of Burke County, N.C. [ad]."
124. C. Happoldt, "The Mineral Springs of Burke," *Wilmington Morning Star* (NC), 17 May 1877; Phifer, "Certain Aspects of Medical Practice," 30; Timothy N. Osment, "Sanitariums," *Digital Heritage*, https://digitalheritage.org/2010/08/sanitariums/.
125. "Piedmont Sulphur Chalybait [sic] Springs of Burke County, N.C. [ad]."
126. "An Act to Authorize the Making of a Turnpike Road from Morganton, in Burke County, to the Cranberry Forge, in Watauga County," Chapter 233, in *Public Laws of the State of North Carolina*, 327–28.
127. Colton, *Mountain Scenery*, 49.
128. R**, "A Trip to the Mountains—The Table Rock," *Western Democrat* (Charlotte), 23 Aug. 1859.
129. "Piedmont Springs [ad]," *Evening Bulletin* (Charlotte), 8 Aug. 1862; "Piedmont Springs, Burke County, N.C. [ad]," *Daily Carolina Watchman* (Salisbury, NC), 21 July 1864; "Piedmont Springs, Burke Co., N.C. [ad]," *Daily Progress* (Raleigh), 18 July 1864; U.S. Population Census 1860. The 1860 census lists Estes' occupation as "Hotel Keeper (Piedmont)." The U.S. Population Census of 1870 gives his occupation as a farmer in the Upper Creek community of Burke County.
130. "Piedmont Springs, Burke County, N.C. [ad]," *Daily Progress* (Raleigh), 29 May 1863; "Piedmont Springs [ad]," *Evening Bulletin* (Charlotte), 8 Aug. 1862.
131. "Piedmont Springs, Burke Co., N.C. [ad]," *Daily Confederate* (Raleigh), 16 June 1864; Abrams, "Western North Carolina Railroad," 12.
132. "The Raid into Burke County," *Western Democrat* (Charlotte), 5 July 1864; "Letter from the Editor, Camp Vance, June 30," *Daily Carolina Watchman* (Salisbury, NC), 1 July 1864; "From Morganton," *Semi-Weekly Standard* (Raleigh), 5 July 1864; Arthur, *Western North Carolina*, 605–08.
133. "From the Salisbury Watchman, July 2," *Fayetteville Semi-Weekly Observer* (NC), 7 July 1864.
134. "Piedmont Springs, Burke County, N.C. [ad]," *Daily Carolina Watchman* (Salisbury, NC), 20 Aug. 1864.
135. "Piedmont Springs, Burke Co., N.C. [ad]," *Daily Progress* (Raleigh), 18 July 1864.
136. "Raid on Piedmont Springs," *Camden Daily Journal* (SC), 8 Dec. 1864.
137. "Piedmont Springs [ad]," *Evening Bulletin* (Charlotte), 8 Aug. 1862; "Piedmont Springs, Burke County, North Carolina [ad]," *Daily Progress* (Raleigh), 6 July 1863; "Piedmont Springs, Burke County, N.C. [ad]," *Daily Carolina Watchman* (Salisbury, NC), 21 July 1864. Walton states that North Carolina pegged the value of a tenpenny nail to five cents to use as currency for a period during the war. A relative's wartime diary from the Goldsboro—Salisbury area gives the price of three dozen eggs at $15. See Walton, *Sketches of the Pioneers*, 88–89. Lerner notes that the general price index of the Confederacy rose at an almost constant rate of 10% / mo. from Oct. 1861 to Mar. 1864. See Eugene M. Lerner, "Money, Prices, and Wages in the Confederacy, 1861–65," *Journal of Political Economy* 63 (Feb. 1955): 23.
138. *Weekly Era* (Raleigh), 26 June 1873.
139. *Raleigh Christian Advocate*, 27 Aug. 1873.

140. E.C., "Editor Observer," *Observer* (Raleigh), 13 July 1879.

141. *Blue Ridge Blade* (Morganton, NC), 20 Mar. 1880; U.S. Population Census 1860. Pearcy's surname is also spelled as Pearcey, Pearsey, Pearsy, or Piercy in various sources.

142. Abrams, "Western North Carolina Railroad," 44, 51.

143. "Piedmont Springs [ad]," *Carolina Mountaineer* (Morganton, NC), 14 May 1884.

144. *Charlotte Home and Democrat*, 17 July 1885; "Death of Miss Nellie Crowson," *Anson Times* (Wadesboro, NC), 13 Aug. 1885.

145. Mabel Lee, "A Racy Letter," *Carolina Mountaineer* (Morganton, NC), 4 Aug. 1883.

146. "To the Mountaineer," *Ibid.*, 30 July 1884.

147. "Western N.C. This Summer," *Raleigh News*, 18 May 1873.

148. E.C., "Editor Observer," *Observer* (Raleigh), 13 July 1879.

149. "Sulphur Springs Hotel, Five Miles West of Asheville, on the Western Branch of the Western N.C.R.R. [ad]," *Asheville Times*, 22 July 1887; "Piedmont Springs Hotel Now Open [ad]," *Morganton Star* (NC), 6 Aug. 1886. Piedmont Springs charged $2 / day; Sulphur Springs, $3 / day.

150. "Mining Matters," *Rutherford Banner* (Rutherfordton, NC), 17 Mar. 1882; *News and Observer* (Raleigh), 2 Feb. 1883; *Charlotte Observer*, 16 Feb. 1883; *Carolina Mountaineer* (Morganton, NC), 12 May 1883; Phifer, *Burke County*, 92–93.

151. *Charlotte Home and Democrat*, 25 Dec. 1885; *State Chronicle* (Raleigh), 28 Jan. 1886; "Sale of Piedmont Springs," *Charlotte Home and Democrat*, 29 Jan. 1886.

152. "Deer Breeding in Burke," *Charlotte Home and Democrat*, 18 Feb. 1887; *Lenoir Topic* (NC), 13 July 1887; *Morganton Star* (NC), 5 Nov. 1886; *Ibid.*, 12 Nov. 1886. Blake also represented an English sporting club that bought 30,000 acres adjacent to the resort property for use as a quail hunting ground. See *Lenoir Topic* (NC), 24 Feb. 1886.

153. *Fisherman & Farmer* (Edenton, NC), 10 Aug. 1888; Williamson, "Seven Ways." The CPI calculator was used for all monetary conversions in this chapter.

154. "Morganton and Burke County," *Morganton Herald* (NC), 11 Dec. 1890.

155. Miller, "Piedmont Springs Hotel"; "Sale of Timber Lands," *News-Herald* (Morganton, NC), 13 Nov. 1902; "The New Wood-Working Plant," *Ibid.*, 16 June 1904.

156. *Morganton Herald* (NC), 16 June 1892.

157. Bell, "Climate and Mineral Springs of North Carolina," 126.

158. Miller, "Piedmont Springs Hotel."

159. *News-Herald* (Morganton, NC), 5 May 1910; Garibaldi, "Happy New Year." Newspapers researched listed no visitors after the late 1800s. Ralph Rives does not show Piedmont Springs of Burke County in his list of mineral spring resorts operating in North Carolina in the early twentieth century. See Ralph Hardee Rives, "Panacea Springs: Fashionable Spa," *North Carolina Historical Review* 42, no. 4 (1965): 430n1.

160. "Great Damage in Burke," *Marion Progress* (NC), 20 July 1916; "Asheville Citizens Claimed by Flood," *Ibid.*; "Reports from Upper Part of County," *News-Herald* (Morganton, NC), 20 July 1916. For information on the tropical systems that caused the flooding, see NOAA, National Centers for Environmental Information, "Investigating the Great Flood of 1916," https://www.ncdc.noaa.gov/news/investigating-the-great-flood-of-1916.

161. Garibaldi.

162. Miller, "Piedmont Springs Hotel."

163. Historic Burke Foundation, R.M. Lineberger Collection, 2003-07-14-013, "Piedmont Springs Hotel, ca 1890," http://pictureburke.bcpls.org/places_2.htm, BCPL; "Piedmont Springs Cemetery," Find a Grave, https://www.findagrave.com/cemetery/2525145/piedmont-springs-cemetery; "Piedmont Springs Cemetery," Cemetery Census: Cemetery Records on the Web, https://cemeterycensus.com/nc/burk/cem189.htm.

164. Phifer, *Burke County*, 109, 129–130; Walton, *Sketches of the Pioneers*, 30.

165. Emmons, *Glen Alpine Springs Hotel*, 11; Phifer, "Saga of a Burke County Family," 316, 323. Phifer documents the Avery family in detail. Emmons is George Thomas Walton's great-great-granddaughter.

166. U.S. Census 1860 (Slave Schedule); U.S. Population Census 1870; *Public Laws of the State of North Carolina* (1870), 117–18; Williamson, "Seven Ways." Walton in 1870 held real estate worth $29K and personal estate estimated at $10K.

167. Oertel, "Mountain Land," 53.

168. *Ibid.*

169. "Waddell, Alfred Moore (1834–1912)," *Biographical Dictionary of the United States Congress, 1774-present*, https://bioguideretro.congress.gov/Home/MemberDetails?memIndex=W000002; "Grand Opening Ball," *Daily Review* (Wilmington, NC), 13 July 1878; "Opening Ball at Glenn Alpine Springs," *Charlotte Observer*, 14 July 1878.

170. "Opening Ball at Glenn Alpine Springs"; "Glen Alpine," *Blue Ridge Blade* (Morganton, NC), 7 Sept. 1878.

171. "'Lithia Alum,' Burke County, N.C., [ad]," *South Atlantic: A Monthly Magazine of Literature, Science, and Art*, 2 (Aug. 1878): 288; "Glen Alpine Springs for Sale," *Morganton Herald* (NC), 9 Aug. 1900.

172. Phifer, *Burke County*, 109.

173. *Charlotte Observer*, 14 Dec. 1878; "Glen Alpine Springs, Burke County, N.C. [ad]," *Raleigh Observer*, 4 July 1879. The *Charlotte Observer* mentioned that George Thomas Walton was the father of Pearson's bride. The ad was published as late as the Sept. 23 issue of the *Raleigh Observer*.

174. Phifer, *Burke County*, 109. Several narratives comment that the hotel was the largest, or one of the largest, frame structures in the state.

175. "Glen Alpine Springs, Burke County, N.C

[ad].," *Raleigh Observer*, 4 July 1879; "'Lithia Alum,' Burke County, N.C., [ad]," *South Atlantic*.

176. Veni Vidi, "Zephyrs from the Blue Ridge," *Farmer and Mechanic* (Raleigh), 24 July 1879.

177. "Glen Alpine Springs," *Newbernian* (New Bern, NC), 6 Sept. 1879.

178. "Glen Alpine Springs, Near Morganton, N.C. [ad]," *Charlotte Observer*, 31 May 1883.

179. "Glen Alpine Springs," *Ibid.*, 12 July 1882.

180. "Zephyrs."

181. "Opening Ball," *Charlotte Observer*, 18 July 1879; "The Opening Ball at Glen Alpine," *Ibid.*, 27 July 1878.

182. "Glen Alpine Springs," *Newbernian* (New Bern, NC), 6 Sept. 1879; Emmons, 13.

183. "Glen Alpine Springs, Burke County, N.C. [ad]," *Raleigh Observer*, 4 July 1879.

184. Veni Vidi, "Glen Alpine Again," *Charlotte Observer*, 25 July 1879.

185. "Glen Alpine Springs [ad]," *Raleigh News*, 17 Nov. 1878.

186. "Mineral Waters [ad]," *Ibid.*, 1 Jan. 1879.

187. Pepper et al., "Report by Committee on Sanitaria and on Mineral Springs," 539–41. The quote is found on page 539.

188. "Glen Alpine Springs [ad]," *Asheville Daily Citizen*, 7 July 1890.

189. "Glen Alpine Springs," *Newbernian* (New Bern, NC), 6 Sept. 1879; "Morganton and Burke County," *Morganton Herald* (NC), 11 Dec. 1890.

190. "Glen Alpine Springs [ad]," *Charlotte Observer*, 4 June 1897. It is not known whether one of the five springs dried up or whether Smith elected to count as one spring a couple of adjacent springs.

191. *Charlotte Observer*, 12 July 1882; F, "Letter from Asheville," *Goldsboro Messenger* (NC), 8 Aug. 1880; *Carolina Mountaineer* (Morganton, NC), 14 May 1884.

192. "Good News from Mr. Morehead," *Tobacco Plant* (Durham, NC), 24 Aug. 1888; "Glen Alpine Springs," *News and Observer* (Raleigh), 5 Sept. 1888. Morehead stayed in late summer 1888 but died several months later in Feb. 1889.

193. *Statesville Record and Landmark* (NC), 3 July 1880; McKesson, "William Simpson Pearson," 375–79.

194. "Morganton and Burke County, North Carolina, *Morganton Herald* (NC), 11 Dec. 1890.

195. *Ibid.*; Emmons, 12; Van Noppen, "On Main Traveled Roads," in Van Noppen, *Western North Carolina since the Civil War*, 33; *Alamance Gleaner* (Graham, NC), 15 Jan. 1878; "The Glen Alpine Springs," *Daily Review* (Wilmington NC), 9 July 1878.

196. "Glen Alpine Springs, A.A. Banks, Prop'r. [ad]," *Durham Daily Globe* (NC), 30 June 1892; Col. T.G. Walton, "Burke County History. Sketches of the Pioneers," *Morganton Herald* (NC), 11 Dec. 1893; "Walton House [ad]," *Raleigh Register*, 26 Jan. 1861.

197. Emmons, 13; *Morganton Herald* (NC), 5 Feb. 1891; Blaylock, "Appalachian Aristocrats," 120–21.

198. "Saturday Night Excursion," *Charlotte Democrat*, 27 July 1888; "Very Cheap Rates to the Mountains," *Asheville Citizen*, 29 July 1888.

199. "Time Table, Western N.C. Railroad," *Carolina Watchman* (Salisbury, NC), 28 Aug. 1879; *Appletons'* (1896), 154.

200. "Glen Alpine Springs for Sale."

201. *Burke County News* (Morganton, NC), 3 Aug. 1900; "Glen Alpine Springs for Sale"; "Valuable Lands and Personal Property for Sale," *Farmer's Friend* (Morganton, NC), 22 Sept. 1898; "Sale of Valuable Hotel and Gold Mine," *Morganton Herald* (NC), 19 Jan. 1899.

202. "Glen Alpine Springs [ad]," *Morganton Herald* (NC), 11 July 1901; *Statesville Record and Landmark* (NC), 6 June 1902.

203. "Glen Alpine Springs School," *News-Herald* (Morganton, NC), 3 May 1906; *News-Herald* (Morganton, NC), 29 Aug. 1912.

204. "Glen Alpine Springs Sold," *Ibid.*, 14 Mar. 1918.

205. Burke County Public Library, "Glen Alpine Springs," *Throwback Thursday* (blog), https://www.facebook.com/bcpls/, Dec. 17, 2020.

206. "My Plantation and Tenements [ad]," *Daily Carolina Watchman* (Salisbury, NC), 21 Jan. 1865; "William Lewis Connelly," Find A Grave, https://www.findagrave.com/memorial/87153990/william-lewis-connelly.

207. Hudson, "Connelly's Springs," 27; "North Carolina, Historical Records Survey, Cemetery Inscription Card Index," FamilySearch, www.familysearch.org.

208. Galvin, *"Early History of Connelly Springs, NC,"* 18, 35; "North Carolina, Historical Records Survey"; "Connelly Springs," *North Carolina Herald* (Salisbury), 5 Aug. 1886; Alpha, "Bits About Burke," *Morganton Star* (NC), 30 July 1886; Chr. O. Nicle, "Connelly's Springs," *State Chronicle* (Raleigh), 22 June 1890; J.W. Long, "Quiet Burke Village Once Drew Vacationers From Many States to Spa's Elegant Hostel: Mineral Spring Was Magnet for Many," *News-Herald* (Morganton, NC), 25 Jan. 1963. Almost all sources consulted erroneously give a year in the mid-1880s as to when Mrs. Connelly "discovered" the spring: She died in 1879. I estimate the year as 1871 because the July 30, 1886, *Morganton Star* writer states that "we have known about the springs for fifteen years" and because the June 22, 1890, *State Chronicle* comments that the discovery occurred "nearly twenty years ago."

209. Galvin, 18.

210. *Carolina Mountaineer* (Morganton, NC) 11 Aug. 1883; Galvin, 18; "Charity Louisiana (Louise) Connelly," Find A Grave, https://www.findagrave.com/memorial/7682030/charity-louisiana-goode. The *Mountaineer* article incorrectly gives Goode's initials as "W.P."

211. "Connelly Springs," *North Carolina Herald* (Salisbury), 5 Aug. 1886; Phifer, *Burke County*, 98–99. Phifer provides a good summary of the somewhat convoluted place name changes in the area.

212. "Quiet Burke Village."
213. *Carolina Watchman* (Salisbury, NC), 17 June 1886.
214. *Morganton Star* (NC), 30 Apr. 1886; *Lenoir Topic* (NC), 21 Apr. 21, 1886; Alpha, "Bits About Burke"; "Connelly Springs," *North Carolina Herald* (Salisbury), 5 Aug. 1886.
215. "Connelly Springs," *North Carolina Herald* (Salisbury), 5 Aug. 1886; "Meroney Bro's Enterprise," *Ibid.*, 20 May 1886.
216. "Meroney Bro's Enterprise," *Ibid.*, 20 May 1886; "'Lithia Alum,' Burke County, N.C., [ad]," *South Atlantic*; Willard, 114. For an illustration of the Meroneys' hotel, see "Connelly's Springs [ad]," *Asheville Citizen*, 22 July 1887.
217. "Connelly Springs," *North Carolina Herald* (Salisbury), 5 Aug. 1886.
218. "Connelly Springs Hotel," *Ibid.*, 24 June 1886.
219. Chr. O. Nicle, "Connelly's Springs," *Daily State Chronicle* (Raleigh, NC), 22 June 1890.
220. *Ibid.*
221. "Connelly Springs," *Carolina Watchman* (Salisbury, NC), 2 Sept. 1886; "Connelly's Springs," *Daily State Chronicle* (Raleigh, NC), 22 June 1890.
222. "Connelly's Springs," *Daily State Chronicle* (Raleigh, NC), 22 June 1890.
223. "Invalid's Home! [ad]," *Asheville Citizen*, 2 Nov. 1887.
224. "Connelly's Springs [ad]," *Asheville Citizen*, 22 July 1887; "Connelly Mineral Springs Hotel [ad]," *Hickory Democrat* (NC), 1 Aug. 1912.
225. "Connelly's Springs," *Daily State Chronicle* (Raleigh, NC), 22 June 1890.
226. *Ibid.*
227. Connelly's Springs [ad]," *Asheville Citizen*, 22 July 1887.
228. "Connelly Springs," *News and Observer* (Raleigh), 23 June 1895.
229. "Medicinal Springs of County Famous Since Colonial Days," *News-Herald* 1924, Prosperity and Publicity Edition [Morganton, NC] [photocopy], Reading Room, BCPL; Fitch, 527.
230. "Connelly's Springs," *Daily State Chronicle* (Raleigh, NC), 22 June 1890; Morganton Herald (NC), 26 Feb. 1891; "Quiet Burke Village."
231. "Quiet Burke Village"; *Hickory Democrat* (NC), 6 June 1912; Galvin, 20; Williamson, "Seven Ways." Galvin includes a non-dated copy of a hotel brochure issued by the Connelly Springs Hotel Company, formed in 1902. The CPI calculator provided almost identical values for 1903 and 1904.
232. Pratt and Berry, 111–15. Waynesville's Haywood White Sulphur Springs was the other Southern Appalachian North Carolina resort.
233. "The Famous Connelly Springs [ad]," *News and Observer* (Raleigh, NC), 1 June 1892. This ad ran for many years with the same text except for modifying the year.
234. "For Health, Pleasure and Comfort, Go to Connelly Springs [ad]," *Savannah Morning News*, 27 June 1900.
235. "Try the Connelly Mineral Springs Resort," *Watchman and Southron* (Sumter, SC), 3 June 1916.
236. *Connelly Mineral Springs Hotel,* North Carolina Room, BCPL. For an example of a nineteenth-century medical article discussing the value of high elevations as a TB therapy, see J. Henry Bennet, "Introduction to a Discussion on the Influence of Mountain Air in the Treatment of Pulmonary Consumption," *British Medical Journal* 2 (July 10, 1880): 42–44, https://doi.org/10.1136/bmj.2.1019.42.
237. "Try the Connelly Mineral Springs Resort," *Watchman and Southron* (Sumter, SC), 3 June 1916.
238. "Great Gathernng at Rutherford College," *Western Sentinel* (Winston-Salem, NC), 11 Aug. 1887; Levi Blanson and R.L. Abernethy, "Local Preachers' Conference and Great Tabernacle Meeting," *Morganton Star* (NC), 25 July 1889. Rutherford College is now a town. The school merged with two others to form Brevard College in the early 1930s. See "History," *Rutherford College, North Carolina*, https://www.rutherfordcollegenc.us/pview.aspx?id=20700&catid=564.
239. F.B. Arendell, "Connelly Springs," *News and Observer* (Raleigh), 2 June 1895.
240. *Ibid.*
241. "Quiet Burke Village."
242. *Asheville Citizen*, 28 Aug. 1888; "Connelly Springs," *News & Observer* (Raleigh, NC), 23 June 1895; *Charlotte Democrat*, 13 July 1888; "Connelly's Springs," *State Chronicle* (Raleigh, NC), 20 July 1888.
243. Cheryl Bollinger, "The healthy history of Connelly Springs," *News-Herald* (Morganton, NC), 28 Aug. 2002. The article and a few other sources erroneously state that Cornelius Vanderbilt may have visited; the Commodore died in 1877.
244. *North Carolina Herald* (Salisbury), 18 June 1890; "Connelly's Springs," *Carolina Watchman* (Salisbury, NC), 3 July 1890; *Charlotte Democrat*, 20 June 1890. A few sources erroneously state that the Salisbury syndicate bought the property after Thomas J.'s death. Thomas J. had been a patient at the Morganton Asylum for three years preceding his death in 1891. See *Union Republican* (Winston-Salem), 3 Feb. 1891.
245. "Connelly Springs [ad]," *News and Observer* (Raleigh), 28 June 1890; "State of North Carolina, Rowan County, in Office Clerk Superior Court," *Carolina Watchman* (Salisbury, NC), 21 Aug. 1890; *Morganton Herald* (NC), 28 Aug. 1890; *Morganton Herald* (NC), 5 Mar. 1891.
246. *Morganton Herald* (NC), 2 Feb. 1899; *Burke County News* (Morganton, NC), 21 July 1899; *Times-Mercury* (Hickory, NC), 12 July 1899; "Sale of Connelly Springs," *Morganton Herald* (NC), 26 Apr. 1900. More research is needed to understand if the Salisbury businessmen had overextended themselves in other ventures.
247. "Connelly Springs Hotel [ad]," *News and Observer* (Raleigh), 23 June 1900; "Big Deal in Furniture," *News-Herald* (Morganton, NC), 29 May 1902; Galvin, 35.

248. Galvin, 35; *Hickory Democrat*, 6 June 1912; "Connelly Mineral Springs Hotel [ad]," *Hickory Democrat* (NC), 1 Aug. 1912.

249. "Fifty years ago: Landmark, March 14, 1913," *Statesville Record and Landmark* (NC), 14 Mar. 1963; "Fifty years ago: Landmark, April 25, 1913," *Ibid.*, 25 Apr. 1963.

250. Fitch, 528.

251. "Quiet Burke Village"; Hudson, 27; "North Carolina Deaths, 1906–1930," FamilySearch, www.familysearch.org; "North Carolina Deaths, 1931–1994," *Ibid.*

Haywood County: Haywood White Sulphur Springs and Eagles Nest

252. Haywood County, NC, "Fast Facts about Haywood County," https://www.haywoodcountync.gov/351/Fast-Facts-About-Haywood-County; Haywood County, NC, "About Haywood County," https://www.haywoodcountync.gov/350/About-Haywood-County.

253. Great Smoky Mountains National Park, NC, TN, "Cataloochee," https://www.nps.gov/grsm/planyourvisit/cataloochee.htm.

254. PeakVisor, "North Carolina: Haywood County," https://peakvisor.com/adm/haywood-county-north-carolina.html; "Fast Facts about Haywood County."

255. H.V.W., "Waynesville, N.C.," *Birmingham News*, 12 Aug. 1905.

256. Arthur, 507; H.B.H., "Waynesville and Haywood County, Where Lofty Mountains Lift their Heads to Kiss the Sky," *Daily State Chronicle* (Raleigh), 28 July 1891.

257. "Sketches of Travel in North Carolina," *North-Carolinian* (Fayetteville, NC), 17 Nov. 1849.

258. "Dear Locum," *Ibid.*, 12 Oct. 1850.

259. U.S. Population Census 1850, FamilySearch, www.familysearch.org; subsequent Census records cited accessed at FamilySearch; Williamson, "Seven Ways." The CPI calculator was used in all relative value calculations in this chapter.

260. U.S. Population Census 1850; U.S. Census 1850 (Slave Schedule); Medford, *Early History*, 35; Starnes, "'The Stirring Strains of Dixie,'" 39; Inscoe, *Mountain Masters*, 116. The decline in the number of enslaved persons in Haywood County between 1850 and 1860 is likely due to the formation of Jackson County in 1851 from sections of Haywood County and Macon County.

261. Brown, "Andrew Jackson," 66; H.A. Chappell, "An Ideal Town in the Land of the Sky," *News and Observer* (Raleigh), 30 June 1901.

262. Allen, *Centennial of Haywood County*, 51–53; Brown, 62–65.

263. *Carolina Messenger* (Goldsboro, NC), 10 Jan. 1876; MSS 80–06, "William Williams Stringfield Collection: Scope and Contents," WCU, https://wcu.lyrasistechnology.org/repositories/2/resources/212.

264. Griffith, *Dr. Samuel Stringfield House*, 5.

265. Griffith, 7; "Sulphur Springs Annex," HCPL, https://cdm16781.contentdm.oclc.org/digital/collection/p16781coll2/id/35/rec/1; Medford, *Middle History*, 4. Medford describes the hotel as "an imposing building" at the time of its opening, an unusual description if indeed it were Springfield's house. Medford also describes a "private" spring that Col. Robert Love used that was separate from the "public" spring. The private spring was filled in during Waynesville construction in the antebellum period. See Medford, *Middle History*, 4–5.

266. U.S. Population Census 1870; Williamson, "Seven Ways."

267. Medford, *Early History*, 62; Allen, 61.

268. W.W. Stringfield, "Western N.C. Railroad," *Asheville Citizen*, 17 Oct. 1878.

269. Bishir, Southern, and Martin, *Guide to the Historic Architecture*, 356; "Haywood White Sulphur and Chalybeate Springs, Season of 1879 [ad]," *North Carolina Citizen* (Asheville), 21 Aug. 1879.

270. L., "Waynesville as a Summer Resort," *Raleigh News*, 29 Aug. 1878; Zeigler and Grosscup, *Heart of the Alleghanies*, 291. The quote is from *Heart of the Alleghanies*.

271. Zeigler and Grosscup, 291; "The Fire at Waynesville," *News and Observer* (Raleigh), 12 Aug. 1885.

272. "Haywood Hotel Burned," *Marion Star* (Ohio), 12 Aug. 1885; "The Fire at Waynesville"; Williamson, "Seven Ways."

273. *Charlotte Home-Democrat*, 13 Nov. 1885.

274. "A Suggestion of Incendiarism," *Asheville Citizen-Times*, 8 Sept. 1885.

275. "The Fire at Waynesville."

276. "Haywood White Sulphur Springs, Waynesville, N.C. [ad]," *Savannah Morning News*, 27 June 1886.

277. *Ibid.*

278. "Must Be Sold [ad]," *Asheville Democrat*, 24 July 1892; H.B.H., "Waynesville and Haywood County."

279. H.B.H., "Waynesville and Haywood County"; "Health Resorts of the South: White Sulphur Springs 001," Haywood County History Collection, HCPL, https://cdm16781.contentdm.oclc.org/digital/collection/p16781coll2/id/2307/rec/6.

280. *Ibid.*

281. H.B.H., "Waynesville and Haywood County"; H.B. Hardy, "Waynesville, Mecca of Tourist and Healthseeker," *News and Observer* (Raleigh), 23 June 1903.

282. "Waynesville, Mecca of Tourist and Healthseeker."

283. *Ibid.*

284. "Haywood White Sulphur and Chalybeate Springs, Season of 1879 [ad]"; "The Haywood White Sulphur Springs Hotel, Waynesville, N.C. [ad]," *Asheville Daily Citizen*, 11 Aug. 1893.

285. Fitch, 530–31.

286. "White-Sulphur-Springs, Waynesville, N.C. [ad]," *Asheville Daily Citizen*, 24 June 1892; "The Haywood White Sulphur Springs Hotel,

Waynesville, N.C. [ad]," *Atlanta Constitution*, 25 May 1898; "Must Be Sold [ad]"; "Relieved of Bright's Disease," *Commonwealth* (Scotland Neck, NC), 12 July 1883; *State Chronicle* (Raleigh), 13 Sept. 1884; Occasional, "Waynesville Notes," *Asheville Daily Citizen*, 16 Apr. 1890.

287. "Must Be Sold [ad]."

288. "Haywood White Sulphur Springs Hotel [ad]," *Asheville Daily Citizen*, 4 June 1895; "Truly the Switzerland of America [ad]," *Ibid.*, 18 June 1895.

289. "Haywood White Sulphur Springs, Waynesville, N.C. [ad]," *News-Observer-Chronicle* (Raleigh), 3 July 1894.

290. "Sulphur Springs Annex"; "Haywood White Sulphur Springs Near Waynesville, N.C. [ad]"; Zeigler and Grosscup, 380. Starnes asserts that the resort largely catered to invalids. I respectfully disagree based on my careful readings of traveler accounts, local boosters' narratives of the resort attributes, and the descriptions of guests who left humid climes to visit the resort, not because they were ill. See Starnes, *Creating the Land of the Sky*, 48.

291. "Mountains. The Finest Scenery in the South Is Up There. Waynesville, The Gem of All," *Morning Times* (Selma, AL), 7 Sept. 1897; "Haywood White Sulphur Springs Near Waynesville, N.C. [ad]"; Zeigler and Grosscup, 292.

292. *News and Observer* (Raleigh), 12 Aug. 1886; "Basket Picnic," *Asheville Daily Citizen*, 23 Aug. 1897.

293. "Haywood White Sulphur Springs, Waynesville, N.C. Under Entire New Management [ad]," *Asheville Daily Citizen*, 20 July 1891.

294. "The Opening Ball," *Daily Citizen* (Asheville), 9 Aug. 1889.

295. H.E.H., "A Brilliant Affair," *Asheville Weekly Citizen*, 6 Aug. 1891.

296. "Waynesville and Haywood County, Where Lofty Mountains Lift their Heads"; *Raleigh Christian Advocate*, 1 Mar. 1893.

297. Rev. P.L. Groome, "A Letter From Waynesville," *Raleigh Christian Advocate*, 20 Jan. 1892.

298. "Must Be Sold [ad]."

299. *Asheville Daily Citizen*, 13 Aug. 1895; *Ibid.*, 3 Oct. 1895.

300. "A Brilliant Affair."

301. "An Interesting Letter from Dallas County's Next State Senator," *Morning Times* (Selma, AL), 2 Sept. 1897.

302. "Mountains. The Finest Scenery in the South Is Up There. Waynesville, The Gem of All," *Ibid.*, 7 Sept. 1897.

303. "Waynesville Old Resort," *Charlotte Observer*, 9 June 1954; "Reception to Mrs. Jackson," *Charlotte News*, 7 July 1911.

304. "Mountains. The Finest Scenery."

305. *Journal and Tribune* (Knoxville), 3 Aug. 1898.

306. *Asheville Daily Citizen*, 3 Aug. 1898.

307. *Journal and Tribune* (Knoxville), 3 Aug. 1898.

308. Newspapers consulted in the week following the walkout published a letter written by a Haywood White Sulphur Hotel clerk commenting on the large crowd at the resort (*Asheville Daily Gazette*, 10 Aug. 1898) but omit any information about the walkout aftermath.

309. Edmonds, *Negro and Fusion Politics*, 204; NC Dept. of Natural and Cultural Resources, *1898 Wilmington Race Riot Commission*, https://www.ncdcr.gov/learn/history-and-archives-education/1898-wilmington-race-riot-commission; LeRae Umfleet, "The Wilmington Massacre—1898," in *NCPedia*, rev. Aug. 2022 by NC Government & Heritage Library, https://ncpedia.org/history/cw-1900/wilmington-massacre-1898.

310. "White Sulphur Springs Hotel," *Asheville Gazette*, 9 May 1900. C.A. Alford accumulated a fortune estimated at $1M at his death around 1908 from his lumber interests and served as Georgia state senator. See Moses Neal Amis, *Historic Raleigh: With Sketches of Wake County (from 1771) And Its Important Towns* (Raleigh: Commercial Printing Co., 1913), 249. Possibly, the B.J. Sloan who was Alford's business partner was the same B.J. Sloan who was an officer in the Tennessee Coal Fields & South Atlantic Transcontinental firm that proposed to build a railroad from Knoxville through Waynesville to Greenville, SC. If true, that might explain the rationale for the firm's purchase of the Haywood White Sulphur. See "Construction," *Railway Age* 43, no. 20 (1907): 788.

311. "White Sulphur Springs Hotel," *Asheville Gazette*, 9 May 1900.

312. "In Sky Land," *Montgomery Advertiser*, 7 Aug. 1900; *Greenville News* (SC), 7 July 1901; "For Health and Pleasure, White Sulphur Springs Hotel [ad]," *Jackson Daily News* (MS), 1 June 1909; "Governor of Florida is at Waynesville," *Asheville Citizen*, 4 Sept. 1913.

313. "Masons Held Enjoyable Celebration Wednesday," *Waynesville Courier*, 26 June 1914; "They Pleased Waynesville," *Gastonia Gazette*, 20 June 1916; "Virginia-North Carolina Press Convention Passes into History as Finest of All Previous Newspaper Meetings," *Asheville Citizen*, 8 July 1905; "Board of Pharmacy Holding Examinations," *News and Observer* (Raleigh), 22 June 1912.

314. "Resort Hotels Are Well Patronized," *Asheville Citizen*, 9 Sept. 1913.

315. "A Trip to the Land of the Sky," *Review* (High Point, NC), 22 June 1916; *Lincoln County News* (Lincolnton, NC), 14 May 1917.

316. *French Broad Hustler* (Hendersonville, NC), 14 Mar. 1918; "Hotel at Waynesville is Now a Sanitarium," *Greensboro Daily News*, 10 May 1918; Rob Neufeld, "WNC Contributed Much in Fight Against Germany," *Asheville Citizen-Times*, 17 Nov. 2018.

317. "A Popular Hotel," *Ocala Evening Star* (FL), 28 Mar. 1919; "Sulphur Springs A Busy Place," *Carolina Mountaineer and Waynesville Courier*, 22 May 1919.

318. "Newspaper Folks Meet," *Beaufort News* (NC), 29 July 1920.

319. "Establish New Vocational Federal Training School at Waynesville March 1," *Asheville Citizen*, 8 Feb. 1921; "Waynesville Selected From Hundreds of Cities As Site for U.S. Vocational School," *Ibid.*, 30 Nov. 1921.

320. "Vocational School Established by Veterans Bureau Expected to Remain at Waynesville for a Year," *Sunday Citizen* (Asheville), 15 June 1924.

321. "Vocational School is Close [sic] on Nov. 15," *News and Observer* (Raleigh), 5 Nov. 1924.

322. "Sulphur Springs Annex"; "Waynesville's Former Mayor Has Had Interesting Career," *Asheville Citizen*, 1 Aug. 1928.

323. Sadie Patton, "Fame of WNC as Major Health Resort Dates from 18th Century," *Asheville Citizen*, 26 Mar. 1950; "Sulphur Springs Annex."

324. "Miss Ethel Craig Is Married To Hugh J. Sloan Saturday Evening," *Waynesville Mountaineer*, 4 Feb. 1943. Blink Bonnie served as the Sloan family home in 1939. See *Waynesville Mountaineer*, 1 June 1939.

325. "Sulphur Springs 002," County Structures, Sulphur Springs, HCPL, https://cdm16781.contentdm.oclc.org/digital/collection/p16781coll4/id/1765/rec/15.

326. Waynesville, NC, Parks and Recreation, "Sulphur Springs Park," https://www.waynesvillenc.gov/departments/parks-recreation/sulphur-springs-park.

327. "Golden Wedding To Be Observed in Atlanta," *Asheville Citizen-Times*, 8 Nov. 1931; "S.C. Satterwait [sic]," *News and Observer* (Raleigh), 23 Mar. 1935; U.S. Population Census 1860; U.S. Population Census 1880; "Bessie B. Satterthwait," Find A Grave, https://www.findagrave.com/memorial/46668560/bessie-b.-satterthwait.

328. "Golden Wedding To Be Observed in Atlanta"; Alex McKay, "Eagles Nest Hotel Fire Remembered at the Tragedy's Centennial," *Mountaineer*, published Apr. 23, 2018, https://www.themountaineer.com/news/eagles-nest-hotel-fire-remembered-at-the-tragedy-s-centennial/article_644caa6c-44d7-11e8-8b20-3f41a4dd889c.html; "Turnpike Hotel, Fifteen Miles West of Asheville [ad]," *Asheville Citizen*, 31 Aug. 1885.

329. "Mrs. S.C. Satterthwaite Dies In Haywood at 93," *Asheville Citizen-Times*, 8 Sept. 1951; Sarah R. Shaber, "Smathers, George Henry," *Dictionary of North Carolina Biography*, published 1994, in NCPedia, https://www.ncpedia.org/biography/smathers-george-henry.

330. McKay, "Eagles Nest Hotel Fire."

331. "Summary Report: North Eaglenest Mountain," in U.S. Dept. of the Interior, USGS, U.S. Board on Geographic Names, https://edits.nationalmap.gov/apps/gaz-domestic/public/search/names/1013987.

332. McKay, "Eagles Nest Hotel Fire"; "J.R. Morgan Recalls Early Days of Establishment of Eagle's Nest Promotions," *Waynesville Mountaineer* (NC), 20 Aug. 1959; "From Waynesville," *Asheville Daily Citizen*, 30 May 1893.

333. "Waynesville," *Western Sentinel* (Winston-Salem), 30 June 1898; "Press Association," *Chatham Citizen* (Pittsboro, NC), 28 June 1898.

334. "Eagle's Nest," *Waynesville Mountaineer*, 2 July 1976.

335. *Ibid.*

336. "Press Association," *Chatham Citizen* (Pittsboro, NC), 28 June 1898.

337. "Waynesville," *Western Sentinel* (Winston-Salem), 30 June 1898.

338. McKay, "Eagles Nest Hotel Fire"; B. Alex McKay, "#throwbackthursday: Eagles Nest Hotel Fire: April 22, 1918," FaceBook, Apr. 19, 2018, https://www.facebook.com/WaynesvilleNC.gov/posts/throwbackthursday-eagles-nest-hotel-fire-april-22-1918originally-built-in-1900-t/1731727580228857/.

339. Louise Frances Dodge, "Miss Dodge at Eagle's Nest," *Morning Tribune* (Tampa), 15 Sept. 1903.

340. "Eagle's Nest"; "Waynesville, Mecca of Tourist and Healthseeker."

341. "Eagle's Nest"; "Popularity of Eagle's Nest Goes Back Half Century," *Ibid.*, 20 Aug. 1959; "Waynesville, Mecca of Tourist and Healthseeker."

342. "Eagle's Nest"; McKay, "Eagles Nest Hotel Fire." The latter article includes an image of a hotel postcard.

343. "Popularity of Eagle's Nest"; "Waynesville, Mecca of Tourist and Healthseeker."

344. "Miss Dodge at Eagle's Nest." Dodge, an influential person in Tampa society, cofounded in 1904 the city's popular Gasparilla festivities. See Nora McGreevy, "The True History and Swashbuckling Myth Behind the Tampa Bay Buccaneers' Namesake," *Smithsonian Magazine*, published Feb. 4, 2021, https://www.smithsonianmag.com/history/true-history-and-swashbuckling-myth-behind-tampa-bay-buccaneers-namesake-180976918/.

345. "'Eagles Nest,' Monarch of the Mountain Peaks," *Asheville Citizen*, 12 June 1904.

346. McKay, "Eagles Nest Hotel Fire"; *Waynesville Courier*, 23 Aug. 1912.

347. H.V.W., "Eagle's Nest, N.C.," *Birmingham News*, 26 Aug. 1905; "Popularity of Eagle's Nest."

348. "Mountain Scenery," *Morning Tribune* (Tampa), 15 Sept. 1901.

349. "Eagle's Nest, N.C."

350. "Miss Dodge at Eagle's Nest."

351. "Missionary from China," *Asheville Weekly Citizen*, 9 Aug. 1901.

352. *St. Petersburg Daily Times*, 14 July 1915.

353. "Returns From Delightful Summer Trip," *Selma Times* (AL), 13 Sept. 1917.

354. "Eagles' Nest [ad]," *Twin City Daily Sentinel* (Winston-Salem), 8 July 1910; Arthur, 503.

355. Scheppegrell, "Hay-Fever Resorts," 524.

356. "No Hay Fever at Eagle's Nest," *Asheville Citizen*, 8 Sept. 1906.

357. "Eagle's Nest, Waynesville," *Asheville Gazette-News*, 11 July 1910.

358. "'Sneezers' Meet This Year at Waynesville," *Asheville Citizen*, 5 Aug. 1915.

359. Ibid.
360. "Eagles Nest [ad]," *Asheville Citizen*, 15 July 1911.
361. "Eagle's Nest and Hay Fever," *Charlotte Daily Observer*, 24 July 1915.
362. "'Sneezers' Meet This Year."
363. *Ibid.* More research is required to determine if the railroad published such a guide.
364. *Henderson Daily Dispatch* (NC), 11 July 1946.
365. "Flames Destroy Famous Hostelry, The Eagle's Nest," *Asheville Citizen*, 23 Apr. 1918.
366. "Regrets for Fire," *Carolina Mountaineer and Waynesville Courier* (NC). 2 May 1918.
367. McKay, "Eagles Nest Hotel Fire."
368. *Knoxville Journal*, 30 June 1925. A heavily advertised camp was the Eagle's Nest Camp for Girls." See "Eagle's Nest Camp for Girls [ad]," *News and Observer* (Raleigh), 30 Apr. 1922.
369. "Potentials of Eagle's Nest Realized," *Waynesville Mountaineer* (NC), 20 Aug. 1959; "Three Florida Real Estate Men Purchase Large Eagle's Nest Tract," *Ibid.*, 20 Aug. 1959; "Popular Mountain Spot Is Coming Back," *Ibid.*, 21 Sept. 1961.
370. McKay, "Eagles Nest Hotel Fire."

South Carolina

Introduction

1. For a variety of topics in each of the four South Carolina regions (Lowcountry, Peedee, Midlands, and Upstate), see *South Carolina Encyclopedia* (Columbia: University of South Carolina Institute for Southern Studies), https://www.scencyclopedia.org/sce/regions/. For overviews on Upstate settlement, see also Timothy P. Grady, "Early White Settlement of Northwestern South Carolina," in *Encyclopedia of Appalachia*, 308; Judith T. Bainbridge, "Greenville, South Carolina," *Ibid.*, 370–71; and Jeffrey R. Willis, "Spartanburg, South Carolina," *Ibid.*, 383–84.
2. Brewster, *Summer Migrations*, 16.
3. *Ibid.*, 27–28.
4. *Ibid.*, 7–8.
5. *Ibid.*, 59, 62.
6. "South Carolina Railroads—Atlanta & Charlotte Air Line Railway," https://www.carolana.com/SC/Transportation/railroads/sc_rrs_atlanta_charlotte_air_line.html.
7. *Palmetto Place Names*, 107 (page citations are to the reprint edition).
8. Chapin, *Health Resorts of the South*, 144, 141.
9. *Ibid.*, 138–40. The Southern Railway system eventually absorbed the Air Line. See Hurley E. Badders, "Oconee County," in *South Carolina Encyclopedia* (Columbia: University of South Carolina, Institute for Southern Studies, updated Aug. 16, 2022), https://www.scencyclopedia.org/sce/entries/oconee-county/. For more information on the Keowee Hotel and its springs as recalled in a 1963 newspaper story, see "Historic Oconee County, South Carolina: Seneca's Mineral Springs," published Jan. 12, 2003, https://sites.rootsweb.com/~scoconee/archived-txt/history/h-29.txt.
10. "Blue Ridge Mineral Springs Hotel," *Keowee Courier* (Pickens Court House, SC), 15 July 1903; Matthew C. Smith, "Blue Ridge Railroad," in *South Carolina Encyclopedia*, updated July 19, 2022, https://www.scencyclopedia.org/sce/entries/blue-ridge-railroad.
11. "Blue Ridge Mineral Springs Hotel (Fronts on Blue Ridge Railroad) [ad]," *Keowee Courier* (Pickens Court House, SC), 20 Mar. 1907; "Blue Ridge Mineral Springs Hotel [ad]," *Augusta Daily Herald* (GA), 23 May 1909. Resort conclusions are drawn from limited information available.
12. "The Mineral Springs Hotel," *Keowee Courier* (Pickens Court House, SC), 19 Apr. 1905.
13. "Blue Ridge Mineral Springs Hotel Arrivals," *Ibid.*, 23 Aug. 1905.
14. "Blue Ridge Mineral Springs Hotel (Fronts on Blue Ridge Railroad) [ad]," *Ibid.*, 20 Mar. 1907.
15. *Ibid.*, 19 May 1909; *Ibid.*, 31 May 1911; "Walhalla, South Carolina," ClemsonWiki, https://www.clemsonwiki.com/wiki/Walhalla,_South_Carolina.
16. "Fort Hill: National Historic Landmark," Clemson University, published Mar. 7, 2012, accessed Aug. 20, 2020, https://www.clemson.edu/about/history/properties/fort-hill/. The website also includes information about the enslaved people held by the Calhoun family.
17. Donna K. Roper, "Pickens County," in *South Carolina Encyclopedia*, updated Aug. 22, 2022, https://www.scencyclopedia.org/sce/entries/pickens-county/ .
18. The *Pickens Sentinel* references the resort as "Ambler's Mineral Springs" in 1877 but as "Griffin Spring" in 1878. "Ambler" had replaced "Griffin" by the turn of the century in publications. See *Pickens Sentinel* (SC), 2 Aug. 1877; *Ibid.*, 22 Aug. 1878.
19. Crook, "Climatology and Health Resorts," 82.
20. *Ibid.*; Crook, *Mineral Waters of the United States*, 422. Crook gives the distance as seven miles in *Mineral Waters* and as six miles in his journal article, perhaps indicating the expansion of Pickens during the period between his two publications.
21. "Climatology and Health Resorts," 82; Crook, *Mineral Waters of the United States*, 422.
22. Crook, *Mineral Waters of the United States*, 422; Matson, "Mineral Waters," 1126. Matson's sales data for South Carolina covers 1911 and does not list Ambler.
23. I located guests' hometowns and descriptions from newspapers retrieved from the Library of Congress's *Chronicling America* website. In particular, the *Pickens Sentinel* proved to be a valuable source for the Ambler House for the period 1886–1903. From the news accounts, I counted over 40 guests for Charleston and about 16 for Greenville.

24. *Pickens Sentinel* (SC), 2 Aug. 1877; *People's Journal* (Pickens, SC), 31 July 1902.
25. For information on the state park, see "Caesars Head State Park," South Carolina State Parks, https://southcarolinaparks.com/caesars-head#jump. The state park website is the source for the elevation; other sources give varying heights.
26. David H. Rembert, Jr., "Caesars Head State Park," in *South Carolina Encyclopedia*, updated July 20, 2022, https://www.scencyclopedia.org/sce/entries/caesars-head-state-park/; Brewster, *Summer Migrations*, 72.
27. "Caesars Head, Mineral Spring, verso," Stereographic Views of South Carolina Collection, https://digital.tcl.sc.edu/digital/collection/stereo/id/1833, USC; Brewster, *Summer Migrations*, 72.
28. W.M.C., "Editorial Correspondence," *Lancaster Ledger* (SC), 18 Aug. 1858.
29. "Gone," *Newberry Herald* (SC), 31 July 1872.
30. "Communications," *Edgefield Advertiser* (SC), 4 Sept. 1844.
31. "Chicks Springs," *Southern Enterprise* (Greenville, SC), 18 Aug. 1854.
32. Louis P. Towles, "Cherokee County," in *South Carolina Encyclopedia*, updated July 20, 2022, https://www.scencyclopedia.org/sce/entries/cherokee-county/.
33. Other minor or short-lived mineral spring retreats in the county were located at Campobello, Cooley Springs, Boiling Springs, and Cedar Springs. See Michael Leonard, *Our Heritage: A Community History of Spartanburg County, S.C.* (Spartanburg: Band & White for Spartanburg Herald and Journal, 1986). For more information on Cedar Springs, see "Our History," South Carolina School for the Deaf and Blind, www.scsdb.org/domain/9.
34. A Visitor, "The Springs of the Spartanburg District," *Edgefield Advertiser* (SC), 22 Aug. 1839.
35. "The Springs of the Spartanburg District," *Ibid.*, 22 Aug. 1839; Myers, "Booker T. Washington, Spartanburg, and the Cherokee Springs Hotel," 26, in Grady and Myers, eds., *Recovering*, vol. 2; U.S. Census 1860 (Slave Schedule), FamilySearch, www.familysearch.org; all subsequent Census citations in this chapter were located in FamilySearch.
36. "Cherokee Springs. F. Cantrell, Proprietor [ad]," *Carolina Spartan* (Spartanburg), 10 July 1856.
37. *Ibid.*; Brewster, *Summer Migrations*, 77.
38. "Cherokee Springs, Spartanburg Dist. S.C. [ad]," *Carolina Spartan* (Spartanburg), 19 June 1862.
39. Myers, 27; Nancy A. Hardesty, "Holiness movement," in *South Carolina Encyclopedia*, updated Aug. 8, 2022, https://www.scencyclopedia.org/sce/entries/holiness-movement/.
40. Myers, 27; "Cherokee Springs [ad]," *Daily Phoenix* (Columbia, SC), 27 July 1871; "Last Sunday at Cherokee," *Carolina Spartan* (Spartanburg), 3 June 1869; Leonard, 217.
41. Marsh, "Notes from Spartanburg," *Charleston Daily News*, 22 Aug. 1872; Myers, 27–28.
42. Myers, 31–32.
43. *Ibid.*, 32–35.
44. Leonard, 216–17.
45. For more information on the location and the main resort owner, see Tina Minty, "William 'The Taylor' Poole Biography," 1–2, https://pacoletmemories.com/PooleFamily.pdf.
46. "The Invalid: Occasioned By His Visit to Pacolet Springs in South-Carolina, for the Recovery of His Health," in Freneau, *Poems Written*, 211–12.
47. Brooks, "Iron Works on Lawson's Fork," 50n26.
48. Drayton, *View of South Carolina*, 49.
49. "Obituary of Col. Robert Coleman Poole"; "Mansion House," *Spartan* (Spartanburg, SC), 14 Aug. 1844; U.S. Census 1860 (Slave Schedule). Poole in 1860 owned three enslaved persons; he may have owned a larger number before his financial loss.
50. *Carolina Spartan* (Spartanburg), 26 Nov. 1857; "New Hotel in Spartanburg," *Ibid.*, 10 Dec. 1857.
51. Writers' Program of the Work Projects Administration in the State of South Carolina, *History of Spartanburg County*, 123.
52. Leonard, 213.
53. "Calybeate [sic] Springs," *Edgefield Advertiser* (SC), 28 June 1848. The article reported the discovery of another chalybeate springs about three fourths of a mile away from the village.
54. "Editorial Correspondence," *Newberry Herald* (SC), 9 Sept. 1874; *Union Times*, 28 May 1880; "Military Hop on the 4th," *Laurens Advertiser*, 29 June 1887.
55. Peale, "Lists and Analyses," 79.
56. "A Chance for Union," *Weekly Union Times* (SC), 21 Nov. 1890; "The Garrett Hydraulic Motor," *Ibid.*, 19 June 1891; U.S. Patent 459,280, "Hydraulic Motor." The background of the invention calls out spring waters, each with a different medicinal property, as an example of the use of the motor.
57. "Garrett Ships Mineral Water," *Weekly Union Times* (SC), 19 June 1891; "Ice Cream Saloon," *Ibid.*
58. "Rocky Cliff Springs," *News and Herald* (Winnsboro, SC), 23 May 1906; *Spartanburg Journal*, 6 Sept. 1906; "Resort for Spartanburg," *Americus Times-Recorder* (GA), 9 May 1906. The resort may have initially been referred to as both "Rocky Cliff" and "Rock Cliff," but most sources consulted use the latter phrase.
59. Racine, *Seeing Spartanburg*, 143.
60. "Harris Lithia Spring Hotel," *Newberry Herald and News* (SC), 25 July 1894; "Harris' Lithia Springs [ad]," *Asheville Daily Citizen*, 23 June 1892; Snowden, *History of South Carolina*, 215. For doubt on the water's therapeutic powers, see "A Miraculous Elixir," Greetings from Greenwood: The Postcard Project, *Greenville Times*, http://greenwoodtimes.com/content/elixir.
61. "Annual Meeting Press Association," *Watchman and Southron* (Sumter, SC), 10 July

1901; *Laurens Advertiser* (SC), 26 May 1886; *Ibid.*, 31 Mar. 1891.

62. Leonard, 214; *Carolina Spartan* (Spartanburg), 30 Apr. 1902.

63. *Carolina Spartan* (Spartanburg), 30 Apr. 1902; *White Stone Lithia Hotel…*[1903], photocopy of original in Mineral Springs file, Caroliniana Library, USC, procured from Kennedy Room, Spartanburg County Public Library, SC. The *Spartan* states the hotel contained 109 rooms; the brochure, "more than two hundred rooms."

64. "White Stone Lithia Water, The Lightest Mineral Water Known [ad]," *News and Herald* (Winnsboro, SC), 9 July 1902.

65. Snowden, ed., *History of South Carolina*, vol. 4, 215.

66. "White Stone Lithia Water is the Lightest Mineral Water [ad]," *Anderson Intelligencer* (Anderson Court House, SC), 2 July 1902.

67. *White Stone Lithia Hotel*.

68. *Newberry Herald and News* (SC), 10 July 1903; "Mystic Shriners in Session," *Bamberg Herald* (SC), 6 Oct. 1904.

69. *County Record* (Kingstree, SC), 18 Aug. 1904; *Watchman and Southron* (Sumter, SC), 3 Aug. 1904; Williamson, "Seven Ways." The CPI calculator was used.

70. "White Springs Stone Hotel Totally Destroyed by Fire," *Union Times* (SC), 16 Mar. 1906.

71. "Harris Buys White Stone," *Herald and News* (Newberry, SC), 15 May 1908; "Buys White Stone Springs," *Bamberg Herald* (SC), 6 July 1911; Gary Henderson, "History Springs Forth in White Stone," www.groupstate.com; "Croft State Park," South Carolina State Parks, https://southcarolinaparks.com/croft. More research is needed to determine if "Dugan" was a misspelling of "Dougan" in "Dougan & Sheftall" as both parties hailed from Savannah.

72. A notable exception is Cedar Springs, which in 1849 became an academy for the education of deaf children in the state.

73. Huff, *Greenville*, 104–06.

74. Kidd, "The History of Salt Sulphur Springs," 226; "John C. Calhoun to James Edward Calhoun, Washington, July 29, 1846," in Jameson, *Annual Report*, 702; "Calhoun to Thomas G. Clemson, Washington, Aug. 8, 1846," *Ibid.*, 704; "Calhoun to James Edward Calhoun, Fort Hill, Sept. 15, 1846," *Ibid.*, 706.

75. Megginson, *African American Life*, 130.

76. Huff, 114; "Mr. Alfred Taylor," *Pickens Sentinel* (SC), 31 Oct. 1912.

77. Writers' Program, *History of Spartanburg*, 124.

78. "Sallie Foster to Her Cousin, Elizabeth Cothran, Glenn Springs, Dec. 31 [1861]," in Kennedy, *South Carolina Upcountry Saga*, 176.

79. See, for example, *Charleston Mercury*, 22 July 1861; *Ibid.*, 10 July 1862; *Charleston Daily Courier*, 8 Sept. 1863.

80. "Yellow Fever in Memphis," *Abbeville Press and Banner* (SC), 16 July 1879.

81. *Anderson Intelligencer* (Anderson Court House, SC), 31 July 1879; *Abbeville Press and Banner* (SC), 13 Aug. 1879.

82. "Quarantine," *Abbeville Press and Banner* (SC), 26 Sept. 1888; "The State Board of Health Carefully Guard Against Yellow Jack," *Watchman and Southron* (Sumter, SC), 29 Sept. 1897.

83. K, "A Visit to Georgia," *Keowee Courier* (Pickens Court House, SC), 21 Aug. 1879.

84. *Anderson Intelligencer* (Anderson Court House, SC), 6 Oct. 1897. The article lamented the lack of good transportation because Anderson residents were beginning to favor that part of the Smokies as a summer retreat.

85. "Charleston Families Quarantined," *Abbeville Press and Banner* (SC), 19 Sept. 1888.

86. "Refugees from Yellow Fever," *Asheville Citizen*, 12 Sept. 1888.

Chick Springs

87. B.F Perry, "Reminiscences of the County of Greenville," *Greenville Enterprise* (SC), 11 Oct. 1871.

88. Writers' Program, *Palmetto Place Names*, 15.

89. Brewster, *Summer Migrations*, 58–59; Buckingham, *Slave States*, 175–76.

90. Writers' Program, 34; Brewster, *Summer Migrations*, 77; Huff, *Greenville*, 92–93; S.S. Crittenden, *Greenville Century Book*, 40.

91. *Edgefield Advertiser* (SC), 6 Aug. 1845.

92. Karen Nutt, "The History of the Chick Springs Hotel," *GoUpstate.com*, https://www.goupstate.com/article/NC/20030730/News/605163898/SJ; Williamson, "Seven Ways." The CPI calculator was used.

93. "Chick's Springs [ad]," *Edgefield Advertiser* (SC), 17 June 1852.

94. *Republic* (Washington, D.C.), 14 Mar. 1851.

95. "A Few Items Gathered in Traveling," *Edgefield Advertiser* (SC), 25 Aug. 1852; "The Chicks and Ourselves," *Ibid.*, 15 Sept. 1852.

96. "A Few Items Gathered in Traveling," *Ibid.*, 25 Aug. 1852. The writer's description of Gabe betrays his own prejudice.

97. "From the Greenville Mountaineer, Chick's Springs, Sept. 8 '52," *Ibid.*, 15 Sept. 1852. That the Chicks owned enslaved persons is established through a blurb in which a Greenville newspaper editor rhetorically asks the proprietors if "your negroes [sic] sell as well as they ever did?" See "We are a Doomed People Unless We Resist," *American Telegraph* (Washington, D.C.), 18 Sept. 1851. The U.S. Census (Slave Schedule) for 1850 lists over 20 enslaved people each for Reuben and Pettus Chick of Union County, SC. It is not known if other enslaved persons besides Gabe worked at the resort.

98. "From the Greenville Mountaineer, Chick's Springs, Sept. 8 '52." For description of Scurry as a slaveowner by one of his former slaves, see Federal Writers' Project: Slave Narrative Project, vol. 14,

South Carolina, Part 4, Raines-Young, 1936–1938, "Morgan Scurry, Newberry, South Carolina, May 19, 1937," Manuscript/Mixed Material, https://www.loc.gov/resource/mesn.144.

99. "Chicks' Springs," *Southern Enterprise* (Greenville, SC), 18 Aug. 1854.

100. W.M.C., "Editorial Correspondence," *Lancaster Ledger* (SC), 18 Aug. 1858.

101. J.S.R., "Editorial Correspondence," *Sumter Banner* (SC), 13 Sept. 1854.

102. "Chick Springs, Greenville District. Splendid Summer Resort," *Abbeville Banner* (SC), 4 June 1857; Huff, 93.

103. "Editorial Correspondence," *Lancaster Ledger* (SC), 18 Aug. 1858.

104. "Saint Mary's Greenville Observes 50th Anniversary of Corner Stone Laying," *Bulletin* (Augusta, GA), 30 Sept. 1953.

105. "Religious Notice," *Southern Enterprise* (Greenville, SC), 22 Dec. 1859; Judy Bainbridge, "Catholic Church Faced Prejudice in 1800s Greenville," *Greenville News*, 1 Jan. 2014, www.greenvilleonline.com.

106. Barber and Howe, *Our Whole Country*, 723–24. An illustration of Chick Springs appears on 723.

107. O'Connell, *Catholicity in the Carolinas*, 368.

108. Ibid.

109. "A Few Items Gathered in Traveling," *Edgefield Advertiser* (SC), 25 Aug. 1852.

110. "Chicks Springs," *Southern Enterprise* (Greenville, SC), 18 Aug. 1854; "Editorial Correspondence," *Sumter Banner* (SC), 13 Sept. 1854.

111. "Chick Springs Letter," *Watchman and Southron* (Sumter, SC), 18 July 1914.

112. Paul Christopher Anderson, "Manning, John Laurence," in *South Carolina Encyclopedia*, updated Aug. 11, 2022, https://www.scencyclopedia.org/sce/entries/manning-john-laurence/; Huff, 93.

113. "Chicks' Springs," *Southern Enterprise* (Greenville, SC), 11 June 1857.

114. Merchant, *South Carolina Fire-Eater*, 32. Congress censured Keitt in 1856 for his role in South Carolina Congressman Preston Brooks' caning of Massachusetts Senator Charles Sumner. For a brief narrative of Keitt's role, see Merchant, 45–46.

115. *Camden Journal* (SC), 10 Oct. 1849.

116. Roberta VH Copp, "O'Neall, John Belton," in *South Carolina Encyclopedia*, updated Aug. 16, 2022, http://www.scencyclopedia.org/sce/entries/oneall-john-belton/.

117. "Chick Springs [ad]," *Edgefield Advertiser* (SC), 17 June 1852; Burns, *History of Blount County*, 81.

118. Brewster, *Summer Migrations*, 60, 63.

119. "Chick's Springs [ad]," *Edgefield Advertiser* (SC), 12 June 1861; "Chick Springs Hotel [ad]," *Charleston Mercury*, 2 June 1862.

120. *Yorkville Enquirer* (SC), 12 Nov. 1862.

121. Huff, 209.

122. "Chick's Springs," *Greenville Enterprise* (SC), 12 Oct. 1870; Huff, 209.

123. Sprout, "Greenville Occasional," *Newberry Herald* (SC), 21 May 1873.

124. Huff, 93, 209; "Death of Mr. Reuben S. Chick," *Newberry Herald* (SC), 9 Feb. 1876; "Summer Health Resort. Chick Springs [ad]," *Morning News* (Savannah), 6 June 1900.

125. Huff, 209; *Anderson Intelligencer* (Anderson Court House, SC), 3 Sept. 1902; "Bull Family of Chick Springs," South Carolina Digital Library, https://scmemory.org/collection/bull-family-of-chick-springs/; *Abbeville Press and Banner* (SC), 16 Aug. 1905.

126. "Taylor Station," *Pickens Sentinel-Journal* (SC), 4 Jan. 1905; "Water That Puts Roses on Pale Cheeks [ad]," *French Broad Hustler* (Hendersonville, NC), 31 Aug. 1905. The supposition about the third hotel being built near Westmoreland's establishment comes from a 1907 newspaper ad referencing the "main hotel building." See "Plan to go to Chick Springs, Hotel Opens June 1st [ad]," *Atlanta Georgian*, 4 May 1907.

127. "What More Do You Want? [ad]," *Atlanta Georgian and News*, 6 July 1907; "Plan to go to Chick Springs, Hotel Opens June 1st [ad]," *Ibid.*, 4 May 1907.

128. "Water That Puts Roses on Pale Cheeks [ad]."

129. "On June 1st Chick Springs Hotel Will Be Ready For You [ad]," *Atlanta Georgian*, 13 May 1907.

130. "Plan to go to Chick Springs, Hotel Opens June 1st [ad]," *Ibid.*, 4 May 1907; "Young Cureton Drowned," *Lancaster News* (SC), 7 July 1906.

131. "Festivities at Chick Springs," *Atlanta Georgian and News*, 2 Aug. 1907.

132. "Water That Puts Roses on Pale Cheeks [ad]."

133. "Hotel Destroyed by Fire," *Birmingham Age-Herald* (AL), 15 Dec. 1907; Williamson, "Seven Ways." The CPI calculator was used.

134. "Will Rebuild Hotel," *Atlanta Georgian and News*, 21 Feb. 1908; "To Build at Chick Springs," *Edgefield Advertiser* (SC), 4 Mar. 1908; "If You Were Offered Board For the Month of June [ad]," *Bamberg Herald* (SC), 10 June 1909.

135. "Half Million Loss in Piedmont District," *Douglas Enterprise* (GA), 5 Sept. 1908; *Watchman and Southron* (Sumter, SC), 24 Apr. 1909.

136. "If You Were Offered Board For the Month of June [ad]." The link between *Anopheles* mosquitoes and malarial parasite transmission in humans had been discovered several years earlier.

137. "To Mothers of Sick and Delicate Children," *Bamberg Herald* (SC), 7 July 1904.

138. "Chick Springs [ad]," *Birmingham Age-Herald* (AL), 29 Apr. 1906.

139. "The Proof is in the Results!" *Ocala Banner* (FL), 6 July 1906.

140. "What More Do You Want?" *Atlanta Georgian and News*, 6 July 1907.

141. "Chick Springs, S.C. [ad]," *Athens Daily*

Herald (GA), 22 May 1915; "A Big New Hotel for Chick Springs," *Anderson Daily Intelligencer* (SC), 1 Feb. 1914; *Bamberg Herald*, 12 Feb. 1914.

142. "A Big New Hotel for Chick Springs"; "Develop Chick Springs," *Abbeville Press and Banner* (SC), 11 Feb. 1914; "Rehabilitating Famous South Carolina Resort," *Bamberg Herald* (SC), 12 Feb. 1914; "The Wonderful Transformation at Chick Springs," *Anderson Daily Intelligencer* (SC), 31 May 1914. The May 1914 article erroneously gives the starting date of the resort as 1846. Visitors' home municipalities were determined by looking at newspapers over a thirty-year period, including society columns and published hotel registers.

143. "Chick Springs," *Anderson Daily Intelligencer* (SC), 16 Aug. 1914.

144. The third railroad was the Atlantic Coast Line. See H. Roger Grant, "Railroads," in *South Carolina Encyclopedia*, updated Aug. 23, 2022, https://www.scencyclopedia.org/sce/entries/railroads/.

145. *Greenville Enterprise*, 14 June 1871; "Chick Springs Letter," *Watchman and Southron* (Sumter, SC), 18 July 1914. The latter citation gives the name of the railroad before Southern purchased the line.

146. "Low Summer Rates via Southern Railway from Atlanta [ad]," *Atlanta Georgian*, 18 July 1908.

147. "Something Special! Annual Mountain and Seashore Excursion Fares [ad]," *Athens Daily Herald* (GA), 7 Aug. 1914.

148. "Greenville-Spartanburg Line Planned," *Atlanta Georgian and News*, 31 July 1907; "Trolley Line Commissioned," *Watchman and Southron* (Sumter, SC), 12 Jan. 1910; "At Chick Springs," *Herald and News* (Newberry, SC), 1 Aug. 1913.

149. "Weekend Trips to Chick Springs at Reduced Rates," *Intelligencer* (Anderson, SC), 26 June 1915.

150. "Gaieties at Chick Springs," *Atlanta Georgian and News*, 27 July 1907.

151. *Athens Daily Herald* (GA), 12 Aug. 1916.

152. *Ibid.*, 29 July 1915; *Ibid.*, 21 Aug. 1915.

153. "Summer Visitors Invited," *French Broad Hustler* (Hendersonville, NC), 31 Aug. 1905.

154. "'Oligarchists' in Secret Conclave at Chick Springs—W.W. Ball in *Columbia State*," *Laurens Advertiser* (SC), 15 July 1914.

155. *Walker County Messenger* (LaFayette, GA), 7 July 1911; "Dixie Checker Cracks after Championship," *Atlanta Georgian*, 20 Aug. 1915; "Stenographers Will Meet Chick Springs," *Intelligencer* (Anderson, SC), 6 June 1916; "Chick Springs Next Year," *Union Times* (SC), 4 July 1913.

156. "Press Association at Chick Springs," *Anderson Daily Intelligencer* (SC), 8 July 1914.

157. "Chick Springs Water [ad]," *Greenville News*, 18 June 1916; "Delight [ad]," *Weekly Times-Recorder* (Americus, GA), 15 July 1915.

158. "Opening Ball at Chick Springs," *Intelligencer* (Anderson, SC), 15 June 1915; "Grand Dress Parade of Militia Tomorrow," *Ibid.*, 15 July 1915; "Chick Springs Involved," *Keowee Courier* (Pickens Court House, SC), 1 Mar. 1916.

159. "Receiver for Chick Springs Company," *Keowee Courier* (Pickens Court House, SC), 8 Mar. 1916; "Hotel at Chicks Sold for $48,000," *Greenville News* (SC), 4 Apr. 1916.

160. "Millionaire Says He Has Not Yet Leased Hotel," *Intelligencer* (Anderson, SC), 14 Apr. 1916; "Invests Thousands in Piedmont Lands," *Ibid.*, 27 Apr. 1916. The deal also included a valuation of $65,000 placed on the northern Greenville County property.

161. "Pythians Will Go to Columbia," *Keowee Courier* (Pickens Court House, SC), 29 Mar. 1916; *Herald and News* (Newberry, SC), 4 Apr. 1916.

162. "Hotel at Chick Springs Will Open Soon," *Abbeville Press and Banner* (SC), 17 May 1916; "Military School at Chick Springs," *Ibid.*, 31 May 1916.

163. "Our Southern Saratoga," *Keowee Courier* (Pickens Court House, SC), 2 Aug. 1916.

164. "Chick Springs Military Academy [ad]," *Laurens Advertiser* (SC), 30 May 1917.

165. *Herald and News* (Newberry, SC), 17 Oct. 1916; "Chick Springs Military Academy Growing," *Laurens Advertiser* (SC), 28 Feb. 1917; "Fire at Chick Springs," *Keowee Courier* (Pickens Court House, SC), 3 Oct. 1917.

166. "Chick Springs School Closed," *Keowee Courier* (Pickens Court House, SC), 2 Jan. 1918.

167. *Banner-Herald* (Athens, GA), 3 July 1924; Flynn, *Short History of Chick Springs*, 5-6.

168. "To Train Veterans at Chick Springs," *Fort Mills Times* (SC), 23 Mar. 1922. Steedly continued to operate the sanitarium until his sudden death in early 1932. The U.S. government operated a training center at Chick Springs at least into 1930.

169. South Carolina Appalachian Council of Governments, *Survey of Historic Places*, 65; "Chick Springs," SC Picture Project, https://www.scpictureproject.org/greenville-county/chick-springs.html.

170. "Chick Springs," SC Picture Project; Nan Lundeen, "Springhouse Offers Slice of Taylors [sic] History: Cleanup May Become First Step to Public Park," *Greenville News* (SC), 25 Oct. 2005; Ismael Tate, "Returning Chick Springs' Flow Spurs Bill Wilson," *Ibid.*, 26 Apr. 2006.

Glenn Springs

171. Karen Nutt, "High Spot Lies Next to Hogback Mountain," GoUpstate, www.GoUpstate.com; "Spartanburg County Topo Maps and Elevations," www.AnyplaceAmerica.com. The latter website, which provides USFS topo maps, states that Shuttle Radar Topography Mission data gives the county's high point as 1,309 ft. but does not specify the location within the county.

172. Writers' Program, *Palmetto Place Names*, 19; Landrum, *History of Spartanburg County*, 7-9.

173. *Statistics of South Carolina*, 725. Spartanburg, the county seat, served as an "important demarcation line" for agriculture—gray, rocky soil to its north for grains and fertile clay soil to

its south for cotton. See Bruce W. Eelman, "Entrepreneurs in the Southern Upcountry: The Case of Spartanburg, South Carolina, 1815–1880," *Enterprise & Society*, 5 (Mar. 2004): 80–81.

174. *Statistics of South Carolina*, 26, 724, 730.
175. Ibid., 725, 727.
176. Means, "History of Glenn Springs," 20.
177. Racine, *Seeing Spartanburg*, 36.
178. Russel, "Glenn's Springs," 213.
179. Walker, "Mineral Water, Dancing, and Amusements: The Development of Tourism in the Nineteenth Century Upcountry," 14, in Grady and Walker, eds., *Recovering*.
180. Russel, 213.
181. U.S. Dept. of the Interior, NPS, National Register of Historic Places, "Glenn Springs Historic District, 8. Significance."
182. Means, 22.
183. Brewster, *Summer Migrations*, 78–79; "Glenn's Springs for Sale. Sheriff's Sale," *Daily Chronicle & Sentinel* (Augusta, GA), 27 Nov. 1841.
184. *Edgefield Advertiser* (SC), 9 May 1839.
185. "Glenn's Springs for Sale. Sheriff's Sale," *Daily Chronicle & Sentinel* (Augusta, GA), 27 Nov. 1841. One dollar in 1841 is equivalent to almost $35 in 2022, using the CPI data found at Williamson, "Seven Ways." The CPI calculator was used in dollar conversions in this chapter.
186. Walker, "Mineral Water," 14; Randall E. Parker et al, "Economic Panics," in NCpedia, https://www.ncpedia.org/panics-economic.
187. Edgar, *South Carolina*, 274.
188. Rousseau, "Jacksonian Monetary Policy," 479–80. Rousseau argues that the fall of cotton prices itself was not the major cause of the May panic.
189. Harris, *Piedmont Farmer*, 500, 503. Harris lived near Glenn Springs and was brother-in-law to Camp.
190. Landrum, 443–44; Racine, 27, 38; U.S. Census 1850 (Slave Schedule), FamilySearch, www.familysearch.org/. All subsequent Census records in this chapter were retrieved from FamilySearch.
191. "Glenn's Springs [ad]," *Edgefield Advertiser* (SC), 21 June 1843; Landrum, 67.
192. "Glenn's Springs [ad]," *Edgefield Advertiser* (SC), 1 June 1842.
193. National Register of Historic Places Inventory-Nomination Form, "Glenn Springs, 8. Significance."
194. "Water Cure Institute at Glenn Springs, S.C. [ad]," *Savannah Daily Republican*, 16 Feb. 1852.
195. Diane C. Vecchio, "From Slavery to Freedom: African American Life in Post-Civil War Spartanburg," 109, in Grady and Walker, eds., *Recovering*.
196. Landrum, 445; "Sale of Glenn Springs," *Camden Weekly Journal* (SC), 9 Aug. 1853; Williamson, "Seven Ways."
197. "Episcopal Female School, at Glenn Springs," *Camden Weekly Journal* (SC), 22 Nov. 1853.

198. "Glenn Springs Female Institute," *Southern Enterprise* (Greenville, SC), 26 May 1854.
199. "Glenn Springs for Sale," *Edgefield Advertiser* (SC), 24 Jan. 1855; "Glenn Springs Female Institute"; Brewster, *Summer Migrations*, 79n31.
200. Means, 25.
201. Walker, "Mineral Water," 15; Burges and Chadwick, "Diary of Samuel Edward Burges," 142; Brewster, *Summer Migrations*, 78, 79n31.
202. "Editorial from the Industrial Issue of the *Spartanburg Herald*, Nov., 1886," reprinted in Means, "History of Glenn Springs," 32.
203. Brewster, *Summer Migrations*, 78. Brewster cites as his source a biographical sketch of Moore by Celina E. Means. Means was Moore's daughter.
204. Moore, "Efficacy of the Water of Glenn Springs," 641–45.
205. "Efficacy of the Water of Glenn Springs," 645, 643.
206. Ibid., 642, 645.
207. Ibid., 644–646.
208. Calhoun, "Letters from John C. Calhoun to Francis W. Pickens," 14; *Savannah Daily Republican*, 28 Aug. 1847; Brewster, *Summer Migrations*, 80.
209. Merchant, 111, 140; Brewster, *Summer Migrations*, 80.
210. Brewster, *Summer Migrations*, 79–80.
211. "Glenn's Springs [ad]," *Edgefield Advertiser* (SC), 1 June 1842.
212. "Glenn Springs [ad]," *Lancaster Ledger* (SC), 3 Aug. 1853.
213. Landrum, 40. Brewster describes a rather convoluted route from Columbia on both the Greenville and Laurens railroads and then picking up a stage line four miles from the Laurens Court House to travel to Glenn Springs. See Brewster, *Summer Migrations*, 81.
214. H. Roger Grant, "Railroads," in *South Carolina Encyclopedia*, updated Aug. 23, 2022, https://www.scencyclopedia.org/sce/entries/railroads/; "List of Acts Passed by the Legislature at Its Session of 1848," *Edgefield Advertiser* (SC), 27 Dec. 1848.
215. "Union Rail Road Convention," *Spartan* (Spartanburg), 6 Feb. 1849.
216. Aaron W. Marrs, "Greenville and Columbia Railroad," in *South Carolina Encyclopedia*, updated Aug. 5, 2022, https://www.scencyclopedia.org/sce/entries/greenville-and-columbia-railroad/.
217. "Glenn Springs Hotel [ad]," *Charleston Daily Courier*, 15 June 1861.
218. "Death at Glenn Springs," *Abbeville Press* (SC), 19 July 1861.
219. "Sallie Foster to Her Cousin, Elizabeth Cothran, Glenn Springs, June 22 [1863]," in Kennedy, *South Carolina Upcountry Saga*, 321; "Foster to Cothran, Glenn Springs, July 2 [1863]," *Ibid.*, 323. The Glenn Springs hotel may also have served as a recruitment center. See "Recruiting Service," *Carolina Spartan* (Spartanburg), 19 June 1862.
220. "Summer Resort [ad]," *Charleston Daily News*, 8 Aug. 1866; "Montvale Springs, 1867 [ad]," *Cartersville Express* (GA), 16 Aug. 1867. Montvale

charged $65 monthly in 1867, but deflation in the U.S. following the war renders the 1867 Montvale $65 rate and the 1866 Glenn $60 rate nearly the same. See Williamson, "Seven Ways."

221. Senior, "Glenn's Spring—Our Trip Home—The Next House, etc.," *Newberry Herald* (SC), 4 Aug. 1869. Adjusting the 1866 monthly rate of $60 to 1869 dollars via the CPI gives $55.60, demonstrating that Anderson reduced the rate in real dollars, regardless of the deflation of the times. See Williamson, "Seven Ways."

222. "For the Summer," *Yorkville Enquirer* (SC), 22 July 1869.

223. Senior, "Glen Springs, Shady Side," *Newberry Herald* (SC), 18 Aug. 1869; Senior, "Glenn Springs, August 1869," *Ibid.*, 25 Aug. 1869.

224. *Charleston Daily News*, 12 July 1869.

225. "In Re. John W. Grady, Bankrupt," *Southern Enterprise* (Greenville, SC), 8 Dec. 1869; "Land Sales," *Charleston Daily News*, 1 Jan. 1870.

226. "The Spartanburg Springs," *Newberry Herald* (SC), 1 June 1870; *Daily Phoenix* (Columbia), 23 June 1870.

227. *Charleston Daily News*, 20 June 1870.

228. "Everybody will be Glad to Hear it," *Newberry Herald* (SC), 13 May 1874.

229. *Ibid.*, 14 July 1875; "Correspondence Columbia Phoenix," *Daily Phoenix* (Columbia), 23 July 1875; "Glenn Springs, Spartanburg Co., S.C. [ad]," *Newberry Herald* (SC), 14 July 1875.

230. *Newberry Herald* (SC), 22 Mar. 1876; Landrum, , 645; U.S. Population Census 1880; *Watchman and Southron* (Sumter, SC), 17 May 1893.

231. Landrum, 645; "Death of Dr. J. W. Simpson," *Weekly Union Times* (SC), 22 Apr. 1881; Walter Edgar, "Simpson, William Dunlap," in *South Carolina Encyclopedia*, updated Aug. 23, 2022, https://www.scencyclopedia.org/sce/entries/simpson-william-dunlap/. William D. had also served as briefly as governor upon Wade Hampton's resignation in 1879.

232. U.S. Population Census 1880; "Sunday at Glenns," *Union Times* (SC), 21 July 1899.

233. "Editorial from the Industrial Issue of the *Spartanburg Herald*, Nov., 1886," 31; Mrs. T. Sumter Means, "Glenn Springs. Its History from Its Discovery, With Personal Sketches of Its Habitues," *Watchman and Southron* (Sumter, SC), 7 May 1890. Several illustrations accompany the *Watchman and Southron* article.

234. "Editorial from the Industrial Issue of the *Spartanburg Herald*, Nov.,1886," 31–32; National Register of Historic Places Inventory-Nomination Form, "Glenn Springs, Continuation sheet 5, Item number 8, Page 1."

235. "Glenn Springs," *Evening Bulletin* (Maysville, KY), 16 July 1890.

236. Walker, "Mineral Water," 19; "Glen Springs Hotel, Glenn Springs, S.C. [ad]," *Watchman and Southron* (Sumter, SC), 1 Sept. 1897.

237. "Glenn Springs Hotel, Glenn Springs, S.C. [ad]," *Watchman and Southron* (Sumter, SC), 28 June 1899.

238. "Editorial from the Industrial Issue of the *Spartanburg Herald*, Nov., 1886," 32.

239. Walker, "Mineral Water," 18; Senior, "Glenn Springs—Shady Side," *Newberry Herald* (SC), 11 Aug. 1869; Senior, "Glenn Spring," *Ibid.*, 8 Sept. 1869; "Glen Springs Hotel," *Watchman and Southron* (Sumter, SC), 28 June 1899; *Watchman and Southron* (Sumter, SC), 2 Sept. 1903.

240. "Glenn Springs, Spartanburg County, S.C. [ad]," *Savannah Morning News*, 19 May 1875; "Glenn Springs Hotel [ad]," *County Record* (Kingstree, SC), 24 June 1909; H.G.O., "Letter from Glenn Springs," *Watchman and Southron* (Sumter, SC), 13 Aug. 1890.

241. Russel, 215; Means, "Glenn Springs. Its History"; "Glenn Springs," *Watchman and Southron* (Sumter, SC), 2 Nov. 1886.

242. Russel, 215.

243. Fitch, 588.

244. "Glenn Springs Ginger Ale," *Watchman and Southron* (Sumter, SC), 17 June 1903.

245. *Newberry Herald and News* (SC), 24 July 1903.

246. *Brunswick News* (GA), 13 Aug. 1909.

247. *Newberry Herald* (SC), 27 Sept. 1876.

248. Eelman, "Entrepreneurs in the Southern Upcountry," 88; "Glenn Springs, Spartanburg Co., S.C. [ad]," *Watchman and Southron* (Sumter, SC), 18 July 1888.

249. Racine, 138; "Glenn Springs Hotel [ad]," *Watchman and Southron* (Sumter, SC), 1 Sept. 1897.

250. Walker, "Mineral Water," 19.

251. "Letter from Glenn Springs."

252. Walker, "Mineral Water," 19.

253. "Glenn Springs Sold," *Herald and News* (Newberry, SC), 22 Dec. 1905.

254. E. H. Aull, "The Editor at Glenn's," *Newberry Weekly Herald* (SC), 26 July 1907.

255. *Laurens Advertiser* (SC), 30 June 1909; "The State Quill Pushers: Regular Yearly Meeting of the South Carolina Press Association at Glenn Springs," *Edgewood Advertiser* (SC), 1 June 1910; Fitch, 588.

256. Walker, "Mineral Water," 21; "Old Glenn Springs Burns to Ground in Two Hours," *Charlotte News*, 28 July 1941.

257. South Carolina Dept. of Archives and History, Glenn Springs Historic District.

Tennessee

Introduction

1. Tennessee, Department of State, *Tennessee Blue Book 2019-2020* (Nashville: The Tennessee Secretary of State, 2019), 1, https://publications.tnsosfiles.com/pub/blue_book/19-20/19-20tnhistory.pdf; *Journal of the Convention of the State of Tennessee* (Nashville: Banner & Whig Office, 1834), 105.

2. Edward T. Luther, "Geologic Zones,"

Tennessee Encyclopedia (Nashville: Tennessee Historical Society; Knoxville: University of Tennessee Press, updated Mar. 1, 2018, http://tennesseeencyclopedia.net/entries/geologic-zones/. Many geologists consider the Unaka Mountains to be the overarching name for the mountain ranges on the border, which include the Iron, the Bald, and the Great Smoky mountains.

3. Campbell, *Southern Highlander*, foldout [n.p.]; *Tennessee Blue Book 2019–2020*, 639; Luther.

4. Killebrew, *Introduction to the Resources of Tennessee*, 274–75. My introduction names only some of the many health resorts sprinkled throughout Southern Appalachian Tennessee.

5. Thorne, "Watering Spas of Middle Tennessee," 342–44; Howell, "John Armfield," 58–59.

6. "Montvale Chalybeate and Sulphur Springs, Blount County, East Tennessee [ad]," *Athens Post* (TN), 27 June 1851.

7. "White Cliff and Sulphur Springs [ad]," *Athens Post* (TN), 22 May 1874; "White Cliff Springs [ad]," *Ibid.*, 26 June 1874; Killebrew, *Report of the Bureau of Agriculture, Statistics, and Mines*, 183.

8. "White Cliff Springs [ad]," *Athens Post* (TN), 17 May 1872.

9. "Line Spring [ad]," *Knoxville Daily Journal*, 27 May 1886.

10. "Wildwood Springs [ad]," *Knoxville Journal and Tribune*, 2 June 1914; *Ibid.*, 26 May 1907.

11. Galbraith and Greever, *Season of 1888*, 5,7.

12. T., "A Few Words for Galbraith's Springs," *Morristown Gazette* (TN), 29 Aug. 1883.

13. "Governor Says Corruption Fund is in Existence," *Columbia Herald* (TN), 3 May 1912; "Hooper Here Issues Reprieve," *Newport Plain Talk* (TN), 23 May 1912.

14. Dunaway, "Incorporation," 1104, table 8.5; R.F. Powell, *Season of 1889: Hales's Springs; You Meet Only the Best in the South; the Place for Families; Read what Guests Say* (Knoxville: n.p., 1889?): 3–4.

15. *Tennessean* (Nashville), 5 Sept. 1866; Fitch, 606.

16. "Easley's Spring [ad]," *Herald and Tribune* (Jonesborough, TN), 11 June 1874.

17. As an example of Knoxville parties heading to Clark Spring, see *Herald and Tribune* (Jonesborough, TN), 12 Aug. 1896.

18. "Yeager's Springs," *Greeneville American* (TN), 2 June 1875; East Tennessee, Virginia, and Georgia Railway Company, *Guide to the Summer Resorts (1880)*, 38.

19. Arbuts, "Clark Spring," *Herald and Tribune* (Jonesborough, TN), 21 Aug. 1895.

Austin's Springs

20. Tennessee Dept. of Environment and Conservation, "Upper Tennessee Water Basin, Watauga River Watershed," https://www.tn.gov/environment/program-areas/wr-water-resources/watershed-stewardship/watersheds-by-basin/upper-tennessee-river-basin0/watauga-river-watershed.html; North Carolina Environmental Quality, "Watauga River Basin Documents," https://deq.nc.gov/about/divisions/mitigation-services/dms-planning/watershed-planning-documents/watauga-river-basin.

21. Tennessee Historical Commission, "Daniel Boone: Marker Number 1A27," Historical Marker Database, https://www.hmdb.org/m.asp?m=83060 ; Michael Toomey, "Watauga Association," in *NorthCarolinahistory.org: An Online Encyclopedia*, North Carolina History Project, https://northcarolinahistory.org/encyclopedia/watauga-association/; W. Calvin Dickinson, "Watauga Association," in *Tennessee Encyclopedia*, http://tennesseeencyclopedia.net/entries/watauga-association/); Toomey, "Transylvania Purchase," *Ibid.*, https://tennesseeencyclopedia.net/entries/transylvania-purchase/. All cited *Tennessee Encyclopedia* articles were last updated Mar. 1, 2018, unless otherwise indicated.

22. *Goodspeed's History of East Tennessee*, 899; Bob Robinson, "St. John Milling," *Johnson City Press* (TN), 29 Dec. 2005.

23. Edward A. Johnson, "Railroads," in *Tennessee Encyclopedia*, https://tennesseeencyclopedia.net/entries/railroads/; Watauga Association of Genealogists, *History of Washington County*, 97–98. In 1869, the two railroads merged to form the East Tennessee, Virginia, and Georgia Railroad (ETV&G).

24. Irwin, "Cone and Adler," 49–50. Irwin explores the Cone and Adler families' travels from Bavaria to the U.S. as Jews in context of a larger "chain of migration" where New World opportunities lay in moving away from one's native home in the Old World.

25. Washington County, TN, *Deed Book* 43, 519.

26. Hawkins County relinquished part of its land over the years to be included in the creation of several other Tennessee counties, including Grainger. See Henry R. Price, "Hawkins County," in *Tennessee Encyclopedia*, https://tennesseeencyclopedia.net/entries/railroads/.

27. Box 1, filed alphabetically in the Ca-Cook Folder, Recommendation Orders Series, HCA.

28. "Scott Mass Meeting at Dalton," *Georgia Citizen* (Macon), 11 Sept. 1852; Elizabeth (Betsy) Hoole McArthur, "Civil War Anniversary: The Clisby Austin House: 'I've Got Joe Johnston Dead!,'" *Dalton Daily Citizen Times* (GA), 31 May 2014, https://www.dailycitizen.news/news/local_news/civil-war-anniversary-the-clisby-austin-house-i-ve-got/article_ab2b54a6-bb2a-5414-8d1b-064c3127336f.html; "Tunnel Hill United Methodist Church," https://thumc.org/history/. The Southern conferences withdrew from the Methodist Episcopal Church in 1844 to form the Methodist Episcopal Church, South. See Durwood Dunn, *The Civil War in Southern Appalachian Methodism* (Knoxville: University of Tennessee Press, 2013), 48.

29. "New Advertisements: Limestone Springs," *Albany Patriot*, 11 Aug. 1859.

30. "Limestone Springs, at Tunnell [sic] Hill, GA, [ad]," *Ibid*.

31. *Ibid*.; Marvin Sowder, "Civil War Anniversary: Clisby Austin and Tunnel Hill," *Dalton Daily Citizen*, 10 Sept. 2011, https://www.dailycitizen.news/news/local_news/civil-war-anniversary-clisby-austin-and-tunnel-hill/article_a57599a9-4d8b-5b42-badd-4255f04f5252.html.

32. "Limestone Springs for Sale [ad]," *Georgia Journal and Messenger* (Macon), 1 Feb. 1860.

33. "Come to Tunnel Hill," *Weekly Chronicle & Sentinel* (Augusta), 25 Feb. 1862; Sowder, "Civil War anniversary: Clisby Austin"; "A Good Eating House," *Daily Press and Herald* (Knoxville), 9 Nov. 1869.

34. "Rev. Clisbe Austin," *Daily Press and Herald* (Knoxville), 10 Oct. 1872.

35. "Enterprise," *Ibid.*, 26 Mar. 1873.

36. "Austin Springs [ad]," *Talbotton Standard* (GA), 6 Aug. 1873.

37. "Austin's Springs," *Bristol News* (TN & VA), 23 June 1874.

38. Peale, *Lists and Analyses*, 103–06.

39. "Austins Springs [ad]," *Daily Press and Herald* (Knoxville), 2 May 1873.

40. "Adler Springs," *Herald and Tribune* (Jonesborough), 8 May 1873; "C.W.C.," "Upper East Tennessee. An Unsurpassed Section of Country," *Press and Messenger* (Knoxville), 23 July 1873.

41. E.J.H., "Cholera Near Whitesburg," *Daily Press and Herald* (Knoxville), 13 July 1873; "Cholera Notes," *Ibid*.

42. F.H. Austin, "Bull's Gap. No Cholera there—The Barber-shop Thieves Heard From," *Daily Press and Herald* (Knoxville), 29 Aug. 1873.

43. "Johnson City," *Ibid.*, 3 July 1873.

44. Rev. C. Austin, "A New and Valuable Discovery," *Daily Press and Herald* (Knoxville) 2 Sept. 1873; U.S. Patent 152,939, "Improvements in Medical Compounds."

45. "Austin's Liver Regulator [ad]," *Bristol News* (TN & VA), 12 May 1874; "Austin's Liver Regulator [ad]," *Thomasville Times* (GA), 25 July 1874.

46. U.S. Population Census 1870, U.S. Population Census 1880, both accessed at FamilySearch, www.familysearch.org.

47. East Tennessee, Virginia and Georgia Railroad Co., *Guide to the Summer Resorts* (1879), 37, McClung. The *Guide* contains an illustration of the resort hotel.

48. "On the Watauga!" *Bristol News* (TN & VA), 7 July 1874.

49. "Auction Tea Party," *Comet* (Johnson City), 23 May 1885; *Morristown Gazette*, 28 June 1882; "Annual Picnic," *Comet* (Johnson City), 21 June 1888; "Longfellow Literary Circle," *Ibid.*, 6 June 1889.

50. *Guide to the Summer Resorts* (1879), 37.

51. "Austin's Aluminous Sulphated Chalybeate Springs [ad]," *Memphis Daily Appeal*, 15 June 1877.

52. *Guide to the Summer Resorts* (1879), 37.

53. "Editorial Jottings by the Way," *Thomasville Times* (GA), 19 Sept. 1874.

54. Jack Plane, "Letter from Our Traveling Correspondent," *Savannah Morning News*, 19 Aug. 1878.

55. "Austin's Aluminous Sulphate Chalybeate Springs [ad]," *Knoxville Daily Chronicle*, 30 July 1878; "Montvale Springs, Blount County, East Tennessee [ad]," *Ibid*.

56. "Bon Aqua: "Memphians Not Wanted There," *Public Ledger* (Memphis), 23 July 1879.

57. *Knoxville Daily Chronicle*, 9 July 1879; "East Tennessee: Memphians Sojourning There Testify to Hospitality and Plenty, Knoxville, Tenn., July 18," *Public Ledger* (Memphis), 18 July 1879.

58. J. Harvey Mathes, "East Tennessee Welcomes Refugees with Open Arms," *Memphis Daily Appeal*, 19 July 1879.

59. Adler, untitled unpublished typescript, 5. Jacob Adler's son, Samuel, recalled in his memoir teaching Taylor how to draw his cards.

60. "Wanted [ad]," *Daily Memphis Avalanche*, 16 Aug. 1876; "Ladies! Your Attention [ad]," *Herald and Tribune* (Jonesborough), 6 Jan. 1876; Williamson, "Seven Ways."

61. "Watauga Institute For Young Ladies [ad]," *Herald and Tribune* (Jonesborough), 1 Nov. 1876.

62. Washington County, TN, *Deed Book* 46, 258.

63. Bird, "Tobacco in East Tennessee," 6–7.

64. *Comet* (Johnson City), 19 July 1884; "Banner House, Elk Park, N.C. [ad]," *Ibid.*, 9 Aug 1884; *Ibid.*, 27 May 1886; *Herald and Tribune* (Jonesborough), 21 Jan. 1886; *Chattanooga Daily Chronicle*, 25 Apr. 1885; *Knoxville Daily Chronicle*, 11 Mar. 1882.

65. *Morristown Gazette*, 1 Aug. 1883; Burns, *History of Blount County*, 75; "Death of F.H. Austin," *Comet* (Johnson City), 3 June 1886.

66. *Comet* (Johnson City), 24 Nov. 1887.

67. "Land Sale," *Comet* (Johnson City), 1 Dec. 1887; Washington County, TN, *Deed Book* 53, 560; "Jacob Adler v. C. Austin."

68. "Notice to Creditors to File Claims," *Comet* (Johnson City), 14 Mar. 1889; *Ibid.*, 15 Aug. 1889.

69. "A Beautiful Health and Summer Resort [ad]," *Appeal-Avalanche* (Memphis, 27 July 1892.

70. "Summer Resort," *Herald and Tribune* (Jonesborough), 26 May 1892.

71. "Johnson City—To Be Advertised as a Summer Resort," *Comet* (Johnson City), 28 Apr. 1898.

72. *Comet* (Johnson City), 27 July 1893; "Austin Springs to be Improved," *Ibid.*, 31 Mar. 1898; *Ibid.*, 9 June 1898; "Dr. Walter L. Miller in Luck," *Ibid.*, 8 Apr. 1897; "Gov. Taylor Ill," *Ibid.*, 1 Sept. 1898; *Ibid.*, 22 Sept. 1898; *Ibid.*, 16 Mar. 1899; "An Outing," *Ibid.*, 10 Aug. 1899. A few newspaper announcements used the term "Riverside Inn," but the majority referenced a variation of "Austin's Springs Hotel."

73. *Comet* (Johnson City), 21 Aug. 1902.

74. "Colt Show and Picnic," *Herald and Tribune* (Jonesborough), 16 Aug. 1893; "Fair at Austin Springs," *Chattanooga Daily Times*, 5 June 1897; "Austin Springs: Fourth of July Program," *Comet* (Johnson City), 26 June 1903.

75. Lucy Gump, comp., "Austin Springs Hotel Register: 'Residences,' Summer Seasons, 1902 & 1903," typescript in possession of author; *Austin Springs Hotel Register*, June 1902—Sept. 1903. Interestingly, two visitors recorded their addresses as England and Italy; possibly, they were visiting friends or family in the Johnson City area. Gump graciously provided the author with a copy of her typed notes from the register and allowed the author to take notes directly from the register at her home. In fall 2019, Gump donated the hotel register to ETSU.

76. *Austin Springs Hotel Register*.

77. *Journal and Tribune* (Knoxville), 6 June 1903; "Austin Springs Opened," *Comet* (Johnson City), 22 June 1905.

78. G.C., interview by Lucy Gump, 22 May 2005, handwritten notes by Gump in possession of author. G.C. was born in 1909; therefore, the year he recalled in his interview is estimated to be around 1912–1914 (his earliest memory of going to Austin's).

79. "$250,000 Good Road Bonds Sold," *Kingsport Times* (TN), 20 Apr. 1920; "New Bridge Will Be Opened At Hyder's Bluff on Friday," *Bristol Herald Courier* (TN), 4 Aug. 1921.

80. Adler, 5.

81. "Plan Boys' Camp for Johnson City," *Johnson City Chronicle*, 10 Jan. 1924; "Catalogue of 'Castle Heights on the Watauga' Is Issued Featuring Johnson City; Camp Will Be Opened July 2," *Ibid.*, 15 Apr. 1924; "Castle Heights in Bankrupt Court," *Bristol News Bulletin* (TN), 24 June 1925.

82. "Tourist Camp in Oakland Park is Ordered Closed," *Johnson City Chronicle*, 22 Apr.1927.

83. "To Inaugurate Auto Racing in Johnson City," *Tennessean* (Nashville), 7 June 1931; June Hale Pollock and Nancy Pollock Haga, "Austin Springs," in Joyce and W. Eugene Cox, comps. and eds., *History of Washington County*, 712–13; G.C. interview. G.C. recalled walking through the hotel when it was a shell and that a builder by the name of Jack Wallace constructed the Country Kitchen on the burned-down hotel site.

84. "Fire Completely Destroys Country Kitchen Pavilion," *Johnson City Press and Staff-News*, 1 Aug. 1935.

85. "Riverside Park," Washington County, TN, Plat Book 1, 132, recorded 27 May 1937; Washington County, TN, Deed Book 201, 495, recorded 24 May 1938; "Reunion Notes," 23 Sept. 2005, handwritten notes taken by Lucy Gump with several Austin Springs School alumni, notes in possession of author; G.C. interview.

Cloudland Hotel

86. See, for example, Peter D. Weigl and Travis W. Knowles, "Megaherbivores and Southern Appalachian Grass Balds," *Growth and Change: A Journal of Urban and Regional Policy* 26 (July 1995): 365–382; Atul A. Joshi, Jayashree Ratnam, and Mahesh Sankaran, "Frost Maintains Forests and Grasslands as Alternate States in a Montane Tropical Forest-Grassland Mosaic," *Journal of Ecology* 108 (Jan. 2020): 123.

87. Mitchell, "Notice of the Height of Mountains in North Carolina," 378.

88. Williams, "André Michaux," 16, 18, 20; Williams, *Early Travels*, 331–32, 331n14; "Group Seeks to Save Roan," *Hickory Daily Record* (NC), 6 July 1997.

89. Williams, *Early Travels*, 303–05.

90. Silver, *Mount Mitchell*, 65; Arthur, 513.

91. Michael Joslin, "Lilies on the Roan," *Mitchell News-Journal* (NC), 12 July 1995.

92. Lanman, *Letters from the Alleghany Mountains*, 147.

93. Wyman, "Tennessee Places," 100; Williams, "Early Iron Works," 41.

94. Merritt, *Early History of Carter County*, 63–64.

95. "Iron Making in North Carolina," *Athens Post* (TN), 2 Apr. 1858.

96. Williams, *General John T. Wilder*, 1–3; *Cloudland Hotel On Top of Roan Mountain in East Tennessee and Western North Carolina* ([Cloudland, N.C.?], [1895?], inside back cover.

97. Williams, *General John T. Wilder*, 3, 10, 13, 18–19.

98. *Ibid.*, 35.

99. *Ibid.*, 39–40, 42–43; Govan and Livingood, *Chattanooga Country*, 295–98.

100. Laughlin, *Roan Mountain*, 71; Williamson, "Seven Ways." The CPI calculator was used in all dollar conversions unless otherwise noted.

101. Caldwell, "Folklore Interview."

102. Robbie D. Jones, "Carnegie," in Joyce and W. Eugene Cox, comps. and eds., *History of Washington County*, 736–42.

103. Arthur, 558; Nicely, *Forging a New South*, 287.

104. N.B.B., "Bakersville and Roan Mountain," *Observer* (Raleigh), 29 Aug. 1877.

105. *Ibid.*; Michael Joslin, "Hotel Key Part of Roan's Mythology," *Johnson City Press* (TN), 11 Jan. 1987; The Rambler, "Above the Clouds," *Weekly Public Ledger* (Memphis), 29 July 1884; G., "From North Carolina," *Public Ledger* (Memphis), 30 Sept. 1879.

106. "Above the Clouds."

107. David Gaynes, "Cloudland Hotel: What It Used to Be, and Is Now," *Johnson City Press-Chronicle* (TN), 17 Aug. 1975; *Comet* (Johnson City, TN), 11 Apr. 1885.

108. Laughlin, 83; "Local News," *Lenoir Topic* (NC), 29 July 1885; Williamson, https://www.measuringworth.com/dollarvaluetoday/?amount=40000&from=1885. The construction project calculator was used.

109. *Comet* (Johnson City, TN), 13 June 1889.

110. *Cloudland Hotel; The Great Southern Resort for Hay Fever*, n.p. Later brochures do not mention tennis, so it is not a fact that the courts were actually built.

111. Laughlin, 101; D.W., interview by author,

May 18, 2004, Unicoi, TN. Handwritten notes in possession of author.

112. "An Immence [sic] Hotel," *Comet* (Johnson City, TN), 6 Dec. 1884.

113. *How to Get There* [1885], MCPL; Ashton Chapman, "On Roan Mountain: Former Clerk Recalls Heyday of Cloudland Hotel," *Asheville Citizen-Times*, 5 July 1953.

114. *How to Get There* [1885]; "On Roan Mountain: Former Clerk Recalls"; DW interview; Ruby Ford, "Guests Stayed at Cloudland Hotel for $2.50 per Day—The Price of a Good Steak Now...," *Elizabethton Star* (TN), 9 June 1952; "Ex-Cloudland Hotel Staff Holds Reunion," *Elizabethton Star* (TN), 19 Aug. 1956.

115. S., "Correspondence," 334; Morgan, "The Cloudland Hotel"; John Parris, "Roaming the Mountains: The Cloudland Hotel, Barely a Trace Remains of Cloudland Hotel," *Asheville Citizen*, 29 Oct. 1987; Michael Joslin, "The Bald Road: Pathway to the Top of the Mountain," *Mitchell News-Journal* (Mitchell County, NC), 1 Feb. 1995; Laughlin, 83; J.M., interview by author, 16 Oct. 2004, Mitchell County, NC, handwritten notes in possession of author. All interviewees unless otherwise noted are identified by initials only to preserve confidentiality.

116. Russo, "The Hack Line Road."

117. "Before This Time Next Year We May All Drive to the Top of the Roan in High on Paved Roads: Wages and Prices on Road to the Roan Construction in 1878," *Spruce Pine Tri-County News* (NC), 21 Dec. 1950, SPPL.

118. McKinney, "Cloudland Hotel," 4.

119. Kivette, "The Roan Was Always a Very Special Mountain," 14–15; [Bill Sharpe], "Mitchell," *A New Geography* (n.p.: n.d.), 239, two-page photocopy annotated with book author's name, SPPL.

120. Pippen, interview by Swindell; Russo et al, interview by Fulcher.

121. *Guide to the Summer Resorts* (1879), 36; East Tennessee, Virginia and Georgia Railroad Co., *Guide to the Summer Resorts* (1881), 23, McClung; Chun, *Descriptive Illustrated Guide-Book*, 66.

122. *Cloudland Hotel on Top of Roan Mountain* [1896?].

123. Chun, 66, 69–70; S., "Correspondence: Roan Mountain," 333.

124. J.M. interview.

125. *Roan Mountain Inn, Roan Mountain, Tenn*; Oswald, "Southern Summer Resorts: First Paper," 124; "On Roan Mountain: Former Clerk Recalls."

126. "Cloudland Hotel at the Top of Roan Mountain," *Resources and Enterprises of Upper East Tennessee* (Knoxville?: Enterprise Publishing Co., 1885), in Kozsuch, 68; Williamson, "Seven Ways."

127. P.M.S., interview by author, 12 Nov. 1998, Johnson City, TN, handwritten notes in possession of author.

128. *Comet* (Johnson City, TN), 30 July 1885.

129. Fulcher, "Muir, Michaux, and Gray," 19.

130. Scott, "A Visit to Mitchell and Roan Mountains," 18–19.

131. Warner, *On Horseback*, 51.

132. *Ibid.*, 54.

133. *Cloudland Hotel on Top of Roan* Mountain [1895?], 23.

134. Presbrey, *Empire of the South*, 63–64.

135. Tennessee State Board of Health, *First Report*, 266; P.M.S. interview; *Cloudland Hotel, Top of Roan Mountain, 6,394 Feet Above the Sea, Western North Carolina* [after 1892?], reprinted in Laughlin, 90; Laughlin, 94.

136. Mitman, "Hay Fever Holiday," 601–02, 606–07. The U.S. Hay Fever Association published a list of catarrh-free places, including the entire Alleghany Mountain range, providing the Cloudland with indirect Association endorsement. See "Hay Fever and Its Cure," *New York Times*, 14 Sept. 1884.

137. Blackley, *Experimental Researches*, 7. Blackley attributed the farm laborers' lack of hay fever to either "the absence of the predisposition which mental culture generates" or to an acquisition of a degree of insusceptibility. See Blackley, 155.

138. Beard, *Hay-Fever*, 81–82.

139. *Ibid.*, 87.

140. Mitman, 619–20; "Hay Fever and Hope," *New York Times*, 2 Sept. 1898.

141. "The Hay Fever Delusion," *New York Times*, 17 Sept. 1880.

142. *Ibid.* The Cloudland viewed the White Mountain resorts, particularly the Summit House on Mt. Washington, as rivals. Much of the Cloudland's promotional material proudly proclaimed that it stood an elevation 200 feet higher than Mt. Washington.

143. Mitman, 609.

144. Chapin, *Health Resorts of the South*, 139.

145. Beard, 84; *Cloudland Hotel on Top of Roan Mountain* [1895?], 20.

Tuberculosis or TB—also known in the nineteenth century as wasting disease, consumption, or phthisis—originally was viewed as a fashionable disease. Robert Koch's discovery of the tubercle bacillus in 1882 validated the hypothesis that microbes caused disease (now known as the germ theory). The acceptance of the germ theory led to the societal view associating TB with the lower class. See Tera W. Hunter, *To 'Joy My Freedom: Southern Black Women's Lives and Labors After the Civil War* (Cambridge: Harvard University Press, 1997), 193–94.

146. Caldwell; P.M.S. interview; Morgan, "The Cloudland Hotel"; Pauline Murrell Stone, interview by Norma Myers, 1993, Series II, Folder 4, Murrell Family Collection, ETSU.

147. Ford, "Guests Stayed at Cloudland Hotel for $2.50 per Day"; Caldwell; Fulcher, "Muir, Michaux, and Gray," 19–20; Stone, interview by Myers; Pippen interview by Thomas Swidnell.

148. Starnes, "Creating the Land of the Sky," 48, 74.

149. *Register—Penland House*, property of M.B., Bakersville, NC; M. B., interview by author, 16 May 2004, Bakersville, NC, handwritten notes in possession of author. The Young's Hotel ran a hack through the Valley of the Roan, most probably the old Glen Ayre Road, to the Cloudland.

150. *Asheville Democrat*, 30 June 1892; "Gone to Roan: Geo. W. Vanderbilt and Party Off Early This Morning," *Asheville Citizen-Times*, 24 June 1892.

151. M.B. interview; *Register—Penland House*.

152. Allison, *Address*, 3; *Elizabethton Mountaineer* (TN), 26 June 1896. Williams collected pamphlets and miscellany, which are bound together in *Tennesseeana*.

153. "Guests Stayed at Cloudland Hotel For $2.50"; Chun, 70.

154. "Guests Stayed at Cloudland Hotel For $2.50"; "Cloudland Hotel: Only Memories Remain"; "Cloudland Hotel: What It Used to Be, and Is Now"; "Mitchell County News, 1885," *The Lenoir Topic*, 20 May 1885, reproduced in Bailey, ed., *Heritage of the Toe River Valley*, vol. 4, 99.

155. Mary Abarr, "Were Lost Up in the Clouds: Experience of Two Memphians in the Appalachians," *Memphis Commercial Appeal*, 18 Aug. 1894.

156. "Cloudland Hotel: What It Used to Be"; "Wilder's Cloudland Hotel Brought First Influx to Roan," *Elizabethton Star* (TN), 12 June 1955. Wilder's Carnegie Land and Improvement Co. recruited hundreds of workers, including Italian immigrants and Blacks to help build Johnson City's Carnegie Addition's commercial and residential buildings. In 1890, Johnson City's Black population numbered almost 1,000, nearly 25% of the town's total population. See Jones, "Carnegie," 739. Possibly, Wilder may have recruited a few Johnson City cooks and a barber to work at the Cloudland.

157. "Aunt Eliza Remembers the Cloudland Hotel," reproduced from unannotated newspaper clipping in the scrapbook of Myron Houston, in Bailey, ed., *Heritage of the Toe River Valley*, vol. 4, 344.

158. "Hotel With 166 Rooms Operated on the Roan for Years," *Spruce Pine Tri-County News* (NC), 21 Dec. 1950, SPPL; Williamson, "Seven Ways." For 1905, one of the years that the Gouges lived at the Cloudland, $40 translates in 2022 dollars to $1370 (CPI) and $6,560 (Unskilled Wage).

159. "Hotel Key Part."

160. J.M. interview.

161. *Ibid.*; "The Bald Road: Pathway to the Top of the Mountain"; Morgan, "The Cloudland Hotel"; Ruth Gardner Bledsoe, "Evan and Mary (Polly) Hughes," in Bailey, ed., *Heritage of the Toe River Valley*, vol. 1, 293.

162. H. T. Finck, "Mammoth Cave and Cloudland," *Evening Post: New York*, 27 Aug. 1898; Series I, Folder 2, Murrell Family Collection, ETSU.

163. McKinney, 4.

164. "Business Troubles," *New York Times*, 24 May 1893; "Carnegie Companies Assign.: Unable to Float Bonds, There Was Nothing Else for Them to Do," *New York Times*, 5 June 1893.

165. Carter County, "Quarterly Minutes," 398; Williamson, "Seven Ways."

166. P.M.S. interview.

167. "Hotel With 166 Rooms Operated on the Roan for Many Years"; A.J., "The John Wilson Gouge Family," unpublished typescript, 15 Apr. 1986, 4, photocopy in possession of D.W.

168. Beeson, "Illustrated Record," 1–4, D.R. Beeson, Sr., Papers, ETSU; Fink, *Backpacking*, 16; D.W., interview. D.W. commented that her aunt was born on the Cloudland dining room table. A doctor charged $25 to deliver her; the Gouges in turn charged him $25 to spend the next several days at the hotel because of a snowstorm that stranded him.

169. *Johnson City Staff* (TN), 23 October 1917.

170. "Cloudland Hotel: What It Used to Be"; "Hotel Key Part"; Morgan, "The Cloudland Hotel"; Laughlin, 105.

171. V.C., interview by author, 9 Mar. 2004, Johnson City, TN, audiotape recording in possession of author; M.C., interview by author, 3 Feb. 2003, Carter County, TN, audiotape recording in possession of author; Russo et al, interview by Bob Fulcher; Fulcher, "Hack Line Road," 34.

172. "The Week of April 29, 1941," [*Tri-County News*, 20 April 1971], ASU; Miriam Rabb, "New Road Opens Roan Mountain to Thousands of Auto Travelers," *Journal and Sentinel* (Winston-Salem), 22 May 1955.

173. Norman C. Gibson, "Historic Roan Mountain Inn to Be Re-Opened in a Few Days," *Elizabethton Star* (TN), 8 July 1949; "On Roan Mountain: Former Clerk Recalls."

174. "Muir, Michaux, and Gray," 15.

Montvale Springs

175. Wright, "Montvale Springs," 51; Burns, *History of Blount County*, Tennessee, 82, map. I consider Burns and Wright to be the authoritative sources for Montvale. Both researched deeds, early newspapers, and other sources to provide excellent overviews.

176. Wright, 50, 50n7; Burns, *History of Blount County*, 79–80, 80n40; Bridges et al, *Terra Incognita*, 278.

177. Burns, *History of Blount County*, 80–81, 280; Burns, "*Montvale—The Saratoga of the South*," [*Smoky Mountain Historical Society Newsletter*], 13–14, "Springs—Montvale" Subject File, McClung.

178. "Montvale Springs, Blount County, East Tenn.," *Daily Chronicle and Sentinel* (Augusta), 15 Apr. 1847.

179. *Montvale Springs, Blount County* (1874), 3–4, UTK.

180. Burns, History of Blount County, 80–81; Adele Broady, "Montvale Springs," *Enterprise*, December 29, 1938, "Springs—Montvale" Subject File, McClung; Wright, "Montvale Springs," 55n29.

181. Burns, *History of Blount County*, 80–81; Burns, "Montvale—Saratoga of the South," 14;

Cate and Callaway, *Back Home in Blount County*, 85.

182. Wright, 48; "Lamar House [ad]," *Knoxville Mercury*, 5 Feb. 1857.

183. Burns, *History of Blount County*, 81–82; Wright, 48; Williamson, "Seven Ways." The Consumer Price Index (CPI) calculator was used for all dollar conversions in this chapter.

184. Burns, *History of Blount County*, 82; Wright, 48n2, 49, 55; Sterling Lanier to Jane Lanier Ogburn, March 3, 1861, quoted in Wright, 49.

185. Z, "Correspondence of the Courier," *Charleston Daily Courier*, 29 Aug. 1857; Blount, "Letter from Montvale Springs," *Times & Sentinel Tri-Weekly* (Columbus, GA), 22 Aug 1857; Long Grabs, "Montvale Springs, Aug. 24, 1858," *Lancaster Ledger* (SC), 1 Sept. 1858.

186. "Montvale Springs [ad]," *Daily Morning News* (Savannah), 26 May 1853.

187. Wright, 49–50, 60, 60n44; "Montvale has Great History," *Knoxville Journal*, 30 June 1929; Blount, "Letter from Montvale Springs," *Times & Sentinel Tri-Weekly* (Columbus, GA), 22 Aug 1857. For a rare northern notice of the resort, see "Montvale Springs, June 29, 1854," *New York Herald*, 17 July 1854.

188. Michaux, *Travels*, 93. Michaux noted that the "Tennessee Itch," a dermatological affliction causing pimples on the abdomen, shoulders, arms, and thighs, could be relieved by a "cooling regimen" and bathing.

189. Reniers, *Springs of Virginia*, 74.

190. *Montvale Springs, Blount County* (1867), 14, 20–21, "Montvale Springs, Blount County, An Analysis of the Springs 1867," Tourism Folder 7–8, PAM Tourism Box 7, McClung.

191. Ibid., 17, 21, 23.

192. Wright, 55–56.

193. Burns, "Montvale—The Saratoga of the South," 14; Broady, "Montvale Springs."

194. Burns, "Montvale—The Saratoga of the South," 14; Peggy Swenson, "Montvale Hosts Aristocracy During 1800's," *Maryville-Alcoa Times*, 28 Feb. 1975, "Springs—Montvale" Subject File, McClung.

195. *Peterson Magazine* 53 (1868), 237, quoted in Lanier, *Tiger-Lilies*, i; Wright, 59.

196. Wright, 57.

197. Burns, "Montvale—The Saratoga of the South," 14. Burns notes that Mitchel also wrote that most of the guests during his stay were from Georgia with some families from Louisiana and Alabama.

198. Cate and Callaway, 86.

199. "Montvale—Saratoga of the South," 16.

200. "Famed Old Montvale Springs May Rise Again as Y Boys' Camp," *Knoxville News-Sentinel*, 27 Oct. 1946.

201. Burns, "Montvale—The Saratoga of the South," 16; Cate and Callaway, 86.

202. Dunaway, *Slavery in the American Mountain South*, 84.

203. "Montvale Springs [ad]," *Daily Morning News* (Savannah), 11 June 1861; *Knoxville Daily Register*, June 12, 1862; Fred Brown, "Water from Montvale Springs Would Cure All that Ailed You," *Knoxville News-Sentinel*, 18 Jan. 2000; Wright, 49.

204. Wright, 49. Williamson, "Seven Ways."

205. "Montvale Springs [ad]," *Daily Register* (Knoxville), 10 May 1863; "Montvale Springs [ad]," *Daily Southern Chronicle* (Knoxville), 28 July 1863.

206. "Death of Brig. Gen. Donelson," *Daily Register* (Knoxville), 19 Apr. 1863; Eicher, *Longest Night*, 456; Wright, 60, 61n50.

207. *Montvale Springs, Blount County* (1867), 2.

208. Wright, 49, 62.

209. U.S. Population Census 1880, FamilySearch, www.familysearch.org/; "Montvale Springs, Blount County, Tenn. [ad]," "Montvale Springs, Blount County, East Tennessee [ad]," *Morristown Gazette* (TN), 4 Aug. 1875; *Knoxville Daily Tribune*, 19 Apr. 1876.

210. "Montvale Springs for Sale," *Daily Tribune* (Knoxville), 18 Oct. 1877; *Morristown Gazette* (TN), 14 Nov. 1877; *Daily Tribune* (Knoxville), 9 Jan. 1878.

211. "Notice," *Knoxville Daily Chronicle*, 26 Nov. 1879; "Another Change of Ownership at Montvale," *Ibid*., 18 Dec. 1879; "Montvale Springs, House of Seven Gables [ad]," *Ibid*., 8 June 1882; Burns, *History of Blount County*, 83; "Montvale Springs, Blount Co., East Tenn.," *Maryville Times*, 7 Aug. 1889. Burns states that Joseph L. King in 1875 executed a trust deed to Spencer Munson of Knoxville in favor of David Engel of Baltimore, who eventually obtained the resort. Charles S. King bought the property in 1875 from the executors of Engel's estate. The two Maryland men who had an inheritance claim for Montvale may well have been related to either or both Engels.

212. "A Trip to Montvale," *Knoxville Daily Chronicle*, 23 July 1879.

213. Ibid.; "Regulations at Montvale," *Ibid*., 30 July 1879.

214. "A Letter from Senator Brownlow," *New York Times*, 31 July 1869.

215. Burns, "Montvale—The Saratoga of the South," 17.

216. Lucy Templeton, "Sunday Country Calendar: Old Montvale," *Knoxville News-Sentinel*, 19 June 1955.

217. *Montvale Springs, Blount County* (1874), 35–36; Burns, "Montvale—The Saratoga of the South," 17.

218. Horse Talk," *San Francisco Examiner*, 20 Aug. 1884; *Prominent Families of New York City*, rev. ed. (New York: The Historical Co., 1898), 70; "The Future of Montvale," *Knoxville Tribune*, 25 Nov. 1894. Bonner bought the legendary, world record-setting horse "Maude S." from W.H. Vanderbilt.

219. Burns, *History of Blount County*, 83; "Losses by Fire," *New York Times*, 14 May 1896.

220. Burns, *History of Blount County*, 84–85; "Montvale Springs, A Beautiful and Healthful Summer Resort," *Maryville Times*, 26 Aug. 1899.

221. Callahan, *Montvale*, 55.
222. Burns, *History of Blount County*, 84; "Saratoga of the South," *Savannah Morning News*, 7 Sept 1884.
223. "Hotel Burns at Montvale," *Knoxville News-Sentinel*, 21 Nov. 1933; "Famous Resort Hotel Goes Up in Flames," *Ibid*.
224. "Montvale Springs Inn Ready to Serve You!," *Ibid.*, 27 Nov. 1933.
225. "Death Takes Ludwig Pflanze Before Dreams Are Realized," *Knoxville News-Sentinel*, 29 Oct. 1934; "YMCA Camp Has Large Attendance," *Knoxville Journal*, 31 Aug. 1952; *Harmony Family Center—Montvale*, www.harmonyfamilycenter.org/montvale.

Rhea Springs

226. TVA, "Watts Bar," https://www.tva.gov/Energy/Our-Power-System/Hydroelectric/Watts-Bar-Reservoir; George E. Webb, "The Scopes Trial," in *Tennessee Encyclopedia*, updated Mar. 1, 2018, https://tennesseeencyclopedia.net/entries/the-scopes-trial/. All cited *Tennessee Encyclopedia* articles were last updated Mar. 1, 2018, unless otherwise indicated.
227. Edward T. Luther, "Walden Ridge and Sequatchie Valley," *Ibid.*, http://tennesseeencyclopedia.net/entries/walden-ridge-and-sequatchie-valley/.
228. Musicus, "The Great American Traveler," *Nashville Union and American*, 27 Aug. 1872.
229. J. Pope Dyer, "Rhea Springs, Fountain of Health," *Chattanooga Times*, 28 July 1934; Bettye J. Broyles, "Rhea County," in *Tennessee Encyclopedia*, https://tennesseeencyclopedia.net/entries/rhea-county/ ; Sarah Jackson Martin, "Blythe Ferry," *Ibid.*, https://tennesseeencyclopedia.net/entries/blythe-ferry/; Fred S. Rolater, "Treaties," *Ibid.*, http://tennesseeencyclopedia.net/entries/treaties/.
230. "Rhea, John (1752–1832)," *Biographical Directory of the United States Congress, 1774– present*, https://bioguideretro.congress.gov/Home/MemberDetails?memIndex=R000181; Broyles, "Rhea County."
231. Safford, *Geology of Tennessee*, 456–58, 497.
232. USDA, *Monthly Report*, 124–25; Allen, "Appendix A: Valentine C. Allen, Early History of Rhea County," in Allen and Broyles, comp., *Rhea County History*, 68; Broyles, comp., *History of Rhea County*, 24; "Crops in East Tennessee," *Daily Morning News* (Savannah), 7 July 1857.
233. Seth Tallent, "Sulphur Springs (1807–1878); Rhea Springs (1878–1941)," in Broyles, comp., *History of Rhea County*, 144, 146.
234. *Ibid.*, 144.
235. *History of Tennessee*, 1070–71; U.S. Population Census 1850, U.S. Census 1850 (Slave Schedule), FamilySearch, www.familysearch.org/.
236. Daniel Ferkin email correspondence, 24 Feb. 2020; Tallent, 144.
237. Tallent, 145; W.T. Blackwell, "Rhea County Sulphur Springs," *Athens Post* (TN), 29 May 1857. The *Athens Post* article does not specify whether Horr or Stanton had been cured.
238. "Sulphur Springs, Rhea County," *Athens Post*, 27 June 1856.
239. Tallent, 145.
240. "Rhea ounty [sic] Sulphur Springs [ad]," *Athens Post*, 29 Aug. 1856.
241. Blackwell, "Rhea County Sulphur Springs."
242. "'Rhea Springs'—Rates of Fare Reduced," *Ibid.*, 25 June 1858; Williamson, "Seven Ways." The CPI calculator was used.
243. "Chancery Sale [ad]," *Nashville Patriot*, 5 Nov. 1858.
244. Tallent, 145–46; *History of Tennessee*, 1070–71.
245. "Sulphur Springs Rhea County, Tenn. [ad]," *Athens Post*, 10 Aug. 1860; "Chilhowee Springs [ad]," *Ibid.*, 20 July 1860; "Catoosa Springs [ad]," *Nashville Union and American*, 27 May 1860.
246. Tallent, 145; Works Projects Administration for the State of Tennessee, *Tennessee*, 363.
247. "Party at the Rhea Springs," *Athens Post*, 28 Aug. 1857.
248. "Rhea ounty [sic] Sulphur Springs [ad]."
249. Blackwell, "Rhea County Sulphur Springs."
250. *Ibid.*; "Rhea Springs!," *Augusta Evening Dispatch*, 12 June 1858; Pepper et al, "Report of Committee on Sanitaria and Mineral Springs," 547; Fitch, 600.
251. "More Aid For the Soldiers," *Athens Post*, 28 Feb. 1862; Broyles, *History of Rhea County*, 33–36.
252. Broyles, *History of Rhea County*, 34–36; Campbell, *Records of Rhea*, 36.
253. Allen and Broyles, comp., 35.
254. Broyles, *History of Rhea County*, 38.
255. *History of Tennessee*, 1071; "Farms and House Lots [ad]," *Brownlow's Knoxville Whig, and Rebel Ventilator*, 10 Jan. 1866; Elizabeth Kelly, "The History of the Rhea Springs Church (As Read at the Home-Coming Service on Sunday, July 8th, 1934, at Rhea Springs, Tenn.)," unpublished typescript, Holston Discontinued Box, "Rhea Springs Church, Rhea Springs, TN" folder, HCA.
256. Phil Leigh, "Opinionator: Disunion—Colonel Wilder's Lightning Brigade [blog]," *New York Times*, 25 Dec. 2012, https://opinionator.blogs.nytimes.com/2012/12/25/colonel-wilders-lightning-brigade/; Burkett, ed., *Historical Review*, 6 ; Lizzie Wilson, "Rockwood," *Athens Post*, 14 Aug. 1868; C.A.R., "From Rhea County. Sulphur Springs, Tenn., June 23, 1875," *Knoxville Whig and Chronicle*, 7 July 1875.
257. Allen and Broyles, comp., 41; "Neal, John Randolph (1836–1889)," *Biographical Directory of the United States Congress, 1774– present*, https://bioguideretro.congress.gov/Home/MemberDetails?memIndex=N000013; Bennie McKenzie Fleming, "John R. Neal, Jr.," in Broyles, *History of Rhea County*, 333–34.
258. Sarah Ruth Frazier, "Legend and Romance of Rhea Springs," *Chattanooga Sunday Times*

[magazine section], 4 Oct. 1936; Dyer, "Rhea Springs, Fountain of Health."
259. Anon., "Rhea Springs Letter. The Cincinnati Southern—Good Luck Fishing, &c.," *Knoxville Daily Chronicle*, 4 May 1879.
260. "Rhea ounty [sic] Sulphur Springs [ad]"; Blackwell, "Rhea County Sulphur Springs"; "Pin Hook Ferry," *Athens Post*, 6 Aug. 1858.
261. Broyles, *History of Rhea County*, 24; Charles V. Patton, "Old Timer: Riot Stopped Work on Early Streetcar Line in Knoxville," *Knoxville Journal*, 6 May 1956; "Rhea Springs, Sulphur Springs Post-office [sic], Rhea County, Tenn. [ad]," *Knoxville Daily Chronicle*, 15 July 1875; C.A.R., "From Rhea County"; Townsend A. Thomas, "From East Tennessee: Health-Water-Masonry-Personals," *Nashville Union and American*, 12 Aug. 1871.
262. Anon., "Rhea Springs Letter."
263. "Chattanooga and Return: Queen & Crescent Route [ad]," *Bourbon News* (Paris, KY), 29 June 1909.
264. "Automobile Parties Going for Week-End," *Chattanooga News*, 15 Aug. 1919; "Parties Going to Weekend Dance at Rhea," *Ibid.*, 27 Aug 1919.
265. "Many Late Arrivals at Rhea Springs Hotel," *Chattanooga News*, 8 Sept. 1920.
266. *Horry Herald* (Conway, SC), 21 Aug. 1913.
267. Frazier, "Legend and Romance of Rhea Springs"; *Chattanooga News*, 30 July 1918; "Patriotic Dances at Rhea Springs," *Chattanooga News*, 3 Sept. 1918.
268. Peale, *Mineral Waters*, 540.
269. "Rhea Springs Mineral Water [ad]," *Presbyterian of the South* (Atlanta), 13 Sept. 1911; "Health by the Glass [ad]," *Chattanooga Daily Times*, 3 July 1930.
270. Tallent, 146.
271. *Ibid.*, 146–47; "U.S. Inspectors Are Investigating Big Promotion Scheme," *Dickson County Herald* (TN), 10 July 1914; J.C. Wasson, "Thompson Owen Wasson," in Broyles, *History of Rhea County*, 400.
272. "Rhea Springs Hotel Burns," *McNairy County Independent* (Selmer, TN), 7 Jan. 1916; Dyer, "Rhea Springs, Fountain of Health."
273. *Polk County News* (TN), 1 Dec. 1921.
274. Fitch, 600; Tallent, 147.
275. "Thompson Owen Wasson," in Broyles, *History of Rhea County*, 400; Pat Guffey, "Remembering Rhea Springs: Part 10, Kenneth Jolley Looks Back," *Rhea Herald News*, 28 Nov. 2014, https://www.rheaheraldnews.com/lifestyles/article_0e06b91a-7724-11e4-9ea3-1b44f986455d.html.

Tate Spring

276. Van West, *Tennessee's Historic Landscapes*, 166; Caruthers, "Bean Station," 33.
277. Luckett, "Cumberland Gap National Park," 303.
278. Hilliard, 193; Killebrew, *First and Second Reports*, 493–94. Hilliard page references are to the 2014 edition.
279. Edward T. Luther, "Geologic Zones," in *Tennessee Encyclopedia*, updated Mar. 1, 2018, http://tennesseeencyclopedia.net/entries/geologic-zones/.
280. Killebrew, *First and Second Reports*, 493–94.
281. "Intelligence from American Scientific Stations," 493.
282. *Ibid.*; Works Projects Administration for the State of Tennessee, *Tennessee*, 314.
283. "Intelligence from American Scientific Stations," 493; *Goodspeed's History of East Tennessee*, 1154; Crook, *Mineral Waters of the United States and Their Therapeutic Uses*, 441.
284. Fitch, 596–97; Peale, *Lists and Analyses*, 100.
285. Works Projects Administration for the State of Tennessee, *Tennessee*, 312.
286. U.S. Population Census 1850, U.S. Census 1850 (Slave Schedule), "Samuel Baker Tate Family Tree," Grainger County Deed Book 20, 467–68, all at FamilySearch, www.familysearch.org; Miller, "David Tate (Pioneer)," 209; "Died," *Southern Confederacy* (Atlanta), 10 June 1862; "Died," *Athens Post* (TN), 27 Feb. 1863; "Tate Epsom Spring, Grainger Cty, TN—Annual Circular 1879," 10–11, Tourism Folder 19, PAM Tourism Box 7, McClung.
287. "No Cholera in Morristown," *Knoxville Weekly Chronicle*, 2 July 1873.
288. "Cholera Notes," *Daily Press and Herald* (Knoxville), 26 July 1873; J.B., e-mail message to author, Oct. 7, 2004.
289. Hamer, "Thomas Tomlinson," *Tennessee: A History*, 678; *Goodspeed's History of East Tennessee*, 1159; *Tate Epsom Spring; Grainger County, Tenn.* (1879), 7.
290. "Tate Springs Hotel Will Open May First," *Erwin Magnet* (TN), 27 Apr. 1926. A syndicate of Knoxville and Atlanta capitalists bought the resort and planned to construct a new hotel, which was never built. See "Formal Opening of Tate Spring Hotel Will Occur Saturday Night," *Knoxville Journal*, 30 April 1926.
291. Graves, *Tate Springs*, 15. "Dr. Tomlinson Passes Here: Associate Owner of Hotel at Tate Springs," *Knoxville Journal*, 28 August 1930; "Dr. Oscar R. Tomlinson," *New York Times*, 28 Aug.1930, http://pqasb.pqarchiver.com/nytimes/advancedsearch.html.
292. "Building Condemned: Kingswood School Has Housing Need," *Knoxville News-Sentinel*, 5 Oct. 1958; "Kingswood School President Dies at 76," *Ibid.*, 22 Dec. 1991; "Kingswood to Honor 50 Years," *Ibid.*, 28 May 1995; "Kingswood Home for Children," https://www.kingswoodkids.org/. The newspaper articles are in the "Springs—Tate" Subject File, McClung.
293. East Tennessee, Georgia, and Virginia Railroad Company, *Guide to the Summer Resorts* (1880), 46, McClung.
294. Faulkner, "Industrial Archaeology, 41–42, 48; Fred Brown, "Big Dreams of Corryton's Found

Were Shattered by Panic of 1892," *Knoxville News-Sentinel*, 14 June 1992.

295. *Annual Pamphlet of Tate Epsom Spring Containing Information Relative to Location [...] With Regard to Its Use, Effects, Shipping Directions, etc.* (Knoxville: S.B. Newman & Co., 1898), 9; "Tate Spring: The Carlsbad of America, Tennessee Annual 1898," Tourism Folder 22, PAM Tourism Box 7, McClung.

296. Faulkner, 54; C.L.B., telephone interview by author, 26 Aug. 2004, handwritten notes in possession of author; Carson Brewer, "Tate Spring Still Flows; The Tales It Could Tell!," *Knoxville News-Sentinel*, July 25, 1982.

297. East Tennessee, Virginia, and Georgia Railroad Company, *Guide to Summer Resorts* (1881), 30, 36; "Season 1880. Montvale Springs, Blount County, Tenn. [ad]," *Daily Memphis Avalanche*, 27 June 1880.

298. *Daily Journal and Tribune* (Knoxville), 5 June 1911; *Tate Spring, Tennessee: The Carlsbad of America, Open All the Year* (n.p., [1927?]), 3, "Tate Spring, Tennessee Annual Booklet ca. 190_?" Tourism Folder 23, PAM Tourism Box 7, McClung. I believe the pamphlet dates from after 1926 because it mentions an eighteen-hole golf course.

299. *Tate Epsom Spring; Grainger County, Tenn; Annual Circular of Tate Epsom Spring, Containing Location, Analysis of the Water [...] Together with Many Certificates and List of References, Card of Resident Physician, Shipping Directions, etc.* (Knoxville: Whig and Chronicle Steam Printing Co., 1879), 7, "Tate Epsom Spring, Grainger Cty, TN—Annual Circular 1879" Tourism Folder 19, PAM Tourism Box 7, McClung.

300. *Tate Epsom Spring; Grainger County, Tenn.; Annual Circular of Tate Epsom Spring, Containing Location, Analysis of the Water [...] Together with Many Certificates and List of References, Card of Resident Physician, Shipping Directions, etc.* (Knoxville: Ogden Brothers General Book and Job Printing, 1882), 10–11, "Tate Epsom Spring Annual Circular, Ogden Bros. Gen., Book and Job Printing 1882," Tourism Folder 20, PAM Tourism Box 7, McClung.

301. *Tate Spring; The Carlsbad of America; A Health and Pleasure Resort; Situated in One of the Loveliest Valleys of East Tennessee [...]; Thos. Tomlinson, Owner and Prop'r, Tate Spring, Tenn.* (n.p.: S.G. Newman, [mid-1890s?]), 7. I speculate that this pamphlet dates from the mid-1890s.

302. "Tate Springs, Tenn.," *Houston Post*, 20 May 1906.

303. Ibid., 10–11.

304. *Tate Spring, Tennessee: The Carlsbad of America, Open All the Year* [1927?], 5, 36; Klein, *Discovering Donald Ross*, 182.

305. Bruce, "Bean Station," 7; CLB interview.

306. *Tate Epsom Spring; Grainger County, Tenn.; Annual Circular of Tate Epsom Spring, Containing Location, Analysis of the Water [...] Together with Many Certificates and List of References, Card of Resident Physician, Shipping Directions, etc.* (Knoxville: The Chronicle Co., Steam Book and Job Printers and Binders, 1883), 11; *Annual Pamphlet of Tate Epsom Spring* (1898), 7, 23, 29, 35; "Tate Springs, Tenn.," *Houston Post*, 20 May 1906.

307. C.L.B. recollected that "people put great stock" in the mineral water, that Tate Spring's reputation was based on it.

308. *Tate Epsom Spring; Grainger County, Tenn.* (1879), 11.

309. "Tate Spring Epsom Water [ad]," *Birmingham Post-Herald*, 26 May 1904.

310. *Tate Epsom Spring; Grainger County, Tenn.* (1883), 10.

311. Weiss and Kemble, *Great American Water-Cure Craze*, 100–2, 117.

312. Clarke, *Atlanta Illustrated*, 108. Patients given electric baths sat in a tub as electrical currents passed through the water to them. See Jeremy Agnew, *The Electric Corset and Other Victorian Miracles: Medical Devices and Treatments from the Golden Age of Quackery* (Jefferson, NC: McFarland, 2021), 112.

313. Unfortunately, for Tate, however, eight other mineral spring resorts also claimed that title. See Enno Sander, "The 'Carlsbad Springs' of the United States of North America," *Medical Mirror* 8 (January 1897): 567–76.

314. *Tate Epsom Spring; Grainger County, Tenn.* (1879), 18; *Tate Spring, Tennessee: The Carlsbad of America, Open All the Year* [1927?], 13.

315. B., "Tate Spring. Important Announcement," *Knoxville Daily Tribune*, 23 Sept. 1881.

316. *Annual Pamphlet of Tate Epsom Spring* (1898), 18–19; *Tate Spring, Tennessee: The Carlsbad of America, Open All the Year* [1927?], 13.

317. *Tate Epsom Spring; Grainger County, Tenn.* (1883), 11.

318. I counted the number of testimonials and references from the 1879, 1882, 1883, and 1886 Tate Spring promotional pamphlets. I tried to avoid double-counting, as the same testimonials and references appeared season after season. Although the publication of testimonials and references does not give a total picture of the resort's total guest breakdown by state, it suggests interesting trends. See *Tate Epsom Spring; Grainger County, Tenn.* (1879), 9–17; *Tate Epsom Spring; Grainger County, Tenn.* (1882), 36–39; *Tate Epsom Spring; Grainger County, Tenn.* (1883), 30–34; and *Annual Pamphlet of Tate Epsom Spring Containing Location, Analysis of the Water [...] Together with Many Certificates and List of References, Card of Resident Physician, Shipping Directions, etc.* (Knoxville: S.B. Newman and Co., Steam Book and Job Printers, 1886), 16–22, "Tate Epsom Spring Annual Pamphlet, Grainger Co., TN 1886 Knoxville," Tourism Folder 21, PAM Tourism Box 7, McClung.

319. *Tate Epsom Spring; Grainger County, Tenn.* (1879), 10, 12–13, 17; *Tate Epsom Spring; Grainger County, Tenn.* (1882), 33, 36.

320. Jones and Tifft, *The Trust*, 22.

321. New York attendees gave, for example, 1

testimonial or reference in 1879, 12 in 1882, 29 in 1883, and 35 in 1886. South Carolina residents provided 6 testimonials or references in 1879, 10 in 1882, 20 in 1883, and 23 in 1886. These numbers suggest trends only.

322. "Tate Springs [ad]," *South Bend Tribune*, 13 Aug. 1873; *Ibid.*, 15 May 1883; D.S., telephone interview by author, 6 October 2004, handwritten notes in possession of author; Mary Jane Stull Studebaker, "J.M.'s Illness," originally privately printed, but reprinted in 1969 by the Studebaker Family National Assn., in Young, *Studebaker History Corner*, 12.

323. "Tate Spring Hotel Register," MS-198, June 1923, Box 1, Special Collections, UTK. The chemical site today is the headquarters for Eastman Chemical, a Fortune 500 company.

324. Works Projects Administration for the State of Tennessee, *Tennessee*, 312.

325. D.S. interview.

326. Aron, *Working at Play*, 241, caption, 242.

327. Corbett, *Making of American Resorts*, 10, 228, 239–40.

328. C.LB. interview.

Unaka Springs

329. *Herald and Tribune* (Jonesborough, TN), 3 June 1886. No information could be located from sources consulted to provide a definitive starting date for the hotel.

330. "James W. Deaderick," in Moore and Foster, *Tennessee: The Volunteer State, 1769–1923*, vol. 2 (Chicago and Nashville: S.J. Clarke Publishing Co. 1923), 109–10; Goforth, *Building the Clinchfield*, 98; J.G, interview by author, Mar. 14, 2004, Erwin, TN, audiotape recording in possession of author. All interviewees unless otherwise noted are identified by initials only to preserve confidentiality.

331. "Unicoi County—Misc—Unicoi County Postmasters," http://ftp.rootsweb.com/pub/usgenweb/tn/unicoi/misc/unicoipo.txt; J.G. interview.

332. "Three C's Railrord [sic]," *Comet* (Johnson City, TN), 7 Aug. 1890; "The Three C's Road Completed to the North Carolina Line," *Journal and Tribune* (Knoxville), 22 Aug. 1890.

333. "To the Mountains," *Macon Telegraph* (GA), 16 July 1889; "The Charleston, Cincinnati and Chicago Railroad Company is now Open for Business [ad]," *Comet* (Johnson City, TN), 21 Aug. 1890.

334. Unicoi County *Deed Record* 5, 437–42. All *Deed Records* and *Deed Books* cited were found in the Erwin location. Two handwritten dates in the deed give 1895 as the year; two other dates for the same deed appear, however, to be written as 1893.

335. *Ibid.*; Alderman, *All Aboard*, 12.

336. Unicoi County *Deed Record* 5, 437–38, 440.

337. *Ibid.*, 437, 440. A property tax on the springs is still controversial today, per F.T., interview by author, May 1, 2004, Unicoi County, TN, handwritten notes in possession of author for this and subsequent author interviews cited; U.M., interview by author, Sept. 27, 2004, Unicoi County, TN.

338. Lyle, "Unaka Springs Resort," in Unicoi County Heritage Book Committee, *Unicoi County*, 15; "Flood Damages Heavy. Waters in Tennessee Rivers Receding—Traffic Being Resumed," *New York Times*, 25 May 1901; F.T. interview; Lyle, 15; Painting based on photograph, property of F.T.

339. F.T. interview; Lyle, 15; J.H., interview by author, 1 May 2004, Unicoi County, TN; Goforth, 27; H.M. Deaderick, Unaka Springs, Tennessee, to O.K. Morgan, Johnson City, Tennessee, Feb. 23, 1916, transcript in the hand of H.M. Deaderick, property of James A. Goforth, Erwin, TN. Deaderick wrote his letter on stationery that included a photo of the hotel and a hotel ad. Lyle states that the hotel was moved in 1910 to accommodate construction of the mainline Carolina, Clinchfield, and Ohio Railway. Goforth, however, states that all construction work begun in 1905–1908 was finished by 1909 before the CC&O began operations.

340. F.T. interview; J.H. interview; Unicoi County *Deed Book* 74, 1946; Bailey and Bailey, "Lost Cove and Unaka Springs."

341. H.C., interview by author, 1 May 2004, Erwin, TN; J.H. interview; Chester and Carrie Bailey, "Lost Cove and Unaka Springs."

342. Bailey and Bailey.

343. J.H. interview; F.T. interview; U.M. interview; Alderman, *All Aboard*, 12.

344. F.T. interview; J.H. interview; *Erwin Weekly Magnet*, 12 July 1894.

345. Bailey and Bailey; J.H. interview; F.T. interview; "Some Attractive Round Trip Fares Offered by Seaboard Air Line Railway [ad]," *Atlanta Constitution*, 14 July 1915; "Annual Mountain Excursion Southern Railway [ad]," *Orlando Evening Star*, 7 Aug. 1913; "Spend Your Vacation in Cool Comfort [ad]," *Fort Worth Star-Telegram*, 8 July 1914.

346. A.W., interview by author, 27 Sept. 2004, Unicoi County, TN; F.T. interview.

347. *Erwin Weekly Magnet*, 12 July 1894; "Hike to Unaka Springs," *Ibid.*, 11 June 1926; *Erwin Times*, 26 July 1926; "Family Picnic at Unaka Springs," *Erwin Record*, 24 August 1928; T.L., interview by author, 21 May 2004, Erwin, TN; J.G. interview.

348. H.C. interview; U.M. interview.

349. F.T. interview; H.C. interview; A.W. interview; U.M. interview; J.H. interview.

350. H.C. interview; F.T. interview; A.W. interview; T.L. interview.

351. F.T. interview.

352. A.W. interview; J.H. interview; J.G. interview; T.L. interview. Unicoi County had tried as early as 1923 to construct a road from the south end of the county bridge to Unaka Springs. A newspaper article noted that the road "will be a great convenience in getting to Unaka Springs." See "Road to Unaka Springs Soon," *Erwin Weekly Magnet*, 11 Apr. 1923.

353. J.H. interview; A.W. interview; F.T. interview; U.M. interview; H.C. interview.

354. Unicoi County, TN Deeds: "Trustee's Deed," 152–53; "Warranty Deed from Dr. Aura Barrowman," 320–22; "Warranty Deed from Stella Hopson," 130–31.

355. J.H. interview; Bailey and Bailey. For more on Lost Cove, see Alderman, *All Aboard*, 14, and Christy A. Smith, *Lost Cove, North Carolina: Portrait of a Vanished Appalachian Community, 1864–1957* (Jefferson, NC: McFarland, 2022).

356. Bailey and Bailey; F.T. interview; A.W. interview; J.G. interview; J.H. interview; Jim Wozniak, "Unaka Springs Eternal," *Johnson City Press* (TN), 24 Dec. 2007.

Virginia

Introduction

1. Switzer, *Report on the Internal Commerce*, 162.

2. For an overview of the spring region, see John Alexander Williams, "Virginia and West Virginia Springs," in *Encyclopedia of Appalachia*, ed. Ruby Abramson and Jean Haskell (Knoxville: University of Tennessee Press, 2006), 679–80.

3. Fitch, 629, 670; Cohen, *Historic Springs*, v.

4. Boyd, *Resources of South-West Virginia*, 166; "Iron Lithia Springs [ad]," *Tazewell Republican* (VA), 11 June 1903.

5. Amory, *Last Resorts*, 452 (page citation is to the reprint edition).

6. Burke, *Mineral Springs of Western Virginia*, 126, 154.

7. Moorman, *Virginia Springs* (1847), iii, 84, 100, 92–93. Burke, among many denigrations, called Moorman "biased in favour of the creation of his own imagination" and criticized the White's "glaring want of *design* [italics original] in the arrangement of the buildings." See Burke, *Mineral Springs of Western Virginia*, 100, 112.

8. Blanton, *Medicine in Virginia*, 342–44.

9. A wealth of social history sources exists on the more popular Virginia springs. One antebellum source, an early postbellum book, and one current example are Mark Pencil [Mary M. Hagner], *The White Sulphur Papers, Or Life at the Springs of Western Virginia* (New York: Samuel Colman, 1839); Edward Alfred Pollard, *The Virginia Tourist. Sketches of the Springs and Mountains of Virginia* (Philadelphia: J.R. Lippincott & Co., 1870); Lewis, *Ladies and Gentlemen on Display*.

10. Amory, 455; Fishwick, *Springlore*, 80.

11. Hale, *Four Valiant Years*, 367.

12. Fishwick, 84.

13. Mayo, "Henry Clay," 301–03; Williams, *Appalachia*, 133.

14. Genovese, *Sweetness of Life*, 212; Belinda Anderson, "Salt Sulphur Springs," *e-WV: The West Virginia Encyclopedia*, updated Sept. 22, 2023, https://www.wvencyclopedia.org/articles/170.

15. "Mr. Webster," *Lynchburg Virginian*, 14 July 1851.

16. University of Mary Washington, "The Papers of James Monroe," https://academics.umw.edu/jamesmonroepapers/biography/calendar/august/; "The President at the Springs," *Madisonian* (Washington, D.C.), 1 Sept. 1838; "The President—Democratic Party," *Independent Press* (Abbeville Court House, SC), 21 Sept. 1855; Fishwick, 121. Buchanan, from PA, spent much time at that state's Bedford Springs.

17. Monroe, "Extracts from Dr. Burke's New Book on the Virginia Springs," *Richmond Enquirer*, 12 July 1853.

18. Virginia Center for Digital History and University of Virginia Library, "Valley of the Shadow: Civil War-Era Newspapers," "The Virginia Springs," *Staunton Vindicator*, 12 Aug. 1859, https://valley.lib.virginia.edu/news/rv1859/va.au.rv.1859.08.12.xml#02; *Alexandria Gazette*, 15 Sept. 1856; "Fauquier White Sulphur Springs," *Ibid.*, 18 July 1857.

19. "A New Line," *Charleston Courier*, 27 Mar. 1839; "Stages [ad]," *Constitutional Whig* (Richmond), 26 Sept. 1831; Amory, 452; Myer, "The Trail System of the Southeastern United States." For an illustration of routes to the Virginia Springs, see Ashton W. Reniers, cartographer, "The Springs of Virginia and the Routes Leading Thereto," in *The Springs of Virginia: Life, Love, and Death at the Waters, 1775–1900* (Chapel Hill: University of North Carolina Press, 1941), inside of cover.

20. Moorman, 218; "Western Mail Line," *Constitutional Whig* (Richmond), 14 May 1828.

21. "Bath Coffee-House [ad]," *Martinsburg Gazette* (VA), 19 Sept. 1838.

22. "Stage Accident," *Richmond Enquirer*, 28 Sept. 1838.

23. "Augusta Springs [ad]," *Ibid.*, 11 July 1826; Charles Culbertson, "Historic Stribling Springs Was One of the Top U.S. Resorts," *News Leader* (Staunton, VA), 30 May 2015, https://www.newsleader.com/story/news/history/2015/05/30/historic-stribling-springs-one-top-us-resorts/28240213/.

24. Prolix, *Letters Descriptive of the Virginia Springs*, 73.

25. Moorman remarked in his 1847 mineral springs treatise that "routes have all been greatly improved.... [P]ersons can now reach our mountains with far greater ease, safety and expedition than they could have done some years ago." See Moorman, 216.

26. Theriault, "Shannondale Springs," 4.

27. "Shannondale Springs," *Martinsburg Gazette* (VA), 23 May 1838.

28. "Summer Resort. Helpful Attractions of the Washington Springs, VA. [ad]," *Brownlow's Knoxville Whig*, 6 June 1866; "Virginia and Tennessee Railroad. Red Sulphur Springs [ad]," *Lynchburg Daily Virginian*, 21 July 1854; "Va. and Tenn. Railroad. Buchanan, Natural Bridge, Lexington, and Rockbridge Alum Springs [ad]," *Ibid.*

29. "The Virginia Springs," *Daily Dispatch* (Richmond), 21 June 1860.

30. "Virginia Central Railroad [ad]," *Savannah Daily Georgian*, 20 July 1853; "The Mineral Springs of Virginia," *Alexandria Gazette*, 19 June 1858.

31. Wilson, "From Enslavement to Entrepreneurship," 162; "Our Watering Places," *Winchester Virginian*, 14 Aug. 1850.

32. For examples of the labor and services that enslaved persons provided at the Virginia Springs, see Wilson, 164, 169; Dunaway, *Slavery in the Mountain South*, 82–83; Lewis, 41–42, 196–97.

33. Dunaway, 82; Wilson, 164.

34. *Daily Dispatch* (Richmond), 8 Mar. 1860; Bratton, "Fields's Observations, 76, 91.

35. LaFauci, "Taking the (Southern) Waters, 16–17; Lewis, 42.

36. "35 New Historical Markers Approved in June: Fauquier White Sulphur Springs," https://www.dhr.virginia.gov/press_releases/35-new-historical-markers-approved-in-june/; Lewis, 43.

37. Fain, *Black Huntington*, 34; *Daily Dispatch* (Richmond), 8 Mar. 1860.

38. Fain, 35. Fain provides a thoughtful discussion of the implications of the use of free Black waiters at the White Sulphur on page 35.

39. *Ibid.*, 29–33, 35; Lewis, 42–43.

40. Fain, 28.

41. Lewis gives an example of a slaveowner haggling with the superintendent of the Fauquier White Sulphur Springs over the terms of payment, period of time, and use of the slaveowner's pastry cook. See Lewis, 42.

42. Williams claims without attribution that White Sulphur Springs upon the 1858 reorganization of its stock company shifted entirely to free Black employees. See Williams, *Appalachia*, 134. The reorganized stock company shareowners were principally Virginians (not northerners who might have been abolitionists); at least one, Jeremiah Morton, owned enslaved persons. See Moorman, 82; Lewis, 42. Lewis comments that one unidentified hotel in the vicinity before 1850 hired only free servants. See Lewis, 224n14.

43. Cohen, 80, 156.

44. Quarles, *Occupied Winchester*, 123. The approximate count includes movements when one calvary moved into Winchester as the opposing calvary was leaving.

45. Cohen, 56, 143, 156; "Taking the Waters: 19th Century Medicinal Springs of Virginia: Medicinal Springs of Virginia in the Nineteenth Century, Warm Springs: Letter from the Medical Director of the Army of West Virginia to Dr. J. H. Hunter, December 16, 1861," http://exhibits.hsl.virginia.edu/springs/warmmedicaldirectorletter; U.S. War Dept., *War of the Rebellion*, 984.

46. Cohen, 172; U.S. War Dept., 1026; David Bard, "Battle of White Sulphur Springs." in *e-WV: The West Virginia Encyclopedia*, Nov. 19, 2010, https://www.wvencyclopedia.org/articles/1240.

47. Guerrant, *Headquarters Diary*, 592–95.

48. Cohen, 143; Country Zest and Style, "Historic Fauquier White Sulphur Springs Remembered," https://issuu.com/uncoveringthevalley/docs/cz_fall20_issuu/s/11108711.

49. Brian Katen interview by Sarah McConnell, Virginia Humanities, With Good Reason Radio, "African-American Heritage Tourism," Mar. 27, 2010, https://www.withgoodreasonradio.org/episode/african-american-heritage-tourism/ . To understand the context of Black society at the Virginia springs originating in antebellum times, see National Park Service, "Yellow Sulphur Springs: Historic American Landscape Survey: Written Historical and Descriptive Data," HALS VA-55, 2–3, https://tile.loc.gov/storage-services/master/pnp/habshaer/va/va2200/va2213/data/va2213data.pdf .

Holston Springs

50. For more information on the Carter Family, see "Carter Family," https://countrymusichalloffame.org/artist/carter-family and "The Carter Family Fold," http://www.carterfamilyfold.org/.

51. "Scott County VA Peaks List," https://listsofjohn.com/searchres?c=953.

52. Michael Joslin, "Time, Elements Carve Tunnel Into Wonder," *Johnson City Press* (TN), 30 Aug. 1993.

53. J.W., email to author, Feb. 6, 2007; K.S., email to author, July 9, 2021; D.B. Palmer, "From D.B. Palmer: Tells of a Plesant [sic] Trip through the East," *Barton Beacon* (Great Bend, KS), 4 Aug. 1898; "Mountain Springs Hotel [ad]," *The Post* (Big Stone Gap, VA), 20 Sept. 1905.

54. Jim Hall, "Scott County Residence was Showplace of Mountain Empire," *The Post* (Big Stone Gap, VA), 4 June 1959; "Remembered ... Hagan Hall—Rufus Ayers Estate," *Scott County Herald-Virginian*, 2 July 1980, Scott County Historical Society, Scott County, Virginia, "Documents: Remembering," http://sites.rootsweb.com/~vaschs2/remembering.htm; Addington, *History of Scott County*, 345–46.

55. Peale, *Lists and Analyses of the Mineral Springs of the United States,* 56.

56. "Holston Springs," *Charleston Courier*, 25 Jan. 1810; "Holston Springs [ad]," *Savannah Daily Republican*, 21 July 1856.

57. Sullivan County Historical Commission and Associates, *Historic Sites of Sullivan County*, xvii, 7; Summers, "In the Heart of the Holston Country," 128; King, "Early Abingdon Taverns," 13; "Wilderness Road," http://www.virginiaplaces.org/transportation/wildernessroad.html; R Jackson Marshall III, "Great Wagon Road," in *NCPedia*, https://www.ncpedia.org/great-wagon-road.

58. "Holston Springs," *Charleston Courier*, 25 Jan. 1810.

59. *Ibid.*; Southwestern Virginia Genealogical Society, Roanoke, Virginia, "Martin D. McHenry," contributed by Miss Aileen McHenry (typed copy of the original), *Virginia Appalachian Notes* (Feb.

1986): 28, http://www.virginiaroom.org/digital/files/original/50/4917/VANv10n1.pdf

60. Summers, *History of Southwest Virginia*, 465.

61. *Acts Passed*, 64–66.

62. Sullivan County Historical Commission and Associates, 7.

63. U.S. Population Census 1830, FamilySearch, www.familysearch.org; subsequent Census records cited accessed at FamilySearch.

64. Southwestern Virginia Genealogical Society, Roanoke, Virginia, "Martin D. McHenry," contributed by Miss Aileen McHenry (typed copy of the original), *Virginia Appalachian Notes* (Feb. 1986): 26, http://www.virginiaroom.org/digital/files/original/50/4917/VANv10n1.pdf; "Maj. Thomas Goodson, Sr.," 304, FamilySearch, https://www.familysearch.org/photos/artifacts/30888425.

65. Brad Scott, "By the Waters of Possum Creek: A More Comprehensive History of Weber City, Virginia," https://drbrop.wordpress.com/2021/02/20/a-more-comprehensive-history-of-weber-city-virginia/.

66. M.C., telephone interview by author, Kingsport, TN; H.G., unpublished typescript, *History of Exchange Place* (2017); B.M., interview by author, Kingsport, TN; Bud Phillips, "Most Slave Quarters Are Gone With the Wind," *Bristol Herald-Courier* (TN), 1 Feb. 2009, https://heraldcourier.com/news/most-slave-quarters-are-gone-with-the-wind/article_1145bc96-b444-54f5-a923-1527ad02b925.html; L.P. Summers, "Walnut Grove Cemetery Is Among Section's Most Historical Spots," *Bristol Herald Courier* (TN / VA), 5 July 1936.

67. Summers, 659-60; Stevenson, *Increase in Excellence*, 40.

68. Summers, 642; Virginia Department of Historic Places, "086-0003 Preston House," https://www.dhr.virginia.gov/historic-registers/086-0003/; Mary Widener, "World Traveler, Author Opens Trading Post in Historic House," *Richmond Times-Dispatch*, 2 Aug. 1950.

69. David Hunter Strother, *Holston Springs*, [1857?], pencil drawing, 17.3 cm. x 24.8 cm., West Virginia and Regional History Center, David Hunter Strother Collection, West Virginia University Library, Morgantown, WV, https://strother.lib.wvu.edu/catalog/W1995030192; "Tales of Pluck and Adventure," *Beatrice Evening News* (NB), 17 Oct. 1899. Strother, who used the pseudonym "Porte Crayon," illustrated a series of fictious articles he wrote for *Harper's Magazine* in the mid-1850s based on his travels, which included SW VA. For more background on Strother's trip, see Robins, "Illustrating Appalachia," 1–3. The 1899 article, reprinted across the country, describes an incident at Holston Springs involving a young Cherokee male. Although the article contains errors, such as the location of Holston Springs, and likely exaggerations, it is plausible that a Cherokee boy may have been employed. Interestingly, the article mentions the employment of young white males but does not reference the use of Black enslaved laborers.

70. Pollard, *Virginia Tourist*, 118.

71. U.S. Population Census 1840.

72. Sullivan County Historical Commission and Associates, 79; Owens, "Exchange Place," 19. John Strother Gaines associated with Holston Springs is not the same as John Strother Gaines, a Sullivan County cousin, who served as an influential federal trade agent in Choctaw negotiations. See James P. Pate, "George Strother Gaines," *Encyclopedia of Alabama*, updated Oct. 12, 2015, http://www.encyclopediaofalabama.org/article/h-1476.

73. National Register of Historic Places, "The Preston Farm"; B.M. interview.

74. M.C. interview. M.C. interviewed a descendant of John S. Gaines about 2016.

75. Sullivan County Historical Commission and Associates, 79.

76. "Addendum to contract between John Gaines and John Preston exchanging Holston Springs for Exchange Place," Aug. 20, 1845 (typescript by H.G.of photocopy of original, EP).

77. Owens, 10.

78. *Knoxville Register*, 21 July 1847.

79. "Holston Springs [ad]," *Savannah Daily Republican*, 21 July 1856. No Gaines are found in Scott County in either the 1850 or 1860 U.S. Censuses.

80. *Knoxville Register*, 21 July 1847.

81. Disturnell, *Springs*, 124.

82. N.L.E., "A Summer Retreat," *Knoxville Register*, 17 July 1856.

83. Ibid.

84. Garland, "Economic Survey," 9.

85. Addington, 183; "Norfolk Southern Promotes Railroad Safety at Virginia's Natural Tunnel," July 9, 2013, http://www.nscorp.com/content/nscorp/en/news/norfolk-southern-promotes-railroad-safety-at-virginias-natural-tunnel.html.

86. Owens, 10.

87. M.C. interview.

88. "Holston Springs Hotel Register," photocopy of the original, EP. I created the title for the photocopied pages. The photocopy consists of about 33 ledger-size sheets dating from 1853 through 1858 (none for 1855). Cursive writing is difficult to decipher at times; ink on some pages is faded on the photocopy. The page that recorded the Wetumpka, AL, visitor's 1856 sojourn could not be found. From calculating expenses for some guests, I determined that a 2-wk. stay cost $10.

89. "Holston Springs Hotel Register."

90. Ibid. Antebellum resorts in Southern Appalachia in general charged half rates for children and servants (slaves) plus possibly 50 cents daily for a horse. The Russell County family consisted of parents, 3 children, 1 servant, 2 horses; Cummings was by herself with 3 servants and 6 horses.

91. Ibid.

92. I cross-referenced several recurring hotel register guest names and their home locations against the 1850 and 1860 U.S. Censuses to determine occupations. I was unable to determine the profession of the Baltimore guests, who stayed

for a night and then re-registered 3 wks. later for another night or so. I presume that they were merchants or businessmen.

93. Robins, 2.

94. For example, the 1856 season of ~16 weeks welcomed ~280 guests, a few of whom I may have double-counted, or an average of 2–3 guests per day. Guests included "Mr. Somebody" on Aug. 15. In 1858, 77 guests registered Apr. 30—June 24 for an average of 1–2 guests per day. The hotel clerks recorded "lady" if a wife accompanied her husband although the clerks may have erred in that detail on occasion, thus under-counting the true guest number.

95. "Holston Springs Hotel Register."

96. Ibid. I counted the number of guests who were charged $10 or more (at least 2 wks.' stay).

97. Ibid. No location was listed for two groups. Lynchburg was listed for three groups, two of which consisted of the same three men. More research is needed to determine why the Mississippians chose Holston Springs over other antebellum resorts.

98. *Richmond Dispatch*, 4 Aug. 1889.

99. "Holston Springs Hotel Register."

100. "Sale of Springs," *Daily Dispatch* (Richmond), 30 Aug. 1858; "Death of a Minister," *Richmond Dispatch*, 28 July 1860; "A Card—Female Education: Holston Springs Female Boarding School," *Weekly Mississippian* (Jackson), 29 Dec. 1858. The quote is from the *Weekly Mississippian*.

101. "Holston Springs for Sale," *Charleston Daily Courier (TN)*, 13 Apr. 1860; "By the Waters of Possum Creek"; Works Project Administration, "Ex-Slave Stories (Texas): William Davis," *Federal Writers' Project, Slave Narratives: A Folk History of Slavery in the United States From Interviews with Former Slaves* (Washington: 1941), 289, https://memory.loc.gov/mss/mesn/161/161.pdf; Guerrant, *Headquarters Diary*, 14, 213–16.

102. Guerrant, 222.

103. "Ex-Slave Stories (Texas): William Davis," 289, 291.

104. Ibid., 291–92. After his father's death, Davis joined the army and was stationed in Texas.

105. "Holston Springs Property for Rent [ad]," *Abingdon Virginian*, 4 Mar. 1870.

106. Pollard, 118.

107. "General Ayers Is Dead; Won Fame By State Bond Fight," *Daily Press* (Newport News, VA), 15 May 1926; Addington, 339–40. The title of "General" refers to Ayers' elected position, not to a military rank.

108. "Holston Springs [ad]," *Richmond Dispatch*, 9 June 1892; *The Big Stone Gap Post* (VA), 2 Mar. 1893. Ayers' home in Big Stone Gap now serves as the museum. See Virginia State Parks, "Southwest Virginia Museum," https://www.dcr.virginia.gov/state-parks/southwest-virginia-museum. Ayers may have added the impressive columned portico shown in later photographs when he remodeled the hotel. See Pat Jones, "Career of a Southwestern Virginian," *Richmond Times-Dispatch Magazine*, 30 Apr. 1939, 8–10.

109. "Gen. Ayers' Residence Burned," *Big Stone Gap Post* (VA), 17 Dec. 1913.

110. "Picnic," *Bristol Herald Courier* (TN), 6 June 1919; *Kingsport Times* (TN), 28 May 1920; "Bacon Bat," *Ibid.*, 6 June 1922.

111. "Well-known and Historic Virginia Farm to be Broken Up and Sold," *Kingsport Times* (TN), 1 May 1941.

Montgomery County: Yellow Sulphur Springs, Alleghany Springs, Montgomery White Sulphur Springs

112. Virginia's New River Valley: Our Region, https://www.newrivervalleyva.org/our-region/.

113. *Lists and Analyses of the Mineral Springs of the United States*, 56.

114. "Welcome to Alta Mons!," https://www.altamons.org/our-history.html; Cohen, *Historic Springs*, 38–39; Virginia Dept. of Historic Resources, "060–0487 Crockett Springs Cottage," https://www.dhr.virginia.gov/historic-registers/060-0487/.

115. "Montgomery White Sulphur [ad]," *Richmond Enquirer*, 24 July 1855; Fishwick, *Springlore*, 153; "Yellow Sulphur Springs," https://yellowsulphursprings.com/historic-yellow-sulphur-springs-the-area/.

116. Cohen, 123.

117. Pollard, *Virginia Tourist*, 127–28.

118. Moorman, *Mineral Springs of North America*, 172.

119. Lewis, 87.

120. Viator, "To the Editor of the Enquirer," *Enquirer* (Richmond), 23 Nov. 1810.

121. "For Sale or Rent [ad]," *Virginia Argus* (Richmond), 9 Apr. 1814; "Yellow Springs [ad]," *Richmond Enquirer*, 7 July 1818; "Yellow Springs [ad]," *Ibid.*, 31 Jan. 1826.

122. "Yellow Springs [ad]," *Richmond Enquirer*, 17 May 1833; "Yellow Springs [ad]," *Ibid.*, 12 June 1835.

123. Fishwick, 155. The 1850 federal census does not list Forrest's occupation or value of his real estate or personal estate. The 1860 federal census lists $21,800 and $9,200 respectively for the value of real estate and personal estate. Forrest's worth in 1840 is unknown. See U.S. Population Censuses 1850, 1860, FamilySearch, www.familysearch.org; subsequent census data in this chapter accessed at FamilySearch.

124. U.S. Dept. of the Interior, NPS, National Register of Historic Places Inventory—Nomination Form, "Yellow Sulphur Springs," 2.

125. Fishwick, 155.

126. Virginia Museum of Fine Arts, "Yellow Sulphur Springs, Montgomery Co., Va. (Primary Title), Album of Virginia (Series Title)," https://www.vmfa.museum/piction/6027262-8052041/.

127. Mann, "Mountains," 415; George McLean, "The Virginia and Tennessee Railroad during the

Civil War," in *Encyclopedia Virginia*, Virginia Humanities, June 8, 2023, https://encyclopediavirginia.org/entries/the-virginia-and-tennessee-railroad-during-the-civil-war/.

128. *Daily Dispatch* (Richmond), 22 Jan. 1856; "Virginia and Tennessee Railroad [ad]," *Ibid.*, 7 Aug. 1854; "Yellow Sulphur Springs in Montgomery County, VA. [ad]," *Ibid.*, 25 July 1854.

129. Fishwick, 228; National Register of Historic Places, 3.

130. "Montgomery White Sulphur Springs [ad]," *Lynchburg Daily Virginian*, 21 June 1856.

131. "Alleghany Springs [ad]," *Daily Herald* (Wilmington, NC), 14 June 1860.

132. "Visitors to the Virginia Springs [ad]," *Charleston Daily Courier*, 13 June 1854.

133. Lewis, 73; "Alleghany Springs [ad]," *Richmond Daily Whig*, 16 June 1854.

134. "Public Sale of the Alleghany Springs [ad]," *Richmond Enquirer*, 29 Mar. 1859.

135. Pollard, *Virginia Tourist*, 89.

136. Moorman, *Virginia Springs*, 278.

137. "Alleghany Springs [ad]," *Richmond Daily Whig*, 16 June 1854.

138. "Alleghany Springs, Montgomery County, VA.," *New Orleans Daily Crescent*, 16 June 1860.

139. "Montgomery County, Virginia," *The Farmer* 1 (July 1866): 303.

140. U.S. Population Censuses 1850, 1860, 1870; Williamson, "Seven Ways." The CPI calculator was used.

141. Cohen, 75; Thorp, "The Beginnings of African American Education in Montgomery County," 331.

142. "Montgomery White Sulphur Springs [ad]," *Daily Dispatch* (Richmond), 27 May 1856.

143. *Acts of the General Assembly of Virginia*, 236–37.

144. "To Carpenters [ad]," *Daily Dispatch* (Richmond), 15 Feb. 1855; Cohen, 76; Boyd, *Resources of South-West Virginia*, 21.

145. A.B.C., "The Springs," *Daily Dispatch* (Richmond), 31 Aug. 1858.

146. "Montgomery White Sulphur Springs [ad]," *Daily Dispatch* (Richmond), 27 May 1856.

147. Cohen, 76.

148. "Montgomery White Sulphur Springs [ad]," *Richmond Enquirer*, 24 July 1855.

149. Pollard, 121.

150. Moorman, *Virginia Springs*, 336.

151. Pollard, 121.

152. "Montgomery White Sulphur Springs [ad]," *Daily Dispatch* (Richmond), 27 May 1856.

153. A.B.C., "The Springs."

154. "Coyner's Spings [sic], Va., July 19th, 1859," *Wilmington Journal* [NC], 22 July 1859.

155. Ibid.

156. "The Montgomery Alum Springs," *Richmond Enquirer*, 3 Aug. 1858.

157. K., "Montgomery White Sulphur Springs, August 23d, 1856," *Richmond Enquirer*, 2 Sept. 1856.

158. National Register of Historic Places, 2; *Lynchburg Daily Virginian*, 5 Aug. 1856.

159. Fishwick, 157; Shirley P. Thomas, "Montgomery White Sulphur Springs," *United Daughters of the Confederacy Magazine* 60 (Mar. 1997): 26.

160. *Richmond Daily Whig*, 26 Apr. 1861; Somers, "War and Play," 10. Newspapers that publicized the resort included the *Nashville Union and American*, the *Memphis Daily Appeal*, the *Charleston Mercury*, and the *New Orleans Daily Crescent*.

161. "Alleghany Springs [ad]," *Alexandria Gazette*, 25 May 1862.

162. "Alleghany Springs [ad]," *Richmond Whig*, 2 July 1862.

163. "Montgomery White Sulphur Springs [ad]," *Daily Avalanche* (Memphis), 22 May 1861; *Daily Dispatch* (Richmond), 6 June 1862.

164. Schaller, *Soldiering for Glory*, 94–95.

165. *New York Times*, 27 July 1862; *Yorkville Enquirer* (SC), 15 Oct. 1862.

166. Chitwood, "Confederate Surgeons of Wythe County," 13; Virginia Center for Civil War Studies, "Montgomery White Sulphur Springs," https://civilwar.vt.edu/montgomery-white-sulphur-springs/.

167. "Alleghany Springs For Sale [ad]," *Richmond Whig*, 6 Nov. 1863; *Daily Dispatch* (Richmond), 25 Jan. 1864; Virginia Center for Civil War Studies, "Montgomery White Sulphur Springs."

168. Pollard, 120.

169. Fishwick, 157, 159; *Alexandria Gazette*, 16 Nov. 1870.

170. "Alleghany Springs [ad]," *Nashville Union and Dispatch*, 16 June 1887; Grattan, *Reports of Cases Decided*, 640, 643.

171. Pollard, 120.

172. "Virginia Agricultural and Mechanical College," *Daily Dispatch* (Richmond), 26 July 1872; Fishwick, 157; "Appendix," in *Annual Reports*, 2.

173. "Alleghany Spring Water [ad]," *Daily Dispatch* (Richmond), 6 June 1866; *Clarksville Weekly Chronicle* (TN), 20 July 1866; "Letter from the Alleghany Springs of Virginia," *New Orleans Crescent*, 21 June 1868.

174. Cohen, 1; "Montgomery White Sulphur Springs [ad]," *Memphis Daily Appeal*, 25 May 1869.

175. French, *Two Wars*, 376–77.

176. "General Longstreet Avoided Like a Leper," *Edgefield Advertiser* (SC), 11 Sept. 1873; Starnes, "Forever Faithful," 187–88.

177. Fishwick, 232–33; Starnes, "Forever Faithful," 178.

178. Fishwick, 233.

179. "Tournament Ball," *Norfolk Virginian*, 5 Sept. 1868; "Montgomery White Sulphur Springs [ad]," *Tri-Weekly Clarion* (Meridian, MS), 5 Aug. 1869.

180. "Montgomery White Sulphur Springs for Rent [ad]," *Richmond Dispatch*, 18 Dec. 1877; "Sale of the Montgomery White Sulphur Springs [ad]," *Baltimore Sun*, 2 July 1881; *Evening Visitor* (Raleigh), 1 Sept. 1881.

181. Fishwick, 159; Norfolk and Western, 26.

182. Newspapers from Newspapers.com and

from the Library of Congress Chronicling America website were browsed.

183. The Yellow Sulphur Springs ledger existing pages' daily entries were analyzed from the ledger's first recorded date of Aug. 26, 1887, through Aug. 31, 1890; were randomly browsed from July 1891-July 1893; and analyzed daily from June 3, 1894 through the last entry of July 10, 1895. See "Yellow Sulphur Springs Hotel Account Book," VPI. The Montgomery White Sulphur Springs ledger existing pages' daily entries were analyzed from Aug. 26, 1887, through Aug. 31, 1888, and then browsed at random through 1890. See "Montgomery White Sulphur Springs Guest Book," VPI. Unless otherwise indicated in endnotes, the discussion of visitors for these timeframes is based on the ledger entries.

184. Fishwick, 232–33; "Yellow Sulphur Springs... Finding Aid," VPI.

185. Cyrus Adler, "New Orleans," *JewishEncyclopedia.com: The unedited full-text of the 1906 Jewish Encyclopedia*, https://www.jewishencyclopedia.com/articles/11496-new-orlean.

186. "Fire at Alleghany Springs," *Richmond Dispatch*, 13 Feb. 1900.

187. *Richmond Dispatch*, 25 Nov. 1902; Fishwick, *Springlore*, 236; Cohen, 77.

188. Fishwick, 159.

189. U.S. Dept. of the Interior, NPS, "Yellow Sulphur Springs: Historic American Landscape Survey," 3–4. Professor Brian Katen of Virginia Tech discovered the Black affiliation to Yellow Sulphur Springs when researching Virginia Black newspapers; see Virginia Tech, School of Architecture and Design, Landscape Architecture, "Brian Katen, ASLA," https://archdesign.caus.vt.edu/faculty/brian-katen-asla/.

190. U.S. Dept. of the Interior, NPS, "Yellow Sulphur Springs: Historic American Landscape Survey," 4.

191. *Ibid.*; John Davis, "Black Roanoke: Our Story—February 3, 2014," 3–4, 2021, https://www.roanokeva.gov/DocumentCenter/View/1537/Black-Roanoke-Our-Story?bidId= ; Harrison Museum of African American Culture, "Henry Street Music Festival," https://harrisonmuseum.com/henry-street-heritage-festival/ .

192. Sean Kotz, "Piece of Black History comes to Light," *Roanoke Times*, 16 Dec. 2010, www.roanoke.com; "Yellow Sulphur Springs: Historic American Landscape Survey," 4–5.

193. C.S., email to author, Sept. 15, 2021.

194. Shari Dragovich, "Roanoke, Henry Street, and All that Jazz," *The Roanoker* (May / June 2016), https://theroanoker.com/magazine/features/roanoke-henry-st/.

195. Kotz, "Piece of Black History comes to Light."

196. "Yellow Sulphur Springs: Historic American Landscape Survey," 4.

197. Fishwick, 160.

198. Cohen, 124.

199. *Ibid.*; "Charles A. Crumpacker," *Richmond Times-Dispatch*, 19 Sept. 1942; "Obit—Linkous, Charlise Crumpacker Lester," *Roanoke Times*, 12 Feb. 1994 [typescript provided by Virginia Tech Libraries Scholarly Communications], https://scholar.lib.vt.edu/VA-news/ROA-Times/issues/1994/rt9402/940212/02140183.htm.

200. "Yellow Sulphur Springs Medicine," *Baltimore Sun*, 5 Nov. 1998; "Yellow Sulphur Springs," https://yellowsulphursprings.com/read-the-press-release/ .

201. A.B.C., "The Springs"; "Editorial Correspondence: Salt Sulphur Springs," *Richmond Enquirer*, 22 July 1859; "New Route for Summer Travel," *Richmond Dispatch*, 21 May 1859; "New River White Sulphur Springs [ad]," *Ibid.*, 4 July 1859.

202. *Season of 1875, Warm Springs, Bath County, Virginia*, 3.

203. "Yellow Sulphur Springs, Va.,—From Our Fair Correspondent," *Daily Commercial Herald* (Vicksburg), 7 Aug. 1888.

204. "The Alleghany Springs—Sympathy for France—Distinguished Ex-Confederates Enjoying Themselves," *New York Herald*, 27 Aug. 1870.

205. U.S. Census 1850 (Slave Schedule); U.S. Census 1860 (Slave Schedule).

206. U.S. Census 1860 (Slave Schedule).

207. Early, *Lieutenant General Jubal Anderson Early*, x.

Shannondale, Jordan White Sulphur Springs, Rock Enon

208. Paul Anderson, "Shenandoah Valley during the Civil War," in *Encyclopedia Virginia, Virginia Humanities,* updated Dec. 7, 2020, https://encyclopediavirginia.org/entries/shenandoah-valley-during-the-civil-war; Howard G. Adkins, "Ridge and Valley Province," in *e-WV: The West Virginia Encyclopedia*, updated Oct. 22, 2010, https://www.wvencyclopedia.org/articles/80.

209. Fitch, 670–71; West Virginia State Parks, Berkeley Springs State Park, "History," https://wvstateparks.com/park/berkeley-springs-state-park/. Carved out of Virginia during the Civil War, West Virginia gained statehood in 1863.

210. Fitch, 673. Capon Springs even today caters to vacationers. See Capon Springs and Farms, https://www.caponsprings.net/.

211. "The Mineral Springs of Virginia," *Daily Dispatch* (Richmond), 16 June 1858; "For the Springs: Baltimore and Ohio Railroad [ad]," *Daily Exchange* (Baltimore), 5 Aug. 1858.

212. Rock Enon, or Capper's Springs as it was known in the antebellum period, probably used Black enslaved labor, but more research is needed to support that hypothesis.

213. Cohen, 70; Historic Jordan Springs, "History: 1549," https://historicjordansprings.com/year-1549/ ; Cartmell, *Shenandoah Valley Pioneers*, 207. Sources credit the Catawbas with the first known use of the water although the Catawbas

generally are associated with the Piedmont of the Carolinas. The Monacans, members of the Catawba tribe of the Sioux, controlled areas of the Blue Ridge Mountains and the Shenandoah Valley at the time of the Jamestown landing in 1607. This tribe may be the one that sources reference. See VA Dept. of Education, "Virginia's First People, Past & Present: Culture—Language," https://www.doe.virginia.gov/instruction/history/virginias-first-people/culture/language/index.shtml.

214. Cartmell, 207.

215. *Ibid.* In 1790, the *Winchester Gazette* published an essay on a nearby medicinal spring with no name, which therefore must have predated Duvall's purchase. See Frederic Morton, *The Story of Winchester in Virginia: The Oldest Town in the Shenandoah Valley* (Strasburg: Shenandoah Publishing House, 1925), 227.

216. "Sulphur Spring Near Winchester (VA.) [ad]," *Phenix Gazette* (Alexandria), 18 June 1831; "White Sulphur Spring, Near Winchester [ad]," *Ibid.*, 1 Aug. 1832; "Frederick White Sulphur Springs [ad]," *Ibid.*, 4 Aug. 1837; Cartmell, 207.

217. I was unable to determine the name of the physician brother to Allen and the relationship of Leroy to Allen.

218. "The Frederick White Sulphur Spring [ad]," *Phenix Gazette* (Alexandria), 16 July 1833; "Frederick White Sulphur Springs for Sale or Rent [ad]," *Alexandria Gazette*, 5 Apr. 1836.

219. "Frederick White Sulphur Springs for Sale or Rent [ad]"; U.S. Population Census 1850, U.S. Census 1850 (Slave Schedule), both at FamilySearch.org, www.familysearch.org; subsequent census records cited in this chapter accessed at FamilySearch.

220. "White Sulphur Spring, Near Winchester [ad]."

221. "Frederick White Sulphur Springs for Sale or Rent [ad]"; Cohen, 70; Cartmell, 207. Several sources give either 1832 or 1834 as the year in which Branch Jordan acquired the mineral spring resort. Newspapers advertising the resort for sale were published in 1836.

222. "Cash for Negroes [ad]," *Winchester Republican* (VA), 13 June 1832; "Frederick White Sulphur Springs," *Alexandria Gazette*, 4 Aug. 1837; Cartmell, 297, 299.

223. "Frederick White Sulphur Springs," *Alexandria Gazette*, 4 Aug. 1837; "Frederick White Sulphur Springs [ad]," *Richmond Enquirer*, 22 May 1838; "The Watering Places," *New York Herald* (New York City), 13 July 1852; "Fire at Jordan's White Sulphur Springs," *Spirit of Jefferson* (Charlestown, WV), 22 Feb. 1876.

224. "Jordan's White Sulphur Springs [ad]," *Spirit of Jefferson* (Charles Town, VA), 3 Aug. 1852; "Jordan's Springs [ad]," *Alexandria Gazette*, 13 July 1854; "Jordan's White Sulphur Springs [ad]," *Daily Exchange* (Baltimore), 6 July 1859; "Jordan's W.S. Springs [ad]," *Ibid.*, 23 July 1860; *Spirit of Jefferson* (Charlestown, WV), 23 July 1889.

225. "The Watering Places."

226. Cohen, 72; The Watering Places"; "History: Years 1855–1861."

227. "The Watering Places."

228. Theriault, "Shannondale Springs," 2–3.

229. Theriault, 3; U.S. Dept. of the Interior, NPS, National Register of Historic Places, "Shannondale Springs."

230. "Shannondale Springs. An Act to Incorporate the Shannondale Springs Company in the County of Jefferson," *Virginia Free Press* (Charlestown, VA), 26 Apr. 1838; U.S. Census 1850 (Slave Schedule); "Cash for Negroes [ad]," *Martinsburg Gazette* (VA), 28 Oct. 1851; Theriault, 6, 12; Slave Trade Letters to William Crow, Accession #12890, Special Collections, University of Virginia Library, Charlottesville, Va., http://ead.lib.virginia.edu/vivaxtf/view?docId=uva-sc/viu03972.xml. The slave trade letters website provides a detailed scope note on Crow but no specific information on Shannondale enslaved persons.

231. Theriault, 11–12; "Shannondale Springs For Sale [ad]," *Richmond Enquirer*, 2 Mar. 1847; *Daily Dispatch* (Richmond), 4 Aug. 1855.

232. *Alexandria Gazette*, 26 Mar. 1858.

233. Theriault, 4; "Shannondale Springs For Sale [ad]"; Howe, *Historical Collections of Virginia*, illustration on unnumbered page following page 340.

234. "Shannondale Springs For Sale [ad]"; "Shannondale Springs," *Martinsburg Gazette*, 10 June 1841.

235. Howe, 343; Moorman, *Mineral Springs of the United States and Canada*, 313.

236. Theriault, 23fn27; "Shannondale Springs, in Jefferson County, Va. [ad]," *Virginia Free Press* (Charlestown, VA), 22 Aug. 1839; "National Register of Historic Places Continuation Sheet, Section number 8, Page 2."

237. Mary J. Windle, "Summer Sketches—No. 12," *Daily Republic* (Washington, D.C.), 22 Aug. 1853.

238. "An Anti-Somnambulist," *Richmond Enquirer*, 1 Dec. 1843.

239. Theriault, 7n27.

240. Calvert, "To Isabelle van Havre, Sept. 24, 1820," *Mistress of Riverdale*, 362.

241. "Frederick White Sulphur Springs," *Alexandria Gazette*, 4 Aug. 1837; "Capper Springs [ad]," *Winchester Republican*, 24 Sept. 1858; "Capper Springs [ad]," *Ibid.*, 17 Aug. 1860.

242. Bell, *Mineral and Thermal Springs*, 16; "Capper Springs [ad]," *Winchester Republican*, 17 Aug. 1860.

243. "White Sulphur Spring, Near Winchester [ad]."

244. "Hie to the Mountains: Random Thoughts and Pleasant Wanderings," *Richmond Daily Whig*, 13 June 1845.

245. "The Virginia Springs," *Alexandria Gazette*, 7 May 1856.

246. *Winchester Gazette*, 12 May 1821; Moorman, 312; Everett House, Capper Springs, Frederick County, Virginia [ad]," *Winchester Republican*, 5 Aug. 1859.

247. "Shannondale Springs," *Richmond Enquirer*, 24 Aug. 1821; Theriault, 4.
248. *Staunton Spectator*, 28 Sept. 1843; Theriault, 12; "The Presidential Tour," *American Telegraph* (Washington, D.C.), 8 Aug. 1851.
249. "Fort Mountains, Va.," *New York Herald* (New York City), 13 Oct. 1844; "White Sulphur Springs, Frederick Co., Va., Aug. 30, 1851," *Ibid.*, 8 Sept. 1851.
250. "Winchester, Sept. 6," *Richmond Enquirer*, 12 Sept. 1843; "Winchester, Va.," *New York Herald* (New York City), 18 Aug. 1844. Much more research is required to determine if political views helped to determine the choice of resort. Theriault notes that Shannondale was a "Whig enclave" for years. See Theriault, 6.
251. "Winchester, Sept. 6."
252. Resources consulted provide scant information on antebellum amusements at Capper's. A ten-pin alley was constructed in 1857 or 1858. See "Capper Springs [ad]," *Winchester Republican*, 24 Sept. 1858.
253. "Frederick Co., Va., Feb.. [sic] 10, 1840," *Alexandria Gazette and Virginia Advertiser*, 20 Mar. 1840.
254. Lewis, 203; "The Tournament at Capon," *Alexandria Gazette*, 5 Sept. 1854; "Tournament," *Daily Dispatch* (Richmond), 15 Sept. 1856; *Indiana State Sentinel* (Indianapolis), 27 Sept. 1849; "Our Watering Places: Fashion in Virginia," *New York Herald*, 8 Sept. 1851; Theriault, 9–10.
255. "Shannondale Springs," *Martinsburg Gazette* (VA), 23 May 1838; Mary J. Windle, "Summer Sketches—No. 4," *Daily Republic* (Washington, D.C.),16 July 1853; "Sulphur Spring Near Winchester (Va.), *Phenix Gazette*, Alexandria, 18 June 1831.
256. "Shannondale Springs," *Martinsburg Gazette*, 10 June 1841.
257. "Capper Springs, Frederick County, Va. [ad]," *Alexandria Gazette*, 17 July 1869; "The Season at Rock Enon," *Evening Star* (Washington, D.C.), 9 July 1878; "In the Country: A Trip to Rock Enon Springs," *National Republican* (Washington, D.C.), 7 July 1874.
258. Cohen, 104; "Michael Lohr Capper Family Tree," Familysearch, https://www.familysearch.org/tree/pedigree/landscape/K88R-BFT; "Corrections and clarifications in red ink by William Emerson Capper," 211–12, SBA.
259. "Caper Springs for Sale," *Winchester Republican*, 25 July 1828.
260. U.S. Population Census 1850; Cohen, 104; "Capper Springs," *Winchester Republican*, 17 July 1857; "Capper Springs [ad]," *Ibid.*, 7 Aug. 1857. Sources consulted do not indicate whether Marker owned or hired enslaved persons to construct the buildings or to work otherwise at Capper's.
261. "By Yesterday's Evening Mails," *Alexandria Gazette and Virginia Advertiser*, 30 July 1859.
262. U.S. Population Census 1860.
263. Theriault notes that little information is available for Shannondale during the Civil War. See Theriault, 13. No source consulted contains information on Capper's status during the war.
264. Brown, *Retreat from Gettysburg*, 365; Historic Jordan Springs, https://historicjordansprings.com/during-civil-war/; Hale, *Four Valiant Years in the Lower Shenandoah Valley*, 61.
265. Douglas, *I Rode with Stonewall*, 242. Jerry Oppenheimer provides an interesting piece of trivia: E.C. Jordan's young niece who stayed with his family during the war was Ethel Skakel Kennedy's paternal grandmother. See Jerry Oppenheimer, *The Other Mrs. Kennedy* (New York: St. Martin's Press, 1994), 4.
266. Brown, 365.
267. "The Southern Watering Places. Where Not to Go for the Summer," *New York Herald* (New York City), 27 June 1865.
268. *Ibid.*
269. "Jordan's White Sulphur Springs [ad]," *Baltimore Daily Commercial*, 11 Apr. 1866.
270. Cartmell, 207.
271. Jordan's White Sulphur Springs," *Virginia Free Press* (Charlestown, WV), 27 May 1869.
272. "Jordan's W. Sulphur Springs, Frederick Co., VA.," *Virginia Free Press* (Charlestown, WV), 10 June 1871.
273. "Fire at Jordan's White Sulphur Springs," *Spirit of Jefferson* (Charlestown, WV), 22 Feb. 1876; "Jordan's White Sulphur Springs [ad]," *Ibid.*, 8 Aug. 1876.
274. *Spirit of Jefferson* (Charlestown, WV), 23 July 1889; Cohen, 70; Bill Garrad, "Once-Gay Resort Has Grim Task of Fighting Communism," *Richmond Times-Dispatch*, 15 July 1951; "Jordan White Sulphur Springs [ad]," *Evening Star* (Washington, D.C.), 7 June 1895; *Times Dispatch* (Richmond), 19 March 1911.
275. "Sale of Jordan Alum [sic] Springs," *Times* (Richmond), 2 Mar. 1902; *Times Dispatch* (Richmond), 19 March 1911.
276. *Shepherdstown Register* (WV), 25 May 1888.
277. *Martinsburg Herald* (WV), 8 Mar. 1890.
278. *Shepherdstown Register* (WV), 25 Sept. 1902; Theriault, 15.
279. Theriault, 17–18; Bushong, *History of Jefferson County*, 3 (page reference is to the reprint edition); U.S. Dept. of the Interior, "Shannondale Springs."
280. *Shepherdstown Register* (WV), 21 Aug. 1869.
281. "Rock Enon Springs Company," *Richmond Dispatch*, 9 Dec. 1871; "Rock Enon Springs [ad]," *Evening Star* (Washington, D.C.), 25 June 1877.
282. Norris, *History of the Lower Shenandoah Counties*, 793–94; "For Sale or Rent [ad]," *National Republican* (Washington, D.C.), 22 March 1875; "Sale of Rock Enon Springs," *Evening Star* (Washington, D.C.), 23 April 1875. Pratt paid $9,750 for the grounds and building and $1,300 for the furniture.
283. "Rock Enon Springs [ad]," *Evening Star*

(Washington, D.C.), 25 June 1877; B.B., "Life at Rock Enon," *Ibid.*, 22 June 1877.

284. B.B., "Life at Rock Enon"; "The Season at Rock Enon."

285. "Jordan White Sulphur Springs [ad]," *Evening Star* (Washington, D.C.), 7 June 1895; "Rock Enon Springs, Va." *Ibid.*; *Virginia Free Press* (Charlestown, WV), 10 Aug. 1892; *Spirit of Jefferson* (Charlestown, WV), 16 July 1895.

286. "Summering at Rock Enon"; "Sale of Rock Enon Springs" *Times* (Washington, D.C.), 26 Mar. 1899.

287. *Alexandria Gazette*, 11 May 1872; "Capper Springs, Frederick Co., Va. [ad]," *Ibid.*, 17 July 1869.

288. "Editorial Excursion," *Cecil Whig* (Elkton, MD), 14 Aug. 1869.

289. *West Virginia Democrat* (Charlestown, WV), 17 Aug. 1888; "Falls Church," *Evening Star* (Washington, D.C.), 24 Sept. 1895; *Spirit of Jefferson* (Charlestown, WV), 21 Aug. 1888; *Ibid.*, 23 June 1891; *Ibid.*, 28 May 1895; *Ibid.*, 8 Aug. 1893.

290. "What I See in Washington," *Daily State Gazette* (Green Bay, WI), 20 June 1872. I researched digitized newspapers, which typically covered the more prominent citizens' travels. It is possible that others with less financial means, such as clerks, could afford travel to the resorts for a day or two.

291. "Personal," *Evening Star* (Washington, D.C.), 23 Aug. 1878.

292. *Ibid.*, 9 July 1887.

293. *Evening Star* (Washington, D.C.), 22 Aug. 1890; *Spirit of Jefferson* (Charlestown, WV), 2 Sept. 1890.

294. *Evening Star* (Washington, D.C.), 30 Aug. 1883.

295. *Shepherdstown Register* (WV), 13 July 1905.

296. *Evening Critic* (Washington, D.C.), 1 July 1884; "Life at Rock Enon," *Evening Star* (Washington, D.C.), 22 June 1877. Sousa was known at the time for a recent opera; "Stars and Stripes Forever" would not be created for another 12 years. For more information on Greatorex, the "the most famous woman American artist you've probably never heard of," see New York Public Library, Meredith Mann, "Work/Cited Episode 5: Excavating the Art and Life of Eliza Pratt Greatorex," https://www.nypl.org/blog/2021/04/26/workcited-episode-5-excavating-art-and-life-eliza-pratt-greatorex.

297. "Rock Enon Springs and Mineral Baths [ad]," *Evening Star* (Washington, D.C.), 11 May 1885.

298. "Rock Enon's Fountain of Youth," *National Republican* (Washington, D.C.), 16 Aug. 1875; "Bunker Hill Letter," *Martinsburg Independent* (WV), 13 Sept. 1884; Theriault, 15; *Shepherdstown Register* (WV), 7 July 1904; *Evening Star* (Washington, D.C.), 14 Aug. 1896).

299. *Virginia Free Press* (Charlestown, WV), 20 June 1874.

300. "Shannondale Springs Now Open [ad]," *Spirit of Jefferson* (Charlestown, WV), 23 June 1891.

301. Pepper et al, "Report of Committee on Sanitaria and on Mineral Springs," 553, 558.

302. "Rock Enon Springs and Mineral Baths [ad]," *Sun* (Baltimore), 10 June 1889; "Rock Enon Springs, Va. [ad]," *Evening Star* (Washington, D.C.), 5 July 1895.

303. Crook, *Mineral Waters of the United States and their Therapeutic Uses*, 509.

304. *Aegis & Intelligencer* (Bel Air, MD), 22 Aug. 1890.

305. *Spirit of Jefferson* (Charlestown, WV), 12 Aug. 1890.

306. *Virginia Free Press* (Charlestown, WV), 16 Sept. 1871; *Spirit of Jefferson* (Charlestown, WV), 21 July 1885; Peale, *Mineral Waters*, 541; Theriault, 18.

307. Garrad, "Once-Gay Resort"; Richmond Times-Dispatch, 8 June 1954; Historic Jordan Springs, https://historicjordansprings.com/category/history/page/2/.

308. Historic Jordan Springs, https://historicjordansprings.com/category/history/page/2/.

309. "Scout Trustees Named," *Richmond Times-Dispatch*, 27 Feb. 1944; Onofrio Castiglia, "Camp Rock Enon Celebrating Its 75th Anniversary," *Winchester Star*, updated July 19 2010, https://www.winchesterstar.com/winchester_star/camp-rock-enon-celebrating-its-75th-anniversary/article_871afb60-116a-5d2d-a31d-287b9ac7ce0f.html; Boy Scouts of America, Shenandoah Area Council, "Camp Rock Enon," https://www.sac-bsa.org/CampRockEnon.

310. WV Dept. of Natural Resources.

Bibliography

Selected Newspapers Consulted

Abbeville Banner (SC)
Abbeville Press (SC)
Abbeville Press and Banner (SC)
Abingdon Virginian
Abingdon Weekly Virginian
Advertiser and Appeal (Brunswick, GA)
Aegis & Intelligencer (Bel Air, MD)
Alabama Enquirer (Hartselle, AL)
Alabama State Sentinel (Selma)
Alamance Gleaner (Graham, NC)
Albany News (GA)
Albany Patriot (GA)
Alexandria Gazette (VA)
Alexandria Gazette and Virginia Advertiser
American Israelite (Cincinnati)
American Telegraph (Washington, DC)
Americus Times-Recorder (GA)
Anderson Daily Intelligencer (SC)
Anderson Intelligencer (Anderson Court House, SC)
Anniston Evening Star
Anniston Star
Appeal-Avalanche: Memphis
Asheville Citizen-Times
Asheville Daily Citizen
Asheville Daily Gazette
Asheville Democrat
Asheville Gazette-News
Asheville Times
Asheville Weekly Citizen
Athens Banner (GA)
Athens Daily Banner (GA)
Athens Daily Herald (GA)
Athens News Courier (AL)
Athens Post (TN)
Athens Weekly Banner (GA)
Athens Weekly Georgian
Atlanta Constitution
Atlanta Daily Herald
Atlanta Daily Intelligencer
Atlanta Daily Sun
Atlanta Georgian
Atlanta Georgian and News
Atlanta Weekly Intelligencer
Atlanta Weekly Intelligencer and Cherokee Advocate (Atlanta and Marietta)
Augusta Chronicle (GA)
Augusta Evening Dispatch (GA)
Baltimore Daily Commercial
Baltimore Sun
Bamberg Herald (SC)
Banner-Herald (Athens, GA)
Banner-Watchman (Athens, GA)
Barnesville Gazette (GA)
Beaufort News (NC)
Big Sandy News (Louisa, KY)
Big Stone Gap Post (VA)
Birmingham Age-Herald (AL)
Birmingham Iron Age
Birmingham News
Blue Ridge Blade (Morganton, NC)
Bourbon News (Millersburg, KY)
Bourbon News (Paris, KY)
Bristol Herald Courier (TN / VA)
Bristol Herald Courier (TN)
Bristol News (TN & VA)
Bristol News Bulletin (TN)
Brownlow's Knoxville Whig
Brownlow's Knoxville Whig, and Rebel Ventilator
Brunswick Advertiser (GA)
Brunswick News (GA)
Brunswick Times (GA)
Bulletin (Augusta, GA)
Burke County News (Morganton, NC)
Camden Daily Journal (SC)
Camden Journal (SC)
Camden Weekly Journal (SC)
Carolina Mountaineer (Morganton, NC)
Carolina Mountaineer and Waynesville Courier (NC)
Carolina Spartan (Spartanburg)
Cedar Rapids Evening Gazette (IA)
Cedartown Standard (GA)
Central Record (Lancaster, KY)
Charleston Courier (SC)
Charleston Daily Courier (SC)
Charleston Daily Courier (TN)
Charleston Daily News (SC)
Charleston Mercury (SC)
Charlotte Chronicle
Charlotte Democrat
Charlotte Home and Democrat
Charlotte News
Charlotte Observer
Charlotte Sunday Observer
Chatham Citizen (Pittsboro, NC)

Chattanooga Daily Chronicle
Chattanooga Daily Times
Chattanooga News
Chattanooga Sunday Times
Chattanooga Times
Chattooga News (GA)
Chronicle & Sentinel (Augusta, GA)
Cincinnati Commercial Gazette
Cincinnati Commercial Tribune
Cincinnati Post
Cincinnati Tribune
Clarion-Ledger (Jackson, MS)
Clarksville Weekly Chronicle (TN)
Cleveland Morning Leader (OH)
Cleveland Progress (GA)
Climax (Richmond, KY)
Columbia Herald (TN)
Columbus Daily Enquirer-Sun (GA)
Columbus Democrat (MS)
Columbus Enquirer (GA)
Columbus Enquirer-Sun (GA)
Columbus Times (GA)
Comet (Johnson City, TN)
Commonwealth (Greenwood, MS)
Commonwealth (Scotland Neck, NC)
Constitutional Whig (Richmond)
Corbin Times Tribune (KY)
County Record (Kingstree, SC)
Courier-Journal (Louisville)
Cullman Southern Immigrant (AL)
Cullman Times Democrat (AL)
Dahlonega Nugget
Daily American (Nashville)
Daily Avalanche (Memphis)
Daily Carolina Watchman (Salisbury, NC)
Daily Chronicle & Sentinel (Augusta)
Daily Citizen (Asheville)
Daily Columbus Enquirer (GA)
Daily Commercial Herald (Vicksburg)
Daily Confederate (Raleigh)
Daily Constitutionalist and Republic (Augusta)
Daily Dispatch (Richmond)
Daily Exchange (Baltimore)
Daily Georgian (Savannah)
Daily Leader (Lexington, KY)
Daily Memphis Avalanche
Daily Morning News (Savannah)
Daily Phoenix (Columbia, SC)
Daily Press (Newport News, VA)
Daily Press and Herald (Knoxville)
Daily Progress (Raleigh)
Daily Public Ledger (Maysville, KY)
Daily Republic (Washington, DC)
Daily Review (Wilmington, NC)
Daily Southern Chronicle (Knoxville)
Daily State Chronicle (Raleigh, NC)
Daily State Gazette (Green Bay, WI)
Daily State Sentinel (Montgomery)
Daily Times (Chattanooga)
Daily Times (Richmond)
Daily Times-Enterprise (Thomasville, GA)
Daily Tribune (Knoxville)
Daily Tribune (Winfield, KS)

Dalton Daily Citizen (GA)
Dalton Daily Citizen Times (GA)
Danbury Reporter and Post (NC)
Danville Weekly Kentucky Tribune
Dawson County Advertiser (GA)
Democrat (Huntsville, AL)
Democratic Watchtower (Talladega)
Dickson County Herald (TN)
Douglas Enterprise (GA)
Durham Daily Globe (NC)
Edgefield Advertiser (SC)
Elizabethton Star (TN)
Elkin Tribune (NC)
Erwin Magnet (TN)
Erwin Times (TN)
Erwin Weekly Magnet (TN)
Evening Bulletin (Charlotte)
Evening Bulletin (Maysville, KY)
Evening Critic (Washington, DC)
Evening Star (Washington, DC)
Evening Visitor (Raleigh)
Farmer's Friend (Morganton, NC)
Fayetteville Semi-Weekly Observer (NC)
Fayetteville Weekly Observer (NC)
Federal Union (Milledgeville)
Fisherman & Farmer (Edenton, NC)
Forest News (Jefferson, GA)
Forsyth County News (Cumming, GA)
Fort Mills Times (SC)
Fort Payne Journal (AL)
Fort Worth Star-Telegram
Frankfort Commonwealth (KY)
Frankfurt Roundabout (KY)
French Broad Hustler (Hendersonville, NC)
Gainesville Eagle (GA)
Gainesville News (GA)
Gainesville Times (GA)
Gastonia Gazette (NC)
Georgia Citizen (Macon)
Georgia Constitutionalist (Augusta)
Georgia Cracker (Gainesville)
Georgia Journal and Messenger (Macon)
Georgia Telegraph (Macon)
Georgia Weekly Telegraph and Georgia Journal & Messenger (Macon)
Goldsboro Messenger (NC)
Greeneville American (TN)
Greensboro Daily News (NC)
Greenville Enterprise (SC)
Greenville Journal (OH)
Greenville News (SC)
Hartwell Sun (GA)
Hattiesburg News (MS)
Henderson Daily Dispatch (NC)
Herald and News (Newberry, SC)
Herald and Presbyter (Cincinnati)
Herald and Tribune (Jonesborough, TN)
Hickory Democrat (NC)
Highland Messenger (Asheville),
Holmes County Republican (Millersburg, OH)
Home Journal (Perry, GA)
Home Journal (Winchester, TN)
Hornets' Nest (Charlotte, NC)

Horry Herald (Conway, SC)
Independent Monitor (Tuscaloosa)
Independent Press (Abbeville Court House, SC)
Intelligencer (Anderson, SC)
Interior Journal (Stanford, KY)
Jackson Herald (Jefferson, GA)
Janesville Gazette (WI)
Jasper Dubois County Daily Herald (Jasper, IN)
Johnson City Chronicle (TN)
Johnson City Press (TN)
Johnson City Press and Staff-News (TN)
Johnson City Press-Chronicle (TN)
Johnson City Staff (TN)
Journal and Sentinel (Winston-Salem)
Journal and Tribune (Knoxville)
Journal-Patriot (North Wilkesboro, NC)
Kentucky Advocate (Danville)
Kentucky Tribune (Danville)
Keowee Courier (Pickens Court House, SC)
Kingsport Times (TN)
Knoxville Daily Chronicle
Knoxville Daily Journal
Knoxville Daily Register
Knoxville Daily Tribune
Knoxville Journal
Knoxville Journal and Tribune
Knoxville Mercury
Knoxville News-Sentinel
Knoxville Register
Knoxville Weekly Chronicle
Knoxville Whig and Chronicle
La Grange Reporter (GA)
Lancaster Ledger (SC)
Lancaster News (SC)
Laurens Advertiser (SC)
Ledger Independent (Maysville, KY)
Lenoir Topic (NC)
Lexington Herald (KY)
Lexington Leader (KY)
Lincoln County News (Lincolnton, NC)
Lincoln Courier (Lincolnton, NC)
London Sentinel Echo (KY)
Louisville Daily Courier
Louisville Daily Journal
Louisville Journal
Louisville Morning Courier
Lynchburg Daily Virginian
Lynchburg Virginian
Macon Telegraph
Macon Telegraph and Messenger
Marion Progress (NC)
Martinsburg Gazette (VA)
Martinsburg Herald (WV)
Martinsburg Independent (WV)
Maryville Times (TN)
Maryville-Alcoa Times (TN)
Maysville Evening Bulletin (KY)
McNairy County Independent (Selmer, TN)
Memphis Commercial Appeal
Memphis Daily Appeal
Milledgeville Federal Union
Minneapolis Tribune
Mississippi Free Trader (Natchez)

Mitchell News-Journal (NC)
Montgomery Advertiser
Montgomery Daily Advertiser
Morganton Herald (NC)
Morganton Star (NC)
Morning Courier (Louisville)
Morning News (Savannah)
Morning Sun (Savannah)
Morning Times (Selma, AL)
Morning Tribune (Tampa)
Morristown Gazette (TN)
Mount Sterling Advocate (KY)
Mount Vernon Signal (KY)
Nashville Patriot
Nashville Union and American
Nashville Union and Dispatch
National Republican (Washington, DC)
National Tribune (Washington, DC)
New Albany Daily Ledger (Albany, IN)
New Orleans Crescent
New Orleans Daily Crescent
New York Herald
New York Times
Newbernian (New Bern, NC)
Newberry Herald (SC)
Newberry Herald and News (SC)
Newport Plain Talk (TN)
News and Herald (Winnsboro, SC)
News and Observer (Raleigh)
News-Herald (Hillsboro, OH)
News-Herald (Morganton, NC)
Norfolk Landmark (VA)
North Carolina Herald (Salisbury)
North Georgia Citizen (Dalton)
North Wilkesboro Hustler (NC)
North-Carolinian (Fayetteville, NC)
Observer (Raleigh)
Ocala Banner (FL)
Ocala Evening Star (FL)
Orlando Evening Star
Our Mountain Home (Talladega, AL)
Pascagoula Democrat-Star (MS)
People's Journal (Pickens, SC)
Philadelphia Inquirer
Pickens Sentinel (SC)
Pickens Sentinel (SC)
Pickens Sentinel-Journal (SC)
Polk County News (TN)
Portsmouth Daily Times (OH)
Portsmouth Times (OH)
Post (Big Stone Gap, VA)
Presbyterian of the South (Atlanta)
Press and Messenger (Knoxville)
Public Ledger (Maysville, KY)
Public Ledger (Memphis)
Raleigh Christian Advocate
Raleigh News
Raleigh Register
Raleigh Register and North-Carolina Gazette
Richmond Daily Whig
Richmond Dispatch
Richmond Enquirer
Richmond Times-Dispatch

Roanoke Daily Times (VA)
Roanoke Times
Rome Tri-Weekly Courier (GA)
Rutherford Banner (Rutherfordton, NC)
Spartan (Spartanburg)
San Antonio Light (TX)
Sandersville Herald (GA)
Sandusky Daily Commercial Register (OH)
Savannah Daily Georgian
Savannah Daily Republican
Savannah Georgian
Savannah Morning News
Scott County Herald-Virginian
Semi-Weekly Interior Journal (Stanford, KY)
Semi-Weekly Standard (Raleigh)
Semi-Weekly Times-Democrat (New Orleans)
Sentinel-Echo (London, KY)
Shepherdstown Register (WV)
South Bend Tribune
Southern Argus (Columbus, MS)
Southern Banner (Athens, GA)
Southern Confederacy (Atlanta)
Southern Enterprise (Greenville, SC)
Southern Federal Union (Milledgeville)
Southern Literary Gazette (Charleston)
Southern Press (Washington, DC)
Southern Recorder (Milledgeville)
Southern Sentinel (Columbus, GA)
Southern Watchman (Athens, GA)
Spartanburg Journal
Spirit of Jefferson (Charles Town, VA)
Spirit of Jefferson (Charlestown, WV)
Springs Herald (AL)
Spruce Pine Tri-County News (NC)
State Chronicle (Raleigh)
Statesville Daily Record (NC)
Statesville Record and Landmark (NC)
Staunton Spectator
Summerville News (GA)
Summit County Beacon (Akron)
Sumter Banner (SC)
Sunday Citizen (Asheville)
Sunday Leader (Lexington, KY)
Sunday Tribune (Minneapolis)
Sunny South (Atlanta)
Tazewell Republican (VA)
Telegraph and Messenger (Macon)
Temperance Banner (Penfield, GA)
Tennessean (Nashville)
Terre Haute Saturday Evening Mail
Thomasville Times (GA)
Times (Richmond, VA)
Times & Sentinel Tri-Weekly (Columbus, GA)
Times-Picayune (New Orleans)
Tri-Weekly Clarion (Meridian, MS)
Tri-Weekly Nashville Union
Troy Messenger (AL)
Tuscaloosa News
Tuscaloosa Weekly Times
Tuskegee Republican
Twin City Daily Sentinel (Winston-Salem)
Union Banner (Clanton, AL)
Union Springs Herald (AL)
Union Times (SC)
Vicksburg Herald
Virginia Free Press (Charlestown, VA)
Walker County Messenger (LaFayette, GA)
Washington Court House Herald (OH)
Washington Gazette (GA)
Washington Weekly Progress (NC)
Watauga Democrat (NC)
Watchman and Southron (Sumter, SC)
Waynesville Courier (NC)
Waynesville Mountaineer (NC)
Weekly Advertiser (Montgomery)
Weekly Banner-Watchman (Athens, GA)
Weekly Chronicle & Sentinel (Augusta)
Weekly Constitution (Atlanta)
Weekly Constitutionalist (Augusta)
Weekly Era (Raleigh)
Weekly Georgia Telegraph (Macon)
Weekly Mississippian (Jackson)
Weekly News and Advertiser (Albany, GA)
Weekly Public Ledger (Memphis)
Weekly Republic (Augusta, GA)
Weekly Sumter Republican (Americus, GA)
Weekly Sun (Atlanta)
Weekly Times-Recorder (Americus, GA)
Weekly Union Times (SC)
West Virginia Democrat (Charlestown, WV)
Western Democrat (Charlotte)
Western Sentinel (Winston, NC)
Wilmington Journal (NC)
Wilmington Morning Star (NC)
Winchester Republican (VA)
Winchester Virginian
Yorkville Enquirer (SC)

Archival and Special Collections

Archival and special collections institutions cited in notes and in bibliography are abbreviated as found in the parenthetical expressions below the full name of the institution.

Archives of Appalachia, East Tennessee State University, Johnson City, Tennessee (cited as ETSU)

Austin Springs Hotel Register
D.R. Beeson, Sr., Papers
Murrell Family Collection
Roan Mountain Project Collection
WSJK-TV Collection

Burke County Public Library, North Carolina Room, Burke County, North Carolina (cited as BCPL)

Connelly Mineral Springs Hotel, Connelly Springs. N.C., Season: Open May 15th—Nov. 1st, No Consumptives Taken, Wm. Jeff Davis, Owner and

President [pamphlet] [n.p.: n.d.], "Copied 1967 (Collection of Mrs. Paul Smith—Rutherford College)."

Picture Burke: Selected Historical Photographs of Burke County, https://pictureburke.bcpls.org/ North Carolina Room

Calvin M. McClung Historical Collection, Branch of the Knox County Public Library System, Knoxville, Tennessee (cited as McClung)

East Tennessee, Virginia, and Georgia Railway Company guides
"Springs—Montvale" Subject File
"Springs—Tate" Subject File
Tourism Pamphlet Collection

Exchange Place, Kingsport, Tennessee (cited as EP)

Holston Springs Hotel Register
Contract Addendum Between John Gaines and John Preston

Haywood County Public Library, Waynesville, North Carolina (cited as HCPL)

County Structures
Haywood County History Collection

Holston Conference Commission on Archives and History, Holston Conference Archives, Tennessee Wesleyan University, Athens, Tennessee (cited as HCA)

Holston Discontinued Box, "Rhea Springs Church, Rhea Springs, TN" Folder
Recommendation Orders Series

Hunter Library Special Collections, Western Carolina University, Cullowhee, North Carolina (cited as WCU)

William Williams Stringfield Collection, https:// wcu.lyrasistechnology.org/repositories/2/ resources/212

Huntsville History Collection: A Portal to Huntsville's Past, Huntsville and Madison County, Alabama (cited as HCC)

HHC (huntsvillehistorycollection.org)

Mitchell County Public Library, Bakersville, North Carolina (cited as MCPL)

How to Get There [1885]. "Cloudland Hotel" Descriptive Folder.

Pack Memorial Public Library, Asheville, North Carolina

George and Eleanor Stephens Collection
"Western North Carolina" Folder, Folder 281, Vertical Clipping File

South Caroliniana Library Digital Collections, University of South Carolina, Columbia, South Carolina (cited as USC)

Stereographic Views of South Carolina: Chibarro Stereograph Collection http://library.sc.edu/ digital/collections/stereographs.html
Special Collections and University Archives, University Libraries, Virginia Polytechnic Institute and State University, Blacksburg, Virginia (cited as VPI)
Regional History and the Appalachian South Collection
"Montgomery White Sulphur Springs Guest Book (MS2003–007)," http://digitalsc.lib.vt.edu/ Appalachia/Ms2003_007_WhiteSulphurSprings_ Ledger_1886
"Yellow Sulphur Springs Hotel Account Book (Ms1940–033)," http://digitalsc.lib.vt.edu/ Appalachia/Ms1940_033
"Yellow Sulphur Springs Hotel Account Book (Ms1940–033) Finding Aid," https://ead. lib.virginia.edu/vivaxtf/view?docId=oai/VT/ repositories_2_resources_1180.xml

Special Collections Library, James D. Hoskins Library, The University of Tennessee, Knoxville, Tennessee (cited as UTK)

MS-198, "Tate Spring Hotel Register"

Spruce Pine Public Library, Spruce Pine, North Carolina (cited as SPPL)

"Roan Mountain" Folder

Stewart Bell, Jr. Archives, Handley Regional Library and Winchester-Frederick County Historical Society, Winchester, Virginia (cited as SBA)

"Corrections and clarifications in red ink by William Emerson Capper." Special Staff of Writers.

History of Virginia. Vol. 4, *Virginia Biography*. Chicago and New York: American Historical Society, 1924.

Tennessee State Library and Archives, Nashville, Tennessee (cited as TSLA)

Tennessee State Parks Folklife Project Collection

Washington County—Jonesborough Library, Jonesborough, Tennessee

Samuel Adler untitled unpublished typescript

William Leonard Eury Appalachian Collection, Appalachian State University, Boone, North Carolina (cited as ASU)

"Roan Mountain, North Carolina" Folder

Books, Articles, Government Documents, Dissertations, Theses, and Websites

Abrams, William Hudson. "The Western North Carolina Railroad, 1855–1894." Master's thesis, Western Carolina University, 1976. https://libres.uncg.edu/ir/wcu/f/1976 AbramsWilliamHudson.pdf.

Acts of the General Assembly of the Commonwealth of Kentucky. Vol. 2. Frankfurt: J.B. Major, 1860.

Acts of the General Assembly of the State of Georgia, Passed at An Annual Session, in November and December, 1841. Milledgeville: William S. Rogers, State Printer, 1841.

Acts of the General Assembly of Virginia, Passed in 1855.6, in the Eightieth Year of the Commonwealth. Richmond: William F. Ritchie, Public Printer.

Acts of the Seventh Biennial Session of the General Assembly of Alabama Held in the City of Montgomery, Commencing the Second Monday in November, 1859. Montgomery: Shorter & Reid, State Printers, 1860.

Acts Passed at a General Assembly of the Commonwealth of Virginia. Richmond: Thomas Ritchie, 1821.

Adams, George I. "A Century of Gold Mining in Alabama." *Alabama Historical Quarterly* 1, no. 3 (Fall 1930): 271–79. Alabama Department of Archives and History. ADAH Digital Collections. https://digital.archives.alabama.gov/.

Adams, Noah. *Far Appalachia: Following the New River North*. New York: Delacorte Press, 2001.

Addington, Robert M. *History of Scott County, Virginia*. Kingsport, TN: Kingsport Press, 1932.

Adler, Samuel. Untitled unpublished typescript. Washington County—Jonesborough, Tennessee, Library.

Alderman, Pat. *All Aboard*. Erwin, TN: Y's Men's Club of Erwin, 1969.

Allen, William B. *A History of Kentucky*. Louisville: Bradley & Gilbert, 1872.

Allen, William Cicero. *Centennial of Haywood County and Its County Seat, Waynesville, N.C.* Waynesville, NC: Courier Printing Co., 1908.

Allen, William G., and Bettye J. Broyles, comp. *Rhea County History as Recorded by William G. Allen*. Spring City, TN: Rhea County Historical and Genealogical Society, 2003.

Allison, John. *Address of John Allison, on East Tennessee a Hundred Years Ago... Delivered at Seventeenth Annual Meeting Tennessee Press Association, at Cloudland (Roan Mountain, Tenn.) N.C., July 14–16, 1887* (Nashville: Hasslock & Ambrose, 1887).

"American Springs: The Mineral Springs of Georgia." *Chicago Clinic and Pure Water Journal* 19 (Aug. 1906): 265–67.

Amerson, Anne Dismukes. "Joseph Whitner Remembers Spending Summers at Porter Springs." In *I Remember Dahlonega*. Vol. 3, *Memories of Growing Up in Lumpkin County As Told to Anne Dismukes Amerson*. 2d. ed. Dahlonega: Chestatee Publications, 1993.

Amerson, Anne Dismukes. "Porter Springs Was Known as 'The Queen of the Mountains.'" In *I Remember Dahlonega*. Vol. 4, *Stories about the People and History of Lumpkin County*. Dahlonega: Chestatee Publications, 1997.

Amory, Cleveland. *The Last Resorts*. New York: Harper and Brothers, 1952. Reprint, Westport, Conn.: Greenwood Press, 1973.

Anderson, Michael. "'Cora Porter,' *Daily Home, Talladega-Sylacanga-Pell City, Ala.*, 13 Aug 1987." Reprinted in *Talladega County Historical Association newsletter* (Aug. 1989): 3. https://digital.archives.alabama.gov/digital/collection/hgpub/id/19166/rec/16.

Annual Reports of Officers, Boards and Institutions of the Commonwealth of Virginia for the Year Ending September 30, 1872. Richmond: R.F. Walker, Superintendent, Public Printing, 1872.

Appletons' Hand Book of Summer Resorts: With Principal Routes of Travel.... New York: D. Appleton & Co., 1896.

Appletons' Illustrated Hand-book of American Travel: A Full and Reliable Guide By Railway, Steamboat, and Stage.... New York: D. Appleton & Co., 1857.

Armes, Ethel. *The Story of Coal and Iron in Alabama*. Cambridge [U.S.]: University Press, Ethel Armes, 1910.

Aron, Cindy. *Working at Play: A History of Vacations in the United States*. New York: Oxford University Press, 1999.

Arthur, John Preston. *Western North Carolina: A History (1730–1913)*. Raleigh: Edwards & Broughton Printing Co.; published by Edward Buncombe Chapter of the Daughters of the American Revolution, of Asheville, N.C., 1914.

Bailey, Chester, and Carrie Bailey. "Lost Cove and

Unaka Springs." Interview by Pat Alderman, [1970s?], videocassette recording, WSJK-TV Collection. ETSU.

Bailey, Lloyd Richard, Sr., ed. *The Heritage of the Toe River Valley: Avery, Mitchell, and Yancey Counties, N.C.* Vol. 1. Marceline [Mo.]: Walsworth Publishing Co., 1994.

Bailey, Lloyd Richard, Sr., ed. *The Heritage of the Toe River Valley: Avery, Mitchell, and Yancey Counties, N.C.* Vol. 4, *Area News (1777–1949)*. Marceline [Mo.]: Walsworth Publishing Co., 2004.

Baldwin, Thomas, and J. Thomas, *A New and Complete Gazetteer of the United States.* Philadelphia: Lippincott, Grambo & Co., 1854.

Barber, John Warner, and Henry Howe. *Our Whole Country: Or the Past and Present of the United States, Historical and Descriptive.* Vol. 1. Cincinnati: George F. Tuttle and Henry M'Cauley, 1861.

Barclay, Hugh G. "Reminiscences of Rousseau's Raid." *The Confederate Veteran Talladega County Historical Association Newsletter* no. 209 (March 1990): 7. Alabama Department of Archives and History. ADAH Digital Collections. https://digital.archives.alabama.gov/digital/collection/hgpub/id/19191/rec/216.

Barrett, W.T. "Lewis County." *Twenty-Second Biennial Report of the Bureau of Agriculture, Labor and Statistics of Kentucky for 1916–1917.* Frankfurt: State Journal Co., [1918].

Bassett, John Y. "On the Climate and Diseases of Huntsville, Ala., and Its Vicinity, for the Year 1850." *Southern Medical Reports* 2 (1850): 315–23.

Bassett, John Y. "Report on the Topography, Climate and Diseases of Madison County." *Southern Medical Reports* 1 (1849): 256–81.

Batteau, Allen. *The Invention of Appalachia.* Tucson: University of Arizona Press, 1990.

Beale, Charles Currier. *Marcus T.C. Gould, Stenographer.* Reprinted from *Phonographic Magazine and National Shorthand Reporter*, Cincinnati, Ohio, 1904. [Cincinnati]: Phonographic Institute Co., 1904.

Beard, George M. *Hay-Fever; or Summer Catarrh: Its Nature and Treatment; Including the Early Form, or "Rose Cold"; The Later Form, or "Autumnal Catarrh"; and a Middle Form, or July Cold, Hitherto Undescribed; Based on Original Researches and Observations, and Containing Statistics and Details of Several Hundred Cases.* New York: Harper and Brothers, 1876.

Bell, A.N. "The Climate and Mineral Springs of North Carolina." *Transactions of the American Climatological Association for the Years 1893 and 1894.* Philadelphia: American Climatological Association, 1895.

Bell, John. *The Mineral and Thermal Springs of the United States and Canada.* Philadelphia: Parry and McMillan, 1855.

Berney, Saffold. *Hand-Book of Alabama.* 2d rev. ed. Birmingham: Roberts & Son, 1892.

Berry, Chad. "Developing Appalachia: The Impact of Limited Economic Imagination." In *Studying Appalachian Studies: Making the Path by Walking.* Edited by Chad Berry, Phillip J. Obermiller, and Shaunna L. Scott. Urbana: University of Illinois Press, 2015.

Bird, Elsie Taylor. "Tobacco in East Tennessee." Master's thesis, University of Tennessee, 1948. https://trace.tennessee.edu/utk_gradthes/2989.

Bishir, Catherine W., Michael T. Southern, and Jennifer F. Martin. *A Guide to the Historic Architecture of Western North Carolina.* The Richard Hampton Jenrette Series in Architecture and the Decorative Arts. Chapel Hill: University of North Carolina Press, 1999.

Blackley, Charles H. *Experimental Researches on the Causes and Nature of Catarrhus Æstivus (Hay-Fever or Hay-Asthma).* London: Baillière, Tindall & Cox, 1873.

Blackmun, Ora. *Western North Carolina: Its Mountains and Its People to 1880.* Boone, NC: Appalachian Consortium Press, 1977.

Blanton, Wyndham E. *Medicine in Virginia in the Nineteenth Century.* Richmond: Garrett & Massie, 1933.

Blaylock, Matthew Robert. "Appalachian Aristocrats: How Tourists, Elites, and Mountaineers Created a New Western North Carolina, 1880–1920." Ph.D. dissertation, The University of Tennessee, 2017. https://trace.tennessee.edu/cgi/viewcontent.cgi?article=6169&context=utk_graddiss.

Boyd, Charles Rufus. *Resources of South-West Virginia: Showing the Mineral Deposits of Iron, Coal, Zinc, Copper and Lead.* 3rd ed. New York: John Wiley & Sons, 1881.

Bratton, Mary J. "Fields's Observations: The Slave Narrative of a Nineteenth-Century Virginian." *The Virginia Magazine of History and Biography* 88, no. 1 (1980): 75–93. JSTOR.

Brewster, Lawrence Fay. *Summer Migrations and Resorts of South Carolina Low-Country Summer Planters.* Historical Papers of the Trinity College Historical Society. Series XXVI. Durham: Duke University Press, 1947.

Brewster, Willis. *Alabama, Her History, Resources, War Record, and Public Men: From 1540 to 1872.* Montgomery: Barrett & Brown, 1872.

Bridges, Anne, Russell Clement, and Kenneth Wise. *Terra Incognita: An Annotated Bibliography of the Great Smoky Mountains, 1544–1934.* Knoxville: University of Tennessee Press, 2013.

Brockington and Associates. *Gainesville, Georgia Community-Wide Historic Structural Survey Prepared for the City of Gainesville, Community Development Department.* Atlanta: Brockington, 2011. https://www.gainesville.org/fullpanel/uploads/files/gainesville-historic-structural-survey-final-low-res-00001.pdf.

Brockway, D.S. "Hemorrhagic Malarial Fever and Its Successful Treatment Without Quinine." *Transactions of the Medical Association of the State of Alabama, Meeting of 1912, Birmingham, April 16–19.* Montgomery: Brown Printing Co., 1912.

Brooks, Jim S. "The Iron Works on Lawson's Fork."

Piedmont Historical Society: 1–54. http://www.piedmont-historical-society.org/records/pdf/TheIronworksonLawsonsFork.pdf.

Brown, Kent Masterson. *Retreat from Gettysburg: Lee, Logistics, and the Pennsylvania Campaign*. Chapel Hill: University of North Carolina Press, 2005.

Brown, Rosalie B. "Andrew Jackson and the Greasy Cove Race Track." *Tennessee Historical Magazine* Series II, 2, no. 1 (Oct. 1931): 62–66. JSTOR.

Broyles, Bettye J., comp. *History of Rhea County*. Spring City, TN: Rhea County Historical and Genealogical Society, 1991.

Buckingham, J.S. *The Slave States of America*. Vol. 2. London: Fisher, Son, & Co., [1842].

Burden, Greg. *Blount Springs, Alabama's Fountain of Youth*. Blountsville, AL: Fifth Estate, 2014.

Burges, Samuel Edward, and Chadwick, Thomas W. "The Diary of Samuel Edward Burges, 1860–1862 (Continued)." *South Carolina Historical Magazine* 48, no. 3 (July 1947): 141–63. JSTOR.

Burke, Emily P. *Reminiscences of Georgia*. [n.p.]: James M. Fitch, 1850.

Burke, William. *The Mineral Springs of Western Virginia: With Remarks on Their Use, and the Diseases for Which They are Applicable*. New York: Wiley & Putnam, 1842.

Burkett, Elsie Staples, ed. *Historical Review: Rockwood's Centennial Year, 1868–1968*. http://cityofrockwood.com/wp-content/uploads/2019/01/Rockwood-100-1868-1968-History-1.pdf.

Burns, Inez E. *History of Blount County, Tennessee: From War Trail to Landing Strip, 1795–1955*. Nashville: Benson Printing Co., 1957.

Busey, John W., and Travis W. Busey. *Confederate Casualties at Gettysburg: A Comprehensive Record*. Jefferson, NC: McFarland, 2017.

Bushong, Millard Kessler. *History of Jefferson County, West Virginia (1719–1940)*. 1941. Reprint, Westminster, MD: Heritage Books, 2007.

Cain, Andrew W. *History of Lumpkin County for the First Hundred Years, 1832–1932*. With new index by Margaret H. Cannon, Ph.D. 1932. Reprint, Spartanburg: Reprint Co., 1978.

Caldwell, Julian. "Folklore Interview." Interview by Matthew Lane, 6 Mar. 1992. Box 1. Transcript. Roan Mountain Project Collection. ETSU.

Calhoun, John C. "Letters from John C. Calhoun to Francis W. Pickens." *The South Carolina Historical and Genealogical Magazine* 7, no. 1 (Jan. 1906): 12-19. JSTOR.

Callahan, Gertrude E. *Montvale: A Narrative of the People Who Lived in the Foothills of the Smoky Mountains*. 2d ed. n.p.: Gertrude E. Callahan, 1978.

Calvert, Rosalee Stier. *Mistress of Riverdale: The Plantation Letters of Rosalee Stier Calvert, 1795–1821*. Edited and translated by Margaret Law Callcott. Baltimore: Johns Hopkins University Press, 1991.

Campbell, John C. *The Southern Highlander and His Homeland*. New York: Russell Sage Foundation, 1921.

Campbell, T.J. *Records of Rhea: A Condensed County History*. With reprint of V.C. Allen, *Rhea and Meigs Counties (Tennessee) in the Confederate War*. 1940. Reprint, Dayton, TN: Unigraphic, 1976.

Carter County, Tennessee. "Quarterly Minutes Carter County Court (1889–1899)." Book 2. Carter County Courthouse, Elizabethton, Tennessee.

Cartmell, T.K. *Shenandoah Valley Pioneers and Their Descendants: A History of Frederick County, Virginia, From Its Formation in 1738 to 1908*. [n.p.]: T.K. Cartmell, 1909.

Caruthers, Amelia Leer. "Bean Station." *National Historic Magazine* 77 (January 1943): 31–35.

Cashin, Herschel V., Charles Alexander, and William T. Anderson. With an introduction by Major-General Joseph Wheeler. *Under Fire. With the Tenth U.S. Calvary. Being a Brief, Comprehensive Review of the Negro's Participation in the Wars of the United States*. New York: F. Tennyson Neely, 1899.

Cate, Herma R., and Martha H. Callaway, eds., and Anne M. Anderson and Sarah B. McNiell, project cochairmen. *Back Home in Blount County: An Illustrated History of Its Communities*. Maryville, TN: Blount County Historic Trust, 1986.

Chapin, George H. *Health Resorts of the South; Containing Numerous Engravings Descriptive of the Most Desirable Resorts of the Southern States*. Boston: Geo. H. Chapin, 1893.

Chitwood, W.R. "Confederate Surgeons of Wythe County, Part III," *Wythe County Historical Review* 34 (July 1988): 12–18.

Chun, Ida F. *Descriptive Illustrated Guide-Book to North Carolina Mountains. Their Principal Resorts*. New York: E.J. Hale and Son, Publishers, 1881.

Clark, Richard H. *Memoirs of Judge Richard H. Clark*. Edited by Lollie Belle Wylie. Atlanta: Franklin Printing and Publishing Co., 1898.

Clark, Thomas D. *A History of Laurel County*. London, KY: Laurel County Historical Society, 1989.

Clarke, Edward Young. *Atlanta Illustrated*. 3rd ed. Atlanta: Jas. P. Harrison & Co., 1881.

Clay-Clopton, Virginia. *A Belle of the Fifties: Memoirs of Mrs. Clay, of Alabama, Covering Social and Political Life in Washington and the South, 1853–66, Put into Narrative Form by Ada Sterling*. New York: Doubleday, Page & Co., 1905.

Cloudland Hotel On Top of Roan Mountain in East Tennessee and Western North Carolina; 6394 Feet Above Sea Level; The Highest Human Habitation East of the Rocky Mountains. [Cloudland, N.C.?], [1896?].

Cloudland Hotel On Top of Roan Mountain; In East Tennessee and Western North Carolina; 6,394 Feet Above Sea Level; The Highest Human Habitation East of the Rocky Mountains. [Cloudland, N.C.?], [1895?].

Cloudland Hotel; The Great Southern Resort for Hay Fever; 6,394 Feet Above Sea Level; Top of

Roan Mountain; Highest Habitation East of Rocky Mountains; W.E. Ragsdale, Sole Manager ([Cloudland, N.C.?], 1885?-1888?.

"Coca Cola Bottled in Talladega." *Talladega Historical Association Newsletter* (July 1991): 4. https://digital.archives.alabama.gov/digital/collection/hgpub/id/20397/rec/243.

Cohen, Stan. *Historic Springs of the Virginias*. Charleston, WV: Pictorial Histories Publishing Co., 1994.

Coleman, J. Winston, Jr. "Old Kentucky Watering Places." *The Filson Club History Quarterly* 16 (1942): 1–26.

Coleman, J. Winston, Jr. *The Springs of Kentucky: An Account of the Famed Watering-Places of the Bluegrass State, 1800–1935*. Lexington: Winburn Press, 1955.

Collins, Lewis. *Collins' Historical Sketches of Kentucky: History of Kentucky*. Vol. 2. Covington, KY: Collins & Co., 1874.

Colton, Henry E. *Mountain Scenery: The Scenery of the Mountains of Western North Carolina and Northwestern South Carolina*. Raleigh: W.L. Pomeroy; Philadelphia: Hayes & Zell, 1859.

Corbett, Theodore. *The Making of American Resorts: Saratoga Springs, Ballston Spa, Lake George*. New Brunswick: Rutgers University Press, 2001.

Cox, Joyce, and W. Eugene Cox, comps. and eds. *History of Washington County, Tennessee: A Contribution to the Bicentennial Celebration of Tennessee Statehood*. Johnson City, TN: Overmountain Press, 2001.

Crittenden, S.S. *Greenville Century Book: Comprising an Account of the Settlement of the County, and the Founding of the City of Greenville, S.C.* Greenville, SC: Press of Greenville News, 1903.

Croft, M.G. "Geology and Ground-Water Resources of Bartow County, Georgia." *U.S. Geological Survey Water-Supply Paper 1619-FF*. Washington, D.C.: U.S. Government Printing Office, 1963. https://doi.org/10.3133/wsp1619FF.

Crook, James King. "The Climatology and Health Resorts of South Carolina." *Archives of Physiological Therapy* 4, no. 2 (August 1906): 71–83. Internet Archive.

Crook, James King. *The Mineral Waters of the United States and Their Therapeutic Uses; With an Account of the Various Mineral Spring Localities, Their Advantages as Health Resorts, Means of Access, etc.; to Which is Added an Appendix on Potable Waters*. New York and Philadelphia: Lea Brothers and Co., 1899.

Cunyus, Lucy Josephine. *History of Bartow County, Georgia: Formerly Cass*. 1933. Revised reprint, Easley, SC: Southern Historical Press, 1983.

Curry, J.L.M. "Reminiscences of Talladega." *Alabama Historical Quarterly* 8, no. 4 (Winter 1946): 349–68. Alabama Department of Archives and History. ADAH Digital Collections. https://digital.archives.alabama.gov/.

Dean, Lewis S. "Alabama Gold: Golden Harvest of the Piedmont." *Alabama Heritage* 21 (Summer 1991): 20–29.

De Land, T.A., and A. Davis Smith. *Northern Alabama: Historical and Biographical*. Birmingham, AL: De Land & Smith, 1888.

Derry, Joseph T., and R.F. Wright. *Advantages of Georgia for Those Desiring Homes in a Genial Climate: 1906-7*. Prepared Under the Direction of O.B. Stevens, Bulletin of Georgia Department of Agriculture—Serial Number 43A. Atlanta: Franklin-Turner, [1907?].

Disturnell, J. *Springs, Water-Falls, Sea-Bathing Resorts, and Mountain Scenery of the United States and Canada, Giving An Analysis of the Principal Fashionable Watering Places, Mountain Resorts, &tc., with Illustrations*. New York: J. Disturnell, 1855.

Dixon, D.P. "Epidemic of Jaundice in Talladega," *Transactions of the Medical Association of the State of Alabama, Meeting of 1908, Montgomery, April 21-24*. Brown Printing Co.: 1908.

"Dr. Thomas Fearn." Huntsville History Collection: A Portal to Huntsville's Past. http://huntsvillehistorycollection.org.

Donald, J.M., Walter P. Reese, and John P. Furness. "Report on Medical Topography and Epidemics of Dallas County." *Transactions of the Medical Association of the State of Alabama, Annual Session, 1869, Held in Mobile, Ala....* Mobile: Mobile Register Office, 1869.

Dorsey, James E. *The History of Hall County, Georgia*. Vol. 1, *1818–1900*. Gainesville, GA: Magnolia Press, 1991.

Douglas, Henry Kyd. *I Rode with Stonewall*. Chapel Hill: University of North Carolina Press, 1940 and 1968.

Drayton, John. *View of South Carolina, As Respects Her Natural and Civil Concerns*. Charleston: W.P. Young, 1802.

The Dublin University Calendar for the Year 1899. Dublin: Dublin University Press; Hodges, Figgis, and Co., 1899.

Dunaway, Wilma. *The First American Frontier: Transition to Capitalism in Southern Appalachia, 1700–1860*. Chapel Hill: University of North Carolina Press, 1996.

Dunaway, Wilma. "Incorporation of Southern Appalachia into the Capitalist World Economy, 1700–1860." Ph.D. diss., The University of Tennessee, 1994.

Dunaway, Wilma. *Slavery in the American Mountain South*. Cambridge: Cambridge University Press, 2003.

Dunn, C. Frank. "Gen. Green Clay in Fayette County Records." *Register of Kentucky State Historical Society* 44, no. 147 (1946): 146–47. JSTOR.

Dyer, Frederick H. *A Compendium of the War of the Rebellion*. Vol. 3. Des Moines: Dyer Publishing Co., 1908.

Early, Jubal Anderson. *Lieutenant General Jubal Anderson Early, C.S.A.: Autobiographical Sketch and Narrative of the War Between the States*.

With notes by R.H. Early. Philadelphia: J.B. Lippincott, 1912.

East Tennessee, Virginia, and Georgia Railroad Company. *Guide to the Summer Resorts and Watering Places of East Tennessee, North Georgia, and Alabama; Including a Brief Historical Sketch and Description of Its Topography, Climate, Agricultural and Mineral Resources.* Memphis: S.C. Toof & Co., 1881.

East Tennessee, Virginia, and Georgia Railway Company. *Guide to the Summer Resorts and Watering Places of East Tennessee.* Memphis: S.C. Toof & Co., 1879.

East Tennessee, Virginia, and Georgia Railway Company. *Guide to the Summer Resorts and Watering Places of East Tennessee.* Memphis: S.C. Toof & Co., 1880.

Edgar, Walter. *South Carolina: A History.* Columbia: University of South Carolina Press, 1998.

Edmond, Helen G. Edmonds. *The Negro and Fusion Politics in North Carolina, 1894–1901.* Chapel Hill: University of North Carolina Press, 1951; copyright renewed 1979 by Helen G. Edmonds.

Eichner, David J. *The Longest Night: A Military History of the Civil War.* With a foreword by James M. McPherson. New York: Simon & Schuster, 2001.

Ellwanger, Ella Hutchinson. "Estill Springs: A Celebrated Summer Resort in Estill County, Kentucky, with Brief History of the County and Its Early Settlers." *Register of Kentucky State Historical Society* 9, no. 25 (Jan. 1911): 45–53. JSTOR.

Emmons, Louisa. *Glen Alpine Springs Hotel: A History of Burke County's Finest Accommodation.* Morganton, NC: Hollow Tree Press, 2015.

Ervin, Sam J. *Humor of a Country Lawyer.* Chapel Hill: University of North Carolina Press, 1983.

Estill Development Alliance. "Green Clay." https://www.estill.org/green-clay.html.

Fahs, C.F. "Report on Medicinal Properties of the Sulphites and Hyposulphites," *Transactions of the Medical Association of the State of Alabama, Annual Session, 1869, Held in Mobile, Ala....* Mobile: Mobile Register Office, 1869.

Fain, Cicero M., III. *Black Huntington: An Appalachian Story.* Urbana: University of Illinois Press, 2019.

FamilySearch. www.familysearch.org.

Faulkner, Charles H. "Industrial Archaeology of the 'Peavine Railroad': An Archaeological and Historical Study of an Abandoned Railroad in East Tennessee." *Tennessee Historical Quarterly* 44, no. 1 (Spring 1985): 40–58. JSTOR.

Federal Writers' Project: Slave Narrative Project. Vol. 11, North Carolina, Part 1, Adams-Hunter, 1936, Manuscript/Mixed Material, "Interview with W.L. Bost." https://www.loc.gov/item/mesn111/.

Ferguson, John Hill. *On to Atlanta: The Civil War Diaries of John Hill Ferguson, Illinois Tenth Regiment of Volunteers.* Edited by Janet Correll Ellison with assistance from Mark A. Weitz. Lincoln: University of Nebraska Press, 2001.

Fickey, Amanda, and Michael Samers. "Developing Appalachia: The Impact of Limited Economic Imagination." In *Studying Appalachian Studies: Making the Path by Walking.* Edited by Chad Berry, Phillip J. Obermiller, and Shaunna L. Scott. Urbana: University of Illinois Press, 2015.

Fink, Paul M. *Backpacking was the Only Way: A Chronicle of Camping Experiences in the Southern Appalachian Mountains.* Johnson City, TN: East Tennessee State University, Research Advisory Council, 1975.

Fishwick, Marshall. *Springlore in Virginia.* [Bowling Green, Ohio]: Popular Press, Bowling Green State University, 1978.

Fitch, William Edward. *Mineral Waters of the United States and American Spas.* Philadelphia and New York: Lea & Febiger, 1927.

Fleming, Walter Lynnwood. *Civil War and Reconstruction in Alabama.* New York: Columbia University Press, 1905.

Fletcher, Arthur L. *Ashe County: A History.* Jefferson, NC: Ashe County Research Association, Inc, 1963.

Flynn, Jean Martin. *A Short History of Chick Springs.* Travelers Rest, SC: Loftis Printing Co., 1972.

Foscue, Virginia. *Place Names in Alabama.* Tuscaloosa: University of Alabama Press, 1989.

Freemon, Frank R. "The Medical Support System for the Confederate Army of Tennessee During the Georgia Campaign, May-September 1864." *Tennessee Historical Quarterly* 52, no. 1 (Spring 1893): 44–55. JSTOR.

French, Samuel G. *Two Wars: An Autobiography of Gen. Samuel G. French.* Nashville: Confederate Veteran, 1901.

Freneau, Phillip. *Poems Written and Published During the American Revolutionary War... And Other Pieces Heretofore Not in Print.* 3d ed. Vol. 2. Philadelphia: Lydia R. Bailey, 1809.

Frost, William G. "Our Contemporary Ancestors in the Southern Mountains." *The Atlantic Monthly* 83 (Mar. 1899): 311–19.

Fulcher, Bob. "Hack Line Road: The Route to Roan." *Tennessee Conservationist* 67, no. 3 (May-June 2001): 33–36.

Fulcher, Bob. "Muir, Michaux, and Gray on Roan." *Tennessee Conservationist* 64, no. 5 (Sept.-Oct. 1998): 14–20.

Gaines, George S. *The Reminiscences of George Strother Gaines: Pioneer and Statesman of Early Alabama and Mississippi, 1805–1843.* Edited and with an introduction and notes by James P. Pate. Tuscaloosa: University of Alabama Press, 1998.

Gainesville: The Great Health Resort of the South. The Business Center of Northeast Georgia. Its Advantages and Resources. With a foreword by Gordon Sawyer. 1888. Reprint, Gainesville, GA: Georgia Mountain History Museum, Brenau University, 2004.

Galbraith and Greever. *Season of 1888: Annual Announcement of Galbraith's Springs Giving Location, Description ... with Extracts from*

Letters and References, Galbraith's Springs, Hawkins Co., Tenn. Knoxville: Tribune Job Office, [1888].

Galvin, Lynn. *An Early History of Connelly Springs, NC: From Stagecoach Tavern at Happy Home to Famous Connelly Mineral Springs Hotel.* [Morganton, NC]: Lynn Galvin, 2019.

Garibaldi, Lynda. "Happy New Year 1996!, For the News Herald, Friday, January 1, 1996." Typescript. BCPL.

Garland, Jack R. "An Economic Survey of Southwest Virginia During the Ante-Bellum Period." *Washington County Historical Society of Abingdon, Virginia* Series II, no. 24 (1957): 9–15.

Garrett, Franklin M. *Atlanta and Environs: A Chronicle of Its People and Events, 1880s-1930s.* Vol. 2. Athens: University of Georgia Press in association with the Atlanta History Center, 1969.

Gatewood, Willard B. *Aristocrats of Color: The Black Elite, 1880–1920* (Bloomington and Indianapolis: Indiana University Press, 1990.

Gayle, Sarah Haynsworth. *The Journal of Sarah Haynsworth Gayle, 1827–1835: A Substitute for Social Intercourse.* Edited by Sarah Woolfolk Wiggins with Ruth Smith Truss. Tuscaloosa: University of Alabama Press, 2013.

Genovese, Eugene D. *The Sweetness of Life: Southern Planters at Home.* Edited by Douglas Ambrose. Cambridge: Cambridge University Press, 2017.

"George Fearn." Huntsville History Collection: A Portal to Huntsville's Past. http://huntsvillehistorycollection.org.

Goff, John H. [no title]. *Georgia Mineral Newsletter* 11 (1958): 57–58. Reprinted in Utley, Francis Lee and Marion R. Humperley. *Placenames of Georgia: Essays of John H. Goff.* Athens: University of Georgia Press, 2007.

Goforth, James A. *Building the Clinchfield: A Construction History of America's Most Unusual Railroad.* Erwin, TN.: Gem Publishers, 1983.

Goodspeed's History of East Tennessee Containing Historical and Biographical Studies of Thirty East Tennessee Counties. Reprinted from *Goodspeed's History of Tennessee 1887*. Nashville: Charles and Randy Elder Booksellers, 1972.

Govan, Gilbert E., and James W. Livingood. *The Chattanooga Country, 1540–1976: From Tomahawks to TVA.* 3rd ed. Revised and updated by James W. Livingood. Knoxville: University of Tennessee Press, 1977.

Grady, Timothy P., and Andrew H. Myers, eds. *Recovering the Piedmont Past.* Vol. 2. *Bridging the Centuries in the South Carolina Upcountry, 1877–1941.* With a foreword by Melissa Walker. Columbia: University of South Carolina Press, 2019.

Grady, Timothy P., and Melissa Walker, eds. *Recovering the Piedmont Past: Unexplored Moments in Nineteenth-Century Upcountry South Carolina History.* With a foreword by Orville Vernon Burton. Columbia: University of South Carolina Press, 2013.

Grainger County, Tennessee. *Deed Book* 20. FamilySearch.org.

Grainger County Heritage Book Committee. Grainger County, Tennessee and Its People, 1796- 1998. [Grainger County, TN]: Grainger County Heritage Book Committee and Don Mills, Inc., 1998.

Grattan, Peachy R. *Reports of Cases Decided in the Supreme Court of Appeals of Virginia.* Vol. 27, from January 1, 1876 to January 1, 1877. Richmond: Clemmitt & Jones, 1877.

Graves, Mary. *Tate Springs: Home of Kingswood School.* Rutledge, TN: Bill Shirley Publishing Co., [1981?].

Grayson County, Virginia, Heritage Foundation. "A Wonderful Spring!—Thompson's Bromine Arsenic Water Springs in Ashe County, N.C." New River Notes. https://www.newrivernotes.com/ashe_ag_industry_1887_healingsprings.htm.

Green, Fletcher M. "Georgia's Forgotten Industry: Gold Mining. Part I." *Georgia Historical Quarterly* 19 (June 1935): 93–111. JSTOR.

Green, Fletcher M. "Georgia's Forgotten Industry: Gold Mining. Part II." *Georgia Historical Quarterly* 19 (Sept. 1935): 210–28. JSTOR.

Griffith, Clay. *Dr. Samuel Stringfield House, 28 Walnut Street, Waynesville, North Carolina. Waynesville Historic Preservation Committee Local Designation Report.* Asheville: Acme Preservation Services, August 2012. https://www.rowancountync.gov/DocumentCenter/View/11785/Waynesville-Dr-Samuel-Stringfield-House-Designation-Report-PDF.

Guerrant, Edward O. *The Headquarters Diary of Edward O. Guerrant.* Edited by William C. Davis and Meredith L. Swentor. Baton Rouge: Louisiana State University Press, 1999.

Gump, Lucy, comp. "Austin Springs Hotel Register: 'Residences,' Summer Seasons, 1902 & 1903." ETSU. https://archives.etsu.edu/repositories/2/accessions/2415.

Hale, Laura Virginia. *Four Valiant Years in the Lower Shenandoah Valley, 1861–1865.* Strasburg: Shenandoah Publishing House, 1968.

Hall, Chrales Gilbert, ed. Cincinnati, New Orleans & Texas Pacific Railway Company. *The Cincinnati Southern Railway: A History. A Complete and Concise History of the Events attending the Building and Operation of the Road.* Cincinnati: McDonald Press, 1902.

Hamer, Philip M., ed. "Thomas Tomlinson." *Tennessee: A History, 1673–1932.* New York: American Historical Society, 1933.

Hanes, Hiram. *The State of Alabama, United States of America: Its Mineral, Agricultural and Manufacturing Resources Embracing A Sketch of Its Early History and Progress.* Paris: Simon Raçon and C., 1867.

Harney, Will Wallace. "A Strange Land and a Peculiar People." *Lippincott's Magazine* 12 (Oct. 1873): 429–38.

Harris, David Golightly. *Piedmont Farmer: The*

Journals of David Golightly Harris, 1855–1870. Edited and With an Introduction by Philip N. Racine. Knoxville: University of Tennessee Press, 1990.

Harris, W. Stuart. *Dead Towns of Alabama.* Tuscaloosa: University of Alabama Press, 1977.

Harrison, Lowell H. "The Anti-Slavery Career of Cassius M. Clay." *The Register of the Kentucky Historical Society* 59, no. 4 (Oct. 1961): 295–317. JSTOR.

"Health Resorts of the South: White Sulphur Springs 001." HCPL. https://cdm16781.contentdm.oclc.org/digital/collection/p16781coll2/id/2307/rec/6.

Hébert, Keith Scott. "Civil War and Reconstruction Era: Cass/Bartow County, Georgia." PhD diss., Auburn University, 2007. http://hdl.handle.net/10415/1373.

Hill, James B., Jr. "History of the Development of Monte Sano." *Huntsville Historical Review* 34, no. 1 (Winter-Spring 2009): 65–83. Huntsville History Collection: A Portal to Huntsville's Past. http://huntsvillehistorycollection.org.

Hilliard, Sam Bowers. *Hog Meat and Hoe Cake: Food Supply in the Old South, 1840–1860.* With a foreword by James C. Cobb. Athens: University of Georgia Press, 1972. Reprinted, Athens: University of Georgia Press, 2014.

Historic Jordan Springs Event & Cultural Centre. https//historicjordansprings.com.

Horsman, Reginald. *Josiah Nott of Mobile: Southerner, Physician, Racial Theorist.* Baton Rouge: Louisiana State University Press, 1987.

Howe, Henry. *Historical Collections of Virginia.* Charleston, SC: Babcock & Co., 1847.

Howell, Isabel. "John Armfield of Beersheba Springs." *Tennessee Historical Quarterly* 3, no. 1 (March 1944): 46–64. JSTOR.

Hsiung, David C. *Two Worlds in the Tennessee Mountains: Exploring the Origins of Appalachian Stereotypes.* Lexington: University Press of Kentucky, 1997.

Hudson, Edmond. "Connelly's Springs." In Burke County Historical Society, *The Heritage of Burke County, 1981.* Morganton, NC: Burke County Historical Society, 1981.

Huff, Archie Vernon, Jr. *Greenville: The History of the City and County in the South Carolina Piedmont.* Columbia: University of South Carolina Press for Greenville County Historical Society, 1995.

Inscoe, John C. *Mountain Masters: Slavery and the Sectional Crisis in Western North Carolina.* With a new preface to the paperback edition. Knoxville: University of Tennessee Press, 1989.

"Intelligence from American Scientific Stations. Government Organizations. Geological Survey. Mineral Springs in Eastern Tennessee." *Science* 3, no. 63 (1884): 493–94.

Inzer, John Washington. *The Diary of a Confederate Soldier: John Washington Inzer, 1834–1928.* Edited and annotated by Mattie Lou Teague Crow. Huntsville: Strode Publishers, Inc., 1977.

"Irish Potatoes [sic] from Slips." *Western Horticulture Review: Devoted to Horticulture, Pomology, Grape Culture, Wine Manufacture, Rural Architecture, Landscape Gardening, Entomology, Meteorology, etc.* 3 (Oct. 1852): 63–64.

Irwin, Ned L. "Cone and Adler: Old World Ways and a New World Business." *Journal of East Tennessee History* no. 74 (2002): 38–57.

Jamison, J. Franklin, ed. *Annual Report of the American Historical Association for the Year 1899.* Vol. 2, *Calhoun Correspondence.* Washington, D.C.: Government Printing Office, 1900.

Jobe, Abraham. *A Mountaineer in Motion: The Memoir of Dr. Abraham Jobe, 1817–1906.* Edited by David C. Hsiung. Knoxville: University of Tennessee Press, 2009.

Johnson, Leland R. "Epidemic Cholera at Huntsville, 1873." *Huntsville Historical Review* 2, no. 1 (Jan. 1972): 20–31. Huntsville History Collection: A Portal to Huntsville's Past. http://huntsvillehistorycollection.org.

Johnston, William Henry. "The Antipyretic Treatment of Fevers." *Transactions of the Medical Association of the State of Alabama, Thirty-Third Session—1880, Huntsville, April 13th to 16th, 1880.* Montgomery: Barret & Brown, 1880.

Jolly, Clyde. "Old Rowland Springs Resort." *Etowah Valley Historical Society* 22 (1996): 3–4. http://evhsonline.org/wp-content/uploads/2017/11/Volume-22-1996.pdf.

Jones, Alex S., and Susan E. Tifft. *The Trust: The Private and Powerful Family Behind the New York Times.* Boston: Little, Brown, 1999; Boston: Back Bay Books, 2000.

Katz, F.J. *Mineral Resources of the United States 1923, Part II, Nonmetals.* Washington, D.C.: U.S. Government Printing Office, 1926.

Kennedy, A. Gilbert, ed. *A South Carolina Upcountry Saga: The Civil War Letters of Barham Bobo Foster and His Family (1860–1863).* Columbia: University of South Carolina Press, 2019.

Kentucky Geological Survey. *Report of the Progress on the Survey for the Years 1908 and 1909.* Lexington: Continental Printing Co., 1910.

Kidd, James Reginald. "The History of Salt Sulphur Springs." *West Virginia History* 15, no. 3 (Apr. 1954): 187–257.

Kiener, John B., ed. *The Kentucky Encyclopedia.* Lexington: University Press of Kentucky, 2014.

Killebrew, J.B. *Introduction to the Resources of Tennessee, First and Second Reports of the Bureau of Agriculture for the State of Tennessee.* Assisted by J.M. Safford, to whom local assistance was rendered by C.W. Charleton of East Tennessee and H.L. Bentley of West Tennessee. Nashville: Tavel, Eastman & Howell, 1874.

Killebrew, J.B. *Report of the Bureau of Agriculture, Statistics, and Mines for 1876.* Nashville: Tavel, Eastman, & Howell, 1877.

King, Edward. *The Great South: A Record of Journeys in Louisiana, Texas, The Indian Territory, Missouri, Arkansas, Mississippi, Alabama, Georgia, Florida, South Carolina, North Carolina,*

Kentucky, Tennessee, Virginia, West Virginia, and Maryland. Hartford, CT: American Publishing Co., 1875.

King, Moses, ed. *Where to Stop: A Guide to the Best Hotels in the World*. Boston: Moses King, 1894–1895.

King, Nanci. "Early Abingdon Taverns, Inns, Ordinaries and Houses of Entertainment. *Washington County Historical Society of Abingdon, Virginia*. Bulletin Series II, No. 38 (2001): 11–17.

Kivette, Everett M. "The Roan Was Always a Very Special Mountain." *Our State*, 1 May 1972: 14–16. North Carolina Department of Natural and Cultural Resources. North Carolina Digital Collections. https://digital.ncdcr.gov/Documents/Detail/state/1037500?item=1037578.

Klein, Bradley. *Discovering Donald Ross: The Architect and His Golf Courses*. Chelsea, MI: Sleeping Bear Press, 2001.

Kozsuch, Mildred, ed. *Historical Reminiscences of Carter County*. Johnson City, TN: Overmountain Press, 1985.

Kumpe, G.E., and R.T. Abernathy. "Report on Climatology and Diseases of North Ala." *Transactions of the Medical Association of the State of Alabama, Annual Session, 1869, Held in Mobile, Ala…*. Mobile: Mobile Register Office, 1869.

LaFauci, Lauren E. "Taking the (Southern) Waters: Science, Slavery, and Nationalism at the Virginia Springs." *Anthropology & Medicine* 18, no. 1 (Apr. 2011): 7–22.

Landrum, John Belton O'Neall. *History of Spartanburg County*. Atlanta: Franklin Printing & Pub. Co., 1900.

Lanier, Sidney. *Tiger-Lilies: A Novel*. With an introduction by Richard Hartwell. Chapel Hill: University of North Carolina Press, 1969.

Lanman, Charles. *Letters from the Alleghany Mountains*. New York: George P. Putnam, 1849.

Laughlin, Jennifer Bauer. *Roan Mountain: A Passage of Time*. 2d ed. Johnson City, TN: The Overmountain Press, 1999.

Leonard, Michael. *Our Heritage: A Community History of Spartanburg County, S.C.* Spartanburg: Band & White for Spartanburg *Herald and Journal*, 1986.

Lewis, Charlene M. Boyer. *Ladies and Gentlemen on Display: Planter Society at the Virginia Springs, 1790–1860*. Charlottesville: University of Virginia Press, 2001.

Lindsey, T.H. *Lindsey's Guide Book to Western North Carolina*. Asheville: Randolph-Kerr Printing Co., 1890.

Livingston, John. *Circular: American Portrait Gallery: Containing Portraits of Men Now Living: With Biographical and Historical Memoirs of Their Lives and Actions*. Vol. 3. Part 4. New York: John Livingston, 1854.

"Local News in Alabama, 1877–1879." *Alabama Historical Quarterly* 8 (Spring 1946): 48–51. Alabama Department of Archives and History. ADAH Digital Collections. https://digital.archives.alabama.gov/.

Luckett, William W. "Cumberland Gap National Park." *Tennessee Historical Quarterly* 23, no. 4 (December 1964): 303–20. JSTOR.

Luttrell, F. Alex, III. "Society Wins Award from Historic Huntsville Foundation for Work in Erecting Historical Markers." *Huntsville Historical Review* 25 (Summer-Fall 1998): 23–30. Huntsville History Collection: A Portal to Huntsville's Past. http://huntsvillehistorycollection.org.

Mabry, A.G. "Miasmatic Fevers." *Transactions of the Medical Association of the State of Alabama, Annual Session, 1869, Held in Mobile, Ala…*. Mobile: Mobile Register Office, 1869.

Mann, Ralph. "Mountains, Land, and Kin Networks: Burkes Garden, Virginia, in the 1840s and 1850s." *Journal of Southern History* 58, no. 3 (Aug. 1992): 411–34. JSTOR.

Martin, C. Brenden. *Tourism in the Mountain South: A Double-Edged Sword*. Knoxville: University of Tennessee Press, 2007.

Matson, George Charlton. "Mineral Waters." United States Department of the Interior. United States Geological Survey. *Mineral Resources of the United States, Calendar Year 1912, Pt. 2, Nonmetals*. Washington, D.C., Government Printing Office, 1913.

Matson, George Charlton. *Water Resources of the Blue Grass Region, Kentucky*. Washington: Government Printing Office, 1909.

Mattheson, A.C. "Treatment of Relapses of Malarial Fevers." *Transactions of the Medical Association of the State of Alabama, Annual Session, 1869, Held in Mobile, Ala., March 2d, 3d, and 4th, with Proceedings of the Meeting held for Reorganization, in Selma, Ala., March 3d and 4th, 1869*. Mobile: Mobile Register Office, 1869.

Mayo, Bernard. "Henry Clay, Patron and Idol of White Sulphur Springs: His Letters to James Calwell." *Virginia Magazine of History and Biography* 55, no. 4 (Oct. 1947): 301–17. JSTOR.

McCallie, S.W. *Preliminary Report of the Mineral Springs of Georgia*. Geological Survey of Georgia. Bulletin No. 20. Atlanta: Chas. P. Byrd, 1913.

McCallie, S.W. *Preliminary Report on the Mineral Resources of Georgia*, Geological Survey of Georgia. Bulletin No. 23. Atlanta: Chas. P. Byrd, 1910.

McCord, Howard F. *Baptists of Bibb County, Alabama, 1817–1974: In Two Parts*. [n.p.:] Howard F. McCord, 1979.

McDaniel, E.D. "Report Topography, Climatology and Diseases of Wilcox County." *Transactions of the Medical Association of the State of Alabama, Annual Session, 1869, Held in Mobile, Ala…*. Mobile: Mobile Register Office, 1869.

McKesson, Charles F. "William Simpson Pearson." In *Biographical History of North Carolina from Colonial Times to the Present*. Vol. 7. Edited by Samuel A'Court Ashe, Stephen B. Weeks, and Charles L. Van Noppen. Greensboro: Charles L. Van Noppen, 1908.

McKinney, Clint. "Cloudland Hotel." In *Stories 'Neath the Roan: Memories of the People of*

Yancey, Mitchell, and Avery Counties at the Foot of Roan Mountain in North Carolina. Edited by Blue Ridge Reading Team. n.p., 1993.

McKinney, Veneta, trans. "'Gold—Talladega Mountain Home,' *Vernon Courier,* Lamar County AL, June 6, 1895." *Talladega County, Alabama Genealogy Trails: Industrial News.* http://genealogytrails.com/ala/talladega/news_industrial.html.

McKinney, Veneta, trans. "*Vernon Courier,* Lamar County AL, June 15, 1888." *Talladega County, Alabama Genealogy Trails: Industrial News.* http://genealogytrails.com/ala/talladega/news_industrial.html.

McMillan, James B. "The Name of Shocco Springs." *Talladega County Historical Association Newsletter* (Nov. 1987): 12. https://digital.archives.alabama.gov/digital/collection/hgpub/id/19268/rec/182.

Means, Mrs. T. Sumter. "History of Glenn Springs from Its Discovery, With Personal Sketches of Its Habitues." In *Glenn Springs, So. Ca.: Its Location, Discovery, History, Personal Sketches of Its Habitues, What It Will Cure, etc.* Spartanburg, SC: Trimmier's Printing Office and Bookstore, 1888. http://digitalcommons.wofford.edu/localhist/3.

Medford, W. Clark. *The Early History of Haywood County.* Asheville: Miller Printing Co., 1961.

Medford, W. Clark. *The Middle History of Haywood County, with Story Supplement.* Waynesville, NC: [W. Clark Medford], 1968.

"Medical Intelligence: Notice of the Mineral Springs in the State of Georgia." *Southern Medical and Surgical Journal* 5, no. 7 (New Series, July 1849): 442–44. Georgia Regents University. Robert B. Greenblatt, M.D. Library. Historical Collections & Archives. http://augusta.openrepository.com/augusta/handle/10675.2/907.

Megginson, W.J. *African American Life in South Carolina's Upper Piedmont, 1780–1900.* Columbia: University of South Carolina Press, 2006.

Merchant, Holt. *South Carolina Fire-Eater: The Life of Laurence Massillon Keitt, 1824–1864.* Columbia: University of South Carolina Press, 2014.

Merritt, Frank. *Early History of Carter County, 1760–1861.* Knoxville: East Tennessee Historical Society, 1950.

Michaux, François André. *Travels to the Westward of the Allegany Mountains: In the States of Ohio, Kentucky, and Tennessee, in the Year 1802.* Translated from the French. London: R. Phillips, 1805.

Michel, R.F. "Haemorrhagic Malarial Fever." *Transactions of the Medical Association of the State of Alabama, Annual Session, 1869, Held in Mobile, Ala., March 2d, 3d, and 4th, with Proceedings of the Meeting held for Reorganization, in Selma, Ala., March 3d and 4th, 1869.* Mobile: Mobile Register Office, 1869.

Miller, Alan M. "David Tate (Pioneer)." In *Grainger County, Tennessee and Its People, 1796–1998.* [Grainger County, TN]: Grainger County Heritage Book Committee and Don Mills, Inc., 1998.

Miller, Andrew Jerry. "Piedmont Springs Hotel: Burke's Ante-Bellum Mineral Springs, A Historical Notebook Including Photographs." Unpublished typescript, 1986. [n.p.], BCPL. North Carolina Room.

"Mineral Resources of Georgia." *De Bow's Review and Industrial Resources, Statistics, Etc.* 24 (New Series, 4) (Jan.—June 1858): 58–61.

Mitchell, Elisha. "Notice of the Height of Mountains in North Carolina from Prof. E. Mitchell of Chapel Hill University. (Taken from the *Raleigh Register* of Nov. 3, 1835, and forwarded by Prof. M)." *American Journal of Science and Arts* 35 (Jan. 1839): 377–80.

Mitchell, Samuel Augustus. *An Accompaniment to Mitchell's Reference and Distance Map of the United States: Containing an Index of All the Counties, Districts, Townships, Towns, &c., in the Union.* Philadelphia: Mitchell and Hinman, 1835.

Mitman, Gregg. "Hay Fever Holiday: Health, Leisure, and Place in Gilded-Age America." *Bulletin of the History of Medicine* 77, no. 3 (Fall 2003): 600–35. JSTOR.

Montvale Springs... An Analysis of the Springs by Eminent Chemists, and an Account of their Medical Properties ... With an Appendix, Containing Various Certificates of their Successful Use, and References to Some Who Have Tested their Virtues. Knoxville, Tenn.: Daily Chronicle Steam Print., 1874.

Montvale Springs...An Analysis of the Springs, ... and an Account of their Medical Properties and Applicability to Particular Diseases; with an Appendix, Containing Various Certificates of their Successful Use. Atlanta: Franklin Steam Printing House, 1867.

Moore, John Trotwood, ed., and Austin P. Foster. *Tennessee: The Volunteer State, 1769–1923.* Vol. 2. Chicago and Nashville: S.J. Clarke Publishing Company, 1923.

Moore, M.A. "Efficacy of the Water of Glenn Springs, Spartanburg District, S.C., in Certain Diseases." *Charleston Medical Journal and Review* 10 (Sept. 1855): 641–649. HathiTrust.

Moorman, John J. *The Virginia Springs. With Their Analysis; And Some Remarks on Their Character.* Philadelphia: Lindsay and Blakiston, 1847.

Moorman, John Jennings. *Mineral Springs of North America; How to Reach, and How to Use Them.* Philadelphia: Lippincott's Press, 1873.

Moorman, John Jennings. *The Mineral Springs of the United States and Canada, With a Map and Plates, and General Directions for Reaching Mineral Springs.* Baltimore: Kelly and Piet, 1867.

Morgan, Joe L. "The Cloudland Hotel." "Cloudland Hotel" Descriptive Folder. MCPL.

Myer, William Edward. "The Trail System of the Southeastern United States-Colonial Period." *Forty-Second Annual Report of the Bureau of American Ethnology.* Washington, D.C.:

Smithsonian Institution, Bureau of Ethnology, 1923). Plate 15, Kentucky Historical Society Map Collection, https://www.kyhistory.com/digital/collection/Maps/id/114.

"Mystery of the Sphygmograph: Strange Pulse Likenesses—Chicago Tribune." *Current Literature: A Magazine of Record and Review* 14 (Sept.—Dec. 1893): 407.

Nicely, Maury. *Forging a New South: The Life of General John T. Wilder*. Knoxville: University of Tennessee Press, 2023.

Norfolk and Western Railroad Company. *Virginia Summer Resorts on the Norfolk and Western R.R.* Buffalo: Art-Printing Works of Matthews, Northrup & Co., 1889. Internet Archive.

Norris, J.E., ed. *History of the Lower Shenandoah Counties: Frederick, Berkeley, Jefferson and Clarke*. Chicago: A. Warner & Co., 1890.

North Carolina Department of Natural and Cultural Resources. *1898 Wilmington Race Riot Commission*. https://www.ncdcr.gov/learn/history-and-archives-education/1898-wilmington-race-riot-commission.

Nuermberger, Ruth Ketring. *The Clays of Alabama: A Planter-Lawyer-Politician Family*. Lexington: University of Kentucky Press, 1958.

N.W. Ayer & Son. *American Newspaper Annual: Containing a Catalogue of American Newspapers; A List of All Newspapers of the United States and Canada*. Philadelphia: N.W. Ayer & Son, 1882.

Oakes, Mary Paulinus, and Ignatius Sumner. *Angels of Mercy: An Eyewitness Account of Civil War and Yellow Fever by a Sister of Mercy: a Primary Source by Sister Ignatius Sumner*. Baltimore: Cathedral Foundation Press, 1998.

"Obituary of Col. Robert Coleman Poole," *Carolina Spartan* (Spartanburg), 5 Apr. 1882. Transcribed at *Piedmont Historical Society*. http://www.piedmont-historical-society.org/records/bible-poole.html.

O'Bryant, Jeff. *A Brief History of Catoosa County: Up into the Hills*. Charleston: History Press, 2009.

O'Connell, J.J. *Catholicity in the Carolinas and Georgia: Leaves of Its History*. New York: D.J. & Sadlier & Co., 1879.

Oertel, Mrs. J.A. "The Mountain Land of Western North Carolina." *The Aldine* 5, no. 3 (1872): 52–53. JSTOR.

Official Guide of the Railways. "Queen and Crescent Route, Nov. 3, 1895." Georgia's Railroad History & Heritage. www.RailGo.com.

Oswald, Felix L. "Southern Summer Resorts: First Paper." *The Southern Bivouac* 6 (July 1886): 123–28.

Owens, Dalford Dean, Jr., "Exchange Place: Development of the Commercial Frontier." Master's thesis, University of Tennessee, 1996. https://trace.tennessee.edu/utk_gradthes/1231.

Palmer, "Alabama Notes, Made in 1883–1884." *Alabama Historical Quarterly* 22, no. 4 (Winter 1960): 244–72. Alabama Department of Archives and History. ADAH Digital Collections. https://digital.archives.alabama.gov/.

Parks, Joseph Howard. *Joseph E. Brown of Georgia*. Baton Rouge: Louisiana State University Press, 1977.

Partin, Robert. "Alabama's Yellow Fever Epidemic of 1878." *Alabama Review* 10 (Jan. 1957): 31–51.

Pasquill, Robert. *The Civilian Conservation Corps in Alabama, 1933-1942: A Great and Lasting Good*. Tuscaloosa: University of Alabama Press, 2008.

Patterson, Michael Robert. "Theodore Anderson Baldwin—Brigadier General, U.S. Army." *Arlington National Cemetery*. https://www.arlingtoncemetery.net/tabaldwin.htm."BG Samuel Dickerson Rockenbach," *Military Hall of Honor*, https://militaryhallofhonor.com/honoree-record.php?id=3014.

Peale, Albert C. "Lists and Analyses of the Mineral Springs of the United States (A Preliminary Study)." *Bulletin of the U.S. Geological Survey*, no. 32. Washington, D.C.: Government Printing Office, 1886.

Peale, Albert Charles. *Mineral Waters: Abstract from "Mineral Resources of the United States, Calendar Year 1885"—Division of Mining Statistics and Technology*. Washington, D.C.: Government Printing Office, 1886.

Pepper, William, Henry I. Bowditch, A.N. Bell, Stanford E. Chaillé, and Charles Denison. "Report by Committee on Sanitaria and on Mineral Springs." *Transactions of the American Medical Association* 31 (1880): 537–65.

Perkins, Yvonne Spencer, abs. "Morgan Deed Book 'A' (Part Thirteen)." *Valley Leaves: Tennessee Valley Genealogical Society, Inc.* 14 (June 1980): 43–45. Alabama Dept. of Archives & History. https://digital.archives.alabama.gov/digital/collection/hgpub/id/26100.

Pfifer, Edward W. "Champagne at Brindletown: The Story of the Burke County Gold Rush, 1829–1833." *North Carolina Historical Review* 40, no. 4 (Oct. 1963): 489–500. JSTOR.

Pfifer, Edward W. "Saga of a Burke County Family: Conclusion: The Sons." *North Carolina Historical Review* 39, no. 3 (July 1962): 305–339. JSTOR.

Phifer, Edward W. "Certain Aspects of Medical Practice in Ante-Bellum Burke County," *North Carolina Historical Review* 36, no. 1 (Jan. 1959): 28–46. JSTOR.

Phifer, Edward W. "Slavery in Microcosm: Burke County, North Carolina." *Journal of Southern History* 28, no. 2 (May 1962): 137–65. JSTOR.

Phifer, Edward W., Jr. *Burke County: A Brief History*. Raleigh: North Carolina Division of Archives and History, 1979.

Pine, Allison. "Uncovering Trahlyta: Examining Textual Manifestations of Dahlonega's Cherokee Indian Princess." Master's thesis, Georgia State University, 2016. https://scholarworks.gsu.edu/english_theses/211/.

Pioneers' Society of Atlanta. *Pioneer Citizens' History of Atlanta (1832-1902)*. Atlanta: Pioneers' Society of Atlanta, 1902.

Pippen, Sherman. Interview by Thomas Swindell, Roan Mountain, Tennessee, 9 March [1976?]. Audiocassette recording. Collection of Judy Murray, Stewardship Director Emerita, The Southern Appalachian Highlands Conservancy, Kingsport, Tennessee.

Pollard, Edward A. *The Virginia Tourist: Sketches of the Springs and Mountains of Virginia....* Philadelphia: J.R. Lippincott & Co., 1870.

Posey, John F. "Report upon the Topography and Epidemic Diseases of the State of Georgia." *Transactions of the American Medical Association* 10 (1857): 127–148. American Medical Association Archives. https://ama.nmtvault.com.

Powell, R.F. *Season of 1889: Hales's Springs; You Meet Only the Best in the South; the Place for Families; Read What Guests Say.* Knoxville: n.p., [1889?].

Powell, Richard. "Landreth Inducted into Bandmaster's Hall of Fame." *Talladega County Historical Association Newsletter*, no. 196 (Feb. 1989): 12. https://digital.archives.alabama.gov/digital/collection/hgpub/id/19986/rec/66.

Pratt, Joseph Hyde, and Miss H.M. Berry. *The Mining Industry in North Carolina During 1913–17, Inclusive, Economic Paper No. 49.* Raleigh: Edwards & Broughton Printing Co., 1919.

Presbrey, Frank. *The Empire of the South: Its Resources, Industries, and Resorts.* Washington, D.C.: Southern Railway Co., 1898.

Price, Richard Nye. *Holston Methodism: From Its Origin to the Present Time.* Vol. 5, *From the Year 1870–1897.* With an introduction by Bishop R.G. Waterhouse. Nashville: Publishing House of the Methodist Episcopal Church, South, 1913.

Prolix, Peregrine. [Philip Houlbrooke Nicklin]. *Letters Descriptive of the Virginia Springs; The Roads Leading Thereto, and the Doings Thereat.* Philadelphia: H.S. Tanner, 1835.

Public Laws of the State of North Carolina, Passed by the General Assembly, at its Session of 1858-'9: Together With the Comptroller's Statement of Public Revenue and Expenditure. Raleigh: Holden and Wilson, 1859.

Public Laws of the State of North Carolina, Passed by the General Assembly at its Session, 1869–1870: Together With the Comptroller's Statement of Public Revenue and Expenditure. Raleigh: Jo. W. Holden, 1870.

Purcell, Aaron D. "'A Damned Piece of Rascality.' The Business of Slave Trading in Southern Appalachia." *Journal of East Tennessee History* 78 (2006): 1–22.

Purdon, John E. "Correspondence: Psychical Science Congress during Columbian Exposition." *Virginia Medical Monthly* 19 (Apr. 1892—Mar. 1893): 1049–52.

Quarles, Garland. *Occupied Winchester: 1861–1865.* Winchester, VA: Prepared for Farmers & Merchants National Bank, 1976.

Racine, Philip N. *Seeing Spartanburg: A History in Images.* Spartanburg: Hub City Writers Project and Philip N. Racine, 1999.

Ragan, O.G. *History of Lewis County, Kentucky.* Cincinnati: Press of Jennings and Graham, 1912.

Reniers, Perceval. *The Springs of Virginia: Life, Love, and Death at the Waters, 1775–1900.* Chapel Hill: University of North Carolina Press, 1941.

Rennick, Robert M. *Kentucky Place Names.* Lexington: University Press of Kentucky, 1984.

Riley, Benjamin Franklin. *Alabama As It Is: Or, The Immigrant's and Capitalist's Guide Book to Alabama.* 3rd ed. Montgomery: Brown Printing Co., 1893.

Roan Mountain Inn, Roan Mountain, Tenn.: We Challenge the World for Healthful Climate, S.B. Wood, M.D., Owner and Proprietor, "Roan Mountain, North Carolina" Folder. ASU.

"Robert Fearn (1795)." Huntsville History Collection: A Portal to Huntsville's Past. http://huntsvillehistorycollection.org.

Roberts, Frances C. "The Romance and Realism of Monte Sano." *Historic Huntsville Quarterly* 6, no. 4, article 2 (Summer 1980): 3–11. https://louis.uah.edu/historic-huntsville-quarterly/vol6/iss4/2.

Robins, Alee. "Illustrating Appalachia: The Sketchbooks and Publications of David Hunter Strother, 1833 to 1887." Master's thesis, West Virginia University, 2015. https://researchrepository.wvu.edu/cgi/viewcontent.cgi?article=7556&context=etd.

Rousseau, Peter L. "Jacksonian Monetary Policy, Specie Flows, and the Panic of 1837." *Journal of Economic History*, 62 (June 2002): 457–88. JSTOR.

Royse, Isaac Henry Clay. *History of the Story of the 115th Regiment Illinois Volunteer Infantry.* [Terre Haute]: Isaac Henry Clay Royse, With Authority of the Regimental Association Terre Haute, 1900. https://libsysdigi.library.illinois.edu/oca/Books2009-04/historyof115thre00roys/historyof115thre00roys.pdf.

Ruscin, Terry. *A History of Transportation in Western North Carolina: Trails, Roads, Rails and Air.* With a Foreword by Robert Morgan. Charleston: History Press, 2016.

Russel, William T. "Glenn's Springs." *Second Annual Report of the State Board of Health of South Carolina, for the Fiscal Year Ending October 31, 1881.* Charleston: Walker, Evans & Cogswell, 1881.

Russo, Dan. "The Hack Line Road—Then and Now." *Friends of Roan Mountain* 4 (Fall 2000). https://www.friendsofroanmtn.org/_files/ugd/3cc564_e6f4e0d5a17f446aa4c61dbb5f4ab5ce.pdf.

Russo, Dan, Jennifer Laughlin, Florence Greer Street, Judy Murray, and Rosalee Russo. Interview by Bob Fulcher, June 9, 2000, Carter County, Tennessee. Transcript. Tennessee State Parks Folklife Project collection. TSLA.

S. "Correspondence: Roan Mountain—A Summer Resort [Letter to the Editor]." *Garden and Forest* 5 (July 13, 1892): 333–34.

Safford, James M. *Geology of Tennessee* Nashville: S.C. Mercer, 1869.

The Saratoga of the Confederate States: Catoosa Springs, Catoosa County, Georgia, Harman & Nichols, Proprietors ([n.p.]: [1861]). Internet Archive.

Savitt, Todd Lee. *Medicine and Slavery: The Diseases and Health Care of Blacks in Antebellum Virginia*. Urbana and Chicago: University of Illinois Press, 1978.

Sawyer, Gordon. *Northeast Georgia: A History*. Charleston: Arcadia Publishing, 2001.

Schaller, Frank. *Soldiering for Glory: The Civil War Letters of Colonel Frank Schaller, Twenty-Second Mississippi Infantry*. Edited by Mary W. Schaller and Martin N. Schaller. Columbia: University of South Carolina Press, 2007.

Scheppegrell, William. "Hay-Fever Resorts in the United States and Canada." *Journal of the American Medical Association* 71, no. 7 (Aug. 17, 1918): 523–24.

Schroeder-Lein, Glenna R. *Confederate Hospitals on the Move: Samuel H. Stout and the Army of Tennessee*. Columbia: University of South Carolina Press, 1994.

Scott, A.E. "A Visit to Mitchell and Roan Mountains [read June 11, 1884]." *Appalachia: Journal of the Appalachian Mountain Club* 4 (1884): 12–20.

Sears, John F. *Sacred Places: American Tourist Attractions in the Nineteenth Century*. Amherst: University of Massachusetts Press, 1989.

Season of 1875, Warm Springs, Bath County, Virginia, In New Hands and Greatly Improved. Richmond: Gary's Steam Printing Establishment, 1875.

Sellers, Mamie, trans. "1852 and 1859 Alabama Tax Assessment Records, Montgomery County, Rives Beat Real Estate." *Pintlala Historical Association Newsletter* 4 (Oct. 1990): 7–11. https://digital.archives.alabama.gov/digital/collection/hgpub/id/2454/rec/16.

Shapiro, Henry D. *Appalachia on Our Mind: The Southern Mountains and Mountaineers in the American Consciousness 1870–1920*. Chapel Hill: University of North Carolina Press, 1978.

Shocco Springs Conference Center: Who We Are." www.shocco.org/who-we-are/.

Silver, Timothy. *Mount Mitchell and the Black Mountains: An Environmental History of the Highest Peaks in Eastern America*. Chapel Hill: University of North Carolina Press, 2003.

Smith, Eugene Allen. Geological Survey of Alabama. *Statistics of the Mineral Production of Alabama for 1915*. Bulletin, no. 19. Compiled from *The Mineral Resources of the United States*. Montgomery: University, Alabama, 1917.

Smith, Eugene Allen. Prepared in co-operation with the U.S. Geological Survey. *Underground Water Resources of Alabama*. Montgomery: Brown Printing Co., 1907.

Smith, George Gilman. *The Story of Georgia and the Georgia People, 1732–1860*. Macon: George G. Smith, 1900.

Snowden, Yates, ed. In collaboration with H.G. Cutler, and an Editorial Advisory Board Including Special Contributors. *History of South Carolina*. Vol. 4. Chicago: Lewis Publishing Co., 1920.

Snyder, Kristin M. *Tennessee Army National Guard: Integrated Natural Resources Management Plan: Volunteer Training Site—Catoosa*. Updated and revised by Laura P. Lecher. Nashville: Tennessee Military Dept., 2012. www.tn.gov/content/dam/tn/workforce/documents/ENV_inrmp_catoosa_2012_full.pdf.

Somers, Dale A. "War and Play: The Civil War in New Orleans." *The Mississippi Quarterly* 26, no. 1 (Winter 1972–73): 3–28. JSTOR.

South Carolina Appalachian Council of Governments. *A Survey of Historic Places in the South Carolina Appalachian Region*. rev. ed. Greenville: South Carolina Appalachian Council of Governments' Office, [between 1972 and 1976].

South Carolina Department of Archives and History. National Registry Properties in South Carolina. Glenn Springs Historic District, Spartanburg County (Glenn Springs). http://www.nationalregister.sc.gov/spartanburg/S10817742033/index.htm.

Sprague, Stuart Seely. "Alabama and the Appalachian Iron and Coal Town Boom, 1889–1893." *Alabama Historical Quarterly* 37, no. 2 (Summer 1975): 85–91. Alabama Department of Archives and History. ADAH Digital Collections. https://digital.archives.alabama.gov/.

Starnes, Richard D. *Creating the Land of the Sky: Tourism and Society in Western North Carolina*. Tuscaloosa: University of Alabama Press, 2009.

Starnes, Richard D. "Forever Faithful: The Southern Historical Society and Confederate Historical Memory," *Southern Culture* 2, no. 2 (Winter 1996): 177–94. JSTOR.

Starnes, Richard D. "'The Stirring Strains of Dixie': The Civil War and Southern Identity in Haywood County, North Carolina." *North Carolina Historical Review* 74 (July 1997): 237–59. JSTOR.

Statistics of South Carolina: Including a View of Its Natural, Civil, and Military History, General and Particular. Charleston: Hurlbut and Lloyd, 1826.

Stephenson, Martha. "Old Graham Springs: At Harrodsburg, Kentucky, Once the Most Fashionable Summer Resort in the State—Now Only a Memory of the Past." *Register of Kentucky State Historical Society* 12, no. 34 (Jan. 1914): 25, 27–35. JSTOR.

Sterling, Robin, comp. and ed. *Newspaper Clippings from the Cullman, Alabama, Democrat: 1901–1913*. [n.p.]: Robin Sterling, 2017.

Stevenson, George J. *Increase in Excellence: A History of Emory and Henry College*. New York: Appleton-Century-Crofts, 1963.

Stockdale, J.L. "The Early Days of the Medical Proffession [sic] in Talladega County." *Alabama Historical Quarterly* 8, no. 4 (Winter 1946): 407–09. Alabama Department of Archives and History. ADAH Digital Collections. https://digital.archives.alabama.gov/.

Stoll, Steven. *Ramp Hollow: The Ordeal of Appalachia*. New York: Hill and Wang, 2017.

Strayhorn, Zora Shay. "Mentone Alabama: A History." (Mentone Area Preservation Association, Inc., 2021). http://mentonealabama.org/Strayhorn/StrayhornPostCivilWar.htm.

Sullivan County Historical Commission and Associates, and Muriel C. Spoden, comp. *Historic Sites of Sullivan County*. Kingsport, TN: Kingsport Press, 1976.

Sulzby, James F., Jr. *Historic Alabama Hotels and Resorts*. Tuscaloosa: University of Alabama Press, 1960.

Summers, Lewis Preston. *History of Southwest Virginia, 1746–1786, Washington County, 1777–1870*. Richmond: J.L. Hill Printing Co., 1903.

Summers, L.P. "In the Heart of the Holston Country: Holly Bottom alias Halls Bottom." *Washington County Historical Society of Abingdon, Virginia, Bulletin* 9 (Apr. 1943): 126–32.

Switzer, William F. *Report on the Internal Commerce of the United States, Pt. 2 of Commerce and Navigation, The Commercial, Industrial, Transportation, and Other Interests of the Southern States*. Washington, D.C., Government Printing Office, 1886.

Talley, William M. "Salt Lick Creek and Its Salt Works." *The Register of the Kentucky Historical Society* 64, no. 2 (Apr. 1966): 85–109. JSTOR.

Talley, William M., and Paula Franke. *Lewis County*. Charleston: Arcadia Publishing, 2005.

Tate Epsom Spring…Containing Location, Analysis of the Water, Means of Access, Accommodations, Diseases for Which the Water is Highly Recommended….Knoxville: Chronicle Co., Steam Book and Job Printers and Binders, 1879.

Tate Epsom Spring…Containing Location, Analysis of the Water, Means of Access, Accommodations, Diseases for Which the Water is Highly Recommended….Knoxville: Chronicle Co., Steam Book and Job Printers and Binders, 1882.

Tate Epsom Spring…Containing Location, Analysis of the Water, Means of Access, Accommodations, Diseases for Which the Water is Highly Recommended….Knoxville: Chronicle Co., Steam Book and Job Printers and Binders, 1883.

Tate Spring; The Carlsbad of America; A Health and Pleasure Resort…Where Heat, Dust, Mosquitoes, Malaria and Hay Fever are Unknown…. n.p.: S.G. Newman, [mid-1890s?].

Taylor, Thomas Jones. "Early History of Madison County And, Incidentally of North Alabama," *Alabama Historical Quarterly* 1, no. 2 (Summer 1930): 149–68. Alabama Department of Archives and History. ADAH Digital Collections. https://digital.archives.alabama.gov/.

Tennessee. State Board of Health. *First Report of the State Board of Health of the State of Tennessee; April, 1877 to October, 1880*. Nashville: Tavel and Howell, Printer to the State, 1880.

Tennessee. State Supreme Court Cases. Research and Collections. "Jacob Adler v. C. Austin." TSLA. https://supreme-court-cases.tennsos.org/.

Theriault, William D. "Shannondale Springs." *West Virginia History* 57 (1998): 1–26. JSTOR.

Thorne, Charles B. "Watering Spas of Middle Tennessee." *Tennessee Historical Quarterly* 29, no. 4 (Winter 1970–71): 321–59. JSTOR.

Thorp, Daniel B. "The Beginnings of African American Education in Montgomery County. " *Virginia Magazine of History and Biography* 121, no. 4 (2013): 314–45. JSTOR.

"A Tribute to the Grand Old Lady—The Mentone Springs Hotel (1884–2014)." *The Groundhog* 34 (Apr. 2014). https://www.mapamentone.com/uploads/1/0/9/8/109889080/apr2014-groundhog.pdf.

Tuomey, M. *First Biennial Report on the Geology of Alabama*. Tuskaloosa: M.D.J. Slade, 1850.

Unicoi County, Tennessee. "Report of the Commissioners in the Partition of the Unaka Springs Property." *Deed Record*. Vol. 5. Unicoi County Courthouse, Erwin, Tennessee.

Unicoi County, Tennessee. "Trustee's Deed from Howard Akers to C.B. Rumbley." *Warranty Deed Book* 65. Unicoi County Courthouse, Erwin, Tennessee.

Unicoi County, Tennessee. "Warranty Deed from Dr. Aura Barrowman to Mrs. Stella Hopson." *Deed Book* 74. Unicoi County Courthouse, Erwin, Tennessee.

Unicoi County, Tennessee. "Warranty Deed from Stella Hopson to Rex Lewis." *Deed Book* 80. Unicoi County Courthouse, Erwin, Tennessee.

Unicoi County Heritage Book Committee. *Unicoi County, Tennessee and Its People, 1875–1995*. Waynesville, N.C.: Don Mills, Inc.; [Unicoi County, TN.].: Unicoi County Heritage Book Committee, 1995.

United States Census Bureau. *Population of the United States in 1860: Alabama*. https://www2.census.gov/library/publications/decennial/1860/population/1860a-04.pdf.

United States Department of Agriculture. "Census of Agriculture Historical Archive, 1860." https://agcensus.library.cornell.edu/wp-content/uploads/1860b-05.pdf.

United States Department of Agriculture. *Monthly Report of the Department of Agriculture for March 1868*. Washington, D.C.: Government Printing Office, 1868.

United States Department of Agriculture. Natural Resources Conservation Service. *Soil Survey of Estill and Lee Counties, Kentucky*. (n.p.: 2007). https://www.nrcs.usda.gov/Internet/FSE_MANUSCRIPTS/kentucky/KY616/0/Estill_Lee_KY.pdf.

United States Department of the Interior. National Park Service. "Yellow Sulphur Springs: Historic American Landscape Survey: Written Historical and Descriptive Data." HALS VA-55. https://tile.loc.gov/storage-services/master/pnp/habshaer/va/va2200/va2213/data/va2213data.pdf.

United States Department of the Interior. National Park Service. National Register of Historic Places. Inventory—Nomination Form. "Yellow

Sulphur Springs." Virginia Department of Historic Resources. Interactive Database of the Virginia Landmarks Register & National Register of Historic Places. https://www.dhr.virginia.gov/wp-content/uploads/2018/04/060-0013_Yellow_Sulphur_Springs_1979_Final_Nomination.pdf.

United States Department of the Interior. National Park Service. National Register of Historic Places Inventory-Nomination Form. "Glenn Springs Historic District." South Carolina Department of Archives and History. National Registry Properties in South Carolina. Glenn Springs Historic District, Spartanburg County (Glenn Springs). http://www.nationalregister.sc.gov/spartanburg/S10817742033/S10817742033.pdf.

United States Department of the Interior. National Park Service. National Register of Historic Places Inventory-Nomination Form. "Thompson's Bromine and Arsenic Springs, 7. Description." North Carolina State Preservation Office. North Carolina Listings in the National Register of Historic Places. https://files.nc.gov/ncdcr/nr/AH0020.pdf.

United States Department of the Interior. National Park Service. National Register of Historic Places Inventory—Nomination Form. "The Mentone Springs Hotel. 7. Description." https://npgallery.nps.gov/NRHP/AssetDetail?assetID=096467a7-d161-417a-a214-affbb377170a.

United States Department of the Interior. National Park Service. National Register of Historic Places Inventory—Nomination Form. "The Preston Farm: Gaines-Preston Farm (or plantation) and 'Exchange Place.' Section 8. Significance." https://npgallery.nps.gov/GetAsset/8cb0b7dc-7dd0-406e-a58f-255d1feda993/.

United States Department of the Interior. National Park Service. National Register of Historic Places Registration Form. "Shannondale Springs. Section number 7, Page 2." West Virginia Department of Arts, Culture and History. Shannondale-springs.pdf (wvculture.org).

United States Department of the Interior. United States Geological Survey. Geographic Board on Geographic Names. *Domestic Names.* https://edits.nationalmap.gov/apps/gaz-domestic/public/search/names.

United States Forest Service. Daniel Boone National Forest. "Overview / Background: Ghost Resorts Along the Rockcastle." https://www.fs.usda.gov/generalinfo/dbnf/recreation/picnickinginfo/generalinfo/?groupid=74870&recid=39600.

United States War Department. Secretary of War. Brevet Lieutenant Colonel Robert N. Scott. *The War of the Rebellion: A Compilation of the Official Records of the Union and Confederate Armies.* Series 1. Vol. 5. Washington, D.C.: Government Printing Office, 1881.

University of Maryland, Baltimore. UMB Digital Archive. [M.T.C. Gould]. *Esculapia: or the White Sulphur and Chalybeate Springs, of Lewis County, KY.* Cincinnati: Ben Franklin Printing House, 1846. http://hdl.handle.net/10713/3377.

Vandiver, Wellington. "Pioneer Talladega, Its Minutes and Memories." *Alabama Historical Quarterly* 16, no. 2 (Summer 1954): 163–297, plus five unnumbered pages in appendix [entire issue]. Alabama Department of Archives and History. ADAH Digital Collections. https://digital.archives.alabama.gov/.

Van Noppen, John J., and Ina Woestemeyer Van Noppen. With an Introduction by Cratis Williams. *Western North Carolina Since the Civil War.* Boone: Appalachian State University, 1973. JSTOR.

Van West, Caroll. *Tennessee's Historic Landscapes: A Traveler's Guide.* Knoxville: University of Tennessee Press, 1995.

Vincent, George E. "A Retarded Frontier." *American Journal of Sociology* 4 (July 1898): 1–21.

Virginia Museum of Fine Arts, "Yellow Sulphur Springs, Montgomery Co., Va. (Primary Title), Album of Virginia (Series Title)," https://www.vmfa.museum/piction/6027262-8052041/.

Walton, Col. Thomas George. *Sketches of the Pioneers in Burke County History: Being Reminiscences and Sketches, prepared by the late Colonel T.G. Walton for the old Morganton Herald. A Rich Fund of Historical Incidents Connected with the Early Settlers of Western North Carolina....* Easley, SC: Southern Historical Press [nd].

Walton, George E. *The Mineral Springs of the United States And Canada: With Analyses And Notes On the Prominent Spas of Europe And a List of Sea-side Resorts.* New York: D. Appleton, 1874.

Warmuth, Donna Akers. *Washington County.* Charleston, SC: Arcadia Publishing, 2006.

Warner, Charles Dudley. *On Horseback: A Tour in Virginia, North Carolina, and Tennessee With Notes of Travel in Mexico and California.* Boston: Houghton, Mifflin and Company, 1888.

Washington County, Tennessee. "Riverside Park." Plat Book 1. Washington County Courthouse, Jonesborough, Tennessee.

Washington County, Tennessee. Washington County Deed Book 46. Washington County Courthouse, Jonesborough, Tennessee.

Washington County, Tennessee. Washington County Deed Book 53. Washington County Courthouse, Jonesborough, Tennessee.

Washington County, Tennessee. Washington County Deed Book 201. Washington County Courthouse, Jonesborough, Tennessee.

Watauga Association of Genealogists. Upper East Tennessee, comp., prepared by the Book Committee. *History of Washington County.* [Johnson City, TN]: The Association, 1988.

Webb, Robert Dickens. "The Livingston Artesian Well Water." *Transactions of the Medical Association of the State of Alabama, The State Board of Health, Anniston, April 13–16, 1886.* Montgomery: W.D. Brown & Co., 1886.

Weiss, Harry B., and Howard R. Kemble. *The Great American Water-Cure Craze: A History of Hydropathy in the United States.* Trenton, NJ: Past Times Press, 1967.

West Virginia. Department of Natural Resources. District 2 Wildlife Management Areas. "27. Shannondale Springs." https://wvdnr.gov/lands-waters/wildlife-management-areas/district-2-wildlife-management-areas/.

Western and Atlantic Railroad. *W & A: Marietta, The Gem City of Georgia*. Buffalo: Matthews, Northrup & Co., 1885. https://archive.org/details/mariettagemcity00west.

White, George. *Historical Collections of Georgia: Containing the Most Interesting Facts, Traditions, Biographical Sketches, Anecdotes, etc.* New York: Pudney & Russell, 1855.

Willard, H. Eugene. *Morganton and Burke County*. Charleston, SC: Arcadia Publishing, 2001.

Williams, Charlie. "André Michaux, a Biographical Sketch." *Castanea, Occasional Papers in Eastern Botany: No. 2, Proceedings of the André Michaux International Symposium* (December 2004): 16–21. JSTOR.

Williams, David. "Georgia's Forgotten Miners: African-Americans and the Georgia Gold Rush." *Georgia Historical Quarterly* 75, no. 1 (Spring 1991): 76–89. JSTOR.

Williams, John Alexander. *Appalachia: A History*. Chapel Hill: University of North Carolina Press, 2002.

Williams, Samuel C. "Early Iron Works in the Tennessee Country." *Tennessee Historical Quarterly* 6, no. 1 (March 1947): 39–46. JSTOR.

Williams, Samuel C. *Early Travels in the Tennessee Country, 1540–1800, With Introductions, Annotations, and Index.* Johnson City, TN.: Watauga Press, 1928.

Williams, Samuel C. *General John T. Wilder: Commander of the Lightning Brigade*. Bloomington: Indiana University Press, 1936.

Williamson, Samuel H. "Seven Ways to Compute the Relative Value of a U.S. Dollar Amount, 1790 to present." MeasuringWorth, 2024.www.measuringworth.com/uscompare/.

Wilson, Charles Reagan. *Baptized in Blood: The Religion of the Lost Cause, 1865–1920.* Athens: University of Georgia Press, 2009.

Wilson, Kathleen Curtis. "From Enslavement to Entrepreneurship in Appalachian Virginia." *Virginia Magazine of History and Biography* 129, no. 2 (2021): 156–92. JSTOR.

Works Projects Administration for the State of Tennessee. Tennessee Writers' Project. *Tennessee: A Guide to the State*. American Guide Series. New York: Viking Press, 1939.

Wright, G. Richard, and Kenneth H. Wheeler. "New Men in the Old South: Joseph E. Brown and his Associates in Georgia's Etowah Valley." *Georgia Historical Quarterly* 93, no. 4 (Winter 2009): 363–87. JSTOR.

Wright, Nathalia. "Montvale Springs under the Proprietorship of Sterling Lanier, 1857–1863." *The East Tennessee Historical Society's Publications* no. 19 (1947): 48–63.

Writers' Program of the Work Projects Administration in the State of South Carolina. *A History of Spartanburg County*. Compiled by the Spartanburg Unit of the Writers' Program, *American Guide Series* (Illustrated). Sponsored by The Spartanburg Branch American Association of University Women South Carolina. [Spartanburg]: Band & White, 1940.

Writers' Program of the Work Projects Administration in the State of South Carolina. *Palmetto Place Names*. Columbia: South Carolina Education Association, 1941. Reprint, Spartanburg: Reprint Co., 1975.

Wyman, Thomas S. "Tennessee Places: The British Misadventure in Embreeville." *Tennessee Historical Quarterly* 54, no. 2 (Summer 1995): 98–111. JSTOR.

Young, Jan. *The Studebaker History Corner*. (n.p.: Jan B. Young, 2009).

Young, Otis, Jr. "The Southern Gold Rush, 1828–1836." *Journal of Southern History* 48 (Aug. 1982): 373–92. JSTOR.

Ziegler, Wilbur G., and Ben S. Grosscup. *The Heart of the Alleghanies or Western North Carolina....* Raleigh: Alfred Williams & Co.; Cleveland: William W. Williams, 1883.

Index

Abernethy, B.B. 105
Abingdon, VA 4, 124, 191, 192, 194, 195
abolition 27, 31, 68, 124
Adler, Jacob 147, 150
Adler, Samuel 152
Adler Springs 148
Air Line Railroad, GA 36, 45, 48, 51, 57; *see also* Atlanta and Richmond Air-Line Railway, GA
Alabama: map **8**; physiography 7–9; *see also* visitors, southern
Alabama Baptist Convention 18, 29
Alabama Great Southern Railroad 16, 18
Alabama Mineral Line (railroad) 28
Alabama White Sulphur Springs 8, 11, 15, 16, 18, 19
Album of Virginia 198, 200, **207**
Alford, C.A. 110
Alford & Sloan 110
Alleghany Springs, TN 144
Alleghany Springs, VA 190, 197–202, **203, 204, 205**, 206, 209
Allegheny Mountains, VA 210
All-Healing Springs, NC *see* Healing Springs, Ashe County, NC
Allison, Judge John 150, 159
Ambler Springs, SC 119–120
American Hay Fever Association 115
American Medical Association 34, 101, 170, 217; *see also Journal of the American Medical Association*
American Railroad Times 153
Amicalola Falls State Park, GA 53
amusements 12, 17, 18, 22, 26, 28, 29, 30, 39, 45, 46, 47, 48, 51, 52, 56, 61–62, 70, 72, 73, 76, 77, 82, 87, 98, 100, 103, 109, 110, 119, 120, 121, 126, 127, 129, 135–136, 139, 149, 150, 151, 155, 159, 160, 165, 171, 174, 180, 202, 213, 214, 215, 239*n*18
Anderson, SC 118, 119, 131
Anderson, W.G. 137–138
Ansel, Governor Martin F. 129
Appalachian Mountain Club, Boston 157
Appalachian National Scenic Trail (AT) 53, 146, 162
Appalachian Regional Commission (ARC) 1, 2, 3
Appletons' guidebooks 12, 66, 102
Armfield, J. John 143–144
Asbury, Francis 153
Ashe County, NC 86, 88, 90–91
Asheville, NC 84–86, 98, 99, 102, 105, 106, 109–111, 120, 130, 156, 159, 160
Asheville and Spartanburg Railroad 86
"Ashley's Bromine and Arsenic Water" 90
Astor, John Jacob 159
Athens, GA 35, 48
Athens, TN 144, 164, 169, 171
Atlanta 35, 39, 43, 46–51, 62–64, 125, 131, 148
Atlanta and Charlotte Air Line Railway 117–118, 119, 131
Atlanta and Richmond Air-Line Railway, GA, 35, 48; *see also* Air Line Railroad, GA
Atlanta and Richmond Air Line Railroad, SC 140; *see also* Piedmont Air Line Railroad, SC
Atlanta Health Institute 175
Atlanta National Bank 47
Atlantic Coast Line Railroad 102
Augusta, GA 48
Augusta Springs, VA 187
Austell, Alfred 47
Austin, Clisbe (Clisby, Clysby), Sr. 5, 146–150
Austin, Clisbe, Jr. 147, 150
Austin, F.H. (Frederick H.) 147, 149, 150
Austin, H.C. (Henry Clay) 150
Austin House, Johnson City, TN 148, 149
Austin's Liver Regulator 149
Austin's (Austin) Springs, TN 145, 146, 147–151, **152**, 153
Avery County, NC 86, 94
Avoca Spring, TN 145
Aycock, Governor Charles Brantley 110
Ayers, Attorney General of Virginia Rufus 190, 195–196
Ayers, W.S. 155

Babb, Daniel 214
Bailey, Thomas B. 195
Bailey Springs, AL 26
Baker, Eugene 215
Baker, Colonel Harry H. 215
Bakersville, NC 156, 159
Bald Road, NC 156, 160
Baldwin, General Theodore A. 42–43
balls (dancing) 13, 22, 29, 39, 41, 45, 47, 48, 50, 53, 55, 61, 63, 70, 72, 76, 82, 98, 100, 103, 109, 110, 121, 123, 128, 129, 130, 132, 134, 137, 139, 151, 165, 171, 174, 202, 213; resort as dance hall 182
Ballston 136
Balsam Gap, Jackson County, NC 86
Balsam Inn, Jackson County, NC 86
Baltimore & Ohio Railroad 187
Bandler, Arthur S. 92
Banks, Richard 50
Banner House, NC 150
Barker, Eli 88
Barker, Willie 88
Barnes, Sidney M. 76–77
Barnett, Georgia Secretary of State Nathan C. 57
Barrowman, Aura 182
Barton, Captain E. 97
Bartow, Colonel Francis 59

Index

Bartow County, GA, physiography 59
Bassett, John Y. 9, 10
Bath Alum, VA 5
Bath County, KY 68
Bath County, VA 187–188
Battey, T.W. 38
Battey, W.H. 38, 40
Battle, J.F. 105
Beach, Charles 72, 73
Bean Station, TN 4
Beard, George M. 158–159
Beaufort, SC 124
Beauregard, General P.G.T. 5, 190, 201, 202, 204, 209
Bedford Springs, PA 213, 216
Bee Rock, KY 78, 79, 83
Beersheba Springs, TN 143–144
Behan, William J. 204
Bell, B.W. 26
Bell, John 12, 13
Bell County, KY 66
Bell Tavern, VA 30
Berkeley Springs (Bath), VA (WV) 187, 210, 213, 214, 217
Bethesda Healing Springs, NC *see* Healing Springs, Ashe County, NC
Bethesda Springs, GA *see* Porter Springs, GA
Beyer, Edward 198, 200, **207**
Big Tunnel, VA 198, 200
Biltmore 86, 159
Birks, James 166
Birmingham, AL 7, 13, 14, 19
The Birth of a Nation 92
Blackburn, U.S. Senator Joseph Clay Stiles 77
Blackley, Charles H. 158
Blacks, as enslaved persons *see* slave trade; slave work outside resorts; slaves at resorts
Blacks, as freemen during antebellum period: mine workers 54; release from jail, 128; resort workers, 188
Blacks, post–Civil War resort ownership 190, 206–208; resort waiter strikes 5, 110; resort workers 87, 160; *see also* Jim Crow era; Washington, Booker T.
Blacksburg, VA 197, 202
Bladon Springs, AL 14
Blairsville, GA 55
Blake, Benson 204
Blake, Captain R.H. 98
Blink Bonnie, Haywood White Sulphur Springs, NC 111
Blood Mountain, GA 53–54, 58
Bloomingdale Pike *see* Wilderness Road

Blount County, AL, topography 11
Blount County, TN 143, 162, 164
Blount Springs, AL 12–14, **15**, 47
Blue Lick Springs, KY 80
Blue Ridge Mineral Springs, SC 119
Blue Ridge Mountains, GA 33, 35–36, 43, 44, 53, 54, 58; North Carolina 87; South Carolina 117; Virginia 184, 196, 210
Blue Ridge Railroad 118–119, 148
Blue Sulphur Springs, VA (WV) 184, 187, 189
Boat Yard (Historic Boat Yard District) *see* Kingsport, TN
Bon Aqua, TN 150
Bonner, Robert, Jr. 166
Boone, Daniel 66, 69, 74, 147, 172, 191
Boone Dam (TVA) 146
botanists 145, 153, 156, 157
bottled water 6, 11, 14, 28, 29, 42, 64, 89–90, 92, 93, 101, 104, 106, 120, 122–124, 129–130, 139, 151, 171–172, 175, 197, 199, 202, 217
Boyd, Jesse R. 132
Bradley, Governor William 82
Breck, Daniel 76
Breckinridge, John C. 76
Brewster, William J. 31
Brindle Creek, NC 95
Bristol, TN/VA 90, 145, 147, 152, 198
Bromine Arsenic Healing Spring, NC *see* Healing Springs, Ashe County, NC
Brooks, Albert F. 206
Brooks, Congressman Preston S. 137
Brown, Governor Joseph 63, 176
Brown Mountain, NC 95
Brownlow, Mrs. W.G. 176
Brownlow, William G. "Parson" 164, 166
Brownlow family 159
Bryan, William Jennings 77, 168, 191
Buchanan, James 59, 187
Buckingham, James Silk 84, 126
Buffalo Lithia Springs, VA 90, 101, 104
Buladean, NC 154, 156; *see also* Wilder's Forge, NC
Bull, J.A. 129–130, 132, 133
Bull's Gap, TN 148–149

Bullock, Governor Rufus B. 41
Buncombe County, NC 107, 111, 126
Buncombe Turnpike 84
Burbank Road, TN 155, 162
Burges, Samuel 135
Burke County, NC 84, 86, 87, 95; physiography 94
Burke, Thomas 94
Burke, William 184
Burnside, Anderson & Company 81
Bursey, J. 127
Burwell, William H. 206
Butler, General and U.S. Senator Matthew (M.C.) 101, 202

Caesars Head, SC 120, 158
Caldwell, Frank (Franklin) 16
Caldwell, John H. 150
Calf Pen Road *see* Roan Road
Calhoun, A.W. 52
Calhoun, John C. 54, 119, 124, 186–187, 213
Calhoun, Mrs. John C. 136
Calhoun, Congressman William B. 213
Camp, William C. 135
Camp Croft Military Center, SC 124
Camp Rock Enon, Shenandoah Area Council, BSA 218
Campbell, F.J. (Francis Josephus) 81, 82
Campbell, Secretary of the Treasury George W. 187
Campbell, J. 79
Campbell, John C. 1
Campbell, Josephus 78, 79–80
Canby, William 156
Candler, Allen D. 45
Cantrell, Fielding 121
Capon Springs, VA (WV) 187, 188, 210, 213
Capper, John 213
Capper's Springs, VA *see* Rock Enon, VA
Carolina, Clinchfield & Ohio Railway 131, 145, 156, 178; *see also* CSX Corporation
Carson, C.C. 79
Carter, George L. 179
Carter, R.G. (Robert G.) 70
Carter County, TN 86, 142, 145, 146, 153, 162
Carter's Depot, TN 149
Carter's Springs, Lewis County, KY *see* Esculapia Springs, KY
Cartersville, GA 55, 59, 60, 62
Carver's Gap, TN 153, 162
Cass, Lewis 59
Cass County 59–60

Index

Castle Heights Military Academy 152
Catawba County, NC 87, 94
Catawba Nation 211; *see also* Native Americans
Catawba Trail 172
Catoosa County, GA, physiography 33, 37
Catoosa Springs, GA 3, 35–41, *42*, 43, 47, 148, 169
Cedar Creek Springs, KY 66
Cedar Mountain, GA 53, 54–55, 57
Cedar Mountain Springs, GA *see* Porter Springs, GA
Chandler, James 25–26
Chandler Springs, AL 11, 25–29
Chapman, C. Brewster 130, 132
Charleston 117, 120, 125–128, 137, 191
Charleston, Cincinnati & Chicago Railroad 178
Charleston Medical Journal and Review 136
Chattahoochee National Forest 53
Chattanooga 19, 37, 39, 40, 48, 59, 62, 154, 168, 171, 176
Chattanooga Daily Times 176
Chero-Cola 28
Cherokee County, SC 59, 121
Cherokee Lake, TN 173
Cherokee Springs, GA 35, 37, 38, 40
Cherokee Springs, SC 121–122
Cherokee Springs Hotel Company, SC 121
Cherokee Nation 111, 119, 147; ball games 109; discovery, use of springs 37, 46, 55, 102, 168, 191; removal from Georgia lands 53, 54, 59; road construction 112, 163; *see also* 1830 Indian Removal Act; Native Americans
Chesapeake & Ohio Canal 187
Chesapeake & Ohio (C&O) Railroad 72
Chick, Burrell (Burwell) 126
Chick, Pettus W. 126–127, 129
Chick, Reuben S. 126–127, 129
Chick Springs, SC 111, 118, 120, 121, 122, 123, 124–132, *133*
Chick Springs Company 129, 130
Chick Springs Historical Society 133
Chick Springs Military Academy 132
Chick Springs Water Company 132–133
Chiles, Henry 75
Chiles, John 75
Chiles, William 75, 76

Chilhowee Mountain, TN 162
Chilhowee Springs, TN 169
Chocco Springs, AL *see* Shocco Springs, AL
Choice, William 128
cholera *see* epidemics
Christiansburg, VA 188, 196, 197, 198, 206
Chunn, Lancelot 29–30
Chunn, William Ridgely 30
churches 46, 52, 62, 81, 121, 127, 169, 180, 215
Cincinnati 71, 73, 82
Cincinnati Southern Railway 19, 171
Civilian Conservation Corps (CCC) 29, 83, 119, 181
Civil War 11, 20, 27, 31, 35, 37, 44, 51, 63, 64, 67, 79, 80–81, 97, 99, 102, 121, 124–125, 128–129, 137, 165, 170, 173, 189, 195, 201, 214; Atlanta Campaign 40, 202; Battle of Antietam 40; Battle of Chickamauga 40, 154; Battle of Port Royal Sound 124; resorts as war hospitals, training grounds, or military headquarters 10–11, 40, 76, 165, 189, 195, 201, 214; Second Battle of Winchester 214; *see also* "Lost Cause"
The Clansman 92
Clark, Judge Richard H. 61
Clark (Clark's) Springs, TN 145, 151
Clarksville Road, GA 46, 47
Clay, Brutus 66, 68, 75
Clay, Cassius M. 74
Clay, C.C., Jr. (Clement Claiborne) 9, 20
Clay, C.C., Sr. (Clement Comer) 12, 20
Clay, Green 66, 68, 74–75
Clay, Henry 66, 68, 74, 75, 76, 186
Clemson, Thomas 119
Clemson University, SC 119
Clinch, Duncan L. 62
Clinch River 172, 191
Clinton, Bill 88
Cloudland Hotel 6, 98, 114, 146, 153–160, *161*, 162, 170, 178
Coca-Cola Bottling Company 19
The Coca-Cola Company *see* Pemberton Chemical Company
Cohen, Stan 184
Cohutta Springs, GA 5, 34, 35
Coleman, Alvin L. 206
Coleman, J. Winston, Jr. 66
Coleman-Bush Investment Company 77

Colhoun (Calhoun), C.A. (Charles Alexander) 199, 201–203
Collins, C.L. 93
Colorado State Board of Health 92
Colton, Henry E. 96
Columbia 130, 131, 137
Columbia Hotel 138
Cone, Herman 147
Connelly, Elizabeth 102
Connelly, Emma 103
Connelly, Horace W. 105
Connelly Springs, NC 84, 86, 94, 102–106
Connelly Springs Company 104, 105
Conrad, Secretary of War Charles Magill 213
consumption *see* tuberculosis
conventions, meetings hosted at resorts 110, 111, 123, 131–132, 141, 159, 202, 215
Cook's Springs, AL 11
Cooper, Thomas F. 166
Coosa River, AL 24–25, 29
Corryton, TN 174
Cotton Belt Route 180
Country Kitchen *see* Austin's (Austin) Springs, TN
courtship and flirting 22, 61–62, 76, 108, 128, 139, 165, 185–186, 213; single young ladies 120
Covington, KY 73
Cowan, John T. 201–202
Cox, J.W. 151
Coyner's Springs, VA 188
Crab Orchard Springs, KY 13
Cranberry, NC 86, 99, 150, 154, 156
Cranberry Forge, NC 96
Crawford, Governor George W. 39
Crawford, William H. 213
Creek Nation 25, 28; *see also* Native Americans
Crites, Irene Margaret 99
Crites, Solomon Vance 99
Crittenden, General George B. 82
Crittenden, U.S. Senator John C. 76, 187
Crockett, James C. 206
Crockett Springs, VA 197
Croft State Park, SC 124
Crook, James K. 45, 66, 119, 217
Crow, William 212
Crumpacker, Charles A. 208
Crumpler, NC 88, 90
CSX Corporation 178, 183; *see also* Carolina, Clinchfield & Ohio Railway
Cumberland Gap 4, 80, 172, 190

Index

Cumberland Gap and Louisville Railroad 174
Cumberland National Forest *see* Daniel Boone National Forest
Cumberland Plateau 7, 11, 16, 66, 78, 142, 143, 145, 168, 171
Cumberland River, KY 78
Cumming, Mrs. Montgomery 47

Dahlonega, GA 33, 53, 54, 57
Dalton, GA 35, 37, 41, 147
Daniel Boone National Forest 83
Darrow, Clarence 168
Daughters of the Confederacy 110
David, George 59
Davis, Eunice 106
Davis, Jeff (William Jefferson) 106
Davis, Jefferson 13, 202
Davis, Congressman Thomas B. 216
Davis, Varina 204, 209
Davis, William 195
Dayton, TN 168
Deaderick, Arthur V. 178–179, 182
Deaderick, Henry (Mac) 178–179, 182
Deaderick, Mary Adeline Walker 178
Deaderick family 151, 180, 182
De Bow's Review 5, 33–34, 36
Decatur, AL 13, 31
DeKalb County, AL topology 16
Dickson, Dr. and Mrs. Robert L. 91
disfranchisement amendment, NC 110
Dixie Highway (U.S. Highway 25E) 174
Dixon, U.S. Senator Archibald 71
Dixon, Thomas, Jr. 92
Dobbins, M.G. 63, 64
Dodge, Louise Frances 112–113
Donahoo, Robert and Rebecca 64–65
Donelson, General Daniel Smith 165
Dougan & Sheftall 124
Doyle Springs, TN 144
Drayton, Governor John 122
Drennen, Walter Melville 14
Dropped Stitches in Tennessee History 150
drover roads 4, 128, 172
Duffee, Mary Gordon 13
Duffee, Matthew 12–13
Dugan, E.A. 124

Duke, Benjamin 101
Dunaway, Wilma 3
Duvall (Duval), Rezin 211
Duval's or Duvall's (White) Sulphur Spring *see* Jordan's White Sulphur Springs, VA

Eagle, Governor James Phillip 77
Eagles Nest, NC 84, 86, 111–112, *113*, *114*, 115, 116
Early, General Jubal 5, 190, 202, 204; quote on domestic slavery as improvement for Blacks 209–210
Easley, William King 128
Easley's Springs, TN 47, 145
East Tennessee and Georgia Railroad 147, 164
East Tennessee and Virginia Railroad 147, 174, 198
East Tennessee and Western North Carolina Railroad 86, 150, 154, 156
East Tennessee, Virginia and Georgia Railroad 145, 149, 156
East Tennessee, Virginia and Georgia Railway 89; *see also* East Tennessee, Virginia and Georgia Railroad
Eastern Coal Fields, KY 66, 67, 68, 73
Eastman, George 177
Edmundson, James P. 209
Eggleston Springs, VA *see* New River White Sulphur Springs, VA
1849 Union Rail Road Convention, SC 137
1830 Indian Removal Act 25–26, 37; *see also* Cherokee Nation
1835 Treaty of New Echota 37, 168; *see also* Cherokee Nation
electrical therapy (electrotherapy) 63, 175
"Electro Therapeutic Baths" 175
Elizabethton, TN 146, 153
Elk Park, NC 86, 150
Eller, E.E. 92
Emory University School of Medicine 52
Engel, J.C. (Jesse) 166
epidemics: cholera 5, 10, 14, 20, 66, 71, 148–149, 164, 173; resort as refugee from unspecified epidemics 80, 82, 125; smallpox 201; typhoid fever 19, 166; yellow fever 5, 14, 21, 49, 106, 117, 125, 145, 150, 166, 171; *see also* malaria, malarial-type fevers

Ervin, Senator Samuel J., Jr. 93–94
Erwin, TN 107, 145, 146, 178, 180, 181
Esculapia Mineral Spring Company 70
Esculapia Mountain, KY 69
Esculapia Springs, KY 66, 67, 68, 69–73, *74*, *75*, 76
Esculapia Springs (Hotel) Company 72
Estes (Estis), James C. (E.) 95–98
Estill Springs, KY 66, 67, 68, 73–77, *78*
Etowah River, GA 59, 60, 62
Eureka Springs, AR 88–89
European waters, compared to 38, 90, 101, 104, 108, 175
Everett, T.C. 81
Exchange Hotel, Montgomery, AL 163
Exchange Place, Sullivan County, TN 193

Facing South 92
Fagg, George W. 202
Fagg, J.J. 203
Fain, Thomas 194
Fairfax, Ferdinando 212
Farr, W.R.B 129
Farrow, H.P. (Henry Pattillo) 55–56, 59
Fauquier White Sulphur Springs, VA 187, 188, 189, 213
Faw, W.W. 151
Fayette County, KY 79
Fearn, George 20
Fearn, Robert 20
Fearn, Thomas 20
ferry transportation to resorts 80, 152, 171, 187
fevers of unknown origin 10, 35
Fickey, Amanda 3
Fidelity Bankers Trust 173
Fillmore, Millard 187, 213
fire-eater pro-secessionists 3, 124, 128, 137, 201
Firestone, Harvey 159
First Brooklyn Light and Water Cure Institute, NY 175
Fitch, William Edward 14, 19, 104, 106, 108, 170, 184
Flintstone Springs, MD 2
Flournoy, Congressman T.S. 201
Floyd, Governor John B. 194
Ford, Henry 159
Forrest, Armistead (Armstead) W. 198, 209
Fort Payne, AL 15–16, 18
Fort Wayne, Muncie & Cincinnati Railroad 13
Foulkes, Thomas H. 209

Index

Foute, Daniel D. 163, 164
Fowler, W.D. 138
Fox, John, Jr. 2
Fraser, John 153
Frederick White Sulphur Springs *see* Jordan's White Sulphur Springs, VA
French, General Samuel G. 202
Freneau, Phillip 122
Frick, Henry Clay 160
Froehling, Henry 92
Frost, William G. 3

Gaines, George Strother 9
Gaines, John Strother 193–195
Gaines, Samuel M. 193
Gainesville, GA 5, 35, 36, 43–53, 56, 57
Gainesville Hotel, GA 51
Galbraith's Springs, TN 144–145, 173
Gamble, Andrew 166
Gardner, Charles B. 209
Garland, U.S. Attorney General Augustus Hill 216, 217
Garrett Springs, SC 121, 122–123
Garth, Horace 24
Gayle, Governor John 12
Gayle, Sarah Haynsworth 12
Georgia: map 34; physiography 33; *see also* visitors, southern
Georgia Development Company 52
Georgia State Board of Health 46
German Colonization Society 118
Getzendanner, H.C. 215
Giers, Ernst 32
Giers, Jean Joseph 31–32
Giles County, VA 197
Gilmour, Henry S. 201
ginger ales 123, 125, 132, 139
Glade Springs, VA 86, 88, 89, 189
Glen Alpine Springs, NC 84, 86, 87, 94, 99–102
Glen Alpine Springs Company, NC 99
Glen Ayre, NC 116
Glen Ayre Road *see* Roan Road
Glen Springs, KY 5, 66, 68, 69–73
Glen Springs College 73
Glenn, John B. 134
Glenn Springs, SC 90, 120, 121, 122, 124, 133–139, **140**, 141
Glenn Springs Company 134
Glenn Springs Female Institute, SC 135
Globe Hotel, Augusta, GA 41
Gluck, S.G. 173
gold rush Alabama 25; Georgia 25, 37, 47, 53–54, 59; North Carolina 94
Goode, D.P. (David Parham) and Charity Louisiana Connelly 103
Gordon Springs, GA 35
Gore, Al 88
Gorman & Calnan 138
Gouge, John 160
Gouge, John and Mary 161
Gould, Jay 102
Gould, M.T.C. (Marcus Tullius Cicero) 66–67, 68, 70–71
Gower, E.N. (Ebenezer Norton) 44–45, 51
Gower's Spring, GA 35, 36, 44–46
Grady, Henry W. 36
Graham, C.C. (Christopher Columbus) 79–81
Graham, Montrose 79–81
Graham Springs, KY 66, 79, 80
Grainger County, TN, physiography 172–173
Grant, Marguerite G. 102
Grant, Simpson 70
Grant, Ulysses S. 70, 202
Gray, Asa 153, 156
Great Depression 14, 18, 19, 29, 53, 133, 162, 177, 180, 181, 182, 197, 208
Great Flood of 1916 99
Great North Mountain, VA 210, 213
Great Smoky Mountains 113, 125, 144, 145, 162, 163, 167
Great Smoky Mountains National Park 87, 162
Great Valley of Virginia 187, 190, 210, 213
Great Warriors Path (Great Indian Warpath) 74, 172, 187, 191
Greatorex, Eliza Pratt 216
Greenbrier White Sulphur Springs *see* White Sulphur Springs, VA (WV)
Greene, A.A. 29
Greene, Judge Grafton 159
Greeneville, TN 84, 150
Greenville County, SC 117, 120, 125–126, 132
Greenville, SC 117, 118, 120, 126–132
Greenville Coach Factory 44
Griffin's Springs, SC *see* Ambler Springs, SC
Griffith, D.W. 92
Grimes, J.C. 93
Guerrant, John 197–198
Gump, H.D. 151
Guy, NY Supreme Court Chief Justice Charles J. 92
Guyandotte, VA (Huntington, WV) 4, 187
Guyot, Arnold 165

Hack Line Road, TN 155–156, 157, 160, 162
Hackett, Congressman Thomas C. 62
Hagan, Patrick 191, 194
Hagan Springs, Dungannon, VA 191
Hagood, Colonel Benjamin 120
Hale's Red and White Sulphur Springs, TN 144–145, 150, 173
Hall County, GA, physiography 43
Hanna, Colonel A.B. (Alexander) 18
Hamrick, John 73
Hamrick, Will 73
Hanging Rock Spring, Lancaster County, SC 127
Hanna (Mineral) Springs, AL *see* Alabama White Sulphur Springs
Happoldt, John Michael 96
Harman, J.J. 40
Harmony Family Center, TN 146, 167
Harney, Will Wallace 58
Harper, S.C. 93
Harper, Chancellor William 136
Harpers Ferry 187, 210
Harris, J.T. 123, 124
Harris, James M. 55
Harris, John H. 12
Harris Lithia Springs, Laurens County, SC 123
Harrison, Benjamin 71
Harrodsburg, KY 79, 80
Hart, Thomas 68
Harvey House, Spartanburg, SC 138
Hawkins County, TN 144, 146, 147, 148, 173, 194
hay fever 36, 82, 98, 114–116, 120, 157–158; *see also* mountain air
Hay-Fever; or, Summer Catarrh 158
Hay Fever Prevention Association 116
Hayne, U.S. Senator Robert Y. 164
Haywood County, NC 87, 107, 112; topology 106
Haywood White Sulphur Springs, NC 5, 84, 86, 87, 106–111, **115**, **116**
Healing Springs, Ashe County, NC 84, 86, 87, 88–91
Healing Springs, VA 189, 209

Henderson County, NC 86
Henderson Springs, TN 167
Hendersonville, NC 114, 125, 126, 131, 133
Henery, John T. 127
Hewitt, W.C. 41
Hickman, H.H. 38, 41
Highlands, NC 86
Hill, Napoleon 204
Hilliard, Sam Bowers 4
Historic Jordan Springs 217–218
Historic Springs of the Virginias 184
Hogan, Ben 174
Holland, Ed and Kate B. 49
Holland, E.W. (Edmund Weyman) 46–47, 49
Holloway, J.H. 77
Holston Conference, Methodist Episcopal Church 148
Holston River 144, 146, 172, 173, 191
Holston Springs, VA 4, 189, 190–195, **196**; 268n69
Holt, Captain Ridgway (Ridgeway) 202
Holt, Colhoun & Co. 199
Holzendorf, P.B. (Preston Brooks) 45, 46
Homestead *see* Hot Springs, VA
Hood, General J.B. (John Bell) 176, 202
Hood, R.N. 166
Hopson, Stella 182
Horr, W.S. 169, 171
Hot Springs, Bath County, VA 184, 187, 189
Hot Springs, Madison County, NC 9, 111; *see also* Warm Springs, Madison County, NC
Hotel Carnegie, TN 151
hotel rates 30, 57, 97, 150, 166, 169, 194, 214, 268n90; rate comparisons 32, 41, 47, 51, 56, 98, 121, 128, 137–138, 149, 174
Hotel Roanoke 206
hoteliers (professional hotelmen) 4, 30, 41, 50, 52, 70, 106, 138, 146, 150, 163, 172
Household Remedies 166
Houston, Sam 163
Howe, Henry 212
Hsiung, David 4, 6
Hubble, L.F. 82–83
Hughes, Bill 160
Hughes, J.S. 81
Hummell, H. 82
Humphreys, John 121
Hunt House, NC 102
Huntsville, AL 9, 12, 20, 21, 23, 24, 29, 31

Hurst, Colonel J. Garland 215
hydropathy 9, 63, 135

Indian Springs, GA 35, 63
Irby Springs, SC 123; *see also* White Stone Lithia Springs, SC
iron ore, processing industry 25, 37, 43, 59, 98, 146, 153–154, 168; Cooper & Stroup iron works, GA 62; magnetite iron ore 86, 150; Roane Iron Company 154; Roane Iron Works 170

Jackson, Andrew 26, 59, 107, 165
Jackson, Anna (widow of General Thomas "Stonewall") 110
Jackson, C.C. 81
Jackson, Colonel J.F.B. 13
Jackson, MS 19, 125
Jackson, Rachel 165
Jackson County, AL 15
Jackson House, AL *see* Blount Springs, AL
January, Peter 69
Jarnagin, Mrs. John R. 173
Jarvis, Governor T.J. 105
Jim Crow era: racial intermingling at resorts 208; resorts as safe stop for Black visitors 197, 206–208; *see also* Blacks, post–Civil War; Washington, Booker T.
Jobe, Abraham 86
Johnson City, TN 86, 91, 111, 114, 145, 147–152, 154, 156, 157, 178–180
Johnson, Henry 147
Johnson, Henry C. 206
Johnson, J. Fred 176
Johnson, U.S. Attorney General Reverdy 213
Johnston, General Joseph E. 216
Johnston, Lydia (Mrs. Joseph E.) 11
Jones, William D. 195
Jones, William F. 71
Jones Gap Road 120
Jonesboro (Jonesborough), TN 47, 145, 147, 151, 178
Jonesborough Road, TN 145
Jordan, Branch 188, 211
Jordan, E.C. (Edwin) 211, 214–215
Jordan, E.C., Jr. 214–215
Jordan, G.N. (German) 211
Jordan, Granville 211
Jordan, R.M. (Robert) 211
Jordan's White Sulphur Springs, VA 188, 189, 190, 210–218

Journal of the American Medical Association 114; *see also* American Medical Association
Junaluska Mountain, NC 112–115
Junaluska Mountain Road 109, 112

Katen, Brian 190
Kavanagh, Edward 213
Keitt, Congressman Laurence Massillon 128, 137
Kellogg, W.K. 132
Kent, James 199
Kentucky: map **67**; physiography 66
Kentucky Road *see* Wilderness Road
Keowee Hotel, Seneca, SC 119, 249n9
Killebrew, J.B. 142–143
King, Charles S. 165–166
King, Joseph L. 165–166
King, William Rufus 31
Kings Springs, TN 151
Kingsport, TN 4, 177, 180, 191, 193, 207; *see also* Long Island of the Holston
Kingswood Home for Children 173
Kingswood School 173; *see also* resort school or academy
Kirk, Colonel George W. 97, 99, 107
Kirk's Raiders 97
Kirk's Springs, KY 69
Knoxville, TN 119, 144, 147, 150, 162–167, 171, 172, 174, 198
Knoxville and Bristol ("Peavine") Railroad 174
Knoxville and Charleston Railroad 165

Lackland, Samuel W. 212
La Grange Female Institute, GA 62
Lake Sidney Lanier 166
Lamar House, Knoxville 163
Lamine Hotel, AL *see* Alabama White Sulphur Springs
Lancaster, SC 117, 118, 128
land lottery, Georgia 54, 59
"Land of the Sky" 84, 109
"Land of the Sky and Sapphire Country" 119
Lanier, R.S. (Robert Sampson) 204
Lanier, Sampson 163
Lanier, Sidney (author) 33, 165, 204
Lanier, Sidney (Sterling's son) 163

Index

Lanier, Sterling 5, 61, 146, 163, 164, 165, 204
Lanier, William 163
Lanier House, Macon, GA 163
Lanman, Charles 153
Lansing, NC 90
Laurel County, KY 78, 80
Laurens Rail Road Company, SC 137
Lawton, General A.R. 47, 49
Lea Springs 172–173, 174
Lear, Whittington 79
Lee, Robert E. 202
Lee Highway (U.S. Highway 11W) 174
Letcher, Robert 76
Leucht, I.L. 204
Levy, R.W. 204
Lewis, John W. 63
Lewis County, KY, physiography 69
Lexington, KY 74, 76
The Liberator 31
Lick Springs, Greenville County, SC *see* Chick Springs, SC
Lilly, W.H. 77
limestone 8–9, 20, 29, 33–34, 37, 43, 134
Limestone Springs, Cherokee County, SC 121
Limestone Springs, Hall County, GA *see* New Holland Springs, GA
Limestone Springs, Whitfield County, GA 148
Lindsey, E.C. 97
Line Springs, TN 144, 167
Linville Falls, NC 98, 156
Linville Mountain, NC 94, 98
Linville River 94
Linville Wilderness Gorge, NC 94
livestock roads *see* drover roads
Lloyd, Alice 77
London, KY 80, 82
Long Island of the Holston, TN 172, 191; *see also* Kingsport, TN
Longstreet, General James 44, 45, 56, 202
Lookout Mountain, AL 16
Lookout Mountain Hotel, TN 169
Loring, Charles 17
Loring, General William W. 16–17
"Lost Cause" 5, 40, 190, 197, 202; *see also* Civil War
Lost Cove, NC 183
"Lost Provinces" of NC 91
Louisville, KY 76, 82
Louisville, TN 144, 164

Louisville & Frankfurt Railroad 76
Louisville & Nashville Railroad 28
Louisville Gold Mining Company 98
Love, Colonel Robert (James Robert) 4; 106–107
Love, Colonel Robert (Robert Gustavus Adolphus) 107, 178
Loving v. Virginia 207
Lowcountry planter sojourns in Upstate SC 4, 117, 120, 121, 124, 126, 128, 134, 135; *see also* visitors, by occupation; visitors, southern
Lula, GA 48
Lumpkin, Governor Wilson 54
Lumpkin County, GA, physiography 53
Lupton, John Thomas and Elizabeth 19
Lynchburg, VA 198, 199
lynching averted 13–14

Macon, GA 55, 61, 163
Madison County, AL 19–20
Madison Springs, GA 35, 61
Magic City Building and Loan Association, Roanoke, VA 206
Mahone, General William 202
malaria, malarial-type fevers 10, 46, 91, 117, 130; absence at resorts 14, 17, 35, 36, 57, 80, 105, 118–119, 157; *see also* epidemics
Mammoth Cave, KY 13
Manning, G.F. 30
Manning, Governor John Laurence 128
Manning, P.T. 30
Manning, Robert (James) 30
Mansion House (hotel), Spartanburg, SC 122
Marietta, GA 35
Marion, NC 156
Marion, VA 89, 91
Marker, William F. 214
Marshall, General Humphrey 195
Martin, C. Brenden 87
Maryville, TN 162
Mason, Edward 16
Mason, John 16
Mathews, James B. 51
May Flood of 1901 179
Maysville, KY 68, 71, 139
Maysville and Big Sandy Railroad 72
McAden, Rufus Yancey 105
McAfee, L.A. (Lemuel Austin) 50
McAfee expedition 74

McCallie, S.W. 33, 34
McCamy, Samuel R. 51
McCormick, James 69–70
McCormick's Springs, KY *see* Glen Springs, KY
McDonald, G. 38
McElrath, John W. 97
McHenry, Andrew 191–192
McHenry, David 192
McKee, Joseph 54–55
McKinney, Riley 156
McLean, F.C. 79
McMillan, Frank and Goldie 93
McMillan, Lee 93
McNeill, W.A. 92, 93
meals at resorts 47–48, 56, 72, 89, 93, 100–101, 126, 127, 138, 144, 159–160, 167
Means, James B. 134
Medical Society of Virginia 184
Mellette, A.C. 23
Memphis 73, 125, 150, 166, 198; *see also* visitors, southern
Mentone, AL 11, 15, 16, *17*, 18, 19
Merony, Phillip J. 103, 104, 105
Merony, Thomas J. 103, 104, 105
miasma 10
Michaux, André 153
Michaux, François-André 153, 164
Miller, C.M. 138
Miller, Walter J. 151
Milliken & Company 50
Mills, Aubrey 207
Mills, Robert 133–134
Mineral Hill Springs 173
mineral springs: chemical analysis or types of water 11, 14, 26, 30, 38–39, 45, 55, 73, 75–76, 98, 101, 103, 106, 108, 121, 122, 127, 145, 148, 170, 180, 192, 193, 200, 217; therapeutic uses 12, 14, 17–19, 26, 30, 45, 46, 48, 51, 55, 57, 61, 73, 75–76, 77, 88, 90–91, 92, 93, 96, 98, 101, 103–104, 108–109, 120, 122, 126, 130, 134, 136, 139, 144, 145, 148, 163, 170, 173, 175, 179, 184, 192, 193, 198, 199, 200, 202, 212, 216–217; *see also* weight gain at resorts
Miot, Charles L. 127
Mississippi 4, 143, 163; *see also* visitors, southern
Mississippi River 71
Mitchel, John 165
Mitchel, General O.M. 20
Mitchell, Elisha 153
Mitchell, Judge Henry L. 45
Mitchell County, NC 98, 153, 156
Mobile and Ohio Railroad 13

Index

Moccasin Gap, Scott County, VA 191
Monroe, James 187, 213
Monte Sano, AL 9, 10, 18, 19, 20, **21, 22, 23, 24**
Monte Sano State Park, AL 24
Montgomery County, VA 188, 192, 196–198, 199, 208
Montgomery White Sulphur Company 200
Montgomery White Sulphur Springs, VA 188, 189, 190, 197–205, **206, 207**, 209
Montvale Inn, TN 167
Montvale Springs, TN 5, 32, 41, 47, 61, 128, 137, 143–144, 145, 146, 149, 150, 162–166, **167**, 174, 204
Moore, Maurice A. 134, 136, 137
Mooresburg Springs, TN 144–145
Moorman, John J. 184, 199, 200, 212
Morehead, Eugene 101
Morgan, General Daniel W. 94
Morgan, General John Hunt 76
Morgan, Luther 12
Morgan, Thomas 82
Morgan County, AL: geology 29
Morganton, NC 87, 93, 94, 96, 97, 98, 102, 105
Morganton and Cranberry Turnpike Company 96
Morristown, TN 97, 109, 173, 174
Mount Airy Hotel, GA 36
Mount Airy White Sulphur Springs, NC 86
Mount Jefferson, NC 88
Mount Nebo Springs, TN 167
mountain air: ozone benefits 36, 57, 106; relief from heat or mosquitos 17, 19, 20, 21, 23, 29, 31, 35, 36, 46, 48–49, 57, 63, 73, 82, 100, 103, 105, 109, 113, 115, 117, 118–119, 126, 130, 145, 157, 164, 180, 197; *see also* hay fever
Mountain Lake, VA 208
Mountain Springs Hotel, VA 191
mountaineers near resorts: employment, trade with resorts 160, 165; by mission publication 36; by northern newspapers 89–90; perception by Civil War soldiers 81; perception of resort visitors 180–181; by resort owner 237n156; by resort visitors 36, 58, 160, 180; *see also* Lanier, Sidney; Murfree, Mary Noailles

Muir, John 159, 162
Mullins, A.R. 72
Murfree, Mary Noailles 2, 58, 166, 219n7
Murray, Colonel William (GA) 37–38
Murray, William (SC) 135
Murray Springs, GA *see* Catoosa Springs, GA
Murrell, Nannie Snyder 160, 161

National Highway 131
National Park Service 146
National Soldiers Home, TN 111
Native Americans: discovery or use of springs 18, 26, 27, 60, 74, 126, 162, 168, 173; trails 172; work at resorts 192; *see also* Catawba Nation; Cherokee Nation; Creek Nation; Shawnee Nation
Natural Tunnel, Scott County, VA 191, 194
Neal, Congressman John Randolph 171
Negro Law of the Carolinas 128
Nelson, R.W. 72
New Holland Springs, GA 35, 36, 45, 46–50, 52, 56
New Jackson House, AL *see* Blount Springs, AL
New Orleans 17, 19, 31, 36, 125, 187, 190, 199, 204; *see also* visitors, southern
New River 88, 91
New River Valley 5, 189, 190, 196–197
New River White Sulphur, VA 197, 208
New York City 114
The New York Sun 89
The New York Times 158, 176
New York Tribune 31
New York World 89
Newberry, SC 120, 126, 127, 128, 130, 137
Newport, RI 114, 177
newspaper exhortations for southerners to visit southern resorts 5, 36, 40, 95, 128
Nichols, J.S. 40
1904 Louisiana Purchase Exposition 123
1929 stock market crash 53
Noblett, John 168
Nolichucky River 45, 146, 178, 181
Nolichucky River Gorge 145, 178, 183
Norfolk and Western Railroad 90
Norfolk Journal and Guide 207

North Alabama Improvement Company 21, 23
North Carolina: map **85**; western physiography 94
North Carolina Press Association 112
North Carolina springs 126, 128
North Eaglenest Mountain, NC *see* Junaluska Mountain, NC
North Wilkesboro, NC 92
Northeastern Railroad of Georgia 48
Northern Presbyterian Mission Board 102
northerners 21, 31, 36, 42, 68, 71, 87; *see also* visitors, northern
northerners to resort ruins after Civil War 40–41
Northwestern Land Association (Pierre, SD) 23
Nott, Josiah 9–10

Ochs, Adolph and Effie 175
Oconee County, SC 117, 118
Oconee River, GA 50, 51
Oconee White Sulphur Springs, GA 35, 36, 45, 48, 49, 50–53
Oglesby, J.W. 52–53
Ohio River 68, 71
Old Rockcastle, KY 78, 81; *see also* Rockcastle Springs, KY
Old Sweet Springs, VA *see* Sweet Springs, VA (WV)
Oliver, Robert C. 121
Olympian Springs, KY 66, 68
O'Neall, John Belton 128
Orkney Springs, VA 189
O'Shaughnessy, Michael J. 21, 23
Oswald, Felix L. 166
Owsley, William 76

Pace, Ewsiel (Ensil) 50–51
Pacolet Manufacturing Company, GA 50
Pacolet Springs, SC 121, 122
Padgett, Ray and Sandy 18
Palmer, George W. 89, 90, 91
Panic of 1837 30, 134
Panic of 1857 122
Panic of 1873 63
Panic of 1893 23, 160
Patton, Governor Robert M. 11
Peale, Albert C. 148, 191, 197
Pearcy, Gabriel 98
Pearson, Clifton 102
Pearson, John H. 100, 101
Pearson, U.S. consul William S. 101
Pemberton Chemical Company 49
Pendleton, Edmund 193

Pendleton land grant 193
Pensacola, FL 114
Perrine, James 12
Pettigrew, R.F. 23
Pflanze, Ludwig 166–167
Philadelphia Inquirer 31
Phillips, W.C. 92
Phinizy, Barrett 131
Phinizy, Ferdinand 52, 53, 54
Pickens County, SC 117, 118, 119, 128
Piedmont Air Line Railroad, SC 118–119; see also Atlanta and Richmond Air Line Railroad, SC
Piedmont Hotel, Gainesville, GA 45, 56
Piedmont Lumber, Ranch, & Mining Company 98–99
Piedmont Springs, NC 6, 84–85, 87, 88, 94, 95–99
Piedmont Springs Company 97
Pierce, Franklin 187
Pine Mountain State Park, KY 66
Piney River, TN 144, 168, 169
Pippen, Sherman 156, 159
Pisgah National Forest 94, 99
Pitman, Christopher 81
Planter Hotel, Charleston, SC 127
Plummer, R.E.L. (Robert E. Lee) 90
"Plummer Bromine Arsenic Water" 90
political discussions at resorts 26–27, 28, 55, 62–63, 76, 120, 124, 128, 137, 139, 187, 190, 202, 209, 213
Pollard, Edward A. 197, 200, 201–202
Ponder, Ed 29
Poole, Colonel Robert Coleman 122
Poole's Springs, SC see Pacolet Springs, SC
Pope, Colonel William 185
Porter, Lou Dora Plummer 91
Porter Springs, GA 6, 36, 37, 48, 53–59
Portsmouth, OH 71, 73
Powder Marsh, SC see Glenn Springs, SC
Powell, George 11, 13
Powling, John 69
Powling, William O. 69
Pratt, A.S. (Adam) 215
President's Appalachian Regional Commission Report of 1964 3
Preston, John Montgomery 192–193; extended family 194
Preston, U.S. Senator William C. 137

Pritchard, Esther 99
Pritchard, Richard 204, 209
Prohibition 141
Prolix, Peregrine (Philip Houlbrooke Nicklin) 187
promenades: verandahs 18, 30, 38, 72, 75, 79, 81, 89, 100, 103, 108, 112, 121, 130, 139, 144, 149, 155, 165, 174–175, 179, 211, 214, 215; walks along verandahs or through grounds 35, 76, 103, 112, 144, 165, 214
The Prophet of the Smokies 166
Pulaski Alum Springs, VA 197
Pulaski County, KY 78, 79, 80
Purdon, John E. 16

Qualla (Indian) Boundary 87, 111
Queen and Crescent Route (railroad) 171

Rabun Gap, GA 119
radium 92
Radium Springs Corporation of America 92–93
Radium Springs Distributing Company 92
Ragsdale, Annie M. 173
rail car, private 102, 105, 145, 159, 174
railroad guides, promotions 2, 13, 90, 144, 146, 171, 180
railroads, general 11, 13, 19, 85–86, 98, 102, 117, 131, 137, 139–140, 146, 188, 198–199, 200, 213; lack of infrastructure to reach resorts 35, 64, 82, 86; 125, 137, 193–194
Ransom, U.S. Senator M.W. 101
Rawby Springs, VA 104
Red Sulphur Springs, VA (WV) 101, 121, 184, 187, 189, 208
Redfield, John 156–157
Reedy Creek Road see Wilderness Road
resort as part of vacation circuit or grand tour 52, 62, 114, 121, 124, 126, 128, 131, 136, 158, 166, 184, 185, 187, 189, 193, 201, 203–204, 208, 211, 212–213, 216
resort ban on dancing, drinking, or cards 35, 62, 72, 109, 121, 122, 149, 215
resort grounds, landscaping 38, 39, 48, 52, 60–61, 70, 75, 104, 108, 119, 130, 135–136, 138–139, 163, 165, 169, 198, 199, 200, 211, 212, 214, 215
resort school or academy 135, 150, 173, 195
resort use for soldiers or

veterans, other than Civil War 79, 111, 132
Reynolds, A.D. (Abram) 90
Reynolds, R.J. 90
Rhea, Congressman John 168
Rhea, John II 169
Rhea County, TN, physiography 168
Rhea Springs, TN 4, 5, 144, 146, 167–172
Rice, William 14
Rice, W.P. 16
Richmond, KY 76
Richmond, VA 30, 90, 188, 195, 197–198, 199, 200, 201
Richmond and Danville Railroad 102, 109
Richmond and Irvine Turnpike 76
Richmond Dispatch 213
Riddell, Labe 77
Riley, Benjamin Franklin 8–9, 29
Ringgold, GA 37, 39, 40
Rivers, Joseph 46–47, 50
Rivers Springs, GA see New Holland Springs, GA
Riverside Inn, TN see Austin's (Austin) Springs, TN
Riverside Park TN see Austin's (Austin) Springs, TN
roads to resorts 20, 23, 43, 76, 82, 84, 91, 96, 98, 116, 128, 131, 151, 171, 174, 181, 187, 213; better roads detracting visitors from resorts 177, 181–182; Good Road bonds 152; lack of good roads or turnpikes 70, 71, 96, 187, 193–194; road construction 96, 98, 112, 148, 155–156, 163, 188, 198; use of cars to resorts 131, 152, 171, 174
Roan Mountain, TN/NC 98, 114, 116, 153, 154, 155, 159, 160, 161
Roan Mountain Inn, TN 156, 162
Roan Road 155
Roanoke, VA 90, 206; Henry Street, 206
Roanoke River 198, 199
Robertson, U.O. 63, 64
Robinson, Herndon B. 14
Rock Cliff Lithia Springs, SC 123; see also Garrett Springs, SC
Rock Cliff Park, SC 123
Rock Enon, VA 189, 190, 210, 212–216, **217**, 218
Rock Enon Springs Company 215
Rockbridge, VA 5
Rockbridge Baths, VA 178

Rockcastle River, KY 67, 68, 78, 79, 80, 81, 82, 83
Rockcastle Springs, KY 6, 13, 66, 67, 68, 78–83
Rockcastle Springs Company, KY 81
Rockenbach, General S.D. and Emma 43
Roddey, General Phillip 20
Rolling Stone 93
Ross, Bernard 208
Ross, Donald 174
Rousseau, General Lovell 27
Rousseau's Raid 27
Rowland, John Sharpe 4, 35, 36, 60–64
Rowland, Colonel William L. 63
Rowland Springs, GA 4, 35, 59–63, *64*, 65, 163, 175
Rowland Springs Hygienic Institute 63
Ruffin, Edmund 201
Ruffin, Judge Thomas, Jr. 105
Ruggles Campground, KY 73
Rumbley, C.B. 182
Rumbley, J.E. 182
Russell County, VA 194
Rutherford College, NC 105
Ruthrauff, M.E. 119

Safford, James M. 168
St. Clair Springs, AL 9
Salisbury, NC 85, 97, 102, 103, 104, 105
Salt Lick Creek, Lewis County, KY 69
Salt Sulphur Springs, VA 124, 184, 186, 189, 208
Saltville, VA 88, 89, 192
Saluda Gap Road 128
Samers, Michael 3
Sams Gap, TN/NC 178
sanitarium 57, 87, 132
"Saratoga of the South" 5, 36, 38, 51, 164
"Saratoga of the West" 79
Saratoga Springs, including Congress water 5, 11, 38, 39, 71, 90, 101, 136, 164, 165, 177
Sargent, Charles Sprague 156
Sassafras Mountain, SC 119
Satterthwaite (Satterthwait), Hester Smathers 111
Satterthwaite (Satterthwait), S.C. (Samuel Clement) 111–112, 116
Savannah 9, 36, 40, 49, 90, 105, 114, 124, 128, 191; *see also* visitors, southern
Savannah Morning News 41, 146
Scales, Governor A.M. 105
scandals at resorts 13–14, 72, 108, 121–122

Scenic Eagle's Nest Road 116
Schoonmaker, Dalzell 102
Scopes "Monkey" Trial 168, 171
Scott, Sir Walter 39, 211, 213
Scott, Winfield 76
Scott County, VA 189–191
Scoville, Dabney 19
Scurry, Drury 127
Seaboard Air Line Railway 131, 180
Selma, AL 114
Seneca, SC 118, 119
Senter, Stephen W. 173
Sequatchie (Sequatchee) Valley, AL 11
Seven Mile Ford, VA 89
1798 First Treaty of Tellico 168; *see also* Cherokee Nation
Shannondale Springs, VA (WV) 3, 187, 188, 189, 190, 210, 212–215, *216*, 217, 218
Shannondale Springs Corporation 212
Shatley, Martin 91
Shatley Springs, NC 6, 84, 88, 91–93
Shatley Springs Hotel Company, NC 92
Shawnee Nation 69, 74; *see also* Native Americans
Shawsville, VA 198
Sheftall, Solomon 124
Shelby, NC 99
Shelby Springs, AL 9, 10–11
Shell, Frank 155
Sheltering Arms Orphanage, Atlanta 64
Shenandoah River 187, 212, 215
Shenandoah Valley, northern 189, 210
Sherman, General William T. 102
Shocco Springs, AL 11, 25, 27–29
Shocco Springs Alabama Baptist Conference Center 29
Shockley, J.C. 119
Simpson, John Wells 138
Simpson, J. (John) Wistar (Wister) 138
Simpson, William Dunlap 138
Simpson & Simpson 138–139
Sims, D.H. 166
Sisters of Mercy Roman Catholic order 11, 201
Skyland Springs, Henderson County, NC 86
slave trade: coffles 4, 87, 239n24; Richmond slave exchange 188; slave auction 239n24; slaves as payment for resort property 35, 193
slave work outside resorts: agriculture 20, 60, 135, 147; mines 43, 54, 95
slaves at resorts: attack by hotel manager 108; discovery of mineral spring 106; resort workers 4–5, 26, 36, 51, 61, 68, 70, 79, 87, 97, 124, 135, 165, 188, 195, 211, 213; ridicule by proprietor 127; servants accompanying families 85, 194; slave cabins 63, 122, 198; slave leasing 188–189, 212; slaves as resort patients 136, 164, 169
Sloan, B.J. 110, 111
Sloss, J.W. 14
Sloss, Mack 14
Smathers, George Henry 111, 112
Smith, Cathryn 53
Smith, C.S. 101
Smith, Eugene A. 9
Smith, Congressman Samuel A. 169
Smith, Soule 82
Smith & Fowler 138
Smithdeal, William 104
Smithsonian Institution 170
Snead, Sam 174
Somerset, KY 77, 79, 80, 82
Somerset Journal (KY) 82
Sousa, John Philip 216
South & North Alabama Railroad 13
South and Western Railway 179
South Carolina: map *118*; physiography 117
South Carolina State Board of Health 125, 139
Southern and Western Railroad 99
Southern Historical Society 202
Southern Railway 115, 131, 151, 180
Spartanburg, SC 117, 122, 130, 131, 132, 135, 137–141
Spartanburg & Asheville Railroad 140
Spartanburg and Union Railroad 137, 139–140
Spartanburg County, SC 117, 118, 120, 123, 126, 135; physiography 133–134
Spartanburg springs 121
Spence, W.A. 41
Spring City, TN 168, 171
Spring City Park, TN 172
Spruce Pine, NC 179
Stanton, F.P. 169, 171
Stanton, Colonel George W. 101
Starnes, Richard D. 84, 86
State Road, GA *see* Western and Atlantic Railroad, GA

Index

Statistics of South Carolina 133–134
Staunton, VA 187, 188
steamboat transportation to resorts 68, 71, 72, 144
Steedly, B.B. 132
Stephens, Alexander H. 57, 176
Stevens, J.P. 123
Stoll, Steven 2, 3
Stone Pile Gap, GA 55, 57
Stoneman, General George 124
Stout, Samuel H. 40
Stovall, General M.A. 41
Stratton, H.H. 91
Strayhorn, Zora Shay 18
Stribling, Erasmus 187
Stringfield, Maria Love 107
Stringfield, W.W. (William Williams) 107, 108, 109
Strother, David Hunter 192
Stuart, VA 86
Stucke family 119
Studebaker, J.M. 176
Studebaker family 174
Sturgeon, E.T. 82
Sublimity Springs, KY 4, 6, 66, 67, 68, 78–83
Sullivan County, TN 147, 152, 193, 194
Sulphur Springs, AL *see* Alabama White Sulphur Springs
Sulphur Springs (Deaver's), Buncombe County, NC 84, 95, 98, 127
Sulphur Springs, Rhea County, TN *see* Rhea Springs, TN
Sulphur Springs, Spartanburg County, SC *see* Glenn Springs, SC
Sulphur Springs Camp Ground, Rhea County, TN 169
Sulphur Springs Park, Waynesville, NC 111
Sulzby, James H., Jr. 18, 31
Surry County, NC 86
Sweet Chalybeate (Red Sweet) Springs, VA 41
Sweet Springs, KY *see* Estill Springs, KY
Sweet Springs, VA (WV) 9, 188–189
Sykes, James T. 30

Table Rock, SC 120
Table Rock Mountain, NC 94, 96, 98
Table Rock State Park, SC 117, 119
Talbird, Franklin 127
Talladega County, AL, physiography 24–25
Talladega Springs, AL 11, 25–29

Taney, Supreme Court Chief Justice Roger 187, 213
Tate, Samuel B. 173
Tate Spring, TN 4, 131, 144–146, 150, 172–175, **176**, **177**, 178
Taylor, Governor Alf 151
Taylor, Alfred 124, 128
Taylor, Governor Bob 150, 151
Taylor, Charles 197–198
Taylor, Creed 198
Taylor, E.H., Jr. 77
Taylor, J.W. 102
Taylor, General James 71
Taylor, Victoria 208
Taylor, W.H. 148
Taylor Springs, VA *see* Yellow Sulphur Springs, VA
Tennessee: map **143**; physiography 142–143
Tennessee Army National Guard 43
"Tennessee Itch" 164
Tennessee Press Association 159
Tennessee River 4, 142, 144, 146, 167, 168, 171
Tennessee State Board of Health 125, 151, 157
Thomas, J.M. 77
Thompson, C.W. 206
Thompson, Hiram V. 88, 89, 90
Thompson, Jarrett 28
Thompson, Jessee 162
Thompson's Bromine-Arsenic Springs, NC *see* Healing Springs, Ashe County, NC
Thomson, J. Waddy 122
Thomson's Springs, SC *see* Garett Springs, SC
Three C's railroad *see* Charleston, Cincinnati & Chicago Railroad
Tiernan, Frances 84
Tiger-Lilies 165
Timberlake, J.S.C. 108
tobacco 20, 60, 72, 85, 90, 95, 101, 142, 150, 205
Toccoa, GA 48
Todd, Charles 164
Tollesboro, KY 69, 73
Tomlinson, Clement 173
Tomlinson, Oscar R. 173
Tomlinson, Thomas 173
Toombs, Robert 47, 51
tourism 86, 106, 109, 110, 112, 120
tournaments, chivalrous 3, 39, 139, 202, 213
Towns, Congressman and Governor George W. 62
Trahlyta (Cherokee princess) 55
Trahlyta Lodge, GA 59

Trail of Tears 37, 46, 102, 168; *see also* Cherokee Nation
trolley line to resort 131
Troup, George 62–63
tuberculosis 9, 30, 86, 111, 139, 158–159; prohibition of tubercular patients at resorts 87, 105, 115; scrofula (scrofular, scrofulous) diseases 96, 144, 145, 164
Tunnel Hill, GA 37, 39, 40, 148
Tuomey, Michael 9
Turner, Congressman Henry G. 45
Turnpike, NC (resort) 111
Tutwiler, Julia 31
TVA 146, 167–168, 173
Tyler, John 187, 213
typhoid fever *see* epidemics

Unaka Mountains 6, 142, 143, 145
Unaka Springs, TN 107, 131, 145, 146, 151, 178–180, **181**, **182**, **183**
Unicoi County, TN 142, 151, 178
Unicoi Turnpike 163
U.S. Army 42, 124
U.S., Congress, rumor to buy mineral spring resort 90
U.S. Forest Service 146, 155, 162
U.S. Hay Fever Association 115, 158
U.S. Veterans Bureau 132

Valhermoso Springs, AL 11, 29–32
van Buren, Martin 187, 213
Vance, Governor Zebulon 101
Vanceburg, KY 68–70, 71, 72
Vanderbilt, George W. 86, 102, 105, 159
Vanstory, Henry 105–106
verandahs *see* promenades
Vicksburg Cotton Exchange 204
Viduta *see* Monte Sano
Vincent, George 2
Virginia: map **185**; *see also* West Virginia, map
Virginia Agricultural and Mechanical College (Virginia Tech) 202
Virginia and Central Railroad 188
Virginia and Tennessee Railroad 88, 187–188, 197, 198, 199
Virginia Military Institute 185
Virginia springs 3–4, 9, 10, 11, 31, 39, 41, 55, 62, 68, 71, 76, 77, 121, 124, 126, 131, 136, 164, 165, 184–190, 193, 201; *see also* White Sulphur Springs, VA (WV)
Virginia springs geography and

physiography 184, 190–191, 196, 210
Virginia Transient Bureau 208
visitors, by occupation 16, 47, 51, 82, 105, 119, 137, 140, 155, 157, 166, 180, 190, 194, 203–205, 210–211, 216, 274n290; *see also* visitors, southern; Lowcountry planter sojourns in Upstate SC
visitors, Creole 13
visitors from Ohio River Valley 70, 71, 73, 76, 82, 139
visitors, Jewish 190, 204
visitors, midwestern 73, 82, 174, 176
visitors, northern, antebellum 76, 136, 186–187, 213, 261n187
visitors, northern, postbellum 22, 73, 105, 151, 157, 176–177, 181, 204, 216, 265n321
visitors, southern 12–14, 17, 18, 19, 22, 28, 35, 36, 39, 41, 45, 46, 47, 50, 53, 55, 58, 60, 61, 62, 63, 64, 68, 70–71, 73, 76, 80, 82, 86, 91, 93, 100–102, 105, 106, 109–110, 113, 119, 120, 122, 126, 128, 130–131, 136, 140, 149, 151, 157, 163, 164, 166, 169, 171, 173, 175–177, 186, 189, 190, 191, 194–195, 197, 198, 200–205, 210–211, 213, 215; *see also* Lowcountry planter sojourns in Upstate SC; visitors, by occupation
visitors from outside U.S. 205

Wachtel, A.E. 173
Waddell, Congressman A.M. 100
Wade, James 201
Wade, John 201
Walhalla, SC 118, 119, 125, 148
Walker, I.N. (Isaac Nash) 72
Wallace, Jesse 162
Wallace, Joseph 30
Wallerstein, Immanuel 3
Walton, Thomas 95
Walton, Colonel Thomas George 95, 99–102
Walton, W.M. 102
Walton House, NC 102
Walton Road, TN 171
Warm Springs, Bath County, VA 184, 187, 188, 189, 209
Warm Springs, Madison County, NC 2, 9, 84, 87, 95, 98, 124, 126, 155, 172; *see also* Hot Springs, Madison County, NC
Warm Springs, Meriwether County, GA 38, 39, 61
Warner, Charles Dudley 157
Warren, General Eli 47
Warriors' Path *see* Great Warriors Path

Washington, Booker T. 121–122; *see also* Blacks, post–Civil War; Jim Crow era
Washington, George, Jr. (Newport, KY, attorney) 72
Washington Springs, Washington County, VA 188
Wasson, Chapman 172
Wasson, Edward E. 168–169
Wasson, J.C. (Jeremiah Chapman) 169–171
Wasson, Thompson Owen 172
Watauga County, NC 88, 91
Watauga Dam (TVA) 146
Watauga Institute for Young Ladies 150
Watauga River 146–147
water cure *see* hydropathy
water shipments *see* bottled water
Watson, Asa 163
Watt, Abram 165
Watts Bar Dam (TVA) 167–168, 172
Wayne, General Anthony 107
Waynesville, NC 86, 87, 106–114, 116
Webster, Daniel 164, 186, 187
weight gain at resorts 9, 73, 77, 104, 108, 130, 136, 151, 193; *see also* mineral springs, therapeutic uses
West Springs, SC 122
West Virginia: map **186**; *see also* Virginia, map
West Virginia Wildlife Management Area, Shannondale 216
Western and Atlantic Railroad, GA 35, 39, 41, 60, 62, 63, 148
Western North Carolina Railroad 85, 86, 87, 97, 98, 101–102, 107, 109, 112, 115, 156
Westmoreland, George 129
White Cliff Springs, TN 144, 150
White Mountain health resorts, NH 115, 116, 158
White Stone Lithia Ale 123
White Stone Lithia Springs, SC 121, 123; *see also* Irby Springs, SC
White Sulphur Springs, DeKalb County, AL *see* Alabama White Sulphur Springs
White Sulphur Springs, Hall County, GA *see* Oconee White Sulphur Springs
White Sulphur Springs, Lewis County, KY *see* Esculapia Springs
White Sulphur Springs, Morgan County, AL *see* Valhermoso Springs
White Sulphur Springs, VA

(WV) 2, 3, 4, 39, 41, 68, 70, 71, 99–100, 124, 139, 145, 184, 185–190, 193, 197–201, 203, 208–209, 210, 213; *see also* Virginia springs
Whiteside, James A. 169
Whitner, Joseph 59
Wilbur Dam (TVA) 146
Wilder, General John T. 86, 146, 154–156, 160–162, 170–171, 178
Wilder's Forge, NC 155; *see also* Buladean, NC
Wilderness Road 172, 191, 192
Wildwood Springs, TN 144
Wiley, Helen Palmer 91
Williams, Allen 211
Williams, J.B. 93
Williams, General and U.S. Senator Jonathan S. 77
Williams, Leroy P. 211, 213
Wilmington, NC, 1898 race riot 110
Wilson, G.W. 41–42
Wilson, Woodrow and Ellen Louise 110
Winchester, VA 189, 210–214
Winchester and Potomac Railroad 187
Winston, NC 86
Wofford, Joseph 121
Wood, S.B. 162
Woods, W.C. 119
Woodville 164
Woody, John 55
Works Progress Administration 152
Wrenn, B.W. 41
Wyandotte, VA 68, 71
Wytheville, VA 194, 198

Yankton, Dakota Territory 21
Yeager's Springs, TN 145, 146
yellow fever *see* epidemics
Yellow Springs, VA *see* Yellow Sulphur Springs, VA
Yellow Sulphur Springs, VA 188, 190, 197–207, **208**, **209**, 210
Yellow Sulphur Springs Company 198
Yellow Sulphur Springs, Inc. 206
Yellow Sulphur Springs Recreative Sanatorium 208
YMCA, Knoxville 167
YWCA, Chattanooga 19
Young, General P.M.B. 39
Young's Hotel, Bakersville, NC 159
Yznaga, Consuelo and mother 159

Zimmerman, John C. 135, 137

www.ingramcontent.com/pod-product-compliance
Ingram Content Group UK Ltd.
Pitfield, Milton Keynes, MK11 3LW, UK
UKHW051850210426
5322IPUK00025B/648